Cone Beam Computed Tomography
Oral and Maxillofacial Diagnosis and Applications

Cone Beam Computed Tomography

Oral and Maxillofacial Diagnosis and Applications

Edited by

David Sarment, DDS, MS

WILEY Blackwell

This edition first published 2014 © 2014 by John Wiley & Sons, Inc

Editorial Offices
1606 Golden Aspen Drive, Suites 103 and 104, Ames, Iowa 50010, USA
The Atrium, Southern Gate, Chichester, West Sussex, PO19 8SQ, UK
9600 Garsington Road, Oxford, OX4 2DQ, UK

For details of our global editorial offices, for customer services and for information about how to apply for permission to reuse the copyright material in this book please see our website at www.wiley.com/wiley-blackwell.

Authorization to photocopy items for internal or personal use, or the internal or personal use of specific clients, is granted by Blackwell Publishing, provided that the base fee is paid directly to the Copyright Clearance Center, 222 Rosewood Drive, Danvers, MA 01923. For those organizations that have been granted a photocopy license by CCC, a separate system of payments has been arranged. The fee codes for users of the Transactional Reporting Service are ISBN-13: 978-0-4709-6140-7/2014.

Designations used by companies to distinguish their products are often claimed as trademarks. All brand names and product names used in this book are trade names, service marks, trademarks or registered trademarks of their respective owners. The publisher is not associated with any product or vendor mentioned in this book.

The contents of this work are intended to further general scientific research, understanding, and discussion only and are not intended and should not be relied upon as recommending or promoting a specific method, diagnosis, or treatment by health science practitioners for any particular patient. The publisher and the author make no representations or warranties with respect to the accuracy or completeness of the contents of this work and specifically disclaim all warranties, including without limitation any implied warranties of fitness for a particular purpose. In view of ongoing research, equipment modifications, changes in governmental regulations, and the constant flow of information relating to the use of medicines, equipment, and devices, the reader is urged to review and evaluate the information provided in the package insert or instructions for each medicine, equipment, or device for, among other things, any changes in the instructions or indication of usage and for added warnings and precautions. Readers should consult with a specialist where appropriate. The fact that an organization or Website is referred to in this work as a citation and/or a potential source of further information does not mean that the author or the publisher endorses the information the organization or Website may provide or recommendations it may make. Further, readers should be aware that Internet Websites listed in this work may have changed or disappeared between when this work was written and when it is read. No warranty may be created or extended by any promotional statements for this work. Neither the publisher nor the author shall be liable for any damages arising herefrom.

Library of Congress Cataloging-in-Publication Data

Cone beam computed tomography : oral and maxillofacial diagnosis and applications / [edited by] David Sarment.
     p. ; cm.
   Includes bibliographical references and index.
   ISBN 978-0-470-96140-7 (pbk. : alk. paper) – ISBN 978-1-118-76902-7 – ISBN 978-1-118-76906-5 (epub) – ISBN 978-1-118-76908-9 (mobi) – ISBN 978-1-118-76916-4 (ePdf)
I. Sarment, David P., editor of compilation.
[DNLM: 1. Stomatognathic Diseases–radiography.   2. Cone-Beam Computed Tomography–methods. WU 140]
   RK309
   617.5'22075722–dc23
                                                                  2013026841

A catalogue record for this book is available from the British Library.

Wiley also publishes its books in a variety of electronic formats. Some content that appears in print may not be available in electronic books.

Cover design by Jen Miller Designs

Set in 9.5/11.5pt Palatino by SPi Publisher Services, Pondicherry, India

1 2014

To my wife Sylvie
To my children Lea, Myriam, and Nathanyel

Contents

Contributors ix
Preface xi
Acknowledgments xiii

1 Technology and Principles of Cone Beam Computed Tomography 3
Matthew W. Jacobson

2 The Nature of Ionizing Radiation and the Risks from Maxillofacial Cone Beam Computed Tomography 25
Sanjay M. Mallya and Stuart C. White

3 Diagnosis of Jaw Pathologies Using Cone Beam Computed Tomography 43
Sharon L. Brooks

4 Diagnosis of Sinus Pathologies Using Cone Beam Computed Tomography 65
Aaron Miracle and Christian Güldner

5 Orthodontic and Orthognathic Planning Using Cone Beam Computed Tomography 91
Lucia H. S. Cevidanes, Martin Styner, Beatriz Paniagua, and João Roberto Gonçalves

6 Three-Dimensional Planning in Maxillofacial Reconstruction of Large Defects Using Cone Beam Computed Tomography 109
Rutger Schepers, Gerry M. Raghoebar, Lars U. Lahoda, Harry Reintsema, Arjan Vissink, and Max J. Witjes

7 Implant Planning Using Cone Beam Computed Tomography 127
David Sarment

8 CAD/CAM Surgical Guidance Using Cone Beam Computed Tomography 147
George A. Mandelaris and Alan L. Rosenfeld

9 Assessment of the Airway and Supporting Structures Using Cone Beam Computed Tomography 197
David C. Hatcher

10 Endodontics Using Cone Beam Computed Tomography 211
Martin D. Levin

11 Periodontal Disease Diagnosis Using Cone Beam Computed Tomography 249
Bart Vandenberghe and David Sarment

Index 271

Contributors

Sharon L. Brooks, DDS, MS
Professor Emerita, Department of Periodontics
 and Oral Medicine
University of Michigan School of Dentistry
Ann Arbor, Michigan, USA

Lucia H. S. Cevidanes, DDS, MS, PhD
Assistant Professor, Department of Orthodontics
University of Michigan School of Dentistry
Ann Arbor, Michigan, USA

João Roberto Gonçalves, DDS, PhD
Assistant Professor, Department of Pediatric Dentistry
Faculdade de Odontologia
Universidade Estadual Paulista, Araraquara, Brazil

Christian Güldner, MD
Specialist in ENT, Department of ENT, Head
 and Neck Surgery
University of Marburg
Germany

David C. Hatcher, DDS, MSc, MRCD(c)
Adjunct Professor, Department of Orthodontics
University of the Pacific School of Dentistry
San Francisco, California, USA

Clinical Professor, Orofacial Sciences
University of California–San Francisco School
 of Dentistry
San Francisco, California, USA

Clinical Professor
Roseman University College of Dental Medicine
Henderson, Nevada, USA

Private practice
Diagnostic Digital Imaging
Sacramento, California, USA

Matthew W. Jacobson, MSc, PhD
Senior Research Scientist
Xoran Technologies, Inc.
Ann Arbor, Michigan, USA

Lars U. Lahoda, MD, PhD
Plastic surgeon, Department of Plastic Surgery
University of Groningen and University Medical
 Center Groningen
Groningen, the Netherlands

Martin D. Levin, DMD
Diplomate, American Board of Endodontics
Chair, Dean's Council and Adjunct Associate
 Professor of Endodontics
University of Pennsylvania, School of Dental
 Medicine
Philadelphia, Pennsylvania, USA

Private practice
Chevy Chase, Maryland, USA

Sanjay M. Mallya, BDS, MDS, PhD
Assistant Professor and Postgraduate Program
 Director
Oral and Maxillofacial Radiology
University of California–Los Angeles School of
 Dentistry
Los Angeles, California, USA

George A. Mandelaris, DDS, MS
Diplomate, American Board of Periodontology

Private practice
Periodontics and Dental Implant Surgery
Park Ridge and Oakbrook Terrace, Illinois, USA

Clinical Assistant Professor, Department of Oral
 and Maxillofacial Surgery
Louisiana State University School of Dentistry
New Orleans, Louisiana, USA

Aaron Miracle, MD
Resident physician, Department of Radiology and
 Biomedical Imaging
University of California–San Francisco
San Francisco, California, USA

Beatriz Paniagua, PhD
Assistant Professor
Department of Psychiatry
Department of Computer Science
University of North Carolina
Chapel Hill, North Carolina, USA

Gerry M. Raghoebar, DDS, MD, PhD
Professor, Oral and maxillofacial surgeon
University of Groningen and University Medical
 Center Groningen
Groningen, the Netherlands

Harry Reintsema, DDS
Maxillofacial Prosthodontist, Department of Oral
 and Maxillofacial Surgery
University of Groningen and University Medical
 Center Groningen
Groningen, the Netherlands

Alan L. Rosenfeld, DDS, FACD
Diplomate, American Board of Periodontology

Private practice
Periodontics and Dental Implant Surgery
Park Ridge and Oakbrook Terrace, Illinois, USA

Clinical Professor, Department of Periodontology
University of Illinois College of Dentistry
Chicago, Illinois, USA

Clinical Assistant Professor, Department of Oral
 and Maxillofacial Surgery
Louisiana State University School of Dentistry
New Orleans, Louisiana, USA

David Sarment, DDS, MS
Diplomate, American Board of Periodontology

Private practice
Implantology and Periodontics
Alexandria, Virginia, USA

Rutger Schepers, DDS, MD
Maxillofacial Surgeon, Department of Oral and
 Maxillofacial Surgery
University of Groningen and University Medical
 Center Groningen
Groningen, the Netherlands

Martin Styner, PhD
Associate Professor
Department of Computer Science
University of North Carolina
Chapel Hill, North Carolina, USA

Bart Vandenberghe, DDS, MSc, PhD
Advimago, Center for Advanced Oral Imaging
Brussels, Belgium

Prosthetics Section, Department of Oral Health
 Sciences
KU Leuven, Belgium

Arjan Vissink, DDS, MD, PhD
Professor, Oral and maxillofacial surgeon
University of Groningen and University Medical
 Center Groningen
Groningen, the Netherlands

Stuart C. White, DDS, PhD
Professor Emeritus, Oral and Maxillofacial
 Radiology
University of California–Los Angeles School
 of Dentistry
Los Angeles, California, USA

Max J. Witjes, DDS, MD, PhD
Assistant Professor, Department of Oral and
 Maxillofacial Surgery
University of Groningen and University Medical
 Center Groningen
Groningen, the Netherlands

Preface

Technology surrounds our private and professional lives, improving at ever-accelerating speeds. In turn, medical imaging benefits from general enhancements in computers, offering faster and more refined views of our patients' anatomy and disease states. Although this Moore's law progression appears to be exponential, it has actually been almost a century since mathematician Johann Radon first laid the groundwork for reconstruction of a three-dimensional object using a great number of two-dimensional projections. The first computed tomography (CT) scanner was invented by Sir Godfrey Hounsfield, after he led a team to build the first commercial computer at Electric and Musical Industries. The theoretical groundwork had been published a few years earlier by a particle physicist, Dr. Allan Cormack. In 1971, the first human computed tomography of a brain tumor was obtained. In 1979, the year Cormack and Hounsfield received the Nobel Prize for their contribution to medicine, more than a thousand hospitals had adopted the new technology. Several generations of computed tomography scanners were later developed, using more refined detectors, faster rotations, and more complex movement around the body. In parallel, starting in the mid-1960s, cone beam computed tomography (CBCT) prototypes were developed, initially for radiotherapy and angiography. The first CBCT was built in 1982 at the Mayo clinic. Yet, computers and detectors were not powerful enough to bring CBCT to practical use. It is only within the last fifteen years that CBCT machines could be built at affordable costs and reasonable sizes. Head and neck applications were an obvious choice.

Although the technology allows for outstanding image quality and ease of use, we should not confuse information with education, data with knowledge. Doctors treat disease with the ultimate purpose to provide a good quality of life to patients. To do so, an in-depth knowledge of diagnosis and treatment methods is necessary. This textbook aims at providing detailed understanding of CBCT technology and its impact on oral and maxillofacial medicine. To achieve the goal of presenting a comprehensive text, world renowned engineers and clinicians from industry, academic, and private practice backgrounds came together to offer the reader a broad spectrum of information.

The clinician will want to jump in and utilize images for diagnostic and treatment purposes. However, a basic understanding of CBCT properties is essential to better interpret the outcome. Trying to comprehend electronics and formulas is daunting to most of us, but Dr. Jacobson manages, in the first chapter, to present the anatomy of the machine in an attractive and elegant way. Dr. Jacobson is the magician behind the scene who has been concerned for many years with image quality, radiation, and speed. In his chapter, he opens the hood and makes us marvel at the ingeniousness and creativity necessary to build a small CBCT scanner.

The next three chapters are written by oral and maxillofacial radiologists, as well as head and neck radiologists. These two groups of specialists possess immense expertise in head and neck diseases and should be called upon whenever any pathology might be present. In the second chapter, Doctors Mallya and White address the major issue of radiobiology risks. Their chapter allows us to make sound and confident judgment, so that X-ray emitting CBCT is only used when the clinical benefits largely outweigh the risk. Dr. Brooks, a pioneer and mentor to us all, reviews major relevant pathologies and reminds us that findings can often be incidental. Drs. Miracle and Christian's unique chapter is a first: it introduces the use of CBCT for pathologies usually studied on medical CTs.

The next chapters address clinical applications. Dr. Cevidanes and her team, who have pioneered the study of orthognathic surgeries' long-term stability using three-dimensional imaging, review the state of scientific knowledge in orthodontics. Next, Dr. Shepers and his colleagues share with us the most advanced surgical techniques they have invented while taking advantage of imaging. We introduce the use of CBCT for everyday implantology to make way to Drs. Mandelaris and Rosenfeld, who present the most advanced use of CAD/CAM surgical guidance for implantology, a field they have led since its inception. Dr. Hatcher, an early adopter and leader in dental radiology, is the expert in three-dimensional airway measurement, which he shares for the first time in a comprehensive chapter. Dr. Levine was first to measure the impact of CBCT in endodontics, which he demonstrates in his unique chapter. Finally, Dr. Vandenberghe shows us the way to use CBCT in periodontics, a new field with promising research he has in great part produced.

At the turn of the century, some of us were asked by a small start-up company to estimate the number of CBCT in dental offices in years to come. Our insight was critical to the business plan, and we anticipated the company could expect to sell about fifteen units per year in the United States. Looking back, it is difficult to comprehend how we could have been so wrong! Immersed in existing options, we were unable to imagine how our practices could be quickly transformed. We should also recall that, at the time, many other electronics now woven to our personal lives were to be invented. So today, we wonder what comes next. This book is a detailed testimony of our knowledge and a window to the near future. This time, we should attempt to use our imagination. We are clearly at the beginning of an era where technological advances assist patient care. The thought leaders who wrote this book are showing us the road to our future.

Acknowledgments

I would like to express my gratitude to the many people who have helped bring this book together, and to those who have developed the outstanding core technology around which it revolves. The topic of this text embodies interdisciplinary interaction at its best: clinical need, science, and engineering were intertwined for an outstanding outcome. Behind each of these disciplines are dedicated individuals and personal stories which I was blessed to often share. I hope to be forgiven by those who are not cited here.

I am thankful to the editors at Wiley Blackwell, who had the foresight many years ago to seek and support this project. In particular, Mr. Rick Blanchette envisioned this book and encouraged me to dive into its conception. To Melissa Wahl, Nancy Turner, and their team, I am grateful for their relentless "behind the scenes" editorial work.

I am forever indebted to the co-authors of the book. They are leaders of their respective fields, busy treating patients, discovering new solutions, or lecturing throughout the word. Yet, a short meeting, a phone call, or a letter was enough to have them on board with writing a chapter. They spent countless hours refining their text, sacrificing precious moments with their families in order to share their passion. As always, the work was much greater than initially anticipated, yet it was completed to the finest detail and greatest quality.

At the University of Michigan, I received the unconditional support of several experienced colleagues. In particular, Professors William Giannobile, Laurie McCauley, and Russel Taichman were immensely generous of their time, expertise, and friendship while I struggled as a young faculty member.

Many engineers spend nights and weekends building, programming, and refining cone beam machines. To them all, we must be thankful. I am particularly grateful to my friend Pedja Sukovic, former CEO at Xoran Technologies in Ann Arbor, Michigan. We first met when he was a PhD student and I was a young faculty. He came to the dental school as a patient, and casually asked if a three-dimensional radiograph of the head would be of interest to us. At the time, his mentor Neal Clinthorne and he had built a bench prototype in a basement laboratory. It was only a matter of time before it became one of the most sought-after machines in the world.

This work would simply have been unimaginable without the support of my family. I owe my grandmother Tosca Yulzari my graduate studies. She saw the beginning of this book but will not see its completion. My father, long gone, taught me the meaning of being a doctor. My best mentor and friend is my wife Sylvie, who has supported me unconditionally during almost two decades. Finally, I thank my children Lea, Myriam, and little Nathanyel, for giving me such joy and purpose.

David Sarment, DDS, MS

Cone Beam Computed Tomography
Oral and Maxillofacial Diagnosis and Applications

1 Technology and Principles of Cone Beam Computed Tomography

Matthew W. Jacobson

This chapter aims to convey a basic technical familiarity with compact Cone Beam Computed tomography (CBCT) systems, which have become prevalent since the late 1990s as enablers of in-office CT imaging of the head and neck. The technical level of the chapter is designed to be accessible to current or candidate end users of this technology and is organized as follows. In Section 1, a high-level overview of these systems is given, with a discussion of their basic hardware components and their emergence as an alternative to conventional, hospital CT. Section 2 gives a treatment of imaging basics, including various aspects of how a CT image is derived, manipulated, and evaluated for quality.

Section 1: Overview of compact cone beam CT systems

Computed tomography (CT) is an imaging technique in which the internal structure of a subject is deduced from the way X-rays penetrate the subject from different source positions. In the most general terms, a CT system consists of a gantry which moves an X-ray source to different positions around the subject and fires an X-ray beam of some shape through the subject, toward an array of detector cells. The detector cells measure the amount of X-ray radiation penetrating the subject along different lines of response emanating from the source. This process is called the *acquisition* of the X-ray measurements. Once the X-ray measurements are acquired, they are transferred to a computer where they are processed to obtain a CT image volume. This process is called *image reconstruction*. Once image reconstruction has been performed, the computer components of the system make the CT image volume available for display in some sort of image viewing software. The topics of image reconstruction and display will be discussed at greater length in Section 2.

Cone beam computed tomography refers to CT systems in which the beam projected by the X-ray source is in the shape of the cone wide enough to radiate either all or a significant part of the volume of interest. The shape of the beam is controlled by the use of collimators, which block X-rays from being emitted into undesired regions of the scanner field of view. Figure 1.1 depicts a CBCT system of a compact variety suitable for use in small clinics. In the particular system shown in the figure, the gantry rotates in a circular path about the subject firing a beam of X-rays that illuminates the entire desired field of view. This results in a series of

---

Cone Beam Computed Tomography: Oral and Maxillofacial Diagnosis and Applications, First Edition. Edited by David Sarment.
© 2014 John Wiley & Sons, Inc. Published 2014 by John Wiley & Sons, Inc.

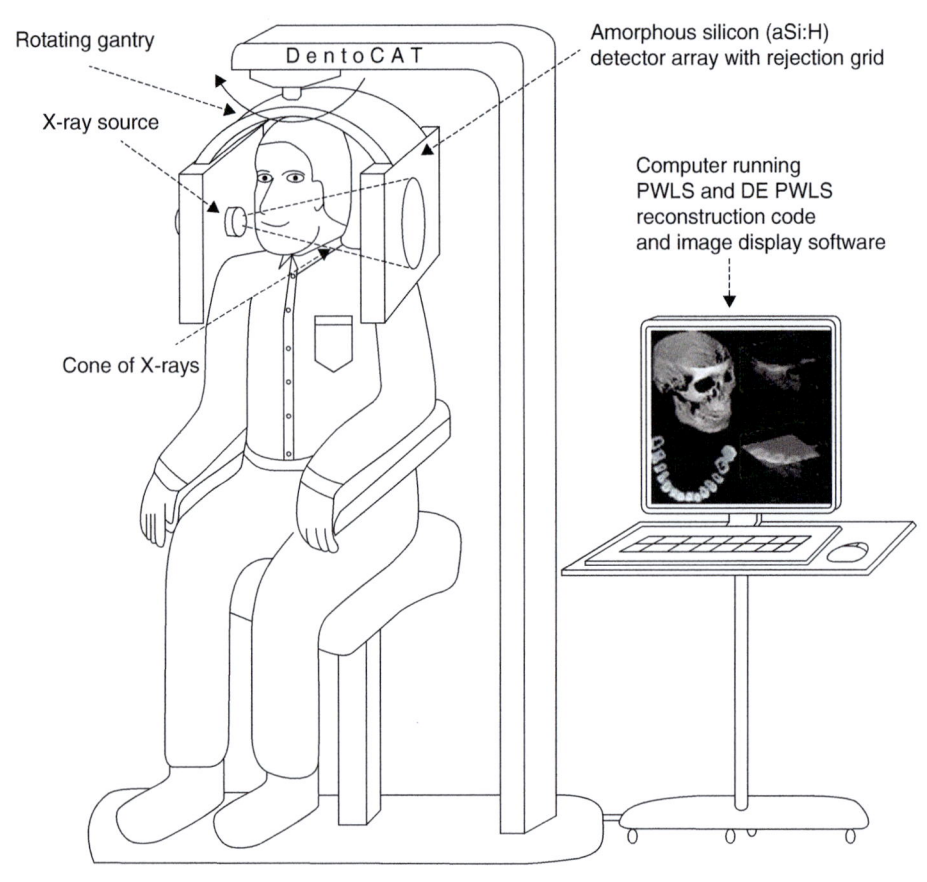

Figure 1.1 The proposed design of DentoCAT. The patient is seated comfortably in chair (the chin-rest is not shown). DentoCAT features cone beam geometry, aSi:H detector array, PWLS and DE PWLS reconstruction methods.

two-dimensional (2D) images of the X-ray shadow of the object that is recorded by a 2D array of detector cells. Cone beam CT systems with this particular scan geometry will be the focus of this book, but it is important to realize that in the broader medical imaging industry, CT devices can vary considerably both in the shape of the X-ray beam and the trajectory of the source.

Prior to the introduction of CBCT, it was common for CT systems to use so-called *fan beam* scan geometries in which collimators are used to focus the X-ray beam into a flat fan shape. In a fan beam geometry, the source must travel not only circularly around the subject but also axially along the subject's length in order to cover the entire volume of interest. A helical (spiral) source trajectory is the most traditional method used to accomplish this and is common to most hospital CT scanners. The idea of fan beam geometries is that, as the source moves along the length of the subject, the X-ray fan beam is used to scan one cross-sectional slice of the subject at a time, each of which can be reconstructed individually. There are several advantages to fan beam geometries over cone beam geometries. First, since only one cross-section is being acquired at a time, only a 1-dimensional detector array is required, which lowers the size and cost of the detector. Second, because a fan beam only irradiates a small region of the object at a given time, the occurrence of scattered X-rays is reduced. In cone beam systems, conversely, there is a much larger component of scattered radiation, which has a corrupting effect on the scan (see "Common Image Artifacts" section). Finally, in a fan beam geometry, patient movement occurring during the scan will only degrade image quality in the small region of the subject being scanned when motion occurs. Conversely, in cone beam systems, where larger regions of anatomy are irradiated at a given time, patient movement can have a much more pervasive effect on image quality.

The disadvantage of fan beam geometries, however, is their inefficient use of X-ray output. Because collimators screen away X-ray output from the source except in the narrow fan region of the beam, much of the X-rays generated by the source go unused. Accordingly, the source must generate more X-ray output than a cone beam geometry for the same region scanned, leading to problems with source heating. Regulating the temperature of the source in such systems requires fast rotating source components, accompanied by a considerable increase in mechanical size, complexity, and expense. As the desire for greater volume coverage has grown in the CT industry, the difficulties with source heating have been found to outweigh the advantages of fan beam scanning, and the CT industry has been gradually moving to cone beam scan geometries. Cone beam geometries have other advantages as well, which have further motivated this shift. The spatial resolution produced by cone beam CT scanners, when used in conjunction with flat panel X-ray detectors, tends to be more uniform than fan beam–based systems.

Although the CT industry as a whole has been trending toward cone beam scanning, the hardware simplifications brought on by CBCT have played a particularly important role in the advent of compact in-office CT systems, of the kind shown in Figure 1.1. Conventional hospital CT scanners are bulky and expensive devices, not practical for in-office use. The reason for their large size is in part due to source cooling issues already mentioned and in part due to the fact that hospital CT systems need to be all-purpose, accommodating a comprehensive range of CT imaging tasks. To accommodate cardiac imaging, for example, hospital CT systems must be capable of very fast gantry rotation (on the order of one revolution per second) to deal with the movement of the heart. This has further exacerbated the mechanical power requirements, and hence the size and expense of the system.

The evolution of compact CT came in part from recognizing how cone beam scanning and other system customizations can mitigate these issues. As discussed, the use of a cone beam scanning geometry increases the efficiency of X-ray use, leading to smaller and cheaper X-ray sources that are easier to cool. Additionally, the imaging needs of dentomaxillofacial and otolaryngological medical offices have generally been restricted to high-contrast differentiation between bone and other tissues in nonmotion prone head and neck anatomy. CT systems customized for such settings can therefore operate both at lower X-ray exposure levels and at slower scanning speeds (on the order of 20–40 sec) than hospital systems. Not only does this further mitigate cooling needs of the X-ray source, it also leads to cheaper and smaller gantry control components.

The emergence of compact CBCT was also facilitated in part by recent progress in fast computer processor technology and in X-ray detector technology. The mathematical operations needed to reconstruct a CT image are computationally intensive and formerly achievable at clinically acceptable speeds only through expensive, special purpose electronics. With the advent of widely available fast computer processors, especially the massively parallel programming now possible with common video game cards, the necessary computer hardware is cheaply available to CT manufacturers and hence also to small medical facilities. Improvements in X-ray detector technology include the advent of flat panel X-ray detectors. Early work on compact CT systems (circa 2000) proposed using X-ray detectors based on image intensifier technology, then common to fluoroscopy and conventional radiography. However, flat panels have provided an alternative that is both cheaply available and also offers X-ray detection with less distortion, larger detector areas, and better dynamic range.

The development of compact CBCT for the clinic has made CT imaging widely and quickly accessible. Where once patients may have had to wait weeks for a scan referred out to the hospital, they may now be scanned and treated in the same office visit. The prompt availability of CT has also been cited as a benefit to the learning process of physicians, allowing them to more quickly correlate CT information with observed symptoms. Some controversy has sprung up around this technology, with questions including how best to regulate X-ray dose to patients. The financial compensation that physicians receive when prescribing a CT scan is argued to be a counterincentive to minimizing patient X-ray dose. In spite of the controversy, CBCT has found its way into thousands of clinics over the last decade and is well on its way to becoming standard of care.

Section 2: Imaging basics for compact cone beam CT systems

This section describes the image processing software components of compact CBCT systems that go into action once X-ray measurements have been acquired. Tasks performed by these components include the derivation of a CT image volume from the X-ray measurements (called *image reconstruction*) and the subsequent display, manipulation, and analysis of this volume. In the subsections to follow, these topics will be covered in a largely qualitative manner suited to practitioners, with a minimum of mathematical detail.

Overview of image processing and display

The volume image data obtained from a CT system is a 3D map of the *attenuation* of the CT subject at different spatial locations. Attenuation, often denoted µ, is a physical quantity measuring the tendency of the anatomy at a particular location to obstruct the flight of X-ray photons. Because attenuation is proportional to tissue density, a 3D map of attenuation can be used to observe spatial variation in the tissue type of the subject anatomy (e.g., soft tissue versus bone). The attenuation applied to an X-ray photon at a certain location also depends on the photon energy. Ideally, when the X-ray source emits photons of a single energy level only, this energy dependence is of minor consequence. In practice, however, an X-ray source will emit photons of a spectrum of different energies, a fact that introduces complications to be discussed later.

Once the X-ray measurements have been acquired, the first processing step performed is to choose an imaging field of view (FOV), a region in space where the CT subject is to be imaged. For circularly orbiting cone beam CT systems, this region will typically be a cylindrical region of points in space that are all visible to the X-ray camera throughout its rotation and that cover the desired anatomy. A process of image reconstruction is then performed in which the X-ray measurements are used to evaluate the attenuation at various sample locations within the FOV. The sample locations typically are part of a 3D rectangular lattice, or reconstruction grid, enclosing the FOV cylinder (see Figure 1.2). The sample locations are thought of as lying at the

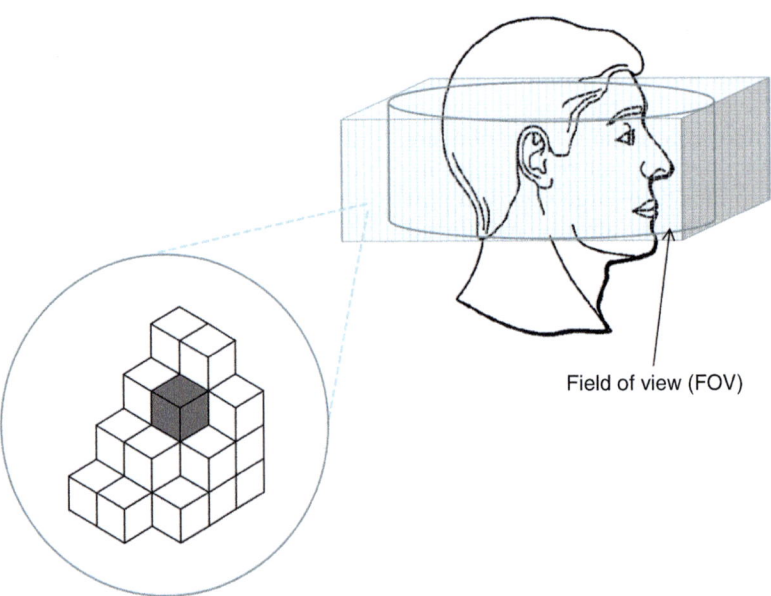

Field of view (FOV)

Figure 1.2 The concept of a reconstruction grid and field of view.

center of small box-shaped cells, called voxels. For image analysis and display purposes, the attenuation of the subject is approximated as being uniform over the region covered by a voxel. Thus, when the reconstruction software assigns an attenuation value to a grid sample location, it is in effect assigning it to the entire box-shaped region occupied by the voxel centered at that location.

The following section will delve into image reconstruction in more detail. For now, we simply note that the selection of an FOV and reconstruction grid brings a number of design trade-offs into play, and must be optimized to the medical task at hand. The selected FOV must first of all be large enough to cover the anatomy to be viewed. In addition, certain medical tasks will require the voxel sizes (equivalently, the spacing between sample points), to be chosen sufficiently small, to achieve a needed resolution. On the other hand, enlarging the FOV and/or increasing the sampling fineness will, in turn, increase the number of voxels in the FOV that need reconstructing. For example, simply halving the voxel size in all three dimensions while keeping the FOV size fixed translates into an eight-fold increase in the number of FOV voxels. This leads in turn to increased computational burden during reconstruction and slows reconstruction speed. Moreover, when sampling fineness in 3D space is increased, the sampling fineness of the X-ray measurements must typically be increased proportionately in order to reconstruct accurate values. This leads to similar increases in computational strain. Finally, as the FOV size is increased, there is a corresponding increase both in radiation dose to the patient, and also the presence of scattered radiation, which leads to a degrading effect on the CT image (see "Common Image Artifacts" section).

Attenuation is measured in absolute units of inverse length (mm^{-1} or cm^{-1}). However, for purposes of analysis and display, it is standard throughout the CT industry to re-express reconstructed image intensities in CT numbers, a normalized quantity which measures reconstructed attenuation relative to the reconstructed attenuation of water:

$$\text{CT No.} = \frac{\mu - \mu_{water}}{\mu_{water}} \times 1000$$

The value of μ_{water} is obtained in a system calibration step by reconstructing a calibration phantom consisting of water-equivalent material. CT numbers are measured in Hounsfield units (HU). In this scale, water always has a CT number of zero, while for air (with $\mu_{air}=0$), the CT number is −1000. Expressing image intensity in HU instead of physical attenuation units provides a more sensitive scale for measuring fine attenuation differences. Additionally, it can help to cross-compare scans of the same object from different CT devices or using different X-ray source characteristics. The effect of the different system characteristics on the contrast between tissue types is more easily observed in the normalized Hounsfield scale, in which waterlike soft tissue is always anchored at a value near zero HU.

Once the reconstructed 3D volume is converted to Hounsfield units, it is made available for display in the system's image viewing software. Typically, an image viewer will offer a number of standard capabilities, among them a multiplanar rendering (MPR) feature that allows coronal, sagittal, or axial slices of the reconstructed object to be displayed (see Figure 1.3). The slices can be displayed as reconstructed, or one can set a range of neighboring slices to be averaged together. This averaging can reduce noise and improve visibility of anatomy at some expense in resolution. Other typical display functions include the ability to rotate the volume so that MPR cross-sections at arbitrary angles can be displayed, a tool to measure physical distances between points in the image, and a tool for plotting profiles of the voxel values across one-dimensional cross-sections.

CT display systems will also provide a drawing tool allowing regions of interest (ROIs) to be designated in the display. The drawing tool will typically show the mean and standard deviation of the voxel values as well as the number of voxels within the ROI to be computed. For CT systems in the U.S. market, this feature is in fact federally required under 21 CFR 1020. Figure 1.4 illustrates a circular ROI drawn in a commercial CT viewer, with the relevant ROI statistics displayed. One function of this tool is to verify certain performance specifications that the CT manufacturer is federally required to provide in the system data sheets and user manual. These metrics will be discussed in greater detail in the "Imaging Performance" section.

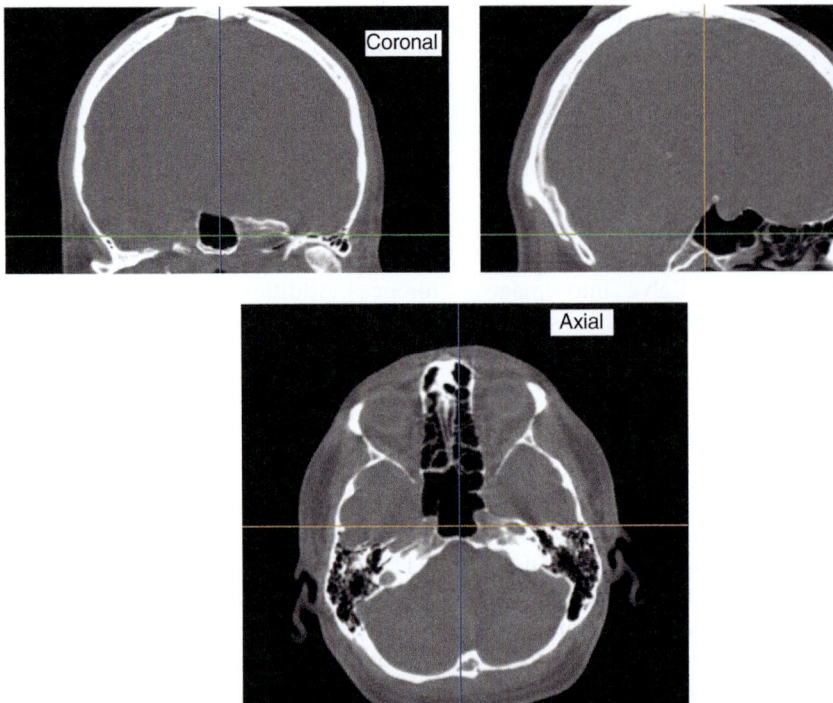

Figure 1.3 Multiplanar rendering of a CT subject.

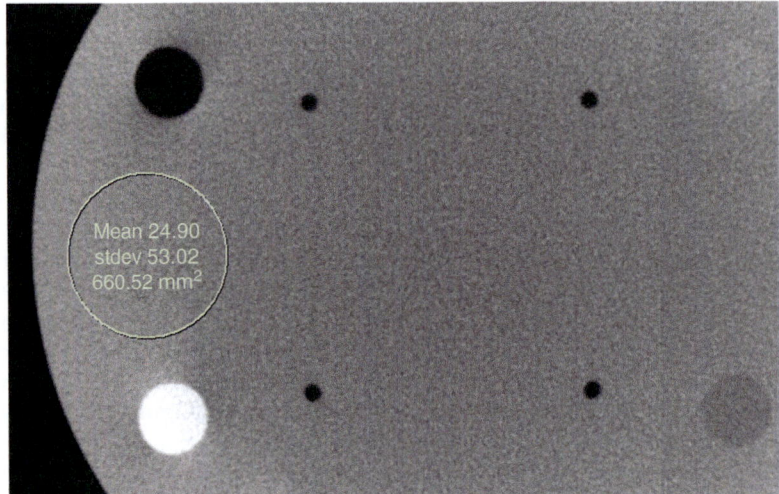

Figure 1.4 Illustration of a region of interest drawing tool in the display of a reconstructed CT phantom.

Another important display capability is the ability to adjust the viewing contrast in the image. Because there are a limited number of different brightness levels that can be assigned to a voxel for display purposes, the viewing software will divide the available brightness levels among the CT numbers in a user-selected range, or window. Image voxels whose CT numbers fall between the

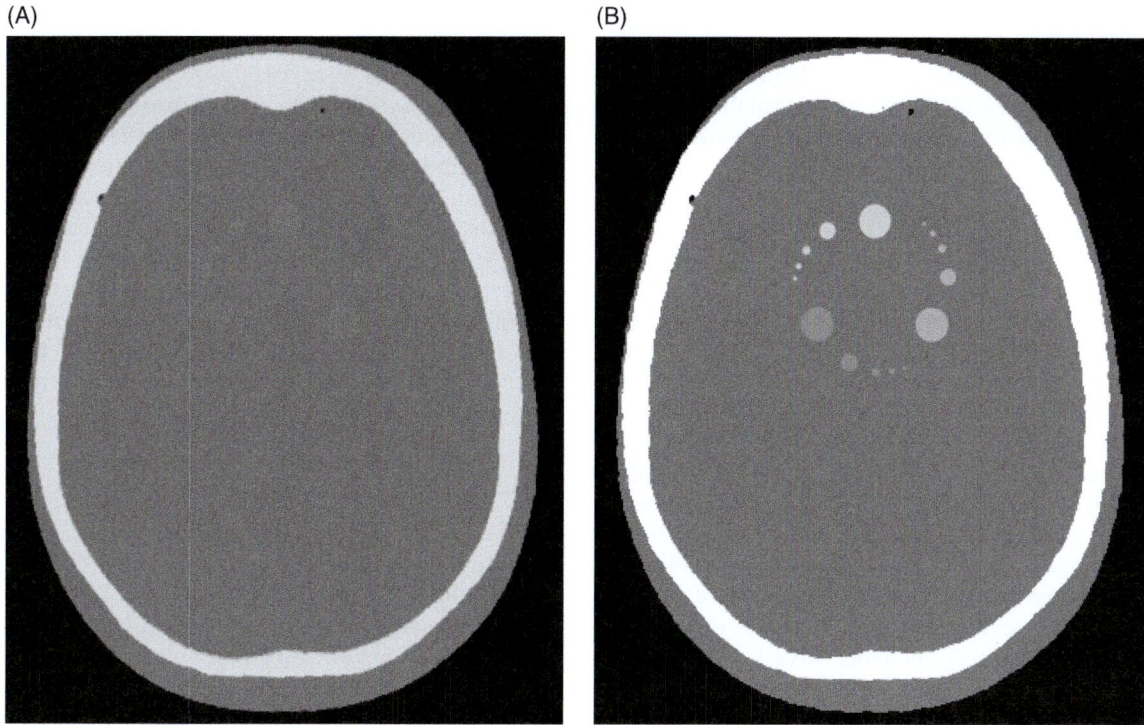

Figure 1.5 Axial slice of computer-generated phantom in (A) a high-contrast viewing window (L/W = 50/1200 HU), and (B) a low-contrast window (L/W = 30/90 HU).

minimum and maximum values set by the window are assigned a proportionate brightness level. If a voxel value falls below the minimum CT number in this range, it will be given zero brightness, whereas if it lies above the maximum CT number, it will be assigned the maximum brightness. It is common to express a window setting in terms of a level (L), meaning the CT number at the center of the range, and a window width (W), meaning the difference between the maximum and minimum CT number in the range. For example, a window ranging between 400 HU and 500 HU would be specified as L=450 HU and W=100 HU.

Narrowing the display window about a particular intensity level allows for better contrast between subtly different image intensities within the window. Figure 1.5 shows an axial slice of a computer-generated head phantom as displayed in both a wide, high-contrast window (Figure 1.5A) and a narrow, low-contrast window (Figure 1.5B). Clearly, the narrower window offers better visibility of the pattern of low-contrast discs in the interior of the slice. At the time of this writing, however, low-contrast viewing windows are more commonly employed by users of compact CBCT systems. This is because certain limitations of the cone beam geometry and of current flat panel technology, to be elaborated upon later, render image quality poor when viewed in high-contrast windows. The industry has therefore been limited to head and neck imaging where often only the coarse differentiation between bone and soft tissue are needed. For these applications, low-contrast viewing windows, such as in Figure 1.5B, tend to be sufficient. The terms *soft tissue window* and *bone window* are commonly used to distinguish between display range settings appropriate, respectively, to soft tissue differentiation and coarse bone/soft tissue differentiation tasks. Soft tissue windows will use window levels of 30–50 HU and window widths of one to several hundred HU. The bone window will use window levels of 50–500 HU and window widths of anywhere from several hundred to over a thousand Hounsfields.

The images in Figure 1.3 and Figure 1.5A are displayed at L/W=50/1200 HU, a setting representative of the bone window. Figure 1.5B is displayed at L/W=30/90 HU, a setting at the narrower end of different possible soft tissue windows.

Image reconstruction

Image reconstruction is the process by which attenuation values for each voxel in the CT image are calculated from the X-ray measurements. This process tends to be the most computationally intensive software task performed by a CBCT system. There are tens of millions of voxels in a typical reconstruction grid and each computed voxel value derives information from X-ray measurements taken typically at hundreds of different gantry positions. A complete image reconstruction task may hence require, at minimum, tens of billions of arithmetic and memory transfer operations. CT manufacturers therefore invest considerable development effort in making reconstructions achievable within compute times acceptable in a clinical environment. Because of the computational hurdles associated with image reconstruction, commercial systems have historically resorted to filtered back projection algorithms. These are among the simplest reconstruction approaches computationally but have certain limitations in the image quality they can produce. As computer processor power has increased over time, however, and especially with the recent proliferation of cheaply available parallel computing technology, the CT industry has begun to embrace more powerful, if more computationally demanding, iterative reconstruction algorithms. The next section will overview conventional filtered back projection reconstruction, which is still the most prevalent approach. The section titled "Iterative Reconstruction" will then give a short introduction to emerging iterative reconstruction methods and some rudimentary demonstrations.

Conventional filtered back projection

To understand conventional image reconstruction, one must first consider a particular line of X-ray photon flight, one that emanates from the X-ray focal spot (see Figure 1.6) to a particular pixel on the detector panel for some particular gantry position. One then considers sample attenuation values of the CT subject along this line, with sample locations spaced at a separation distance, d. If the samples are weighted by this separation distance and summed, then as the separation distance is taken smaller and smaller (making the sampling more and more dense), this weighted sum approaches a

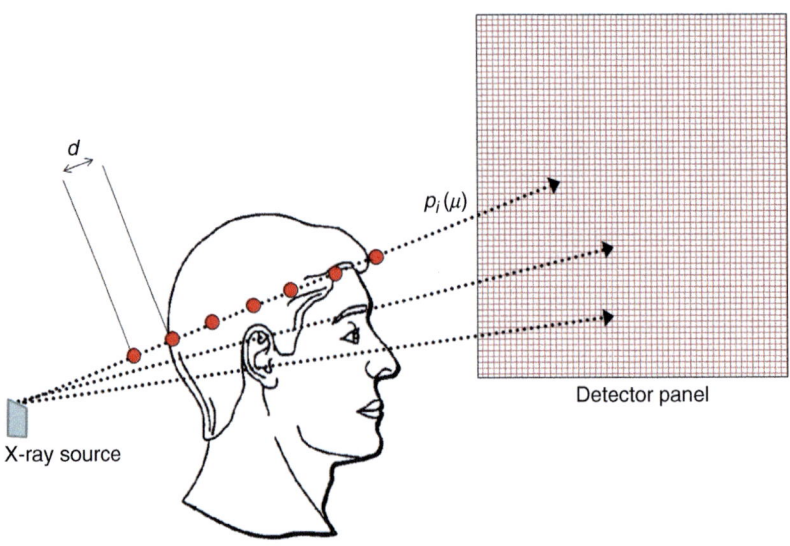

Figure 1.6 The concept of a geometric projection.

limiting value, $p_i(\mu)$, known as the *geometric projection*, or X-ray transform, of the attenuation map, μ, along the i-th measured X-ray path. The idea behind most conventional reconstruction techniques is to extract measurements of the geometric projections from the raw physical X-ray measurements and to then apply known mathematical formulas for inverting the X-ray transform.

The calculation of geometric projections from raw X-ray measurements requires the knowledge of certain physical properties of the source-detector X-ray camera assembly. For example, it is necessary to know the sensitivity of each detector pixel to X-rays fired in air, with no object present in the field of view. It is also necessary to know the detector offset values, which are nonzero signals measured by the detector even when no X-rays are being fired from the source. The offset signals originate from stray electrical currents in the photosensitive components of the detector. These properties are measured in a calibration step performed at the time of scanner installation, by averaging together many frames of an air scan and a blank scan (a scan with no X-rays fired). The air scan and blank scan response will drift over time due to temperature sensitivity of the X-ray detector and gradual X-ray damage, and therefore they must be refreshed periodically, typically by recalibrating the device at least daily.

Once the geometric projections have been calculated, an inverse X-ray transform formula is applied. Commonly, such formulas reduce to a filtering step, applied view-by-view to the geometric projections, followed by a so-called *back projection* step in which the filtered projection values are smeared back through the FOV. Algorithms that implement the reconstruction this way are thus called *filtered back projection* (FBP) algorithms and are used in a range of tomographic systems, both in CT and other modalities. The fine details of both the filtering step and the back projection step are somewhat dependent on the scanning geometry, that is, on the shape of the gantry orbit and the shape of the radiation beam. Generally speaking, however, the filtering step will be an operation that sharpens anatomical edges in the X-ray projections while dampening regions of slowly varying intensity. The smearing action of back projection, meanwhile, will typically be along the measured X-ray paths connecting the X-ray source to the panel, in a sense undoing the forward projecting action of the radiation source. For circular orbiting cone beam CT systems, our primary focus here, a well-known FBP algorithm is the Feldkamp Davis Kress (FDK) algorithm (Feldkamp and Davis, 1984). We will focus on the FDK algorithm for the remainder of this section.

Figure 1.7 illustrates the stages of FDK reconstruction up through filtering, including the data

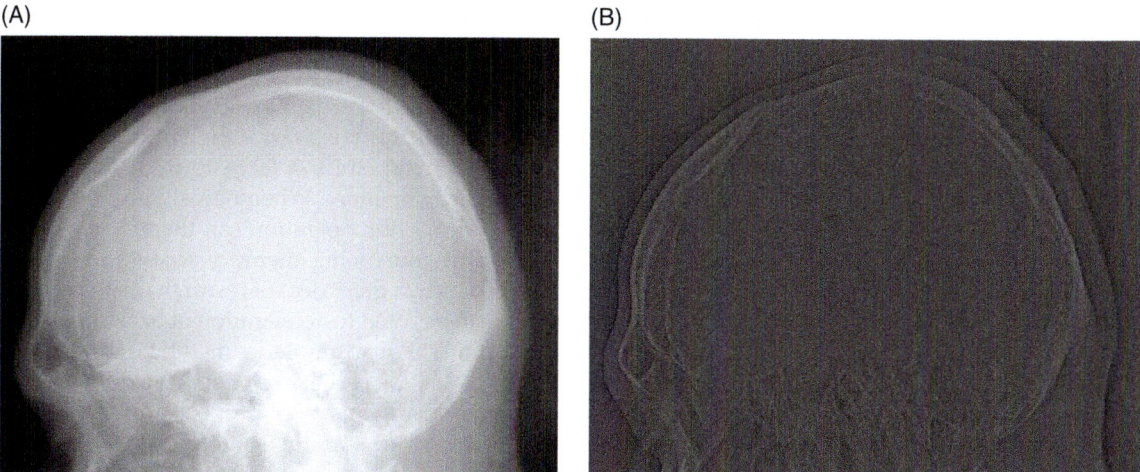

Figure 1.7 Illustration of the precorrection and filtering stages of the FDK algorithm for a CT subject. (A) One frame of precorrected geometric projection measurements. (B) The same frame after filtering.

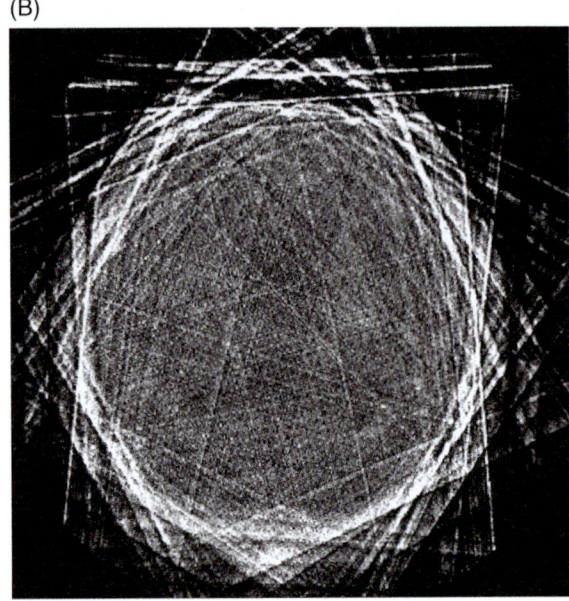

Figure 1.8 The back projection step of the FDK algorithm for progressively larger numbers of frames: (A) 1 frame. (B) 12 frames.

precorrection step, for one frame of a cone beam CT scan. The edge sharpening effect of the filter is clear in Figure 1.7B. Because the sharpening operation can also undesirably amplify sharp intensity changes due to noise, the filtering operation will also employ a user-chosen cutoff parameter. Intensity changes that are "too sharp," as determined by the cutoff, are interpreted by the filter as noise, rather than actual anatomy, and are therefore smoothed. Generally speaking, it is impossible to distinguish anatomical boundaries from noise with perfect reliability, and so applying the cutoff always leads to some sacrifice in resolution in the final image. A judgment must be made by the system design engineers as to the best trade-off between noise suppression and resolution preservation.

Figure 1.8 shows the result of back projecting progressively larger sets of X-ray frames. In Figure 1.8A, where only a single frame is back projected, one can see how smearing the projection intensities obtained at that particular gantry position back through the FOV results in a pattern demarcating the shape of the X-ray cone beam. In Figure 1.8B, C, D, and E, as contributions of more gantry positions are added, the true form of the CT subject gradually coalesces.

As mentioned earlier, image reconstruction is computationally expensive compared to other processing steps in a CT scan. For conventional filtered back projection, most of that expense tends to be concentrated in the back projection step. For the filtering step, very efficient signal processing algorithms exist so that filtering can be accomplished in a few tens of operations per X-ray measurement. Conversely, in back projection, each X-ray measurement contributes to hundreds of voxels lying along the corresponding X-ray path and therefore results in hundreds of computations per data point. Perhaps even more troublesome is that both the voxel array and the X-ray measurement array are too large to be held in computer cache memory. When naively implemented, a back projection operation can therefore result in very time-consuming memory-access operations. Accordingly, a great deal of research over the years has been devoted to acceleration of back projection operations. For example, a method for approximating a typical back projection with greatly reduced operations was proposed by Basu and Bresler (2001). Later, the same group proposed a method that makes memory access patterns more efficient, resulting in strong acceleration over previous methods (De Man and Basu, 2004).

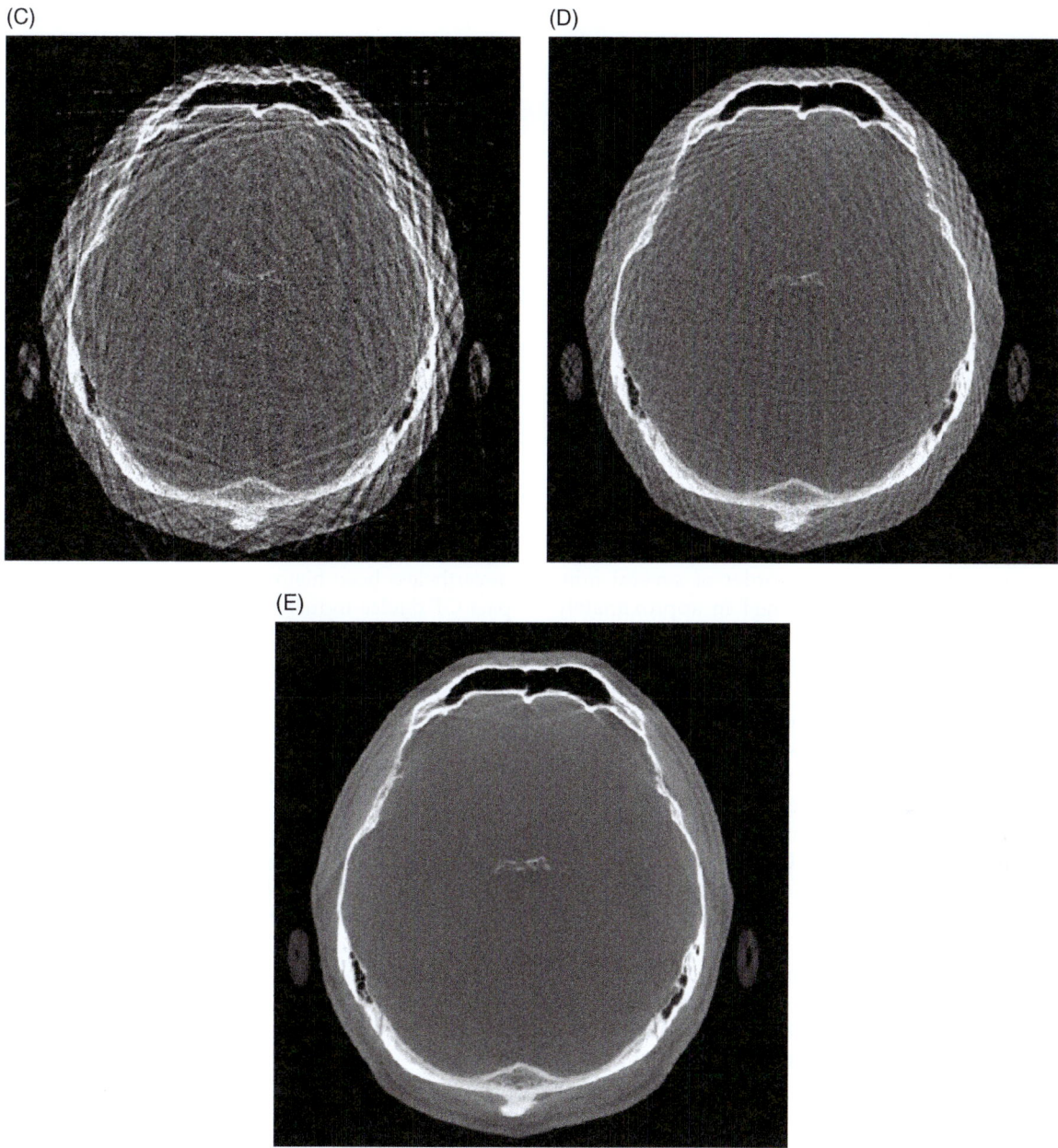

Figure 1.8 (*Continued*) (C) 40 frames. (D) 100 frames. (E) 600 frames.

Much of the acceleration of image reconstruction seen over the years has also been hardware-based. For high-end CT systems, specialized circuit chips known as application-specific integrated circuits (ASICs) have been used in place of software to implement time-consuming reconstruction operations (Wu, 1991). Since the cost of developing such specialized chips can run into millions of dollars, this route has generally been available only to large CT manufacturers. Parallel computing technology has also often been used as an approach to acceleration. Operations like back projection often consist of tasks that are independent and can be dispatched to several processors working in parallel. For example, the contribution of each X-ray frame to the final image can be computed independently of other frames. Similarly, different collections of slices in the reconstruction grid can be reconstructed in parallel.

Although parallel computing has become increasingly available to smaller manufacturers with the emergence of multicore CPUs, it has taken a particular significant leap forward in recent years with the advent of general purpose graphics processing units (GPGPUs). Essentially, it has been found that the massive parallel computing done by common video game graphics cards can be adapted to a variety of scientific computing problems, including FDK back projection (Vaz, McLin, et al., 2007; Zhao, Hu, et al., 2009). This advance has first of all led to a dramatic speed-up in reconstruction time. Whereas five years ago a typical head CT reconstruction took on the order of several minutes, it can now be performed in approximately 10 seconds. Additionally, the use of GPGPU has greatly cut costs of both the relevant hardware and software engineering work. In terms of hardware, the only equipment required is a video card, costs for which may be as low as a few hundred dollars, thanks to the size of the video gaming industry. The necessary software engineering work has been simplified by the emergence of GPGPU programming languages, such as CUDA and OpenCL (Kirk and Hwu, 2010).

While the FDK reconstruction algorithm is the most common choice for circular-orbit cone beam CT systems, there are limitations to a circular-orbiting CT scanner that appear when the FDK algorithm is applied. Specifically, it is known that a circular-orbiting cone beam camera does not offer complete enough coverage of the object to reliably reconstruct all points in the FOV (or at least not by an algorithm relying on the projection measurements alone). Conditions for a point in 3D space to be recoverable in a given scan geometry are well studied and are given, for example, in Tuy (1983). For circular-orbiting cameras, only points in the plane of the X-ray source satisfy these conditions. Because of this, the accuracy and quality of the reconstructed image gradually deteriorate with distance from the source plane. This is illustrated in Figure 1.9, which shows sagittal views of a computer-generated head phantom and its FDK reconstruction from simulated cone beam CT measurements. Comparing Figure 1.9B to Figure 1.9A, one can clearly see an erroneous drop-off in the image intensity values with distance from the plane of the source, as well as the appearance of streaks and shading artifacts. These so-called cone beam artifacts become more pronounced where the axial cross-sections are less symmetric, for example, in the bony region of the sinuses. It is important to emphasize that artifacts such as these can arise from a number of different causes in actual CT scans, such as scatter and beam hardening (see "Common Image Artifacts"). Here, however, the simulation has not included any such corrupting effects. The artifacts we see here are therefore assuredly and entirely due to the limitations of the circular scan geometry and the FDK algorithm.

In spite of this fundamental weakness in circular cone beam scans, the circular scan geometry has nevertheless been historically favored in the compact CT device industry. This is in part because it simplifies mechanical design. It is also because a range of these artifacts are obscured when the phantom is viewed in a high-contrast bone window (as illustrated in Figure 1.9C and Figure 1.9D), and bone window imaging has been an application of predominant interest for compact CT. On the other hand, this can also be seen as one reason why circular cone beam CT has had difficulty spreading in use from bone imaging to lower contrast imaging applications. In the next section, we discuss iterative reconstruction, which among other things offers possibilities for mitigating the problem of cone beam artifacts.

Iterative reconstruction

Although filtered back projection methods have been commercially implemented for many years, the science has continued to look for improvements using iterative reconstruction methods, both in CT and in other kinds of tomography (Shepp and Vardi, 1982; Lange and Carson, 1984; Erdoğan and Fessler, 1999a). With iterative reconstruction, instead of obtaining a single attenuation map from an explicit reconstruction formula, a sequence of attenuation maps is generated that converges to a final desired reconstructed map. While iterative methods are more computationally

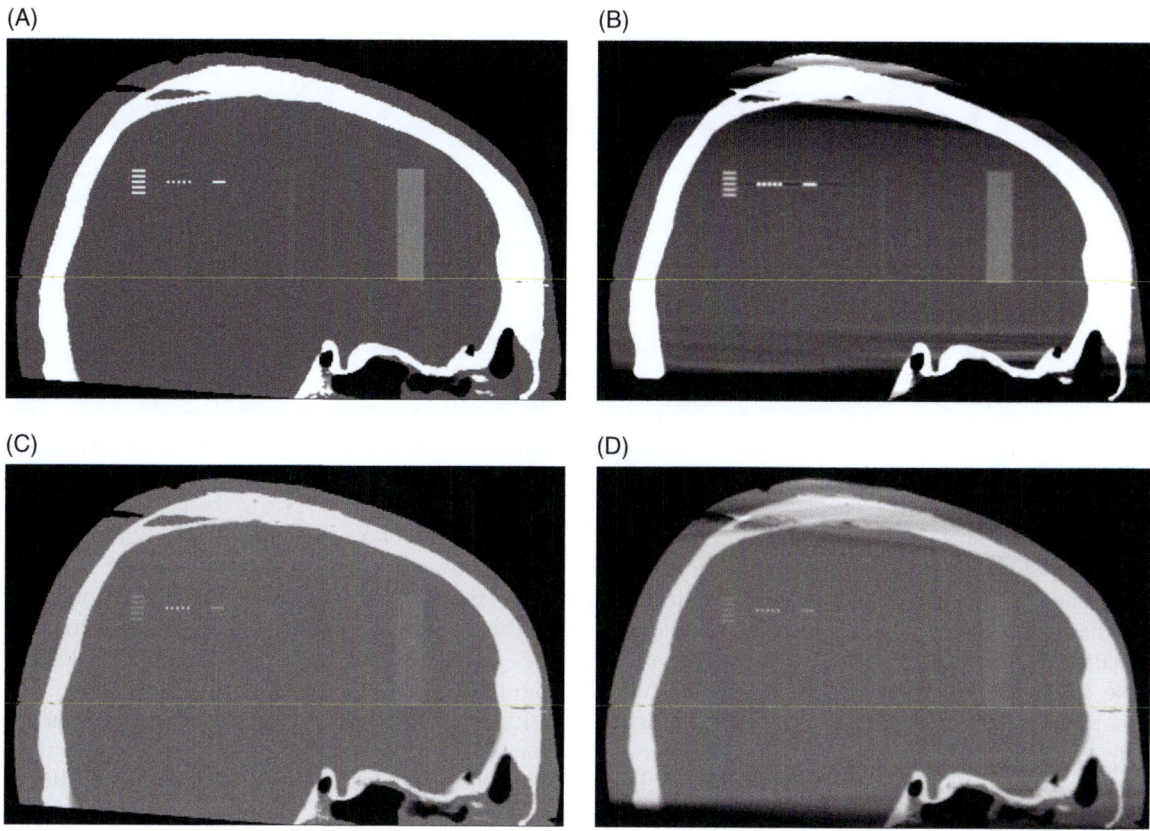

Figure 1.9 Comparison of sagittal views of a computer-generated phantom and its FDK reconstruction in low- and high-contrast viewing window. The dashed line marks the position of the plane of the x-ray source. (A) True phantom, low-contrast window (L/W = 50/200 HU). (B) FDK reconstruction, low-contrast window (L/W = 50/200 HU). (C) True phantom, high-contrast window (L/W = 50/1200 HU). (D) FDK reconstruction, high-contrast window (L/W = 50/1200 HU).

demanding than filtered back projection, they provide a flexible framework for using better models of the CT system, leading to better image quality, sometimes at reduced dose levels. At this writing, iterative methods have also begun to find their way into the commercial CT device market. Notably, the larger medical device companies have commercialized proprietary iterative methods with claims of reducing X-ray dose by several factors without compromising image quality (Freiherr, 2010). Iterative reconstruction software is also marketed by private software vendors such as InstaRecon, Inc., sample results of which are shown subsequently.

In the design of image reconstruction algorithms, there is a trade-off between the amount/accuracy of physical modeling information included in an algorithm, which affects image quality, and the computational expense of the algorithm, which affects reconstruction speed. The previous section overviewed traditional filtered back projection algorithms, which are among the simplest and fastest reconstruction methods. An explicit formula is used to obtain the reconstructed image, and only one pass over the measured X-ray data is required. However, the amount of physical modeling information used in filtered back projection is fairly limited. As an example, filtered back projection ignores statistical variation in the X-ray measurements, leading to higher noise levels in the reconstructed image (or alternatively higher radiation dose levels) than are actually necessary. FBP also ignores the fact that realistic X-ray beams consist of a multitude of X-ray photon energies,

(A) 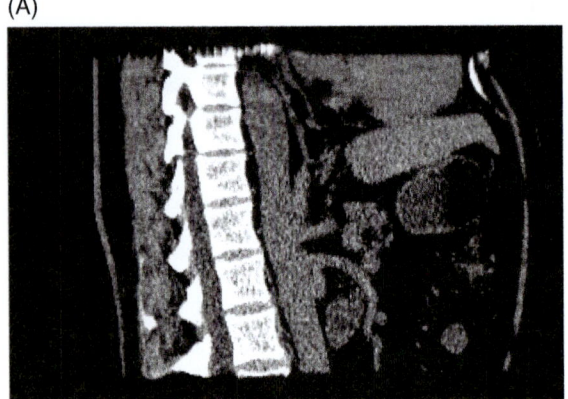 (B)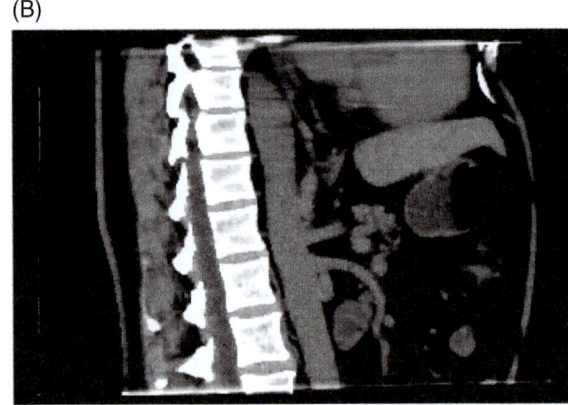

Figure 1.10 Reconstructions of a clinical helical CT scan of the abdomen using (A) filtered back projection and (B) a proprietary iterative algorithm developed by InstaRecon.

approximating the beam instead as a monoenergetic one. This leads to beam hardening artifacts, to be discussed under "Common Image Artifacts." Finally, FBP only incorporates information available in the X-ray measurements, whereas more complicated iterative algorithms can also incorporate a priori knowledge about the characteristics of the patient anatomy. This has important implications for circular-orbit CBCT systems, because for this scanning geometry (see "Conventional Filtered Back Projection" section), the X-ray measurements alone cannot provide enough information to accurately reconstruct the object at all points in the field of view. The FDK algorithm, a variation of FBP specific to circular-orbit systems, produces cone beam artifacts, as a result.

The desire to improve image quality has led many researchers over the years to propose reconstruction algorithms based on more detailed and complicated physical models of CT systems. These more complicated models lead to reconstruction equations that have no explicit solution. Instead, the solution must be obtained by iterative computation, in which a sequence of images is generated that gradually converges to the solution. Generally speaking, every iteration of an iterative reconstruction algorithm tends to have a computational cost comparable to an FBP reconstruction. This extra computation puts a significant price tag on the image quality improvements that iterative reconstruction proposes to bring, a price tag that delayed the clinical acceptability of these methods for many years. Nevertheless, the advantages of iterative reconstruction over filtered back projection are readily demonstrated. Some relevant illustrations are provided in Figure 1.10, Figure 1.11, and Figure 1.12.

Figure 1.10A and Figure 1.10B show a performance comparison of a proprietary iterative algorithm developed by InstaRecon with filtered back projection for a clinical abdominal scan. This particular scan was acquired using a conventional helical CT system, and so the filtered back projection algorithm used was not cone beam FDK. The iterative algorithm achieves reduced image noise and hence more uniform images. Furthermore, since image noise generally trades off with X-ray exposure, noise-reducing iterative algorithms such as these also allow one to scan with reduced X-ray dose, while achieving the same noise levels in the reconstructed image as conventional filtered back projection. Figure 1.11A and Figure 1.11B show a similar comparison for simulated CT measurements of a phantom commonly used to measure low-contrast imaging performance. One sees how the iterative algorithm improves the detectability of low-contrast objects as compared to filtered back projection.

Figure 1.12A and Figure 1.12B show iterative reconstructions of the same computer-generated CBCT phantom scan as in Figure 1.9. This reconstruction algorithm incorporates prior information about the piece-wise smooth structure of the patient anatomy. Reconstruction algorithms

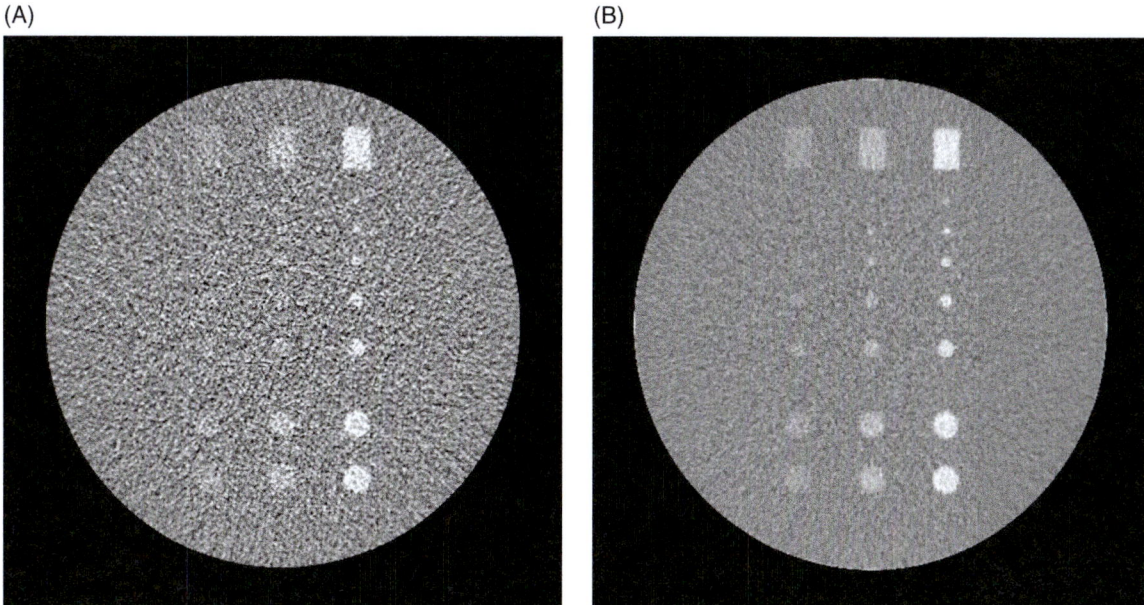

Figure 1.11 Reconstructions of a simulated CBCT scan of a CIRS061 contrast phantom using (A) filtered back projection and (B) a proprietary iterative algorithm developed by InstaRecon.

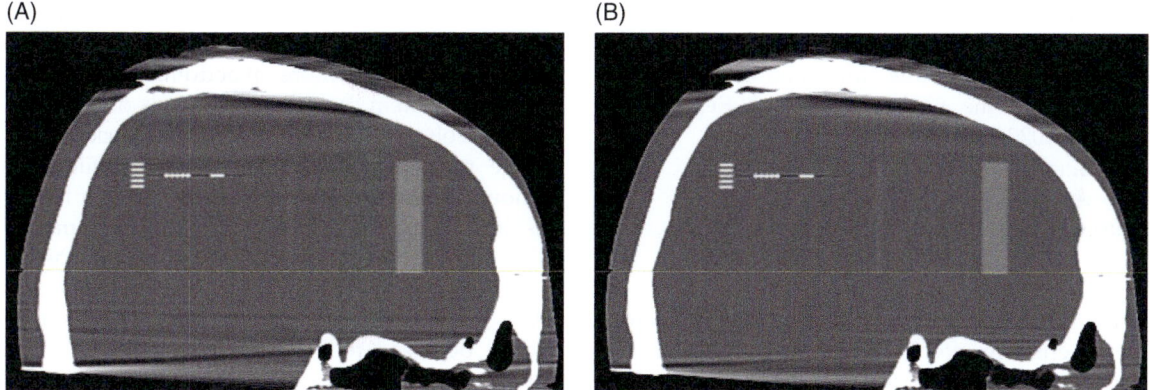

Figure 1.12 Sagittal views of a computer-generated phantom reconstructed using a rudimentary iterative algorithm in a low-contrast viewing window (L/W = 50/200 HU). (A) Result after 30 iterations. (B) Result after 300 iterations.

that incorporate such information (Sukovic and Clinthorne, 2000) are abundant in the medical imaging literature. The reconstruction algorithm used here was more rudimentary than Insta-Recon's algorithm. Among other things, it has not been optimized for speed and it takes many more iterations to converge. However, it was sufficient to show how adding prior smoothness information can mitigate cone beam artifacts. Figure 1.12 shows that the intensity values in the region of the sinuses are much closer to their true value as compared to the FDK results in Figure 1.9B. This occurs because the addition of prior information about anatomical smoothness compensates for the geometric incompleteness of the circular X-ray camera orbit.

Although the image quality benefits of iterative algorithms have been known for many years, it has only recently become possible to run at sufficient speed to make them clinically acceptable for CT imaging. Computing hardware improvements over the years, such as GPGPU discussed earlier, have contributed to reducing computation time per iteration. Additionally, much medical imaging research has been devoted to finding iterative reconstruction algorithms requiring as few as possible iterations to converge (Kamphuis and Beekman, 1998; Erdoğan and Fessler, 1999b; Ahn, Fessler, et al. 2006).

Imaging performance

This section discusses several quantitative measures of image quality that are commonly used to assess the performance of a CT device, namely noise performance, low-contrast detectability, and spatial resolution. CT manufacturers will typically report such quality measurements in the user manuals issued with their devices. Typically also, manufacturers provide customers equipment to repeat these measurements and specify in the user manual how reproducible the measurements should be. For CT manufacturers in the United States, providing this information is legally required by the Code of Federal Regulations (21 CFR 1020.33).

Image noise

The term *measurement noise* refers to random variations in CT measurements. *Image noise* refers to the ensuing effect of these variations on the reconstructed image. In a CT scan, there are several sources of measurement noise that make the measurements not precisely repeatable. When X-rays are fired through a patient along a certain straight-line path, there is randomness in the number of photons that will penetrate through the object to interact with the detector. There is also randomness in the number of photons that, after penetrating the object, will successfully interact with the X-ray detector panel to produce a signal. Finally, there are also elements of random fluctuation in the detector electronics itself, independent of the object and the X-ray source.

Measurement noise leads to sharp discontinuities among the measured values of neighboring detector pixels. When the X-ray measurements are put through the image reconstruction process, the reconstructed CT volume will exhibit correspondingly sharp discontinuities among neighboring voxel values that would otherwise be uniform or gradually varying. This is the visual manifestation of image noise. A common way to measure image noise is to compute the standard deviation of some region of voxels in a phantom of some uniform material (as in Figure 1.4, for example). As mentioned in the "Overview of Image Processing and Display," most CT image viewing software provides this capability. In manuals for a CT device, the noise standard deviation will often be reported as a fraction of the attenuation of water.

CT system engineers make design choices to control noise but must take certain trade-offs into account. Measurement noise can be reduced, for example, by increasing X-ray exposure to the patient, although health concerns place obvious limits on doing so. Certain types of detector panels have better photon detection efficiency than others, giving better resistance to noise. However, such detectors are also more expensive and lead to increased system cost. Other methods of reducing noise involve configuring the X-ray detection and image reconstruction process in a certain way, although these methods entail trade-offs in image resolution. For example, most detector panels allow one to combine neighboring detector pixels to form larger pixels. This "binning" of pixels effectively averages together the signal values that would be measured by the smaller pixels separately and reduces noise. However, projection sampling fineness, and hence resolution, are also reduced as a trade-off. Similarly, the reconstruction software can be designed to include smoothing operations. As mentioned previously, filtered back projection methods include smoothing in the filtering step, while iterative reconstruction methods can enforce image smoothness using a priori anatomical information. These smoothing methods reduce noise but can also blur anatomical tissue borders as a side effect, and so resolution is again sacrificed. Reconstruction algorithms are often compared based on how favorably noise trades off with spatial resolution.

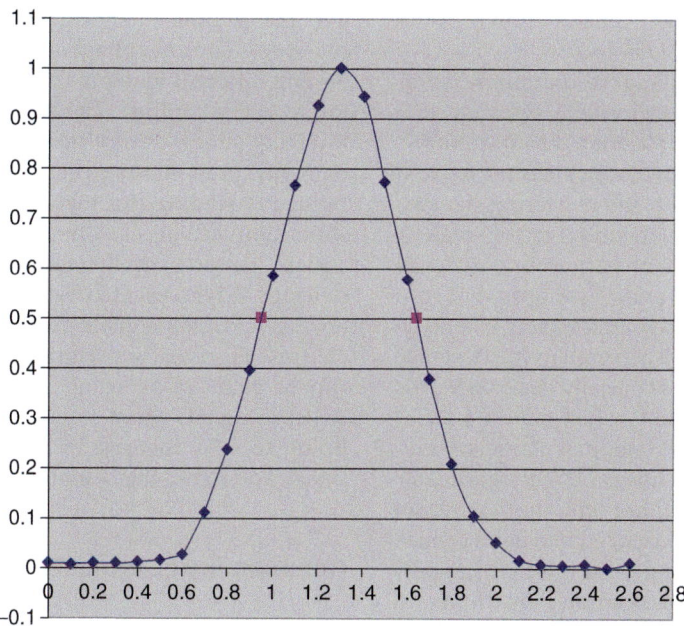

Figure 1.13 Example of a slice sensitivity profile (SSP) illustrated with data from the xCAT-ENT, a commercial mobile cone beam CT scanner for sinus imaging. The profile is plotted on a horizontal axis in units of millimeters.

Spatial resolution

Spatial resolution refers to how well small or closely spaced objects are visualized in an image. Spatial resolution in a cone beam CT system is partly limited by the size of the image voxels used for reconstruction. However, resolution is further limited by various sources of system blur. As discussed in the previous section, certain sources of blur arise as a side effect of various engineering measures taken to reduce image noise. Other sources of blur arise from the physics of the X-ray detection process. Detector glare is an effect whereby X-ray photons striking the detector induce a scattering event that causes a signal to be detected in several neighboring pixels. This leads to a blurring of the projection views and an ensuing blur in the reconstructed image. A similar effect is detector lag, in which the signal detected in one X-ray shot fails to dissipate before the next X-ray shot is taken. This has the effect of blurring together adjacent X-ray shots. Finally, imperfect modeling of the CT system geometry in the reconstruction process can also blur the image. For example, no cone beam CT system produces a perfectly cone-shaped X-ray beam because X-rays are emitted from different points on the surface of the source, rather than from a single apex point. However, this effect is commonly ignored by the reconstruction software, at the expense of spatial resolution.

In conventional helical fan beam CT systems, the amount of blur along the axis of the scanner has historically been significantly different than the blur within an axial slice. This difference has led to common practices, and in some cases regulations, for CT manufacturers to report separate measurements of axial and in-plane spatial resolution. With the advent of cone beam systems, the difference in axial versus in-plane resolution has greatly diminished, but laws designed for helical fan beam systems are so well established that they are still applied to CBCT. To measure spatial resolution axially, an object such as a wire or bead, whose cross-section along the scanner axis is narrow and pointlike, is imaged. Due to blur effects, the cross-section in the image will have a smeared, lobelike profile, such as that shown in Figure 1.12. The amount of blur is reported on a *slice sensitivity profile* such as the one in Figure 1.13. The width of this profile at half its peak value is known as the *nominal tomographic section thickness*.

To measure in-plane spatial resolution, it is traditional to report the *modulation transfer function* (MTF). An MTF is a graph showing how the imaged contrast of densely clustered objects decreases, as a result of system blur, with the clustering density. As a result of blur effects, the intensity of small or narrow objects is diluted with background material in the image, thereby lowering their apparent contrast. Since objects must be of decreasing size to be clustered more densely, an accompanying decrease in contrast with density is typically observed. This is illustrated in Figure 1.14A, which shows a series of progressively denser line pair targets, with the density expressed in line pairs per centimeter (lp/cm). One can see how not only the separation between the more densely spaced line pairs diminishes as a result of blur, but also their percent contrast with the background medium. By measuring the percent contrast of line pair phantoms, one can plot contrast versus line pair density, which is how MTF plots are often expressed. MTFs can also be obtained more indirectly by measuring an in-plane blur profile, similar to the slice sensitivity profile (Boone, 2001). The MTF plots in Figure 1.14B were obtained in such a manner. They show the MTFs for two imaging modes of a commercial ear-nose-throat scanner. The temporal bone mode has a more slowly decreasing MTF, indicative of less blur and higher spatial resolution, than the sinus mode. This is typical, due to the higher resolution needs of temporal bone imaging tasks.

Low-contrast detectability

Low-contrast detectability is a performance parameter of CT systems that measures its overall ability to resolve small differences in intensity between objects. To test low-contrast detectability in a CT system, phantoms such as that in Figure 1.11, containing low-contrast targets of a range of sizes, are often used.

As discussed in the previous section, system blur reduces the contrast of small objects. However, there are other contrast-limiting effects in a CBCT system that can affect the visibility of large objects as well. One contrast-limiting effect in CT systems is the energy spectrum of the X-ray source. At lower average photon energies, obtained by lowering the X-ray source voltage, attenuation differences among different materials generally increase, leading to better contrast. The engineering trade-off in lowering source energy, however, is that the ability of X-ray photons to penetrate the CT subject is reduced, leading to higher noise and photon starvation artifacts. Contrast is also limited by certain features in the electronics of the X-ray detector. When detected X-rays are converted from analog to digital signals, information about tissue contrast is somewhat degraded. This degradation can be reduced by using A/D converters which digitize signals more finely, but the trade-off in doing so is an increase in the cost of the detector panel, and hence the overall system.

Common image artifacts

Image artifacts are visible patterns in an image arising from systematic errors in the reconstruction process. Common kinds of artifacts include streaks and nonuniformity trends, such as in Figure 1.15A. For circular-orbiting CT systems, ring artifacts such as in Figure 1.16A are also commonly encountered. Current use of compact CT systems is often tolerant to artifacts, since bone window viewing of CT images is still very prevalent, and many artifacts are obscured in the bone window. An understanding of artifacts and their causes can still be important, however, for several reasons. First, there are exceptions where artifacts are severe enough to appear even in the bone window viewing applications. When scanning very bony anatomy, for example in dental or skull base imaging, very strong streak artifacts can be present. Artifacts can also be a sign that a CT system is in need of maintenance. Strong ring artifacts can appear when the system is in need of recalibration, for instance. Finally, as practitioners expand their use of compact CT to low-contrast soft tissue imaging applications, the influence of artifacts becomes more noticeable in the less forgiving low-contrast viewing windows. Means of suppressing artifacts will be important to extending compact CT to these applications.

Causes of artifacts can be either advertent or inadvertent. Inadvertent causes include inaccuracies in the calibration of the CT system. When a CT system

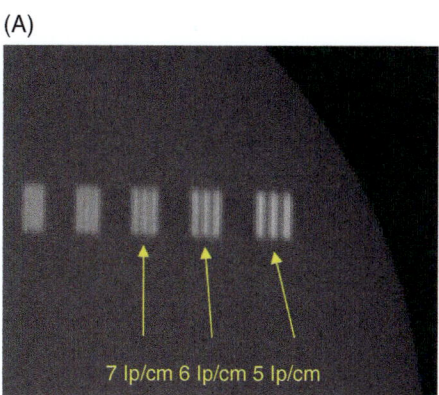

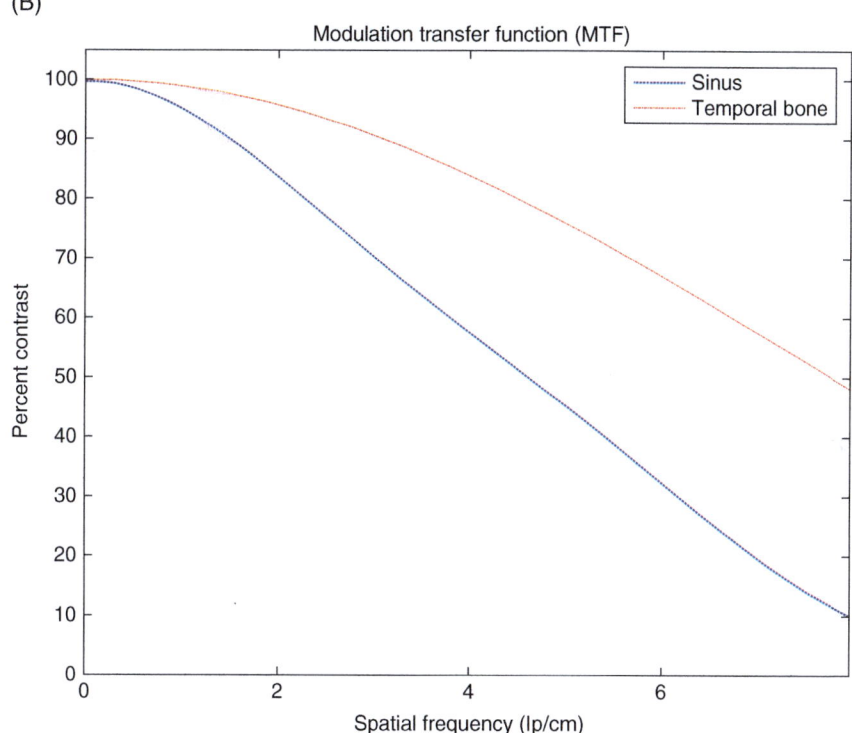

Figure 1.14 Concepts of in-plane resolution measurement illustrated with data from the MiniCAT, a commercial cone beam CT scanner for sinus and temporal bone imaging. (A) Reconstructed image of a phantom containing line pair targets of different densities. lp/cm = line pairs per centimeter. (B) Modulation transfer function for the MiniCAT's sinus and temporal bone scan protocols.

is first installed, and possibly periodically thereafter, certain physical properties of the system must be measured through a calibration procedure. The physical properties to be calibrated are ones that cannot be precisely controlled by the manufacturer, or that may drift over the lifetime of the machine in some uncontrollable way. In the section "Conventional Filtered Back Projection," for example, it was discussed how certain detector pixel parameters must be calibrated periodically using air scans and blank scans. These kinds of calibrated quantities serve as input to the image

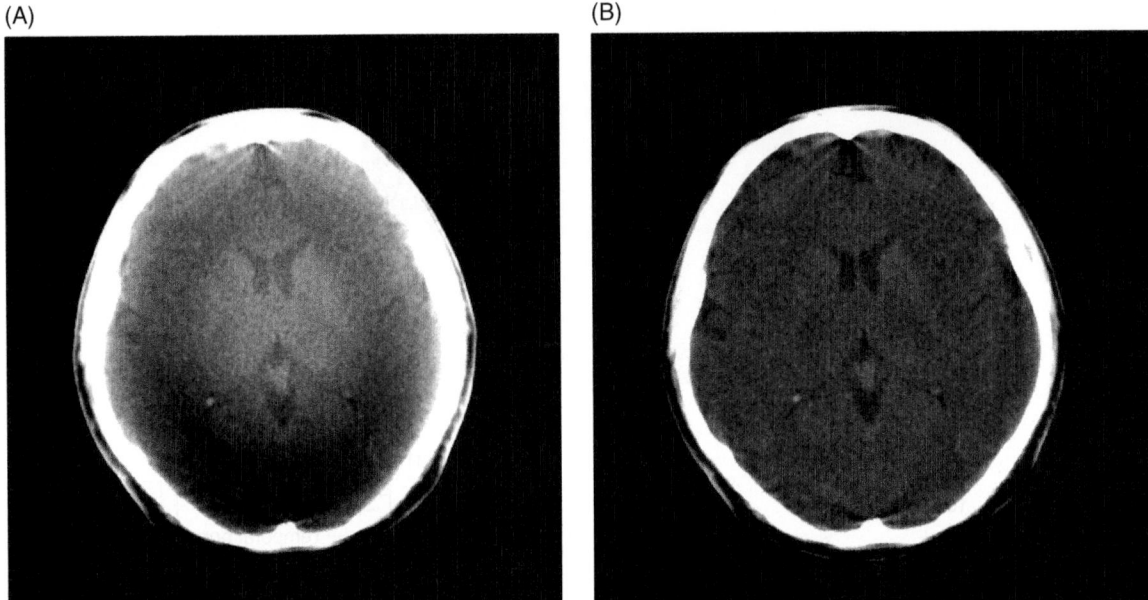

Figure 1.15 (A) Illustration of streaks and nonuniformity artifacts in an axial slice of a low-contrast CBCT scan. (B) The same slice after a postcorrection method is applied.

reconstruction process, which uses them to model system behavior. Inaccuracies in the calibration create disagreement between the true physical X-ray measurements and the mathematical model used by the reconstruction software, resulting in image artifacts. In circular-scanning CBCT systems, inaccuracies in pixel sensitivities and offsets are a typical cause of tree trunk–like ring artifacts, like those shown in Figure 1.16A. Miscalibration of a given pixel will introduce errors in how that pixel's measurement is processed in every X-ray shot. The repetition of these measurement errors throughout the circular orbit of the X-ray camera leads to circularly symmetric artifact patterns in the image, thus showing as rings.

Artifacts can also result from deliberate mathematical errors and approximations made by the reconstruction algorithm to simplify computation. As an example, in the "Conventional Filtered Back Projection" section, it was discussed how cone beam artifacts are an engineering trade-off to the mechanical simplicity of a circular-orbiting CT camera, as well as to the computational simplicity of the FDK reconstruction algorithm. Similar kinds of trade-offs have historically been made in the treatment of other corrupting physical effects such as beam hardening and scatter. Beam hardening is a physical effect whereby the average energy content of an X-ray beam gradually increases as the photons in the beam pass through an object. This occurs because lower energy X-ray photons have a lower probability than higher energy photons of passing through the object unattenuated, and are progressively sifted out of the beam. Scatter is an effect whereby some X-ray photons traveling through the CT subject are deflected from a straight-line path, due to interaction with matter, and generate signal in the wrong detector pixels. When ignored by the reconstruction process, both beam hardening and scatter can contribute to coarse nonuniformity artifacts, such those as shown in Figure 1.15A. Moreover, when scanning bony, asymmetric anatomy, beam hardening and scatter can contribute to streak artifacts, also shown in the figure. Streaks result whenever certain particular X-ray shots contain much more measurement errors than at other positions of the X-ray camera. Beam hardening and scatter effects are a common cause of such errors because their effect varies strongly with the thickness and density of tissue through which the X-ray beam passes.

(A)   (B)

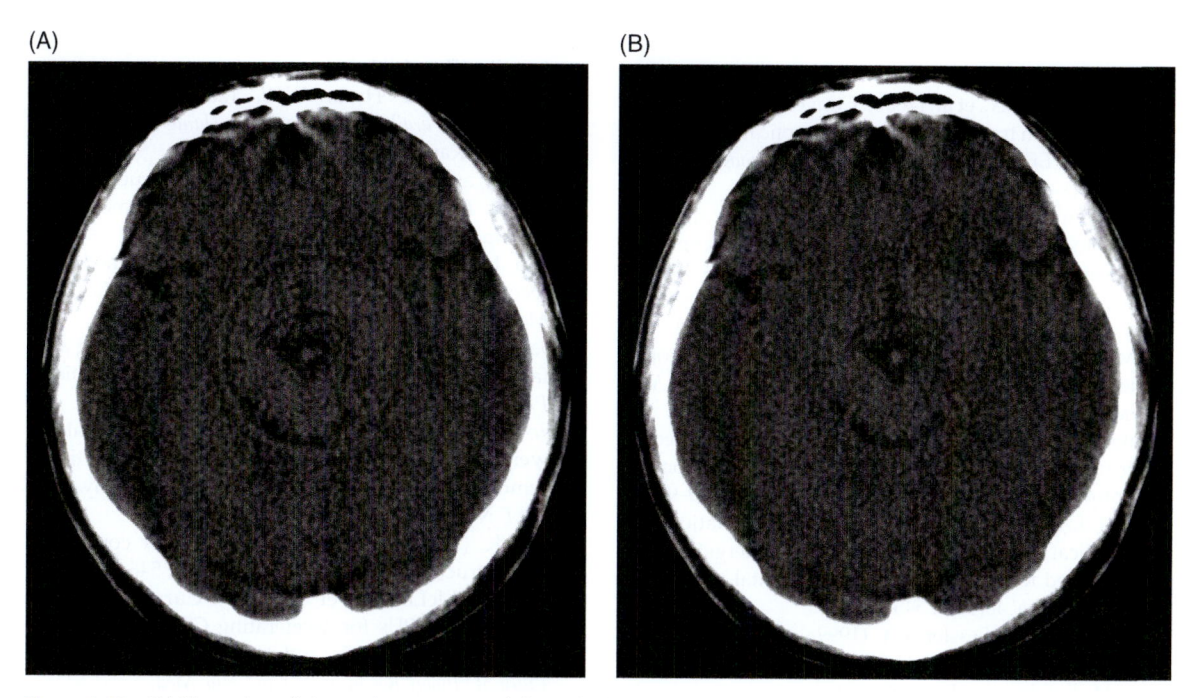

Figure 1.16 (A) Illustration of ring artifacts in an axial slice of a low-contrast CBCT scan. (B) The same slice after a ring correction method is applied.

For asymmetric patient anatomy, these in turn vary strongly with the position of the X-ray camera relative to the patient.

Beam hardening and scatter have historically been computationally expensive to handle in the image reconstruction process in a mathematically precise way, which means that in practice they are either ignored or corrected using computationally cheaper compromises. One of the more mathematically rigorous ways of dealing with beam hardening, for example, is to use an image reconstruction algorithm that models the energy variation of the beam (Elbakri and Fessler, 2002; Elbakri and Fessler, 2003). However, reconstruction algorithms with this level of modeling generally require iterative methods, and only in recent years has computing technology become fast enough to consider using such methods clinically. Similarly, scientific literature has proposed very accurate scatter modeling and correction approaches (Zbijewski and Beekman, 2006). However, achieving clinically viable computation time remains a challenge with these methods.

In situations where rigorous image reconstruction is too expensive computationally, but where the resulting artifacts cannot be tolerated, commercial systems will often remove artifacts from the reconstructed image using fast postcorrection methods. These methods are often proprietary, and therefore it is hard to comment authoritatively on how they work for different CT vendors. However, a variety of postcorrection methods have been proposed in public-domain scientific literature. It is likely that at least some methods used commercially are derived from these. The degree of mathematical or physical modeling rigor on which postcorrection methods are based can vary greatly. There is therefore much ongoing debate in scientific literature over their limitations, as compared to their more computationally expensive, mathematically rigorous alternatives. However, postcorrection methods have certainly proven effective enough to make them popular compromises. Figure 1.15B, for example, demonstrates the reduction of streak and nonuniformity artifacts using a combination of postprocessing approach (Zbijewski and Stayman, 2009; Hsieh, Molthen, et al., 2000). Figure 1.16B demonstrates the reduction of ring artifacts using a postcorrection method (Sijbers and Postnov, 2004).

References

Ahn, S., Fessler, J.A., et al. (2006). Convergent incremental optimization transfer algorithms: Application to tomography. *IEEE Transactions on Medical Imaging* 25(3): 283–96.

Basu, S., and Bresler, Y. (2001). Error analysis and performance optimization of fast hierarchical backprojection algorithms. *IEEE Trans Im Proc* 10(7): 1103–17.

Boone, J.M. (2001). Determination of the presampled MTF in computed tomography. *Med Phys* 28(3): 356–60.

De Man, B., and Basu, S. (2004). Distance-driven projection and backprojection in three dimensions. *Phys Med Biol* 49(11): 2463–75.

Elbakri, I.A., and Fessler, J.A. (2002). Statistical image reconstruction for polyenergetic X-ray computed tomography. *IEEE Transactions on Medical Imaging* 21: 89–99.

Elbakri, I.A., and Fessler, J.A. (2003). Segmentation-free statistical image reconstruction for polyenergetic X-ray computed tomography with experimental validation. *Phys Med Biol* 48(15): 2543–78.

Erdoğan, H., and Fessler, J.A. (1999a). Monotonic algorithms for transmission tomography. *IEEE Transactions on Medical Imaging* 18(9): 801–14.

Erdoğan, H., and Fessler, J.A. (1999b). Ordered subsets algorithms for transmission tomography. *Phys Med Biol* 44(11): 2835–51.

Feldkamp, L.A., and Davis, L.C. (1984). Practical cone-beam algorithm. *J Opt Soc Amer* 1: 612–19.

Freiherr, G. (2010). Iterative reconstruction cuts CT dose without harming image quality. *Diagnostic Imaging* 32(11). Available at www.diagnosticimaging.com.

Hsieh, J., Molthen, R.C., et al. (2000). An iterative approach to the beam hardening correction in cone beam CT. *Med Phys* 27(1): 23–9.

Kamphuis, C., and Beekman, F.J. (1998). Accelerated iterative transmission CT reconstruction using an ordered subsets convex algorithm. *IEEE Transactions on Medical Imaging* 17(6): 1001–5.

Kirk, D.B., and Hwu, W.W. (2010). *Programming Massively Parallel Processors: A Hands-on Approach.* Morgan Kaufman.

Lange, K., and Carson, R. (1984). EM reconstruction algorithms for emission and transmission tomography. *J Comp Assisted Tomo* 8(2): 306–16.

Shepp, L.A., and Vardi, Y. (1982). Maximum likelihood reconstruction for emission tomography. *IEEE Trans Med Imag* 1(2): 113–22.

Sijbers, J., and Postnov, A. (2004). Reduction of ring artefacts in high resolution micro-CT reconstructions. *Phys Med Biol* 49(14): N247-54.

Sukovic, P., and Clinthorne, N.H. (2000). Penalized weighted least-squares as a metal streak artifacts removal technique in computed tomography. *Proc IEEE Nuc Sci Symp Med Im Conf*.

Tuy, H.K. (1983). An inversion formula for cone-beam reconstruction. *SIAM J Appl Math* 43(3): 546–52.

Vaz, M.A., McLin, M., et al. (2007). Current and next generation GPUs for accelerating CT reconstruction: Quality, performance, and tuning. *Proc Intl Mtg on Fully 3D Image Recon in Rad and Nuc Med*.

Wu, M. A. (1991). ASIC applications in computed tomography systems. Fourth Annual IEEE International ASIC Conference and Exhibit.

Zbijewski, W., and Beekman, F.J. (2006). Efficient Monte Carlo based scatter artifact reduction in cone-beam micro-CT. *IEEE Trans Med Imag* 25(7): 817–27.

Zbijewski, W., and Stayman, J.W. (2009). Volumetric soft tissue brain imaging on xCAT: A mobile flat-panel x-ray CT system. *Proc SPIE 7258, Medical Imaging 2009: Phys Med Im*.

Zhao, X., Hu, J.J., et al. (2009). GPU-based 3D cone-beam CT image reconstruction for large data volume. *Int J Biomed Imaging* 2009: 149079.

2 The Nature of Ionizing Radiation and the Risks from Maxillofacial Cone Beam Computed Tomography

Sanjay M. Mallya and Stuart C. White

Configuration of matter

Familiarity with the atomic structure is essential to understanding production of X-rays and their interaction with matter. All matter is composed of atoms. According to the classical view of the atom, as proposed by Niels Bohr, the atom is composed of a positively charged nucleus containing protons and neutrons, with negatively charged electrons that revolve around the nucleus in well-defined orbits. The contemporary view of the atom is described by the Standard Model. As with the classical view, electrons are fundamental particles. But in contrast to the classical view, protons and neutrons are not considered fundamental units; rather, they are composed of quarks. The contemporary model of the atom also differs in its view of the relationship of electrons to the nucleus. Unlike the classical view, which postulates that electrons revolve in a two-dimensional orbit, the modern view considers that electrons are dispersed in three-dimension *orbitals*. Each orbital has a discrete energy state. Within all atoms, the electrons occupy the lowest energy state first. The electrons are held in orbit by an electrostatic attraction to the positively charged nucleus. If an electron absorbs sufficient energy, it can overcome this electrostatic attraction and move to a higher energy state. This energy is termed *binding energy*, and is specific for an orbital and depends on the atomic number (Z) of the element. The higher the atomic number, the more binding energy there is. For any given atom, the binding energy of the outer orbitals is lower than that of the inner orbitals. Some radiations such as ultraviolet light have sufficient energy to remove outer electrons. Other radiations such as X- and gamma rays have enough energy to displace inner electrons. In both these situations, the loss of an electron causes an imbalance between the net charges of electrons and protons in the nucleus, and thus results in *ionization*. These radiations are referred to as *ionizing radiations*.

Nature of ionizing radiation

Radiation is the propagation of energy through space and matter. There are two types of radiation: *particulate* and *electromagnetic* (White and Pharoah, 2009). Particulate radiation is energy transmitted by rapidly moving particles produced primarily by disintegration of unstable atoms. The particles

---

Cone Beam Computed Tomography: Oral and Maxillofacial Diagnosis and Applications, First Edition. Edited by David Sarment.
© 2014 John Wiley & Sons, Inc. Published 2014 by John Wiley & Sons, Inc.

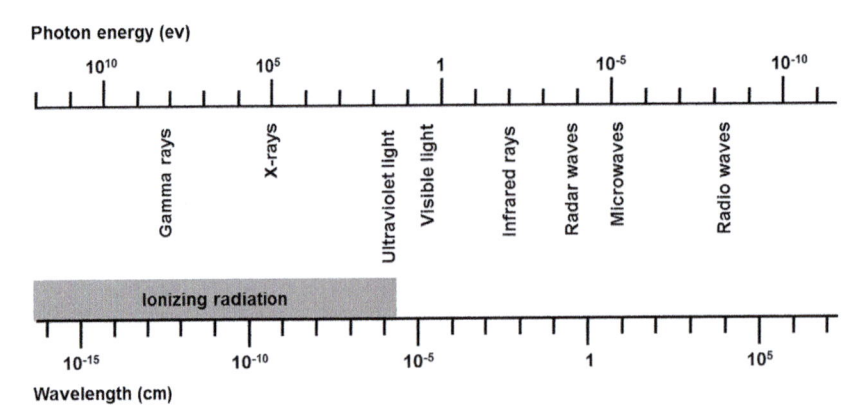

Figure 2.1 The electromagnetic spectrum, showing the relationship between photon energy and wavelength. Note that as photon energy decreases, wavelength increases.

may be charged, for example, α- or β-particles, or may be uncharged particles such as neutrons. Electromagnetic radiation is energy transmitted as a combination of electric and magnetic fields. According to quantum theory, electromagnetic radiation is propagated in small bundles or packets of energy called *photons*. Photons have only energy and no mass are often described in terms of their energy (eV). Some aspects of electromagnetic radiation are better explained by the wave theory, which assumes that these radiations are transmitted as electric and magnetic fields that travel in a wavelike pattern. In this case the radiation is better characterized by its wavelength. Photon energy is inversely proportional to its wavelength.

The term *electromagnetic radiation* refers to a spectrum of radiations that differ in their energies but share some similar properties (Figure 2.1). All electromagnetic radiations travel at the speed of light. The radiations within this spectrum have a broad range of energies ranging from the low-energy (long-wavelength) radio waves to high-energy (short-wavelength) gamma rays. High-energy electromagnetic radiations have sufficient energy to interact with and cause ionization of atoms. These radiations are called ionizing radiations and include γ, X- and ultraviolet radiations. As described below, ionizing radiations have the potential to cause damage to biological molecules, including inducing cancer.

Production of X-rays

X-ray tube

The X-ray tube is the heart of a radiographic imaging system and is housed within the X-ray tube head along with the essential electrical components that supply its power. The X-ray tube consists of a cathode and an anode within an evacuated glass tube. The process of X-ray production starts with the generation of electrons at the cathode. The electrons are accelerated toward the anode by providing a high potential difference between the anode and the cathode. As electrons travel from the cathode to the anode, they accumulate kinetic energy. On striking the anode, this kinetic energy is converted into heat and X-rays. In cone beam computed tomography (CBCT) units, the tube head is linked to the image detector (flat panel or image intensifier) by a C-arm. Control panels on the CBCT unit allow the operator to regulate various parameters of this process and thereby control the nature of the X-ray beam produced. Understanding the impact of these controls on X-ray beam production is important. Selection of the optimal exposure factors influences diagnostic quality of the images as well as the radiation exposure to the patient.

Cathode

The cathode consists of a coil of metallic filament (Figure 2.2). A low-voltage current is used to heat this coil. When the temperature of the filament is

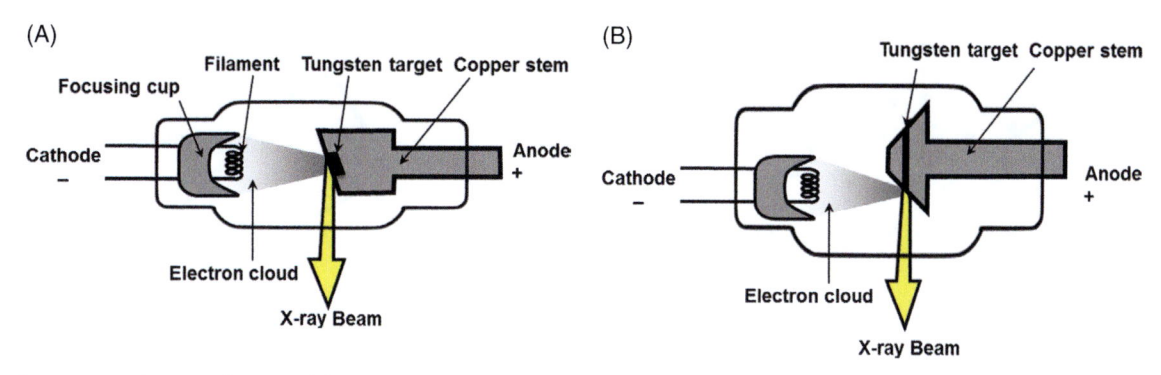

Figure 2.2 Schematic diagram of the components of x-ray tubes with stationary anode (A) or rotating anode (B).

high enough, electrons in the outer orbitals of the tungsten atoms absorb sufficient energy to overcome their binding energy and are released from the filament. The focusing cup is negatively charged and thus electrostatically focuses the electrons to a small area of the anode.

Anode

The anode is composed of a tungsten target embedded into a block of copper (Figure 2.2). As the electrons strike the anode, their kinetic energy is converted into heat and X-rays. The production of X-rays is an inefficient process, with more than 99% of the electron's kinetic energy being converted into heat. The *focal spot*, the area of the target struck by the electrons and from which X-rays are emitted, should be as small as possible. The smaller the focal spot size, the sharper the final images. X-ray tubes have one of two designs. Some machines use a *stationary anode* (Figure 2.2A) like a conventional dental X-ray machine. Others use a *rotating anode* (Figure 2.2B). In this design, the anode is a disc, with an angled surface that serves as the target area. As the anode rotates, successive electrons from the cathode strike sequential regions of the target, and at any given time, the area of the target producing X-rays, the focal spot, is small. However, the heat is dissipated over the larger area of the entire disc. This design allows production of X-rays from small focal spots even at high-energy outputs, or with prolonged exposure times. CBCT units have either stationary or rotating anodes with focal spot sizes ranging from 0.15 mm to 0.7 mm.

X-ray production

Electrons produced at the cathode are accelerated toward the anode by providing a high potential difference between the cathode and anode. As electrons strike the anode, the kinetic energy of the electrons is converted into heat and X-ray photons. This accounts for more than 99% of the energy transfer from the striking electrons to the tungsten atoms. The remainder 1% of energy is converted in X-rays, primarily by bremsstrahlung interactions.

Bremsstrahlung photons

As the electrons course through the tungsten atoms in the target, they may pass close to a nucleus. Due to the electrostatic forces between the positively charged nucleus and the negatively charged electron, the electron is deviated from its course and loses some energy, which is converted into an X-ray photon (Figure 2.3). These photons are called bremsstrahlung photons. Bremsstrahlung photons have a continuous spectrum of energies (Figure 2.4). The maximum energy of the bremsstrahlung photon is determined by the potential difference between the cathode and the anode. For example, an X-ray machine set to operate at 100 kVp will produce bremsstrahlung photons with a maximum energy of 100 keV. Bremsstrahlung photons constitute the majority of the diagnostically useful X-ray beam. From a diagnostic and radiation safety viewpoint, it is important to decrease the numbers of low-energy photons, which increase patient dose

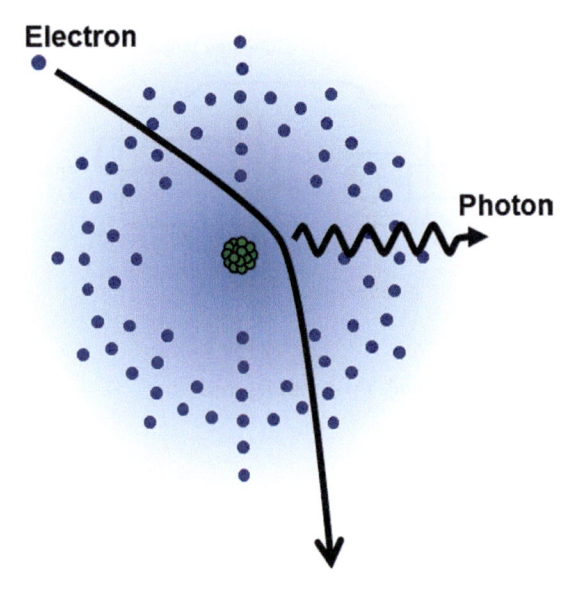

Figure 2.3 Bremsstrahlung photons are produced when an electron is deviated from its path due to electrostatic interaction with the nucleus.

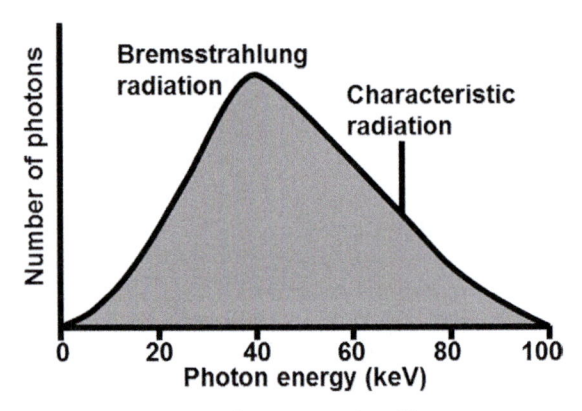

Figure 2.4 Spectrum of photons produced by an x-ray tube operating at 100 kVp. The shaded area under the curve depicts the bremsstrahlung photons. The spike at approximately 69 keV represents characteristic radiation from the tungsten atoms in the target.

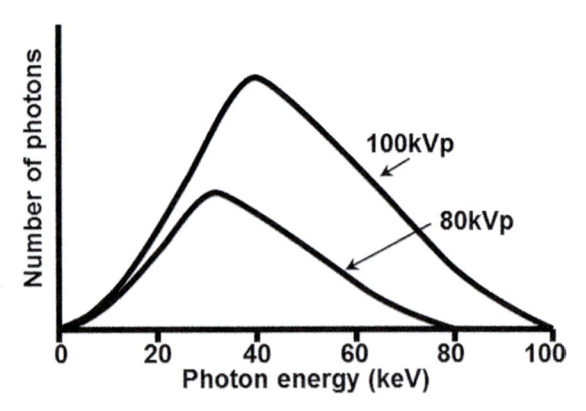

Figure 2.5 Increasing kVp (with constant mA and exposure time) results in more photons, with a higher mean energy and peak energy of the beam.

and decrease image quality. Manufacturers add filters to preferentially absorb low-energy photons.

Parameters of X-ray beams in CBCT units

The controls of X-ray units, including CBCT machines, allow the operator to optimize various aspects of X-ray production. Altering these parameters influences both the image quality and the radiation dose to the patient. Thus, understanding these parameters is of importance to patient care.

Tube voltage (kVp)

Tube voltage refers to the potential difference between the cathode and the anode and is conveyed as peak voltage (kVp). As kVp is increased, there is an increase in the number of photons generated, a higher peak energy, and a higher mean energy of the X-ray beam (Figure 2.5). Increasing the kVp increases the penetrating power of the beam. Increasing kV increases the signal-to-noise ratio but also delivers a higher dose to the patient. Depending on the CBCT unit manufacturer, the kVp is fixed or adjustable. Few studies have examined the effect on kVp on optimization of image quality and patient dose.

Tube current (mA)

The tube current is the flow of electrons from the cathode to the anode and is expressed as milliamperes (mA). It is a reflection of the power delivered to the tungsten filament in the cathode. When the mA setting is increased, the number of electrons liberated at the cathode is increased; this translates into a higher number of X-ray photons produced (Figure 2.6). However, the mean and peak energies of the beam remain same.

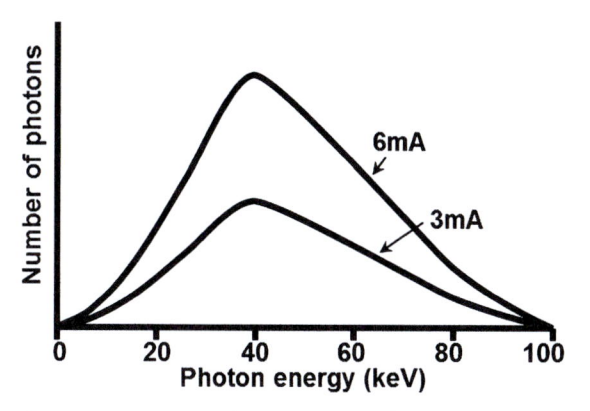

Figure 2.6 Increasing the mA setting (with constant kVp and exposure time) results in more photons but no change in the mean and peak energies of the beam.

Exposure time

The exposure time is the total time during which X-ray production takes place during the CBCT scan. During the CBCT scan, multiple projections of the field of interest are obtained at varying angles. In most CBCT units, the exposure is *pulsed*, so that X-ray production takes place only during acquisition of the basis projections. In some units, the exposure is *continuous*—X-rays are produced and expose the patient even when the detector is not recording images. Using a pulsed beam reduces the radiation exposure to the patient. A second variable is the scan time or exposure time. For some units, the scan time is fixed and cannot be varied by the operator. Many contemporary units allow the operator to choose from a variety of scanning modes, such as "high speed" or "high resolution" modes. With high-speed modes, the number of basis projections is reduced, thereby decreasing scan times and thus radiation exposure to the patient. In high-resolution modes, the number of basis projections is increased, and consequently scan time as well as patient radiation dose is increased.

Field of view

Many CBCT units allow the operator to restrict the beam size to a predetermined area or field of view. Typically, the field of view is described as small (or limited), medium, or large depending on the extent

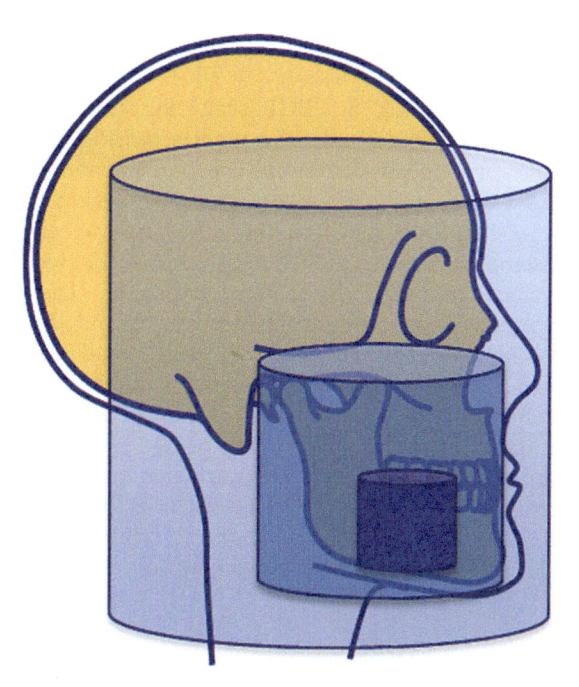

Figure 2.7 Fields of view. Representation of the extent of anatomical coverage for small (limited), medium (dentoalveolar) and large (craniofacial) fields of view.

of anatomic coverage (Figure 2.7). In general, the scan collimations are as below:

a. Small field of view (also referred to as limited or focused fields of view): scan height and width less than 5 cm.
b. Medium field of view (also referred to as dentoalveolar field of view): scan height 5–15 cm.
c. Large field of view (also referred to as craniofacial field of view): scan height greater than 15 cm.

Collimating the beam to as small a region as possible not only reduces patient exposure, it also enhances image quality due to decreased scatter radiation. It is of utmost importance to select the optimal field of view for a particular diagnostic task. For example, when examining teeth for fractures, periapical lesions or accessory pulp canals, a limited field of view CBCT examination acquired at a high resolution is necessary. Similarly, smaller field of view scans have a better diagnostic efficacy for detection of temporomandibular joint erosions.

Rotation angle

Typically during a CBCT scan, the tube and detector move around the patient acquiring multiple projections during a 360-degree rotation. However, some contemporary units provide an acquisition mode where the tube and detector assembly rotate around the patient for 180 degrees, thereby reducing the patient exposure. These modes will use fewer basis projections and thus typically yield images that are lower in resolution than a full 360-degree scan. Depending on the diagnostic task, the images may be of adequate diagnostic quality. The use of 180-degree scans has implications not only in dose reduction but also in situations where patient motion may be an issue. Research comparing the diagnostic efficacies of 360- and 180-degree scans is lacking.

Interaction of X-rays with matter

X-ray photons that strike an object have different potential fates. Some photons pass through the object without any loss of energy. Alternatively, photons may transfer some or all of their energy to the object's molecules. There are three mechanisms whereby diagnostic X-ray photons interact with matter—coherent scatter, Compton scatter, and photoelectric effect.

Coherent scatter

This type of interaction occurs predominantly with X-ray photons with energies less than approximately 10 keV. As a low-energy photon courses adjacent to an atom, it loses all of its energy and causes an outer orbital electron to become excited. As the excited electron returns to its steady state, it emits an X-ray photon, with the same energy as the initial incident photon (Figure 2.8). The scattered photon is typically at an angle to the incident photon. Importantly, coherent scatter does not cause ionization of the atom. At the photon energies used in CBCT imaging, coherent scatter accounts for only a minor proportion of the photon interactions and is of little importance in diagnostic imaging.

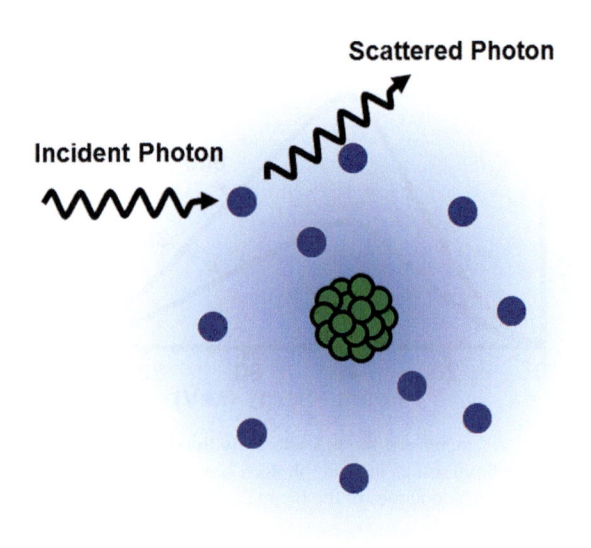

Figure 2.8 Coherent scatter. The incident photon transfers its energy to the atoms, causing the electrons to momentarily vibrate. As the atom returns to the ground state, it emits a photon of the same energy as the incident photon.

Compton scatter

When an incident photon with moderate energy collides with an outer orbital electron, it transfers some of its energy to the electron, which overcomes its binding energy and is ejected from its orbital, causing ionization of the atom. The incident photon retains some of its energy and is scattered at an angle to its initial path (Figure 2.9). Compton scatter has important implications in diagnostic radiology. First, it causes ionization of biological molecules and thus, results in radiation-induced damage. Second, the photons are scattered in all directions. Some of the scattered photons may expose adjacent tissues outside the immediate field of radiation, causing biological damage. Scattered photons may also exit the patient and strike the image receptor, resulting in reduced image contrast. Manufacturers incorporate filters into the X-ray beam to preferentially decrease the number of low-energy photons, thereby decreasing Compton interactions. This added filtration reduces patient dose and also improves image quality. Importantly, during Compton interactions, photons may also be scattered at an angle of 180 degrees—backscatter radiation—and could potentially expose the operator.

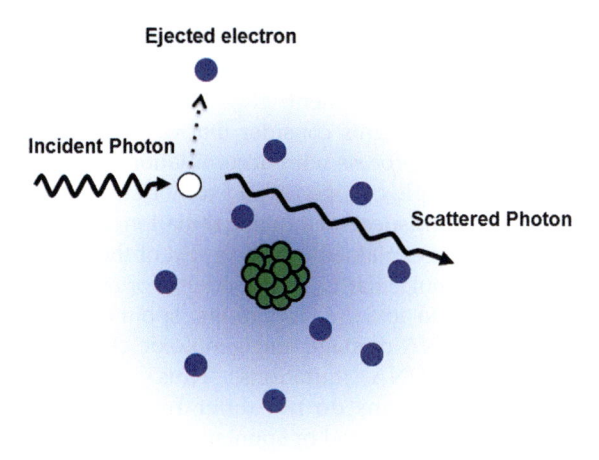

Figure 2.9 Compton scatter. The incident photon transfers some of its energy to an electron, resulting in ionization of the atom. Following this interaction, the photon is deviated from its path as a scattered photon.

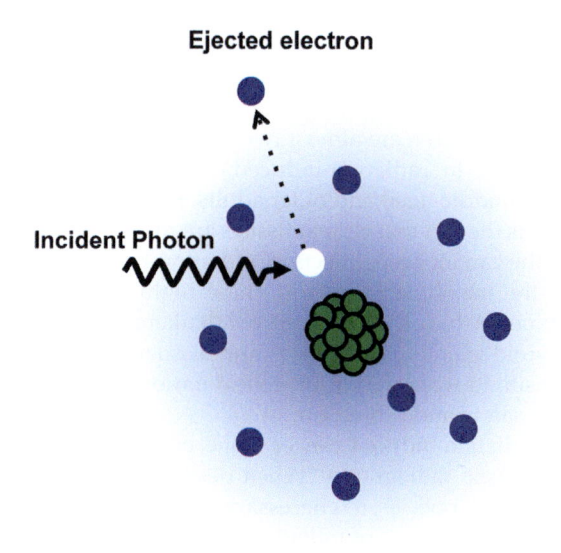

Figure 2.10 Photoelectric interaction. The incident photon transfers all of its energy to the atom, resulting in ionization.

Photoelectric absorption

Photoelectric absorption is an important interaction and is the basis for formation of the radiographic image. In this interaction, the X-ray photon interacts with an inner-orbital electron (Figure 2.10). As the photon collides with the electron, it loses all of its energy to the electron. A part of this energy is used to overcome the binding energy of the electron. The remainder of the energy is converted to kinetic energy of this electron—a photoelectron—that is ejected from the atom. Thus, in a photoelectric interaction, the incident photon loses all of its energy and results in ionization of the atom. Atoms with a high atomic number absorb more photons than atoms with lower atomic numbers; this is the basis for radiographic image formation. Tissues with a higher effective atomic number such as enamel, dentin, and bone absorb more photons than soft tissue and thus are depicted on the radiographic image as radiopaque objects. Likewise, dental materials such as amalgam, gold, and titanium have high atomic numbers and are seen as radiopaque regions on a radiograph.

Biological effects of ionizing radiation

As X-ray photons interact with biological tissues they can cause ionization of atoms in biological tissues. Ionization of biological molecules may manifest as radiation-induced effects. The type and nature of these effects depends on the tissue type exposed as well as the dose. There are two principal types of radiation-induced effects: *deterministic* and *stochastic*.

Deterministic effects

Deterministic effects of radiation are caused when the radiation exposure to an organ or tissue exceeds a particular threshold level. At doses below the threshold, the effect does not occur. All individuals exposed to doses above the threshold will develop deterministic effects. Importantly, at doses above the threshold, the severity of the effect is proportional to the dose. Deterministic effects are typically a result of radiation-induced cell killing. Examples of deterministic radiation-induced effects include cataract formation, skin burns, fibrosis, xerostomia, and mucosal ulcerations. All dentomaxillofacial radiographic examinations are designed so that we do not induce any deterministic effects. However, dentists may often encounter such effects in patients who have received radiation therapy.

Stochastic effects

Unlike deterministic effects, stochastic effects have no minimum threshold for causation. Thus, any dose of radiation has the potential to induce a stochastic effect. While the probability of causing a stochastic effect increases as the radiation dose is increased, the severity of the effect itself is not dependent on dose. Either you get it or you don't. Stochastic effects are caused by radiation-induced damage to DNA. The most important stochastic effect is radiation-induced cancer. The absence of a threshold implies that any amount of radiation carries with it a risk for causing cancer. Although the potential for causing this effect cannot be entirely avoided, minimizing the radiation dose can decrease the possibility of inducing this effect; this is the basis of radiation protection.

Radiation-induced cancer

Cancer induction is the most important stochastic effect from diagnostic radiation. It is well established that exposure to ionizing radiation results in an increase in the incidence of malignancies. These data are largely derived from studies of human populations that were exposed to ionizing radiation, either intentionally or by accident. Examples of such populations include early radiation workers, radium dial painters, uranium miners, individuals irradiated for benign diseases, patients with tuberculosis who underwent repeated chest fluoroscopy, and survivors of the atomic bombings and the radiation disaster at Chernobyl. Studies of these human populations, as well as animal studies, have provided an insight into the mechanistic basis for radiation's cancer-inducing effect. There is strong evidence that radiation-induced carcinogenesis is a consequence of ionizing radiation–induced DNA damage. Ionizing radiation causes several types of DNA damage, including damage to individual bases, single strand breaks, double strand breaks, and DNA–protein cross-links. Misrepair of DNA damage results in mutations of the normal DNA sequence. Such mutations may occur as single base alterations, deletions or insertions of DNA segments, or chromosomal rearrangements such as translocations and inversions. When the mutations involve growth-regulating genes—activation of oncogenes or inactivation of tumor suppressor genes—they can deregulate cell growth and/or differentiation and ultimately lead to neoplastic development.

Current paradigms consider that carcinogenesis is a multistep process with accumulation of mutations in multiple oncogenes and tumor suppressor genes. Several aspects of ionizing radiation–induced cancer can be explained in the context of these contemporary molecular genetic models. For example, in addition to ionizing radiations, spontaneously occurring DNA damage and genotoxic chemicals also cause DNA mutations. Thus, radiation-induced neoplasms do not differ fundamentally from chemical-induced or spontaneous neoplasms. Radiation-induced tumors have no clinical or histological signatures that allow us to differentiate them from sporadically occurring tumors. Second, there is a latent period between radiation exposure and the manifestation of the neoplasm. This is expected given the multistep nature of tumorigenesis. Depending on the tumor type, this may vary from a few years to decades. It is also important to emphasize that there is a wide variation in the risk—young children are almost two to three times more sensitive to radiation-induced cancer, compared with middle-aged and older adults. Equally important is the fact that certain tissues are more sensitive to the carcinogenic effects of radiation than others. In the maxillofacial region, these highly sensitive tissues include the bone marrow (leukemia) and the thyroid glands. These age- and tissue-dependent sensitivities are significant considerations for radiation safety and protection.

Radiation-induced cancer is the principal risk of diagnostic radiography. When designing radiation protection policies, it is necessary to estimate the risk from a given dose of radiation. Currently, these risk estimates are based on the *linear nonthreshold* (LNT) model. The LNT model assumes that cancer risk is directly proportional to radiation dose at all dose levels. The LNT is a hypothesis and has not been scientifically proven or disproven. Nevertheless, there is strong scientific justification that supports this hypothesis. As discussed above, radiation-induced cancer is a consequence of DNA damage. Even when the dose of radiation is small, the possibility of ionizing radiation–induced DNA damage and subsequent DNA mutations exists, and this supports the nonthreshold assumption of this model. Second, cell culture studies have demonstrated that as radiation dose increases, the magnitude of DNA damage also rises, and the probability of DNA mutations increases. This finding provides justification to the assumption of a linear relationship between radiation dose and risk. Most radiation protection agencies around the world, including the International Commission on Radiation Protection and the National Council on Radiation Protection and Measurement, use the LNT to estimate radiation-induced risks. Nevertheless, the LNT model is not universally accepted. The opponents of this model argue that the assumptions do not take into consideration cellular adaptive responses that may be effective at lower doses. Furthermore, the LNT model does not account for age at exposure, and assumes that sensitivity to radiation-induced cancer for a particular organ is the same at all ages. Opponents of the LNT model argue that it overestimates cancer risk from diagnostic radiation.

Risk from CBCT examinations

The basic premise of diagnostic radiology is that the diagnostic benefits from the radiographic examination far outweigh the risks from radiation exposure. When prescribing and performing diagnostic radiological examinations, dentists should ensure that both of these principles are satisfied. To maximize diagnostic benefits, dentists must identify those clinical situations where radiographic examinations would provide additional information that is essential for diagnosis and management of the patient's condition. To minimize risks from radiation exposure, dentists must implement appropriate dose-reduction procedures (White and Mallya, 2012). Importantly, dentists must understand the magnitude of potential risks from radiographic examinations and convey this information in a manner that can be easily comprehended by patients.

Sources of radiation

Background radiation

All individuals are continuously exposed to radiation from various natural and man-made sources (Figure 2.11). Natural radiation sources refer to ubiquitous background radiation. The naturally occurring radionuclides, in particular radon and thoron, contribute to a large part of this background

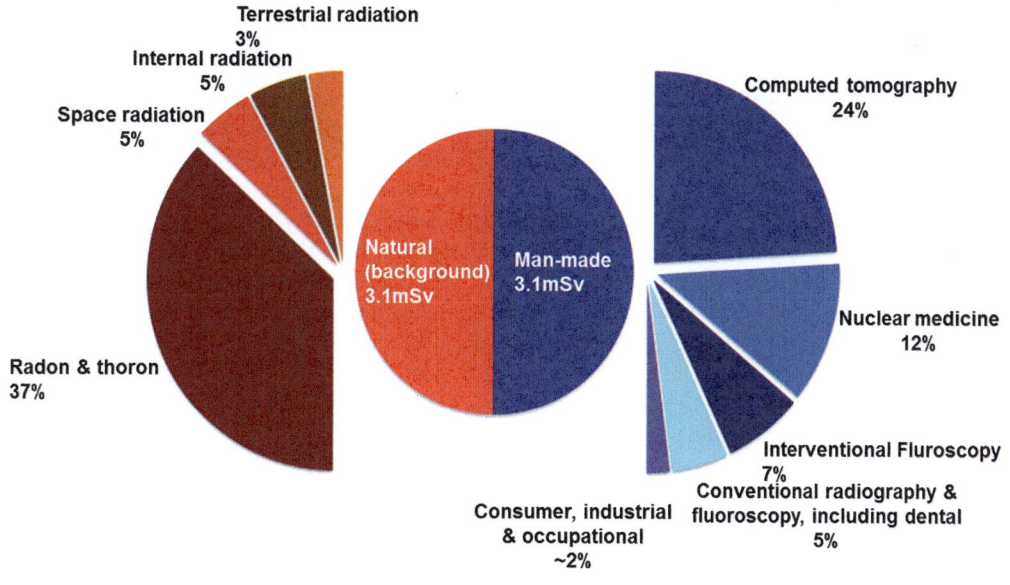

Figure 2.11 Sources of radiation exposure in the United States. The average annual exposure to individuals in the U.S. is approximately 6.2 mSv. Half of this is from background sources and half from man-made sources. The relative contributions of the various sources are shown in the pie chart. Note that diagnostic imaging contributes a large proportion of the total exposure. Data derived from NCRP, 2009.

radiation. Other natural sources include space radiation (cosmic rays and solar energetic particles), terrestrial radiation from radioactive elements in rocks and soil, and internal radiation from radionuclides that are ingested through food and water or inhaled through air. The average annual effective dose from background radiation exposure in the United States is approximately 3.1 mSv (see "Units of Radiation" section for definition of radiation dose units). Background radiation is often used as a basis to convey the magnitude of radiation risks from diagnostic radiological examinations. For example, an examination with an effective dose of 0.31 mSv would result in an exposure equivalent to 36.5 days of background exposure.

Man-made radiation

The major contributor to this category of radiation exposure is from diagnostic radiology and nuclear medicine. Consumer products, occupational exposure, and industrial sources account for a minor component of this category. In the United States there has been a dramatic increase in medical radiation exposure. In 1980 medical radiation exposure was only one-sixth of natural background exposure. In 2006, medical exposures equaled background radiation, increasing the total annual effective dose from all sources to 6.2 mSv. This increase is mainly due to exposures from computed tomography and reflects both an increase in the numbers of examinations as well as the dose per examination. CT now accounts for 24% of the annual total effective dose from all sources. Conventional radiography and fluoroscopy account for 5% of the total dose. Dental radiography accounts for approximately 2.5% of the dose from conventional radiography. It should be emphasized, however, that these data do not include exposure from CBCT, which is being increasingly used in dentistry.

Risk-estimates for CBCT examinations

The principal detriment from diagnostic X-radiation is radiation-induced neoplasia; the magnitude of this risk increases with radiation dose. Thus, knowledge of the dose delivered by a diagnostic radiographic examination is key for its risk-benefit analysis. Several studies have estimated effective doses that result from CBCT examinations (Hirsch et al., 2008; Librizzi et al., 2011; Lofthag-Hansen et al., 2008; Loubele et al., 2009; Loubele et al., 2005; Ludlow, 2011; Ludlow et al., 2003; Ludlow et al., 2006; Ludlow and Ivanovic, 2008; Okano et al., 2009; Pauwels et al., 2012; Roberts et al., 2009; Suomalainen et al., 2009). Typically, these doses are determined using dosimeters placed at multiple sites in a tissue-equivalent anthropomorphic phantom to measure absorbed doses at specific organ sites. The measured absorbed doses are then used to calculate the effective dose from an examination. Such studies provide an estimate of the dose that a patient is likely to receive from a specific CBCT examination.

The striking point that emerges from these studies is that the effective dose, and thus radiation risk, varies significantly between CBCT units from different manufacturers (Figure 2.12 and Table 2.1). Furthermore, different protocol settings of the same unit also result in markedly different radiation doses. This is particularly important because CBCT has often been publicized as a low-dose procedure. However, given the significant variability depending on manufacturer and selected imaging protocol, it is important that dentists fully understand the radiation doses delivered by the specific CBCT exams that they prescribe and make. Given the wide variation in the radiation dose between manufacturers, dentists should give due consideration to this issue when purchasing a unit, or when referring a patient to an imaging facility. Equally important is the increased radiation dose with some high-resolution imaging protocols. Dentists must be familiar with the diagnostic situations that require such high-resolution protocols and appropriately consider the balance between diagnostic benefit and radiation risk.

Often patients who have been prescribed a CBCT examination may inquire about the risks from these procedures. While dentists must be aware of the estimated effective doses from such examinations, it is often useful to convey these to patients, in the context of its equivalent of background exposure. Additionally, it is also useful to provide similar data for commonly used dental and medical radiographic procedures to allow the patient to place the dose to be received in proper perspective. Table 2.1 lists the effective dose from several CBCT, multislice CT, and commonly used dentomaxillofacial radiographic examinations. Figure 2.12 shows these doses grouped by the size of the field of view.

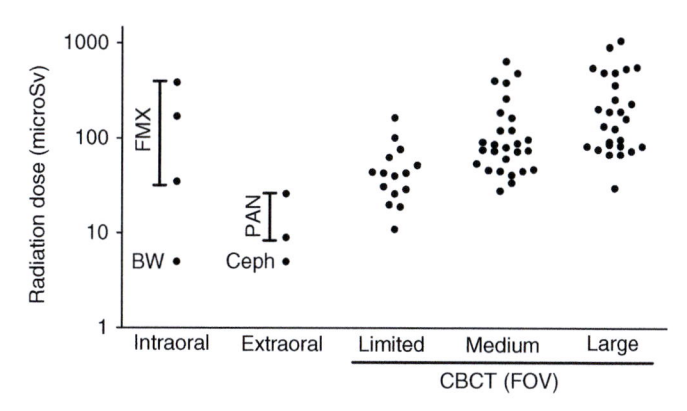

Figure 2.12 Effective doses from dentomaxillofacial examinations. Note that doses are plotted on the y-axis on a logarithmic scale. Data are derived from sources listed in Table 2.1. Note also the striking overlap between limited, medium, and large field of view machines. Thus, in some situations a limited field of view machine can result in a larger effective dose than a large field of view machine from a different manufacturer.

Methods to minimize radiation dose from CBCT exams

While CBCT radiation doses are typically lower than those from multislice maxillofacial CT examinations, it should be remembered that the overarching philosophy of radiation protection is minimizing the radiation dose to the patient while maintaining the diagnostic benefit. This philosophy is embodied in the principle and practice of ALARA—As Low As Reasonably Achievable. This principle aims to reduce the radiation dose of exposed individuals to as low levels as practically achievable. There are several means to satisfy this principle.

Selection criteria

The basic premise of diagnostic radiography is that the diagnostic benefits of radiation far outweigh the risks from radiation exposure. Thus, a fundamental requirement of all diagnostic radiological exams is that they must have the potential to provide information that is valuable for diagnosis and patient management. It must be emphasized that any radiographic examination, including CBCT, be performed after a complete history and clinical examination. Judicious use of diagnostic radiation requires that the dentist identify those clinical situations where the radiological examination is likely to provide this benefit. The term *selection criteria* refers to this process where a dentist, based on the patient's historical and clinical findings, identifies those situations where radiography is needed and prescribes the appropriate radiographic examination that would provide the needed diagnostic examination. Selection criteria are an essential and often overlooked approach to minimizing patient radiation exposure.

Guidelines have been established to help dentists select the appropriate radiographic examination. For example, the American Dental Association has developed guidelines that provide dentists with a framework to prescribe commonly used conventional radiographic modalities, including intraoral, panoramic, and cephalometric imaging (ADA Council on Scientific Affairs, 2001). While these ADA guidelines do not include CBCT imaging, the principles underlying these guidelines apply to prescribing CBCT examinations. These basic principles are clearly outlined in a position paper from the American Academy of Oral and Maxillofacial Radiology (White et al., 2001) and in guidelines from the European Academy of Oral and Maxillofacial Radiology (Horner et al., 2009). Recently, the American Association of Endodontists and the American Academy of Oral and Maxillofacial Radiology (2011) published a joint position statement to provide guidance to the use of CBCT imaging in endodontic treatment. These guidelines emphasize justification of radiographic examinations on an individual basis. CBCT has become increasing popular in orthodontic treatment planning. White and Pae (2009) have suggested guidelines for selection of orthodontic

Table 2.1 Effective doses from selected CBCT and dentomaxillofacial radiographic examinations.

Examination	Effective Dose* (microSv)	Equivalent Background Radiation (days)[‡]
CBCT small (limited) field of view		
3D Accuitomo, 4 × 4 cm	13–44	2–5
Kodak 9000, 5 × 3.7 cm	19–40	2–5
Pax-Uni 3D, 5 × 5 cm	44	5
CBCT medium field of view		
3D Accuitomo170, 10 × 5 cm	54	6
CB Mercuray, 10 cm diameter	279	33
CB Mercuray, 15 cm diameter	548	65
iCAT next generation, 16 × 6 cm	45	5
iCAT classic, 16 × 8 cm	34–77	4–9
iCAT classic, 16 × 8 cm, high-resolution protocol	68–149	8–18
Kodak 9500, 15 × 8 cm	76–166	9–20
NewTom3G, 10 cm diameter	57	7
NewTomVGi, 15 cm × 15 cm, high-resolution protocol	194	23
NewTomVGi, 12 cm × 8 cm, high-resolution protocol	265	31
Picasso Trio, 12 × 7, low dose	81	10
Picasso Trio, 12 × 7, high dose	123	14
Prexion, 8 × 8 cm, low dose	189	22
Prexion, 8 × 8 cm, high dose	389	46
ProMax3D, 8 × 8 cm, low-dose protocol	28	3
Promax3D, 8 × 8 cm, high-dose protocol	122–652	14–77
Scanora 3D, 10 × 7.5 cm	45	5
Veraviewepocs 3D, 8 × 8 cm	73	9
CBCT large field of view		
CB Mercuray, 20 cm diameter	569–1073	67–126
Galileos Comfort, 15 × 15 cm	70–128	8–15
iCat Next generation, 16 × 13 cm	74–83	9–10
Illuma, 21 × 14 cm, low-resolution protocol	98	12
Illuma, 21 × 14 cm, high-resolution protocol	368–498	43–59
Kodak 9500, 20 × 18 cm	93–260	11–31
NewTom 3G, 19 cm diameter	30–68	4–8
NewTom VG, 23 cm × 23 cm	83	10
Scanora 3D, 14.5 × 13.5 cm	68	8
Skyview, 17 × 17 cm	87	10

(Continued)

Table 2.1 (Continued)

Examination	Effective Dose* (microSv)	Equivalent Background Radiation (days)‡
Multislice CT		
Siemens Somatom (64-slice), 12 cm scan length	860	101
Siemens Somatom (64-slice), 12 cm scan length, automatic exposure control protocol	534	63
Siemens Sensation (16-slice), 22.7 cm scan length	1500	177
Siemens Sensation (16-slice), 22.7 cm scan length, low-dose protocol	180	21
Intraoral radiographs		
Bitewings (PSP/F-speed, rectangular collimation)	5	0.6
(PSP/F-speed, rectangular collimation)	35	4
(PSP/F-speed, round collimation)	171	20
Panoramic (digital, CCD-based)	14–24	2–3
Lateral cephalomteric (digital, PSP-based)	6	0.7

* Doses are rounded to the nearest whole number. Dose range is based on data derived from Hirsch et al., 2008; Librizzi et al., 2011; Lofthag-Hansen et al., 2008; Loubele et al., 2009; Loubele et al., 2005; Ludlow, 2011; Ludlow et al., 2003; Ludlow et al., 2006; Ludlow and Ivanovic, 2008; Okano et al., 2009; Pauwels et al., 2012; Roberts et al., 2009; and Suomalainen et al., 2009.
‡ Calculation of background equivalent days is based on an annual exposure of 3.1 milliSv. For doses above 10 microSv, the background equivalent days are rounded to the nearest whole number.

patients who would likely benefit from this imaging, emphasizing its value in assessing craniofacial asymmetry, planning for orthognathic treatment, evaluation of cleft palate patients, localizing impacted and supernumerary teeth, and guiding placement of orthodontic mini-implants. However, its routine use for all orthodontic patients is controversial and has not been substantiated by scientific evidence.

Operator training

Users of CBCT imaging at all levels should have appropriate training in the use of this technology. This is essential both to maximize the diagnostic yield and to minimize the patient dose. The extent of training will depend on the dentist's role in CBCT imaging. All dentists who use CBCT imaging for their patients' care must be familiar with the advantages, applications, and limitations of this technology to ensure that patients selected for these examinations will benefit from the diagnostic information. Furthermore, these individuals must be familiar with viewing and manipulation of multiplanar CBCT images. This includes knowledge of dentomaxillofacial radiographic anatomy and appearances of pathological lesions on CBCT examinations. To maximize diagnostic yield and patient benefit, the entire CBCT volume must be interpreted. This includes navigation through the multiplanar images outside of the region for which the examination was ordered and creating additional reconstructions as appropriate. Where necessary, dentists must consult with an oral and maxillofacial radiologist to report on the entire CBCT image volume.

Dentists who operate CBCT units in their clinics must have adequate training in the principles of CBCT production. All operators of CBCT units,

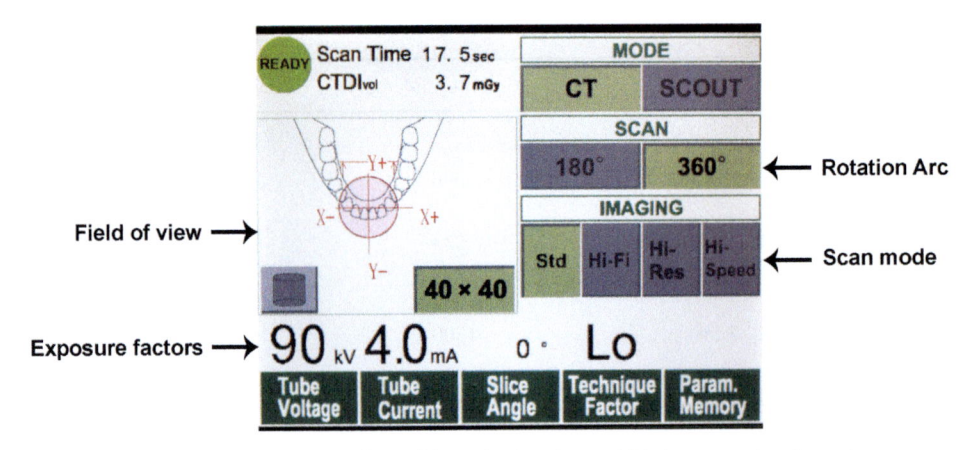

Figure 2.13 Imaging protocol parameters. Control panel from the Accuitomo 170 demonstrating the various parameters to be selected for an imaging examination. These include the exposure factors (kVp and mA), the field of view, the rotational arc, and the scan mode. These parameters must be adjusted to optimize diagnostic quality and minimize radiation dose.

including dentists and their technical staff, must understand the influence of exposure parameters as well as any machine-specific parameters on diagnostic quality and patient dose. These operators must also receive appropriate training in quality assurance protocols and data storage and transfer. Additionally, as with any other radiographic examination, these individuals must understand the principles of radiation protection and implement the following methods to reduce patient dose.

Optimizing imaging protocols

Although performing a CBCT examination appears relatively simplistic, it is essential that operators of CBCT units optimize their imaging protocols to ensure that the radiation dose to the patient is kept as low as reasonably achievable while maintaining adequate diagnostic quality. There are several settings in a CBCT unit that influence both the dose and the image quality (Figure 2.13).

Field of view

The smallest field of view needed for the diagnostic task should be used. Typically, as the field of view increases, the volume of tissue irradiated increases and the radiation dose to the patient is higher (Table 2.1). For example, when imaging the maxilla, collimating the beam to the maxillary region alone will reduce radiation exposure to the thyroid gland and mandibular bone marrow and thus significantly decrease effective dose. In addition to the higher dose, a larger field of view results in more scattered radiation that compromises image quality. To this end, it is important to recognize that a single CBCT unit may not be sufficient to provide field of view sizes that encompass all diagnostic tasks, and this should be a consideration when dentists refer patients for CBCT examinations. Librizzi et al. (2011) showed that diagnostic efficacy to detect temporomandibular joint erosions was significantly impacted by the field of view, with a higher diagnostic accuracy with smaller field of view size. Thus, using a large field of view examination to examine the temporomandibular joints for osteoarthritic changes will not only deliver a higher dose to the patient, it will also result in a lower diagnostic benefit. It should also be emphasized that required diagnostic quality is dependent on the diagnostic task. To this end, clinicians who prescribe CBCT examinations must be familiar with the field of view and select the smallest that will provide an adequate view for each diagnostic task.

Exposure factors

The exposure settings should be optimized for the diagnostic task as well as considering individual patient size and anatomic site to be imaged. This is necessary to get diagnostic quality images and reduce retakes. Typically, this is accomplished by reducing the mA to decrease the number of photons and thus radiation dose. Such optimization is particularly important when imaging a child, due to higher radiosensitivity of the bone marrow and thyroid gland.

One manufacturer, NewTom (Imageworks Corporation), uses a patented "safebeam" technology. In this technology, the amount of radiation received by the image sensor provides feedback to automatically adjust the exposure parameters, thereby customizing exposure for every patient. Such automated adjustments provide an excellent approach to minimizing radiation exposure to patients.

Scan modes

Some contemporary CBCT units allow the operator to select from a variety of scan modes. For example, some units provide the option of a "high resolution" scan mode. These high-resolution modes acquire images at a smaller voxel size. In order to increase the signal-to-noise ratio, these scan modes use an increased mA or more basis projections, both of which increase patient dose (Table 2.1). Prior to using this scan mode, the need for the high resolution for the particular diagnostic task must be evaluated. If the lower resolution mode provides adequate diagnostic information, then the added radiation dose subjects the patient to additional risk while not providing any additional benefit. For example, evaluation of dental and periapical structures and root fractures requires higher resolution, whereas evaluation of craniofacial asymmetry can be satisfactorily accomplished at lower resolutions. For some units, these higher resolution scan modes also increase exposure time, and the clinician must take into consideration the possibility of patient motion, which could degrade image quality and render the examination diagnostically inadequate.

Some manufacturers offer the option of a fast scan mode, where the number of basis projections is reduced, thereby decreasing scan time and lowering radiation dose. Such modes generally yield images with a resolution lower than the standard scan mode. However, depending on the diagnostic task, this image quality may be sufficient. Operators of CBCT units must be familiar with these features of their units and must be adequately trained to select the appropriate scan mode depending on the diagnostic task and the individual patient's circumstances.

Angle of rotation

Some CBCT units allow the operator to select an exposure mode where the rotation arc is 180 degrees instead of 360 degrees. In this mode, the number of basis projections taken for image reconstruction is lower; thus, radiation dose to the patient is lower. Given the decreased number of basis projections, the resolution of the image is lower than when obtained with a full 360-degree rotation. This scan mode will reduce patient dose. However, the adequacy of the diagnostic information with this acquisition mode has not been well studied.

Protective thyroid collars and protective aprons

The use of thyroid shields during maxillofacial CBCT reduces the absorbed dose to the thyroid gland and thus the patient effective dose. However, it is important to ensure that the thyroid collar is not in the path of the primary beam—this would lead to significant artifacts that may compromise the diagnostic quality of the image. When all other procedures are followed, it may not be necessary to use lead aprons during the CBCT exam. However, some states in the United States require the use of lead (or lead-equivalent) aprons for all dentomaxillofacial radiographic examinations.

Units of radiation

Exposure

This unit of radiation conveys the dose of radiation *in air*. The traditional unit of exposure is *Roentgen*. In the SI system, exposure is conveyed as coulombs/kg. From a practical viewpoint, this unit is used to measure the amount of radiation that exits from the X-ray tube head, either at or at various distances from the tube head. These measurements are used to calculate the need for protective shielding. This unit is also used to measure leakage of radiation from the tube head or denote the amount of radiation at the skin surface.

Absorbed dose

As described above, x-radiation interacts with and transfers energy to the patient's tissues. The unit of absorbed dose is a measure of how much energy is transferred to (absorbed by) the exposed tissues. In radiation protection, absorbed doses to the exposed tissues are measured as a first step in estimation of the overall dose from radiographic examinations. In the SI system, absorbed dose is measured in gray. One gray represents 1 joule of energy absorbed per kilogram of tissue. The tradition unit of absorbed dose is *rad*.

Equivalent dose

The type of radiation influences the magnitude of biological damage from the same absorbed radiation dose. The unit of equivalent dose considers the type of radiation that resulted in energy transfer. It is a product of the absorbed dose and the radiation-weighting factor, W_R, and is mathematically summarized as:

$$H_T = \Sigma W_R \bullet D_T$$

where H_T is the equivalent dose, W_R is the radiation-weighting factor, and D_T is the absorbed dose.

For X-rays, the weighting factor is one; thus, absorbed dose is numerically equal to the equivalent dose. Equivalent dose is measured in *Sieverts* (Sv). The traditional unit of equivalent dose is the *rem*.

Effective dose

Different tissues have different sensitivities to radiation-induced stochastic effects. Thus, the total detriment per unit of equivalent dose varies depending on the tissue types exposed. The unit of effective dose accounts for this differential sensitivity. Depending on their sensitivity to radiation-induced stochastic effects, tissues have been assigned a weighting factor. This factor represents the relative contribution of injury to that organ or tissue to total risk of stochastic radiation effect. In the maxillofacial region, tissues with increased risk of stochastic effects include the thyroid gland, active bone marrow, salivary glands, brain, and bone surface. Similar to equivalent dose, the units of effective dose are Sieverts (Sv) or rems. Effective dose is mathematically denoted as:

$$E = \Sigma W_T \bullet H_T$$

where E is effective dose, W_T is the tissue-weighting factor, and H_T is the equivalent dose.

It is important to understand the concept of effective dose. This is the unit that is used to convey the net detriment from a radiographic examination, and it is used to compare radiation risks between different modalities, specific imaging protocols, and radiographic examinations that expose different regions of the body. For example, the risk of a maxillofacial CBCT examination with an effective dose of 100 μSv is ten times higher than the risk from a panoramic radiographic examination with an effective dose of 10 μSv.

References

ADA Council on Scientific Affairs. (2001). An update on radiographic practices: Information and recommendations. *Journal of the American Dental Association*, 132(2): 234–8.

American Association of Endodontists and American Academy of Oral and Maxillofacial Radiology. (2011). Use of cone-beam computed tomography in endodontics: Joint Position Statement of the American Association of Endodontists and the American Academy of Oral and Maxillofacial Radiology. *Oral Surgery, Oral Medicine, Oral Pathology, Oral Radiology and Endodontics*, 111(2): 234–7.

Hirsch, E., Wolf, U., Heinicke, F., et al. (2008). Dosimetry of the cone beam computed tomography Veraviewepocs 3D compared with the 3D Accuitomo in different fields of view. *Dentomaxillofacial Radiology*, 37(5): 268–73.

Horner, K., Islam, M., Flygare, L., et al. (2009). Basic principles for use of dental cone beam computed tomography: Consensus guidelines of the European Academy of Dental and Maxillofacial Radiology. *Dentomaxillofacial Radiology*, 38(4): 187–95.

Librizzi, Z.T., Tadinada, A.S., Valiyaparambil, J.V., et al. (2011). Cone-beam computed tomography to detect erosions of the temporomandibular joint: Effect of field of view and voxel size on diagnostic efficacy and effective dose. *American Journal of Orthodontics and Dentofacial Orthopedics*, 140(1): e25–30.

Lofthag-Hansen, S., Thilander-Klang, A., Ekestubbe, A., et al. (2008). Calculating effective dose on a cone beam computed tomography device: 3D Accuitomo and 3D Accuitomo FPD. *Dentomaxillofacial Radiology*, 37(2): 72–9.

Loubele, M., Bogaerts, R., Van Dijck, E., et al. (2009). Comparison between effective radiation dose of CBCT and MSCT scanners for dentomaxillofacial applications. *European Journal of Radiology*, 71(3): 461–8.

Loubele, M., Jacobs, R., Maes, F., et al. (2005). Radiation dose vs. image quality for low-dose CT protocols of the head for maxillofacial surgery and oral implant planning. *Radiation Protection Dosimetry*, 117(1–3): 211–6.

Ludlow, J.B. (2011). A manufacturer's role in reducing the dose of cone beam computed tomography examinations: Effect of beam filtration. *Dentomaxillofacial Radiology*, 40(2): 115–22.

Ludlow, J.B., and Ivanovic, M. (2008). Comparative dosimetry of dental CBCT devices and 64-slice CT for oral and maxillofacial radiology. *Oral Surgery, Oral Medicine, Oral Pathology, Oral Radiology and Endodontics*, 106(1): 106–14.

Ludlow, J.B., Davies-Ludlow, L.E., Brooks, S.L. (2003). Dosimetry of two extraoral direct digital imaging devices: NewTom cone beam CT and Orthophos Plus DS panoramic unit. *Dentomaxillofacial Radiology*, 32(4): 229–34.

Ludlow, J.B., Davies-Ludlow, L.E., Brooks, S.L., et al. (2006). Dosimetry of 3 CBCT devices for oral and maxillofacial radiology: CB Mercuray, NewTom 3G and i-CAT. *Dentomaxillofacial Radiology*, 35(4): 219–26.

NCRP. (2009). NCRP Report Number 160, Ionizing Radiation Exposure of the Population of the United States. Available at http://www.ncrponline.org/PDFs/2012/DAS_DDM2_Athens_4-2012.pdf.

Okano, T., Harata, Y., Sugihara, Y., et al. (2009). Absorbed and effective doses from cone beam volumetric imaging for implant planning. *Dentomaxillofacial Radiology*, 38(2): 79–85.

Pauwels, R., Beinsberger, J., Collaert, B., et al. (2012). Effective dose range for dental cone beam computed tomography scanners. *European Journal of Radiology*, 81(2): 267–71.

Roberts, J.A., Drage, N.A., Davies, J., et al. (2009). Effective dose from cone beam CT examinations in dentistry. *British Journal of Radiology*, 82(973): 35–40.

Suomalainen, A., Kiljunen, T., Kaser, Y., et al. (2009). Dosimetry and image quality of four dental cone beam computed tomography scanners compared with multislice computed tomography scanners. *Dentomaxillofacial Radiology*, 38(6): 367–78.

White, S.C., and Mallya, S.M. (2012). Update on the biological effects of ionizing radiation, relative dose factors and radiation hygiene. *Australian Dental Journal*, 57(Suppl 1): 2–8.

White, S.C., and Pae, E.-K. (2009). Patient image selection criteria for cone beam computed tomography imaging. *Seminars in Orthodontics*, 15(1): 19–28.

White, S.C., and Pharoah, M.J. (2009). *Oral Radiology: Principles and Interpretation*, 6th ed. St. Louis, MO: Mosby/Elsevier.

White, S.C., Heslop, E.W., Hollender, L.G., et al. (2001). Parameters of radiologic care: An official report of the American Academy of Oral and Maxillofacial Radiology. *Oral Surgery, Oral Medicine, Oral Pathology, Oral Radiology, Endodontics*, 91(5): 498–511.

3 Diagnosis of Jaw Pathologies Using Cone Beam Computed Tomography

Sharon L. Brooks

Clinicians who decide to use cone beam computed tomography (CBCT) for their patients assume the responsibility for the interpretation of the entire volume encompassed in the scan, not just the area that might be the reason for the scan. This means that, in addition to using the scan data to plan implant or orthodontic or temporomandibular joint (TMJ) treatment, the clinician must review all the data to rule out pathologic changes anywhere in the region covered by the scan. Clinicians may elect to do this themselves or have an oral and maxillofacial radiologist or medical radiologist review the scan. However, the person who made the scan—the treating clinician—is ultimately responsible for the complete interpretation of the scan.

This responsibility can present some challenges to the clinician: the scan volume is large and covers structures not typically visualized on standard dental images, such as intraoral and panoramic views; and significant pathologic lesions in the jaws are relatively uncommon and the dentist may not see lesions in the jaws or surrounding structures with enough frequency to feel comfortable diagnosing such conditions.

The best technique for interpreting CBCT scans is to develop a systematic approach to all scans, assuring that all the data are reviewed, before concentrating on the specific area of interest on the scan. For example, if a scan is made to evaluate the edentulous ridge for implant planning, the clinician is not going to forget to make bone measurements if he waits to do so until he has reviewed the rest of the scan. However, it would be easy to forget to read the entire scan if the implant site is evaluated first, because the dentist could get caught up in the excitement of planning treatment for the patient.

In addition to having a standardized way of viewing the CBCT scan, in order to evaluate the scan well the clinician must have a thorough knowledge of anatomy as revealed on the scan. Anatomy of the jaws is well known to all dentists, and the jaw structures seen on CBCT and standard dental images are similar in appearance. However, since the CBCT generally covers a larger field of view, the dentist must review (or relearn) many other structures, including the paranasal sinuses, neck, temporal bone outside the TMJ, skull base, orbits, and many other areas. Limiting the scan field of view to the area of interest reduces the amount of scan volume that must be reviewed. If an abnormality is detected on a CBCT scan, the clinician must make some important decisions. Is the abnormality pathologic or a variation of normal anatomy that is of no clinical significance? If it is considered pathologic, what is it? Does it require further evaluation? Referral to an oral and maxillofacial

---

Cone Beam Computed Tomography: Oral and Maxillofacial Diagnosis and Applications, First Edition. Edited by David Sarment.
© 2014 John Wiley & Sons, Inc. Published 2014 by John Wiley & Sons, Inc.

radiologist or oral and maxillofacial pathologist? Referral to an oral and maxillofacial surgeon for biopsy? Does it need treatment or simply "observation"? If the latter, what is meant by that? Do nothing at all? Reimage later? If so, how often?

The rest of this chapter will help the clinician develop a protocol for reviewing CBCT images and for evaluating lesions detected. An illustrated review of common pathologic lesions in and around the jaws will then be presented. Not all possible lesions can be discussed in the limited space available in this chapter. For that reason, clinicians are strongly encouraged to consult other reference books, such as comprehensive oral pathology and oral radiology texts. Suggested texts are listed at the end of the chapter.

Protocol for reviewing the CBCT volume

There is no single best way to review the entire CBCT volume. However, no matter what protocol the clinician uses, it should be the same for every scan and should permit a thorough evaluation of all the anatomy in all planes. Standard image viewing software allows the clinician to view the data in multiple ways: multiplanar reconstruction (MPR)—the standard axial, coronal, and sagittal planes that can be scrolled through; reconstructed panoramic view; cross-sections perpendicular to the dental arch; specific views of some structures such as the TMJ; and three-dimensional (3D) volumetric renderings (Figure 3.1A, Figure 3.1B, Figure 3.1C, and Figure 3.1D). Some software also permits implant planning and orthodontic analysis, among other functions. The clinician needs to become very familiar with the features available in the software package being used, although all of the packages have many of the same features.

The following protocol is one that the author, an oral and maxillofacial radiologist, finds useful in reviewing CBCT scans for pathology. It is not the only protocol available, but it does cover all

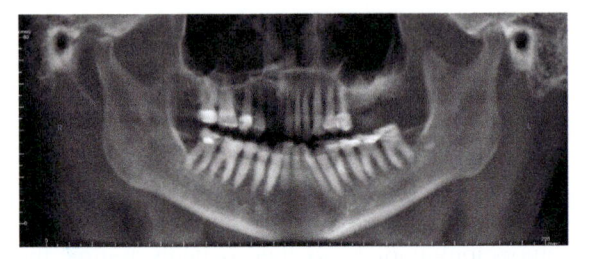

Figure 3.1B Viewing protocol: reconstructed panoramic view.

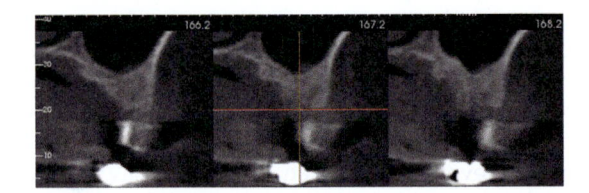

Figure 3.1C Viewing protocol: cross-sections, maxillary arch.

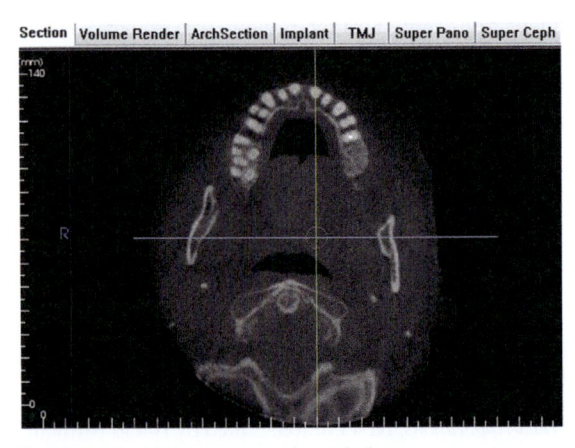

Figure 3.1A Viewing protocol: axial plane.

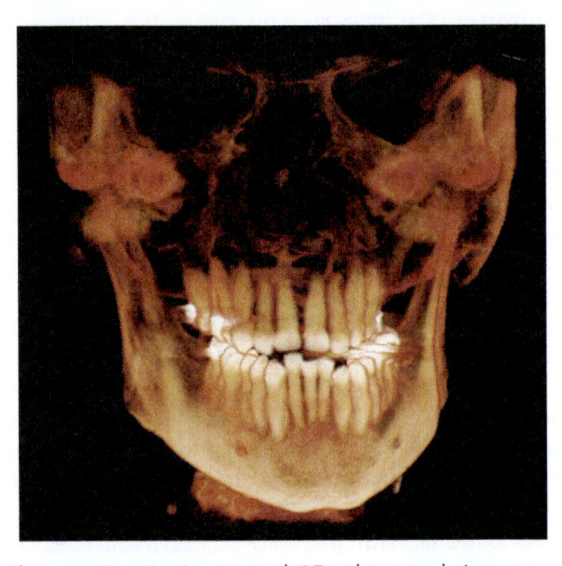

Figure 3.1D Viewing protocol: 3D volume rendering.

the basics. It does not cover implant planning or orthodontic analysis, because these tasks are reserved for the treating clinician.

When the scan volume is first opened, typically the software presents the MPR view: separate panels for the three separate planes, axial (horizontal/occlusal), coronal (frontal), and sagittal (lateral). These planes can be scrolled through (and will be later in this protocol). At this time it is helpful to rotate the scan if necessary to make the mid-sagittal plane vertical and the occlusal plane horizontal. Sometimes the patient's head is not completely straight in the scanner, and straightening the images makes them easier to view and to compare anatomy from one side to the other.

At this point the author likes to view the images in the 3D reconstruction mode because it gives a quick overview of the patient's anatomy and conditions in the jaws: how many teeth are present and major abnormalities visible in the jaws or surrounding areas. The 3D rendering is not used for complete evaluation of the scan because it can be misleading, depending on the protocol used for segmenting the image before viewing, but it can be helpful to get an overall picture of the patient.

A panoramic reconstruction is a useful next step in reviewing the scan because it presents the information in the jaws in a format that is familiar to most dentists and shows relationships between the teeth and adjacent areas. Because the image is a relatively narrow slice through a curved section of anatomy, structures outside that curved plane will not be visible in this view.

The most important part of reviewing the scan is the evaluation of the MPR images. Again, there are different approaches available, but the author prefers to start with the axial view, scrolling from the most inferior slice to the most superior, looking at the anatomy, identifying structures, comparing right with left, and so forth. If an abnormality is noted in the jaws or adjacent structures, the images in the other planes can be scrolled to reveal that structure in all three planes at once, in an effort to determine the nature of the structure, anatomic or pathologic (Figure 3.2). Once the axial slices are reviewed, a similar process is done with the coronal view (anterior to posterior) and sagittal view (one side to the other).

Due to the oblique angle of the mandibular condyles with the mid-sagittal plane, the standard MPR images are not ideal for evaluating the TMJs, and a separate TMJ view is used for this. Finally, cross-sections to the dental arch are viewed to evaluate the teeth and alveolar bone. These views are also helpful in evaluating the relationship of impacted teeth to other teeth and the inferior alveolar canal, the relationship of jawbone pathology to teeth, and bone quantity and quality for implant planning.

Evaluating pathologic lesions

Once an abnormality is detected on a CBCT scan, the next step is to determine the nature of the finding. First is the decision about whether the finding is an actual pathologic lesion or a variant of normal anatomy. Comparison of one side to the other can be helpful in this distinction, but knowledge of normal anatomy and common variations is essential.

Not all abnormalities detected are serious and require treatment, but some may have a great impact on the patient's health and well-being. Thus, the clinician has to determine the nature and importance of the condition detected. While a basic knowledge of pathology is necessary to make this determination, there are some imaging features than can be helpful to the clinician in deciding what to do about the lesion, including when to refer.

Lesions detected on the scan should be evaluated for the following features: location, periphery and shape, internal structure, and effects of the lesion on adjacent structures. With respect to location, is the lesion in the jaws at all or in other bony structures or in soft tissues around the jaws? If it is in the jaws, is it within the tooth-bearing area, thus suggesting an odontogenic origin to the lesion, or outside this area? Is there a single lesion or multiple, similar lesions? Is the lesion localized or generalized? Is it causing jaw expansion?

With respect to the periphery of the lesion, is the border well defined or ill defined (Figure 3.3A and Figure 3.3B)? If it is well defined, is it punched out (no bony reaction), corticated (thin radiopaque line of bony reaction around lesion), or sclerotic (thicker,

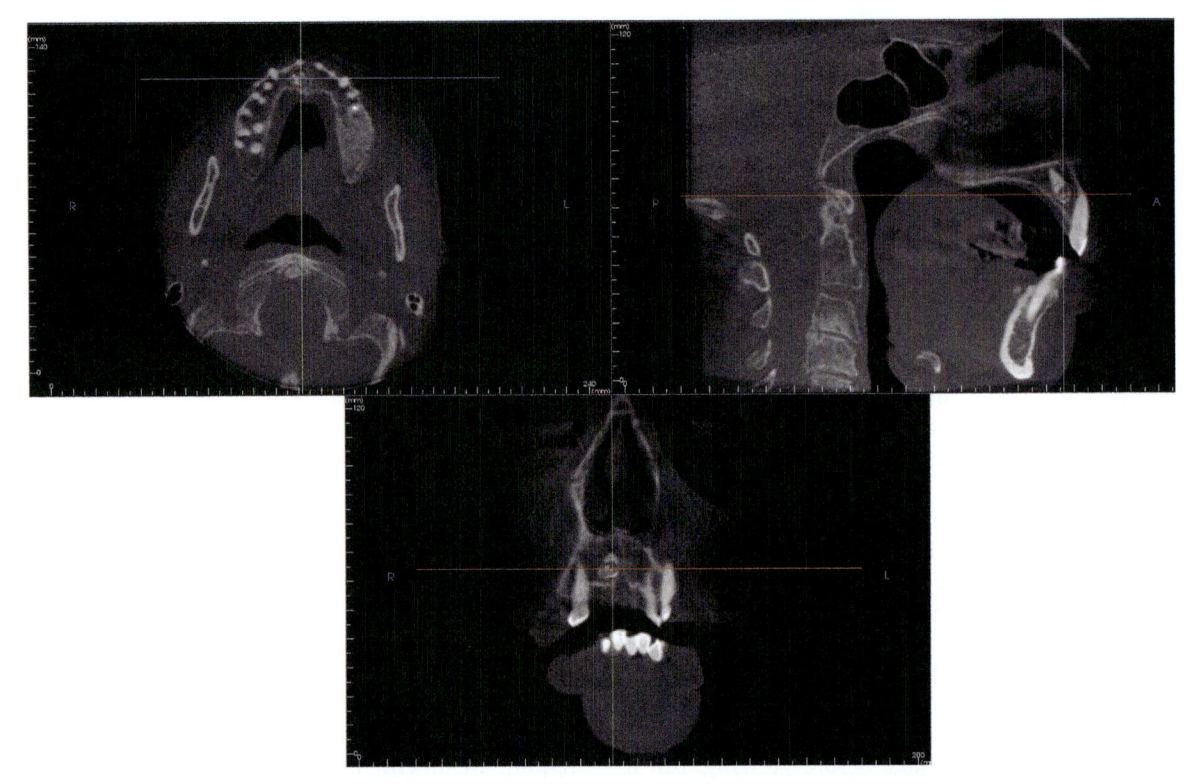

Figure 3.2 Adjusting all planes of multiplanar reconstruction to show the area of interest at the same time can help in diagnosing the condition, such as this resorbing supernumerary tooth in the anterior maxilla.

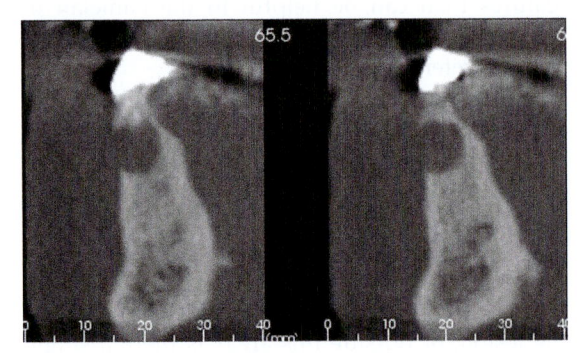

Figure 3.3A Low attenuation (radiolucent) mandibular lesion with well-defined margin, cross-sectional view.

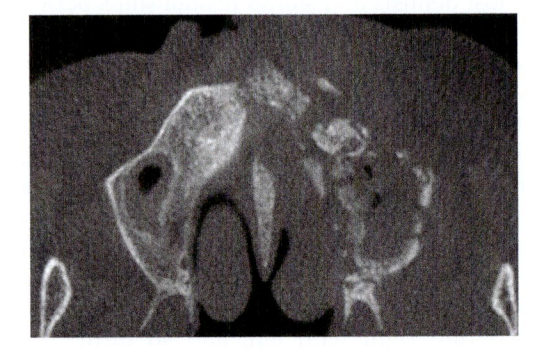

Figure 3.3B Mixed radiolucent-radiopaque maxillary lesion with ill-defined margin, axial view.

nonuniform area of dense bone around lesion)? If the lesion is radiopaque, is there a soft-tissue capsule (radiolucent line or "halo") around the lesion (Figure 3.4A and Figure 3.4B)? If the border is ill defined, does the lesion blend gradually with normal bone or does it permeate ("eat away") at the margin of normal bone?

With respect to the internal structure of the lesion, is it totally radiolucent, totally radiopaque, or mixed radiolucent-radiopaque? If the latter,

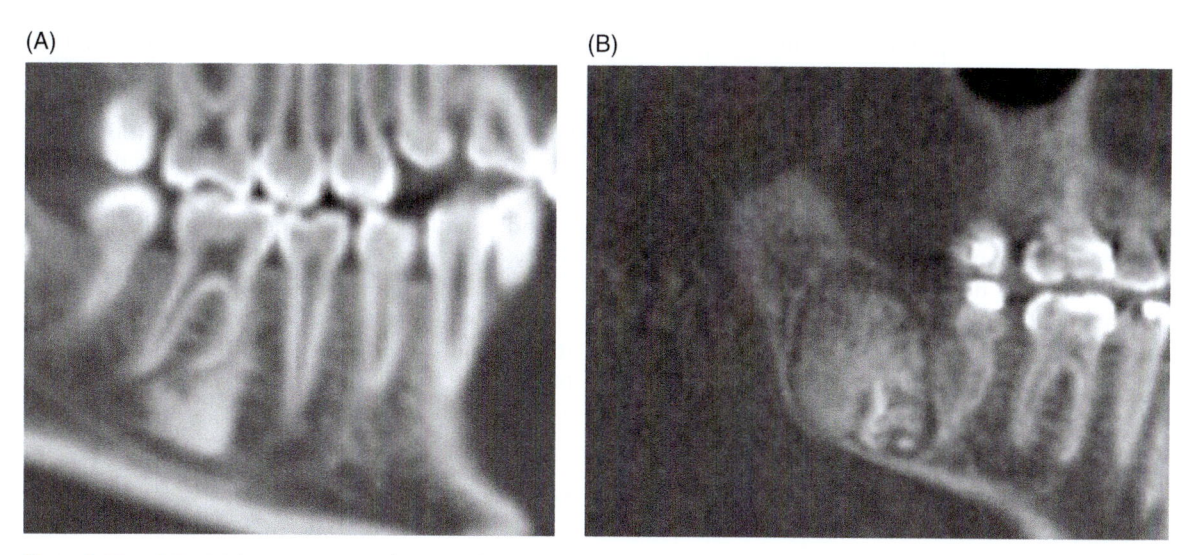

Figure 3.4A and B High attenuation (radiopaque) lesion with (A) well-defined margin but with no radiolucent rim (no "halo"), sagittal view, and (B) well-defined margin, with a radiolucent rim ("halo") separating the lesion from the adjacent normal bone, sagittal view.

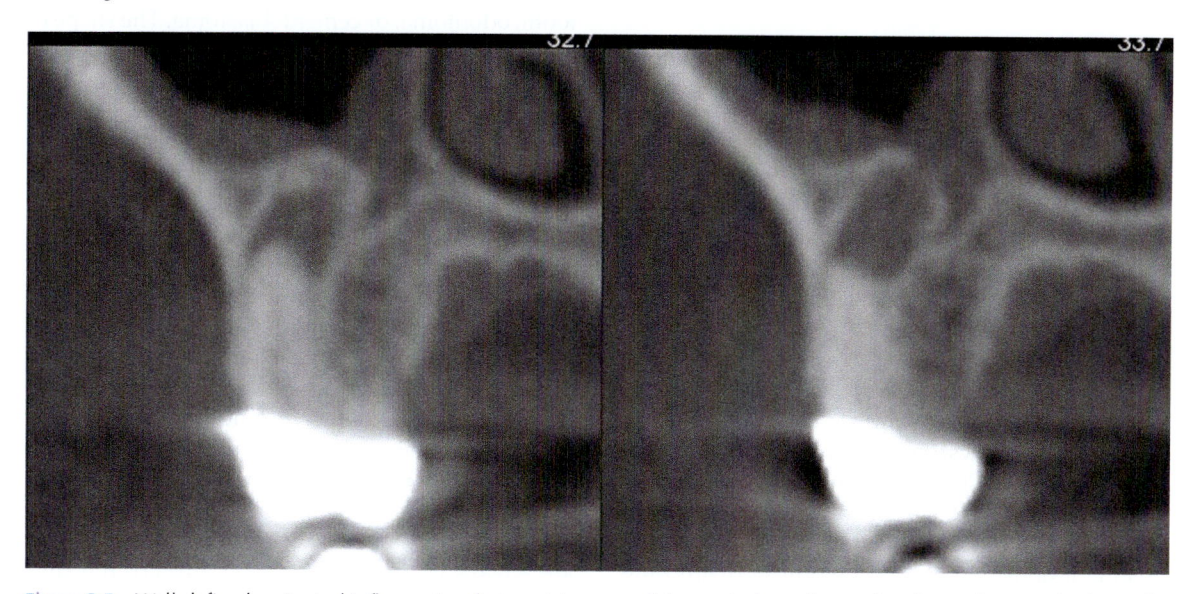

Figure 3.5 Well-defined periapical inflammatory lesion at the apex of the mesio-buccal root of tooth #3, elevating the floor of the maxillary sinus.

what is the relationship between the dense and less dense parts of the lesion?

With respect to the effect of the lesion on adjacent structures, is it displacing teeth? Causing any changes to the periodontal ligament space (PDL) or lamina dura? Widening or displacing the inferior alveolar nerve canal? Altering the floor of the maxillary antrum (Figure 3.5)? Affecting the cortical bone or causing periosteal reactions?

Pathologic lesions of the jaws

After the pertinent features of the lesion have been evaluated, the clinician next needs to make some decisions. Is the lesion developmental or acquired? If acquired, is it most likely a cyst, benign neoplasm, malignant neoplasm, inflammatory lesion, bone dysplasia, vascular abnormality, metabolic disease, or result of trauma? Classifying a lesion is helpful in deciding the next step: further evaluation, possibly including biopsy; treatment; or observation.

The rest of this chapter will be devoted to a review of common lesions that can be found in the jaws, with some lesions in adjacent areas also covered. Most oral pathology and oral radiology texts discuss lesions by major classification, such as cyst or inflammatory condition. Because it is not always easy to determine the classification of a lesion initially, the approach taken in this section of the chapter will be that of guiding the clinician through the thought process of determining the lesion classification—and ultimately in some cases the final diagnosis—by dividing lesions into three major categories: radiopaque lesions, slow-growing radiolucent lesions, and rapidly growing radiolucent lesions.

Radiopaque lesions

A lesion that appears radiopaque on a radiograph is made of a material that absorbs a large proportion of the X-rays hitting it, thus allowing a relatively few to pass through and interact with the X-ray detector. With respect to CT imaging, these lesions are also described as high attenuation or high density. In lesions occurring in the jawbones, radiopaque masses are composed of one (or a combination) of the following materials: enamel, dentin, cementum, bone, ectopic calcification, or foreign material. In standard dental imaging, such as panoramic radiographs, soft tissue may also have a radiopaque appearance if it is replacing air, such as a mucous retention pseudocyst in the maxillary sinus. The same lesion in a CBCT has a density of soft tissue, readily distinguishable from both air and bone.

There are a few general statements about radiopaque lesions that may be helpful in diagnosing something detected on a radiograph. If a lesion contains enamel or dentin, it is some type of tooth tissue: residual root tip, unerupted tooth, supernumerary tooth, or odontoma. Radiopaque objects are not always located where they seem to be in a single plane because their image can be projected. Therefore, it is necessary to localize the lesion in all planes at the same time to determine where the lesion actually is located.

One of the most critical features to observe in radiopaque lesions in the bone is the border: Is there a radiolucent rim or halo around the lesion? If the answer is yes, the lesion is most likely either a tooth or toothlike lesion or a fibro-osseous lesion, both of which have either a developing follicle or a fibrous capsule. If the answer is no, then the lesion is most likely dense bone or foreign material.

Radiopaque lesions in general are benign and many of them do not require treatment after identification. Although sarcomas such as osteosarcoma and chondrosarcoma do produce bone or cartilage, their overall appearance is very different from most radiopaque lesions, having many of the features of a typical malignancy.

Lesions of tooth tissue

If a lesion appears to contain tooth tissue (much denser than bone), the diagnostic choices include tooth fragment, unerupted tooth, supernumerary tooth, odontoma, or cementoblastoma. The shape of the mass and presence of residual PDL and lamina dura or dental follicle generally make identification of teeth or tooth remnants relatively easy.

An odontoma is a benign tumor (or some consider it a hamartoma) composed of tooth tissue (enamel, dentin, cementum, and pulp) in various degrees of morphodifferentiation (Figure 3.6). Compound odontomas contain multiple denticles that can be recognized as small toothlike structures, while the tooth tissues in complex odontomas are all mixed together and do not look like teeth. All odontomas, compound or complex, have a well-defined radiolucent halo and a thin radiopaque (corticated) border, representing a dental follicle. These tumors begin developing at the time of normal tooth development and generally cease growing when tooth development finishes. They are always in the tooth-bearing areas of the jaws and may displace teeth or block them from erupting. Treatment generally is enucleation.

Compound odontomas have a unique appearance that is generally readily identifiable. Complex odontomas must be differentiated from sclerotic bone masses and fibro-osseous lesions. Sclerotic bone masses, discussed more later, do not have a capsule around them and are unlikely to displace or impact teeth. Fibro-osseous lesions, also described later, do have a capsule, but it is frequently larger and less distinct than that of

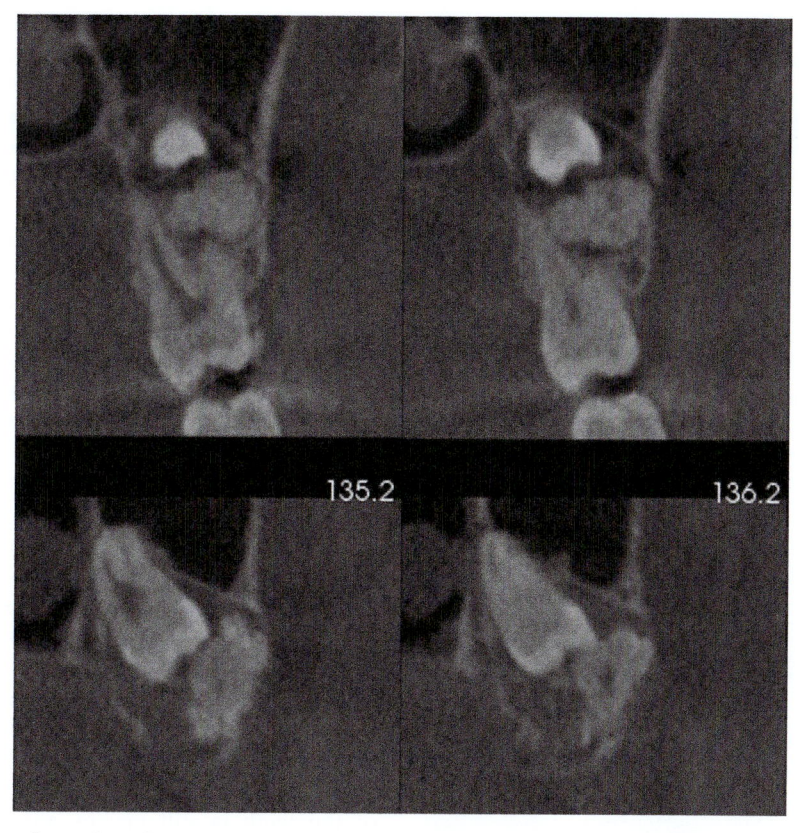

Figure 3.6 Compound-complex odontoma displacing the maxillary left third molar, cross-sectional views. In some sections the lesion resembles teeth, in others the radiopaque mass is more amorphous. There is a radiolucent rim around the radiopaque material, representing the dental follicle.

odontomas and the density of the radiopaque core is generally lower than that of the odontoma.

A cementoblastoma is a benign tumor that produces cementum, occurring usually attached to the root of a mandibular premolar or first molar. It frequently causes root resorption of the affected root and appears to be growing out of the root. It also has a radiolucent capsule and radiopaque border. Pain is a common feature of this tumor, whereas it is not in odontomas. Treatment is extraction of the affected tooth and enucleation of the lesion.

Lesions of bone tissue

Inflammation can lead to bone resorption or bone production or a combination of the two. When inflammation in the dental pulp extends into the surrounding bone, a radiolucent lesion is frequently observed: apical periodontitis, dental granuloma, or radicular cyst. Chronic inflammation can also induce bone formation, leading to a radiopaque bony mass or a thickened radiopaque rim around a radiolucent lesion at the apex of a tooth. This is frequently called sclerosing or condensing osteitis. The border of the mass is generally ill defined and it blends gradually into the adjacent normal bone. There is no radiolucent capsule (Figure 3.7A). Usually the PDL of the affected tooth is widened and pulp vitality testing is negative. Treatment is focused on removing the source of inflammation by endodontic therapy or tooth extraction.

Somewhat similar in appearance is the dense bone island, also called enostosis or idiopathic osteosclerosis. This is generally a well-defined mass of dense bone within the jaws (or other bones of the body) with no radiolucent capsule (Figure 3.7B). It can occur anywhere in the jaws, not just in the tooth-bearing

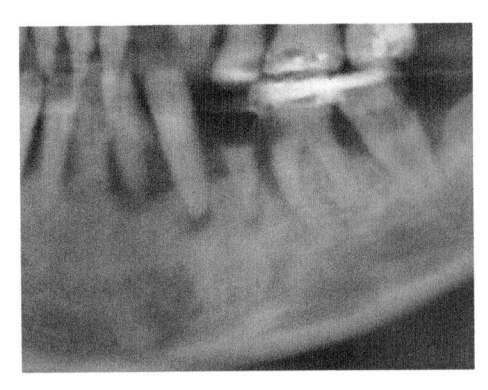

Figure 3.7A Multiple periapical and periodontal inflammatory lesions, reconstructed panoramic view. Peripheral to the radiolucent lesions the bone is very dense, so-called condensing or sclerosing osteitis, with the margins of the altered bone blending into the adjacent unaffected bone.

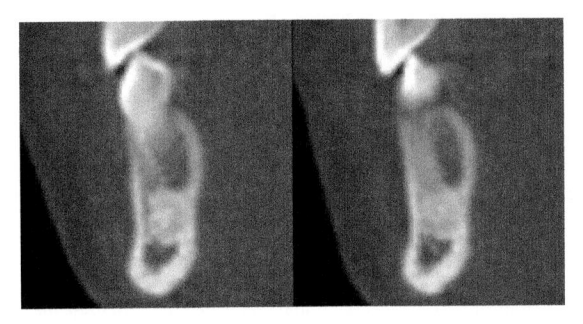

Figure 3.7B Well-defined radiopaque mass inferior to but not associated with a mandibular canine. This dense bone island (enostosis, idiopathic osteosclerosis) appears to arise from the lingual cortical plate.

area, and is considered to be the internal correlate to exostoses or tori. It is benign and requires no treatment. Usually it is quite stable, although growth of the mass has been reported in some cases.

Exostoses, as the name implies, are bony hyperostotic projections from the jawbones. The most common exostoses are mandibular and palatal tori, but they can also occur on the buccal or palatal alveolar ridge and under pontics of fixed prostheses. Diagnosis is not usually in doubt, but the multiplanar images in CBCT may be useful in localizing them.

Fibro-osseous lesions

Fibro-osseous lesion is a general term used for a condition in which normal bone is replaced first by fibrous tissue and later by bony or cementum-like tissue. The radiographic appearance of such lesions depends on the specific lesion and its stage of development. The appearance can range from totally radiolucent, in the fibrous stage, to a mixed radiolucent-radiopaque middle stage, to an almost completely radiopaque mature stage. The lesions designated by the term *cemento-osseous dysplasia* (or simply *cemental dysplasia* or *osseous dysplasia*) have a fibrous capsule, producing a radiolucent rim around the lesion, surrounded by a sclerotic border.

Periapical cemento-osseous dysplasia (PCOD) affects multiple teeth, usually mandibular anterior teeth, and is seen most frequently in women, average age about 40 years, more commonly in African Americans or Asians than in Whites. Single lesions may be designated as focal cemento-osseous dysplasia but are otherwise similar to PCOD.

The PCOD lesions start out as radiolucent lesions at the apices of teeth. Differentiation from inflammatory lesions is done with vitality testing, because teeth affected by PCOD remain vital. Over time, calcified material is deposited within the fibrous lesion, sometimes replacing almost all of the radiolucent part of the lesion, although the radiolucent capsule is usually still visible. The PDL of the teeth is still visible, although the lamina dura may not be distinguishable.

The lesions are asymptomatic and may be found on routine radiographic examination. The imaging features are distinct enough that biopsy is not necessary. In fact, surgical manipulation is discouraged because the lesions can become secondarily infected. No treatment is needed for these lesions.

Similar to PCOD is florid osseous dysplasia (FOD), except the lesions affect multiple quadrants simultaneously and the lesions may grow larger than the typical PCOD lesions (Figure 3.8A and Figure 3.8B). The demographics of this condition are similar to PCOD. Sometimes the lesions are associated with simple bone cysts, giving them a large radiolucent outline. Similar to PCOD, treatment is typically periodic observation only, since these lesions also can become infected if surgery is done.

The major differential diagnosis for FOD is Paget's disease of bone, which is a metabolic condition of abnormal osteoclast activity, not considered to be a fibro-osseous lesion. This condition affects the maxilla more often than the mandible

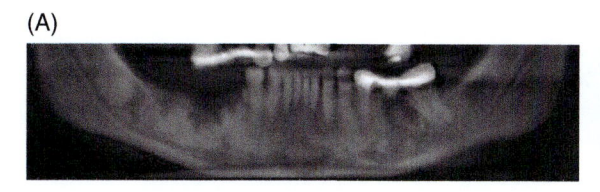

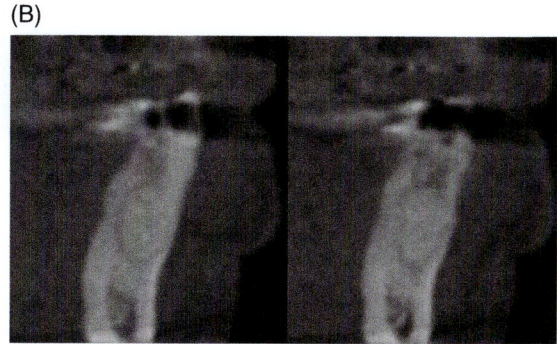

Figure 3.8A and B Florid osseous dysplasia: reconstructed panoramic view (A) and cross-sections through left mandible (B). There are multiple irregular radiopaque lesions throughout the mandible, not associated with any teeth. The radiolucent rim (capsule) is visible around the lesion.

and other bones more often than the jaws. Lesions are not isolated and tend to spread throughout the jaw. The bone pattern may vary, depending on the stage of the disease, from slightly radiolucent, to mixed density, to multiple radiopaque masses without radiolucent capsules. The term *ground glass* is frequently used to describe the irregular bone trabecular pattern of Paget's disease.

Central ossifying fibroma (or cementifying fibroma) is considered to be a true benign tumor, rather than a bone dysplasia. It may have a similar appearance to a focal cemento-osseous dysplasia, but it tends to be much more aggressive, causing significant bony enlargement. Unlike PCOD or FOD, it is a solitary lesion.

Fibrous dysplasia is a fibro-osseous lesion that has an imaging appearance and natural history very different from the other fibro-osseous lesions. It generally appears at a young age and stabilizes at the time of completion of normal bone growth. It most commonly affects one bone (monostotic) but may involve multiple bones (polyostotic), the latter frequently as part of other syndromes. The affected bone starts out radiolucent (fibrous tissue replaces bone), then becomes more radiopaque over time as abnormal bone replaces the fibrous tissue, frequently having a ground glass appearance, although it can also have a mixed radiolucent-radiopaque appearance. Unlike PCOD or FOD, the margins of fibrous dysplasia are generally ill defined, blending in with adjacent normal bone (Figure 3.9A and Figure 3.9B). Fibrous dysplasia can cause significant bone enlargement, fill the antrum in maxillary lesions, and displace the inferior alveolar canal in mandibular lesions. Surgery has been reported to stimulate growth of active lesions. Treatment may include surgical recontouring after the lesion has stabilized and growth has ceased.

Other radiopaque lesions

Calcification of structures outside the jawbones can be seen on CBCT images. The most common ones are calcified carotid atheromas, tonsilloliths, and sialoliths, although calcified lymph nodes are occasionally observed.

Atherosclerosis can lead to the development of plaques within various blood vessels, leading to narrowing of the vessel and occasional embolus formation if parts of the plaque break off. Carotid artery calcifications (CAC) or carotid atheromas occur at the bifurcation of the common carotid artery, which is located in the lateral aspect of the neck at approximately the C3-C4 vertebral junction, an area that is frequently covered in CBCT scans. The CAC may be irregular in shape or show a curved outline suggestive of a vessel wall (Figure 3.10). There is some disagreement about the significance of such calcified atheromas since the calcified plaques tend to be more stable than the noncalcified ones. However, they can be viewed as an indication of generalized cardiovascular disease and referral to a physician for further evaluation is prudent.

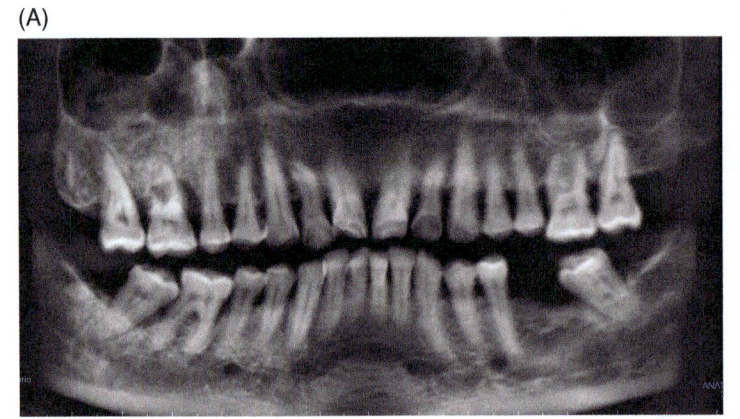

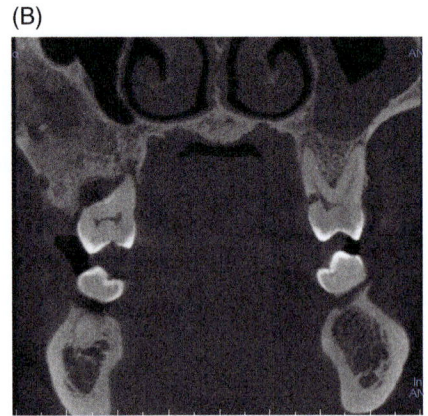

Figure 3.9A and B Fibrous dysplasia: reconstructed panoramic view (A) and coronal view (B). There is a non-uniform radiopaque expansion of right posterior maxilla. In addition, there is periodontitis and dental caries visible, unrelated to the fibrous dysplasia.

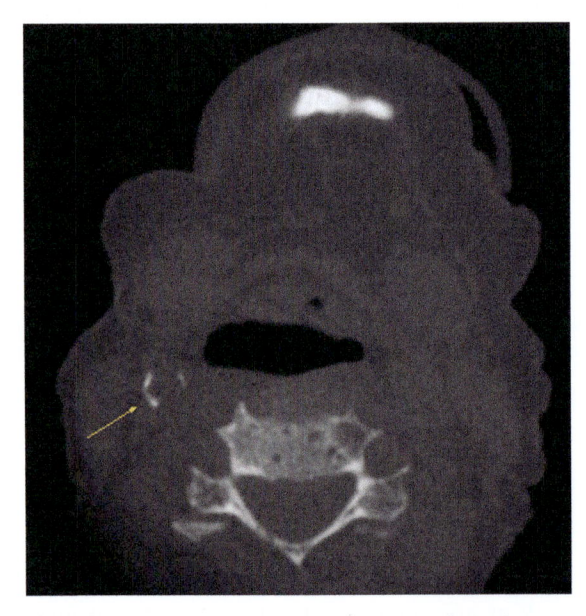

Figure 3.10 Curvilinear radiopaque lines in right neck, at level of C3-C4 vertebral junction, axial view. The appearance and location are correct for a calcified carotid atheroma.

Calcified normal anatomic structures in the same area of the neck can sometimes be confused with CAC, particularly triticeous cartilages (small, oval well-defined calcifications in the thyro-hyoid ligament), superior horn of the thyroid cartilage, and various parts of the hyoid bone.

Small punctate calcifications located in the pharyngeal wall typically suggest the diagnosis of tonsillolith. They are located more superior and more medial than CAC and are frequently multiple. Epithelial and bacterial debris in the crypts of the palatine tonsils can become calcified, leading to the formation of tonsilloliths. Large ones can occasionally be visualized clinically. No treatment is needed, although they have occasionally been implicated in the etiology of halitosis.

Submandibular sialoliths can also occasionally be detected on CBCT scan, located medial and slightly inferior to the mandible, depending on the exact location of the stone. Frequently sialoliths produce symptoms of submandibular swelling and pain. They may be palpable clinically.

A variety of foreign materials can also be observed on CBCT scan, both inside the jaws (typically amalgam fragments and fixation devices such as screws and plates) and in the soft tissues. History of trauma or surgery, particularly cosmetic surgery, may be helpful in differentiating these materials.

Other uncommon radiopaque (or partially radiopaque) lesions that can be seen in the jaws include osteomyelitis (discussed further below), osteopetrosis, osteosarcoma (discussed further below), and bone-producing metastasis. Consultation of a textbook of oral pathology is recommended for more information on all of the conditions discussed above.

Radiolucent lesions

The majority of the lesions occurring in the jawbone are radiolucent in appearance, with normal bone replaced by fluid (cysts) or various soft tissues (tumors, inflammatory cells). Concavities in the surface of the bone can also produce a radiolucent appearance, although the multiplanar imaging of CBCT can distinguish a lesion that is inside the bone from one that is simply indenting it.

While air-filled cavities can be distinguished from fluid- or soft tissue-filled cavities on CBCT, the latter two cannot be separated by CBCT. Conventional CT (medical) and magnetic resonance imaging (MRI) can differentiate various types of soft tissues and may be preferable imaging techniques when soft tissue information is important in the diagnosis or treatment planning of a jaw lesion.

Most of the radiolucent lesions seen in the jaws occur at the apex of teeth as a result of pulpal inflammation and are very familiar to dentists. These lesions can range from a simple widening of the apical periodontal ligament space as the earliest manifestation of the inflammatory process to a definite periapical radiolucent lesion, with well-defined or ill-defined margins, depending on the acuteness or chronicity of the inflammation. History and clinical findings, including vitality testing, along with the imaging appearance, can usually make diagnosis relatively straightforward. Symptoms can precede radiographic changes, however, making diagnosis more difficult in those cases.

Radiolucent lesions occurring away from the apices of teeth are less common and may cause confusion in diagnosis for multiple reasons. Because dentists are not likely to see some of these lesions outside of a textbook, when they do occur it is difficult to identify them. In addition, multiple types of lesions can have similar radiographic appearances, such as cysts and benign tumors. Since some of these lesions may have a significant impact on the patient's life or quality of life, it is important to be able to distinguish which ones are serious and require immediate attention and which ones are less serious and may not even need treatment at all.

To aid in making this determination, radiolucent lesions will be discussed under two broad categories, slow growing and rapidly growing, with emphasis on the radiographic features that distinguish these categories. Examples of the most frequent lesions will also be presented.

Slow-growing radiolucent lesions

Lesions that are relatively slow growing demonstrate some features on radiographs that help to differentiate them from more rapidly growing (and generally more serious) lesions, including borders and effects on adjacent structures.

The borders of slow-growing lesions tend to be distinct and smooth, rather than indistinct and/or irregular, due to the growth pattern of the lesion. These lesions (developmental anomalies, cysts, benign tumors) tend to start with a central nidus and expand outwardly evenly in all directions, although the shape may be constrained by the anatomy of the region.

Benign lesions can get very large, but they are more likely to cause expansion of the bone rather than erosion of the cortical plates and eventual perforation of the bone, as is seen in malignant lesions. This is because the bone has time to remodel around the growing lesion rather than be destroyed by it. Likewise, a slowly growing lesion can cause tooth displacement, similar to orthodontic movement, if it is located in a tooth-bearing area. Teeth can be displaced in rapidly growing malignant lesions also, but that is because the tumor has destroyed the bone holding the teeth and the teeth may seem to float.

Root resorption by itself is not a good clue to the nature of the lesion in the bone because both benign and malignant lesions can cause resorption. The shape and borders of the lesion are much better predictors of the nature of the lesion than the effect on the roots of the teeth.

Slow-growing lesions generally fall into three categories: developmental, cysts, and benign tumors. Developmental anomalies typically include anatomic variants that may be larger than normal or in a slightly different location than expected. Occasionally foramina, such as the incisive or nasopalatine foramen, may be larger than usual and must be differentiated from a cyst occurring in that location, usually on the basis of size. The maxillary sinus may also present with various outpouchings or extensions into the alveolar ridge or maxillary

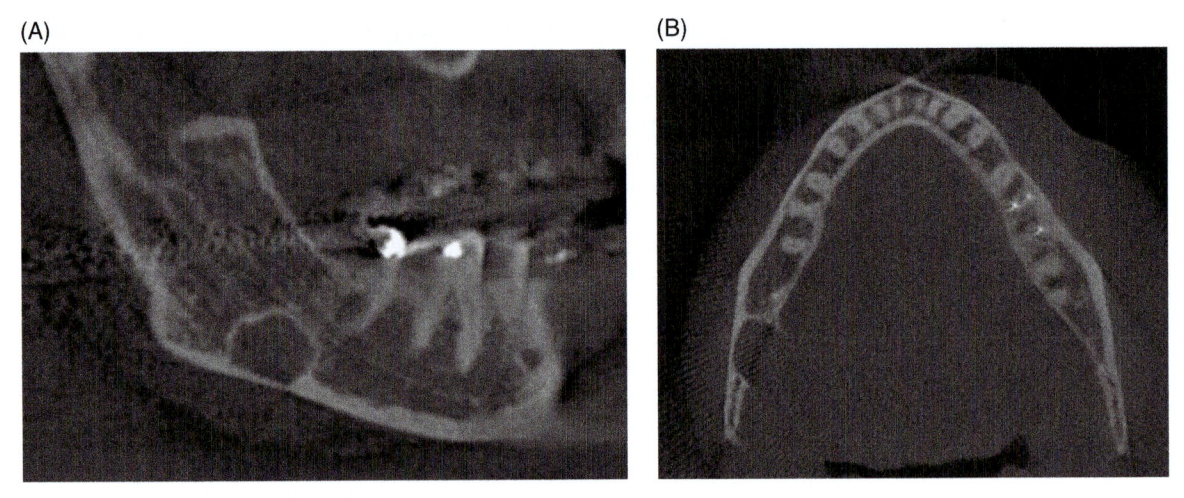

Figure 3.11A and B Lingual salivary gland depression (Stafne bone defect), right mandible. A well-defined depression on the lingual aspect of the mandible is observed on the sagittal (A) and axial (B) views.

tuberosity, simulating disease until they are viewed carefully in all planes. Two examples of a "displaced" anatomic variant is the concha bullosa (ethmoid air cells located within the middle concha of the nose) and the so-called zygomatic air cell defect, in which air cells, similar to those found in the mastoid process, are seen anterior to the TMJ in the articular eminence and the entire zygomatic process of the temporal bone. Neither of these conditions is of clinical significance unless surgery is needed in the area.

The lingual salivary gland depression (Stafne bone defect, static bone cavity) is a developmental anomaly that may be seen occasionally on dental panoramic or CBCT scans (Figure 3.11A and Figure 3.11B). It occurs usually in the posterior mandible, inferior to the mandibular canal and anterior to the gonial angle, and presents as a well-defined and corticated depression or indentation on the lingual surface of the bone. It may or may not involve the base of the mandible, depending on its exact location. It is commonly filled with salivary gland tissue from the submandibular gland but may also contain fat. Other variants of the depression occur in the mandibular premolar region, associated with the sublingual glands, and the buccal surface of the ramus, associated with the parotid gland. The appearance of the condition in the multiple planes of CBCT as a cortical-lined depression on the lingual of the mandible is usually sufficient for diagnosis. No treatment is indicated.

Another developmental anomaly that must be differentiated from pathology is the focal osteoporotic bone marrow. In this situation, one or more radiolucent areas, surrounded by normal trabecular bone, are located within the medullary portion of the jawbone, causing no effect on adjacent teeth or bone. These enlarged bone marrow spaces usually occur in women and are most typically found in the mandibular premolar-molar region, but they may also be seen in the maxillary tuberosity, mandibular retromolar area, edentulous sites, and in the furcation area of molars. They contain normal hematopoietic or fatty marrow and are not considered pathologic, although their exact etiology is not known. If there is doubt about the nature of the condition, follow-up radiographs can be useful to show lack of change over time.

The second major type of lesion falling into the slow-growing category is the cyst. A true cyst is a fluid-filled sac lined by epithelium. It can be developmental in nature, such as a nasopalatine duct cyst that develops within the nasopalatine duct, or inflammatory, such as a radicular cyst forming at the apex of a nonvital tooth. Odontogenic cysts arise superior to the mandibular canal, unlike the lingual salivary gland depression discussed above.

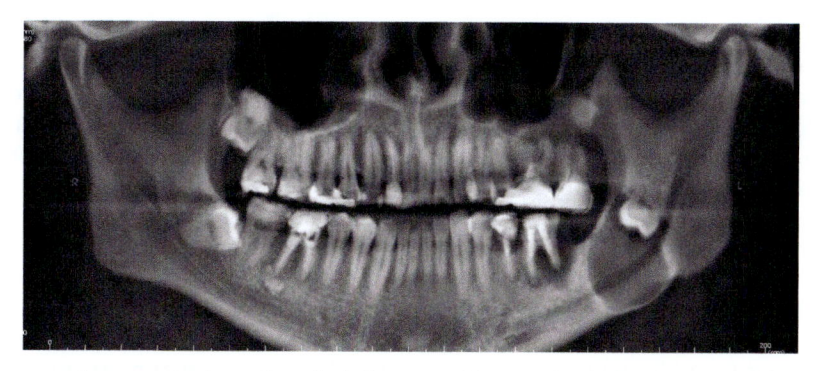

Figure 3.12 Reconstructed panoramic view with multiple lesions visible, including dentigerous cyst around crown of displaced #17; impacted #1, #16, and #32; rarefying osteitis affecting #14, #19, #20, and #30; radiopaque mass at apex of distal root of #30, with a differential diagnosis of complex odontoma, foreign material, or advanced fibro-osseous lesion.

Cysts tend to be round or oval, depending on anatomic constraints, due to the hydrostatic pressure of the fluid within the cyst causing expansion equally in all directions. The border of the lesion is smooth and corticated, although it is possible for a cyst to become infected and lose its smooth margin at that location. Cysts may grow large and cause displacement or resorption of teeth and expansion of the jaw, sometimes thinning the buccal or lingual cortex without perforating it. Cysts are usually totally radiolucent, although dystrophic calcification can occur in older cysts.

The radicular cyst is the most common cyst in the jaws. Differentiating it from a periapical granuloma may not always be possible (or necessary), although radicular cysts tend to be larger than ~1–2 cm. They occur more commonly in the maxilla than the mandible and are centered on the apex (or lateral canal) of a nonvital tooth. The appearance of these lesions on CBCT is similar to their appearance on standard dental radiographs, although the third dimension can frequently be helpful in establishing their exact relationship to adjacent teeth and other structures. In the posterior maxilla, a radicular cyst associated with a maxillary molar can elevate the floor of the maxillary sinus and occasionally can cause a large soft tissue invagination into the sinus that must be distinguished from other causes of sinus disease, such as polyps and mucous retention pseudocysts.

If a cyst is incompletely removed, the remaining epithelium may result in the formation of a residual cyst. History and previous radiographs will be useful in differentiating a residual cyst from other solitary lesions in the jaw.

The dentigerous (follicular) cyst, the second most common cyst in the jaw, occurs around the crown of an unerupted tooth, as a result of fluid accumulating between layers of the reduced enamel epithelium or between the epithelium and the crown of the tooth. It is a well-defined radiolucent lesion that arises from the cemento-enamel junction area of the unerupted tooth (Figure 3.12). Displacement of the affected tooth is a common finding and the cyst may cause appreciable jaw expansion.

Other true cysts in the jaws include the lateral periodontal cyst and the buccal bifurcation cyst. The lateral periodontal cyst arises from epithelial rests in the periodontium and appears as a small well-defined radiolucent lesion lateral to the root of a tooth, usually in the mandible anterior to the molars. Differential diagnosis includes radicular cyst at the foramen of an accessory pulp canal, small neurofibroma, or small keratocystic odontogenic tumor (discussed ahead).

The buccal bifurcation cyst usually occurs in children, buccal to an unerupted first or second molar, with the source of epithelium probably the epithelial cell rests in the bifurcation area. The cyst tends to tilt the roots of the affected tooth lingually and may prevent the eruption of the affected tooth and cause significant bony expansion buccal to the tooth. The cyst is usually treated with curettage without extraction of the tooth.

A pseudocyst in the jaws may look very similar to a true cyst radiographically, but histologically it does not contain an epithelial lining. The most common pseudocyst in the jaws is the simple bone cyst (SBC), also frequently called traumatic bone cyst or solitary bone cyst (Figure 3.13). The SBC is a cavity within bone, most often the posterior mandible, that is lined with connective tissue and may be empty or contain fluid. The etiology of this lesion is not known, but it may represent an aberration in normal bone metabolism or healing. A history of trauma is found in some cases but not all. The lesions may also be seen in association with fibro-osseous lesions.

The border of an SBC may be well defined, like a true cyst, or more diffuse, although in the tooth-bearing area it tends to be well defined. Scalloping of the endosteal surface of the bone is common. It frequently scallops in between the roots of the teeth but usually has no effect on the teeth themselves or on the lamina dura, which remains intact. This lesion is usually asymptomatic and thus is an incidental finding on a radiograph. Management usually consists of conservative opening into the lesion, with curettage of the lining, which both establishes the diagnosis and causes some bleeding into the lesion, which usually initiates healing.

The keratocystic odontogenic tumor (KOT, previously called odontogenic keratocyst) has been reclassified by the World Health Organization from a cyst to a tumor due to its behavior, although it does have an epithelial lining (keratinized) and a cystic cavity within it (Figure 3.14A and Figure 3.14B). The KOT occurs most often in the posterior mandible or ramus, superior to the mandibular canal, but it also is not uncommon in the posterior maxilla, where it may extend into the maxillary sinus and simulate a mucous retention pseudocyst. It may be associated with the crown of a tooth, like a dentigerous cyst, or be a solitary lesion. It may be unilocular or multilocular (single or multiple compartments) and tends to cause less expansion than other lesions of its size due to its propensity to grow longitudinally within the bone

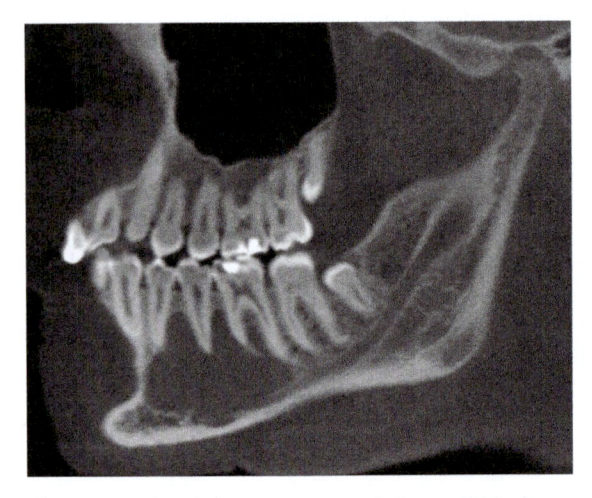

Figure 3.13 Simple bone cyst (traumatic bone cyst) in the left mandible, sagittal view. The lesion, which scallops up in between the teeth, was an empty bone cavity upon curettage.

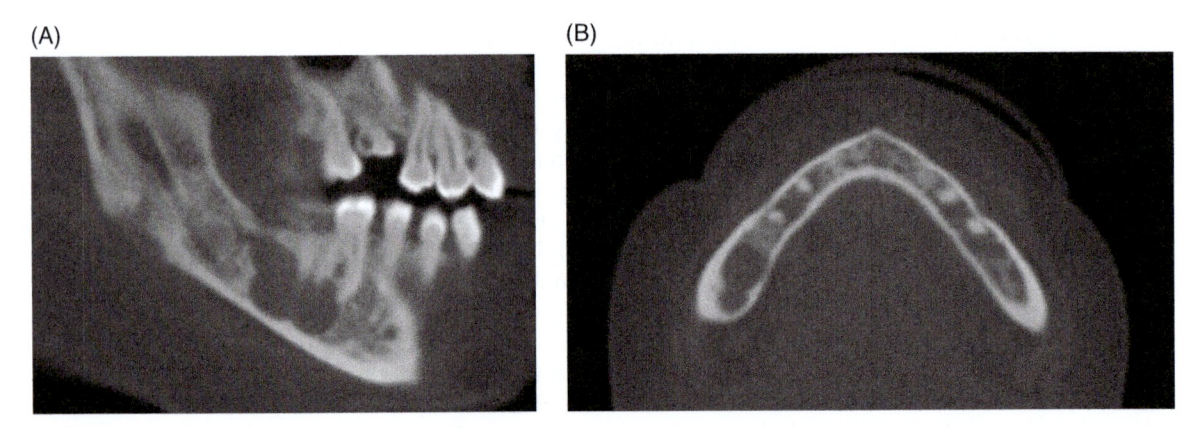

Figure 3.14A and B Keratocystic odontogenic tumor: sagittal (A) and axial (B) views. This is a multilocular radiolucent lesion in the right posterior mandible, with well-defined margins. There is only limited mandibular expansion despite the large size of the lesion.

rather than laterally. The KOT has a high recurrence rate, unlike the true cysts described above.

The margin of a KOT is well defined, unless it becomes infected, and may present a scalloped appearance. If it occurs in association with a tooth, it may be connected to the tooth inferior to the cemento-enamel junction, unlike the dentigerous cyst.

A small percentage of KOTs are associated with the basal cell nevus syndrome, features of which include multiple KOTs, multiple basal cell carcinomas of the skin, and skeletal, eye, and central nervous system abnormalities. This syndrome is inherited as an autosomal dominant trait with variable expressivity.

If a KOT is suspected based on imaging findings, referral for further imaging evaluation is recommended in order to determine the precise boundaries of the lesion prior to treatment, given the propensity of these lesions to recur.

The third major category of slow-growing lesions is the benign tumor. Tumors that occur in the jaws may be of odontogenic origin, that is, arising from cells that form teeth and surrounding structures, or non-odontogenic, including neural and vascular lesions. The odontogenic tumors may be of epithelial origin, such as the ameloblastoma; of mesenchymal origin, such as odontogenic myxoma; or of mixed epithelial and mesenchymal origin, such as odontoma and ameloblastic fibroma. The radiographic appearance and clinical behavior depend on the specific tumor involved.

Various hard tissue calcified or ossified hyperplasias and tumors were discussed above under radiopaque lesions. In this section only totally radiolucent or mixed radiolucent-radiopaque lesions will be discussed.

Benign tumors may be completely radiolucent and present as a single compartment (unilocular) or they may contain radiopaque septa (multilocular) that represent residual bone trapped within the lesion. Some tumors produce bone or other calcified material, causing a mixed appearance.

The ameloblastoma is a benign but locally aggressive tumor of odontogenic epithelium that may present in multiple types: unicystic, multicystic (solid), and desmoplastic (Figure 3.15A and Figure 3.15B). The unicystic type can also occur in the wall of a dentigerous cyst (mural ameloblastoma).

Ameloblastomas are slow-growing tumors that may be asymptomatic and discovered on dental radiographs taken for other purposes or they may cause a slowly expanding swelling that causes the patient to seek treatment. They can occur at any age, although most patients are between 20 and 50 years, and in any part of the jaw, although the majority are in the molar-ramus region of the mandible. The lesions may be totally radiolucent or have multiple septa that remodel into rounded forms such as honeycomb or soap bubble appearance, due to the cystic components of the tumor. They tend to have well-defined, corticated margins. Unlike the keratocystic odontogenic tumor, they frequently cause gross expansion of the jaw, and tooth resorption and displacement are common. The desmoplastic form of ameloblastoma can produce bone and resemble a bone dysplasia instead of a typical radiolucent ameloblastoma. Ameloblastomas

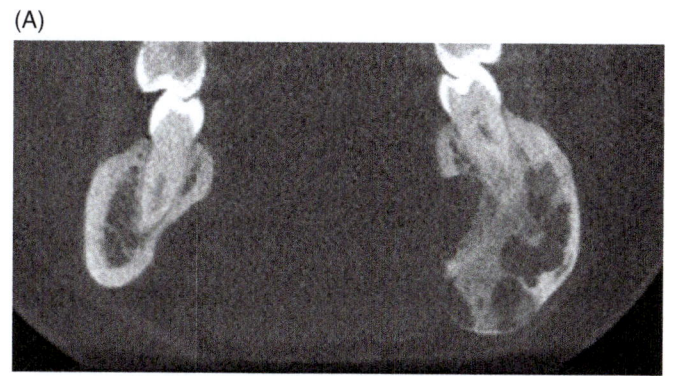

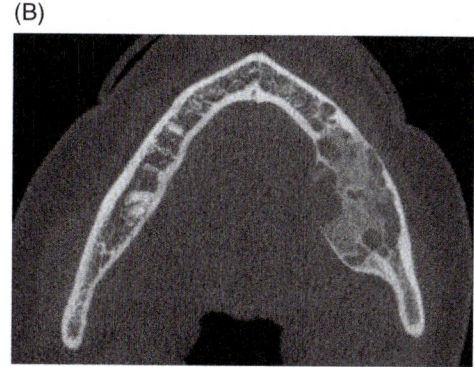

(A)

(B)

Figure 3.15A and B   Ameloblastoma in the left mandible: coronal (A) and axial (B) views. The lesion is multilocular and expansile but still has well-defined margins. (Courtesy of Dr. David C. Hatcher, Sacramento, CA)

can recur following surgery, presenting typically with a multicystic appearance.

Small unicystic ameloblastomas may not be able to be differentiated from true cysts. The differential diagnosis for multilocular ameloblastomas includes keratocystic odontogenic tumor (KOT), central giant cell granuloma (CGCG), odontogenic myxoma (OM), and ossifying fibroma (OF), all discussed elsewhere. There is usually less bone expansion with the KOT due to its longitudinal growth. The CGCG usually occurs in a younger age group and has wispy septa. The septa in OM are frequently straighter ("tennis racket"), and those in OF are usually wider, more granular, and less well defined.

If an ameloblastoma is suspected, especially in the maxilla, additional soft tissue imaging (conventional CT, MRI) is recommended to determine the full extent of the lesion and the degree of extension into other structures, such as the maxillary sinuses and nasal cavity.

OMs arise from odontogenic ectomesenchyme and resemble cells from the dental papilla. They are not encapsulated and thus may have a less well-defined margin than ameloblastomas, although they can have a corticated border. The septa in the OM are variable in shape, but there tends to be at least a few straight septa, which aids in the identification of this tumor. OMs tend to affect the premolar and molar areas of the mandible but also can occur in similar locations in the maxilla. It may scallop in between teeth, like a simple bone cyst, and rarely resorbs teeth. Expansion is generally less than with ameloblastoma. As with ameloblastoma, additional conventional CT and MRI may be helpful in planning treatment, which usually includes block resection.

Other benign odontogenic tumors that can occur in the jaws, albeit with less frequency than the ones discussed above, include calcifying epithelial odontogenic tumor (Pindborg tumor), ameloblastic fibroma, ameloblastic fibro-odontoma, adenomatoid odontogenic tumor, and central odontogenic fibroma. Consultation of a pathology reference book for more details on these tumors is recommended.

Non-odontogenic tumors can also occur in the jaws, primarily of neural or vascular origin. A lesion occurring in an expanded mandibular nerve canal should be suspected to be of neural origin, such as neurilemoma, neuroma, or neurofibroma. Vascular lesions include central hemangioma and arteriovenous fistula (A-V malformation).

Some reactive lesions in the jaws can also present as tumors or cysts radiographically. The central giant cell granuloma (giant cell reparative granuloma, giant cell lesion) is considered to be a reactive lesion to an unknown stimulus. It typically occurs in young individuals (<20 years) in the mandible anterior to the first molars, although it can occur elsewhere in the jaws. Painless swelling is the most common presenting symptom. The lesion grows slowly and thus usually has a well-defined margin. It frequently displaces teeth and may also resorb roots. It can be totally radiolucent but frequently contains wispy septa that are distinctively different from those of odontogenic tumors such as ameloblastoma. An uneven expansion of the jaws occurs in larger lesions. Histologically the lesions contain multiple giant cells, which are also a feature of the brown tumors of hyperparathyroidism. For that reason patients with giant cell lesions need to be evaluated for hyperparathyroidism. Treatment may include enucleation, although there have been reports of successful resolution with intralesional injections of corticosteroids.

Aneurysmal bone cysts are reactive lesions in the bone of unknown etiology, but they may represent an exaggerated response of vascular tissue within bone. They may occur as a solitary lesion or in association with other lesions such as fibrous dysplasia or giant cell granuloma. They are most often found in the posterior mandible in persons under age 30 and may present as a relatively rapidly growing swelling. However, the border of the lesion is usually well defined and there may be multiple wispy internal septa. Because they contain multiple blood-filled sinusoids, aspiration of the lesion has a hemorrhagic appearance.

Cherubism is a rare inherited autosomal dominant disease that presents in children as bilateral facial swelling as a result of multilocular lesions in the posterior mandible or both the mandible and maxilla. When the maxilla is involved, the skin is stretched tightly over the cheeks, causing the lower eyelid to be depressed. This exposes a thin line of sclera, which makes it appear that the child is raising his eyes to heaven, thus displaying a cherubic appearance. The bilateral nature of the disease, occurring in the posterior of the jaws, is generally sufficient to differentiate cherubism from central giant cell granuloma and fibrous dysplasia. Treatment is usually delayed because the disease stabilizes during adolescence, after which cosmetic surgery can be performed if needed.

In making a differential diagnosis of a radiolucent lesion observed on a radiograph, it is frequently helpful to divide lesions by location. Those occurring at the apex of a tooth are most likely to be inflammatory in origin, including periapical abscess, periapical granuloma, radicular (or periapical) cyst, or periapical scar. However, other radiolucent lesions can occur at the apex of a tooth, including the early stage of periapical cemento-osseous dysplasia and simple bone cyst. Pulp vitality testing can be very helpful in distinguishing these lesions, as can the presence or absence of an intact periodontal ligament space and lamina dura. Multiple periapical inflammatory lesions can also be associated with dentin dysplasia.

Lesions that occur around the crown of an unerupted tooth are relatively few in number and include normal dental follicle (normal follicular space is 2–3 mm), dentigerous cyst (follicular space >5 mm), and a few benign tumors, such as adenomatoid odontogenic tumor and ameloblastic fibroma. Biopsy may be needed to differentiate these, although radiopaque flecks within the lesion are not uncommon with adenomatoid odontogenic tumor.

Lesions that occur in other locations within the jaws present more choices and a more difficult differential diagnosis. Knowledge of typical radiographic appearances and typical locations and patient demographics can be helpful in distinguishing between lesions. Although in many cases biopsy is required to establish the final diagnosis, the ability to evaluate the appearance of the lesion and to determine whether it is most likely a slow-growing or a fast-growing lesion can be very helpful in planning the next step for the patient.

Rapidly growing lesions

Rapidly growing lesions have the potential to produce serious consequences for the patient, in terms of pain or other symptoms or destruction of normal tissue and replacement with abnormal cells. There are two major categories of lesions that fall into the "rapidly growing" classification: inflammation and malignancy. It is not always possible to distinguish these lesions radiographically since they can present with similar appearances.

The classical radiographic appearance of these lesions is a radiolucent (or mixed density) lesion with borders that are not well defined. The borders may blend subtly into the adjacent normal bone or may demonstrate a permeative margin, where it appears that the lesion is eating away at the bone.

Other common features include a tendency to erode cortical bone rather than displace it outward as the lesion grows and a tendency to surround the roots of teeth, destroying the bone, rather than displacing the teeth the way a benign lesion might do. In addition, inflammatory and malignant lesions frequently—although not always—cause neurological symptoms, including pain and paresthesia.

The majority of the rapidly growing lesions are inflammatory in nature, usually associated with a devital tooth or advanced periodontitis, making their diagnosis generally relatively straightforward. However, correlation with history and clinical findings is essential in interpreting these lesions correctly, as it is with all lesions seen on radiographs, since malignant lesions occurring in the jawbones can mimic inflammatory ones.

The typical periapical inflammatory lesions are well known to dentists because they are seen frequently in dental practice. A tooth with deep caries or a deep restoration or a history of trauma may develop a pulpal inflammation, which can progress to inflammation in the surrounding bone. The initial radiographic appearance is a widening of the apical periodontal ligament space, followed by loss of a well-defined lamina dura. As the disease process advances, an ill-defined radiolucent lesion may appear at the apex of the tooth, centered on the apical foramen. Frequently the inflammatory process becomes chronic as the body attempts to wall it off and the borders of the lesion become more defined. At this stage typically a microscopic diagnosis would be periapical granuloma or radicular cyst, depending on the specific stage of the lesion.

If the inflammation starts within the periodontium, rather than in the dental pulp, the widest part of the radiolucency will be at the alveolar crest and not at the apex. However, the inflammatory process can continue down the root of the tooth and affect all the bone surrounding the tooth.

Occasionally, however, the body is not successful in walling off the inflammatory process, either because of the virulence of the causative organism or the inadequacy of the immune response to the insult, and the patient may develop an osteomyelitis, an inflammation of the bone that may affect all parts of the bone: marrow, cortex, medullary bone, and periosteum. This occurs most often in the posterior mandible, probably due to the smaller blood supply than in the maxilla.

The course of osteomyelitis is quite variable, and thus the radiographic appearance of the disease is also, ranging from completely radiolucent to completely radiopaque to a mixture of radiolucent and radiopaque (Figure 3.16A, Figure 3.16B, and Figure 3.16C). The bone may contain ill-defined radiolucent areas with radiopaque foci, representing areas of necrotic bone, that will eventually slough and become sequestra. The borders of bone infections are generally diffuse, especially as the disease process continues, extending well beyond the initial nidus of infection. When osteomyelitis becomes chronic, it becomes very difficult to treat because there are many areas of necrotic bone within the diseased area and these are nonresponsive to treatment. In addition to oral and intravenous antibiotics, areas of osteomyelitis are frequently treated with surgical curettage to remove necrotic bone.

It is not uncommon for bone affected by osteomyelitis to demonstrate erosion or perforation of the cortex, with inflammation extending into the

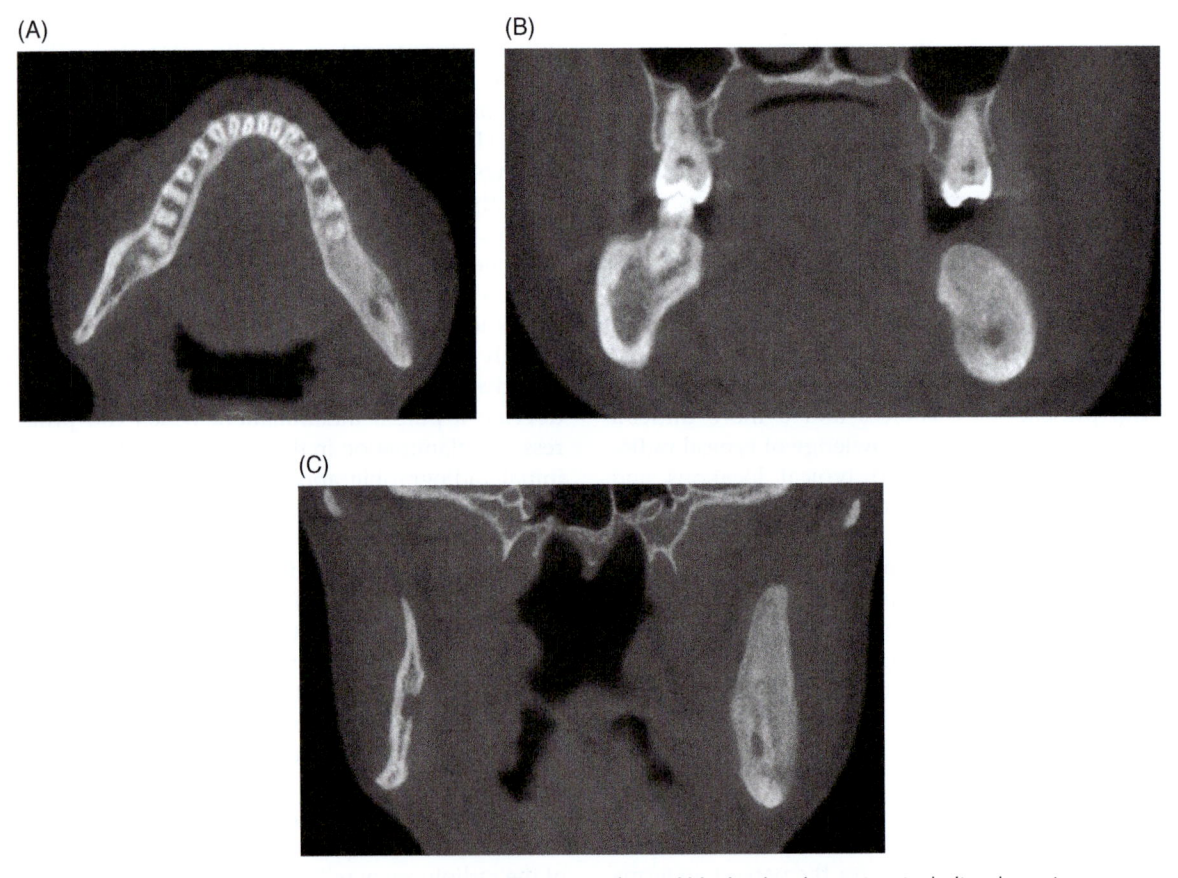

Figure 3.16A, B, and C Severe osteomyelitis affecting the entire left mandible distal to the canine, including the entire ramus except for the condyle: axial (A) and coronal (B, C) views. The bone in the left mandible is sclerotic, with a ground glass appearance and loss of normal trabecular pattern. The body and ramus of the mandible are expanded and there is loss of differentiation between medullary and cortical bone. The right side of the mandible is normal.

surrounding soft tissue. Attempts at bony repair can also be seen as new bone is laid down by the periosteum on the periphery of the diseased bone. This may have the appearance of thin layers of bone over the defect, looking like layers of onion, as the periosteum is lifted and new bone is formed underneath it, stimulated by the inflammation. This type of effect is more common in children than in adults, due to the looseness of the attachment of the periosteum and the greater potential for bone formation.

Osteomyelitis, especially in the acute phase, may produce various signs and symptoms, including rapid onset, pain, swelling of soft tissues, fever, lymphadenopathy, purulent drainage, and paresthesia of the lower lip. Chronic osteomyelitis, which may occur if the acute phase is inadequately treated or arise without an acute phase, usually has a longer course, with intermittent episodes of pain, swelling, fever, and other classic signs of inflammation or infection.

Differential diagnosis of osteomyelitis includes fibrous dysplasia, Paget's disease of bone, and osteosarcoma. Typically, fibrous dysplasia does not present with the acute inflammatory symptoms and the pattern of bony enlargement is different (within the bone rather than on the surface with periosteal new bone). Paget's disease tends to affect the entire mandible and does not present with sequestra, as does osteomyelitis. Bone destruction is usually seen in osteosarcoma, along with other bony changes.

Other inflammatory changes can occur in the bone besides those associated with pulpal pathology and trauma, including osteoradionecrosis. When bone receives a high dose of radiation, such as during radiotherapy for a malignancy, the bone suffers damage, either as a result of cell death or loss of cell repair ability due to changes in the vasculature in the bone. When such irradiated bone is traumatized, such as through tooth extraction, the bone lacks an adequate healing response and part of the bone may become necrotic. Radiographically, the bone affected by osteoradionecrosis can appear very similar to acute or chronic osteomyelitis. Differentiation is via history of radiation therapy. However, it is also possible that a recurrence of the original neoplasm may invade the bone and cause a similar appearance; thus, a thorough examination is mandatory.

Necrotic, exposed bone has also been reported in the jaws of patients who have taken bisphosphonate drugs, which are used to inhibit osteoclasts and reduce bone metabolism, either as treatment for bone involvement in a number of malignancies or in the prevention of osteoporosis. Most of the cases reported in the literature have occurred in patients taking potent bisphosphonates intravenously for malignancies. The radiographic appearance may vary widely, resembling classic osteomyelitis in some cases, but typically there is exposed bone visible clinically.

The other major category of lesions that fits into the "rapidly growing" class is the malignancy, either a primary or a metastatic tumor. Radiographically they can be very similar to inflammatory lesions, although if the tumor arises in the soft tissues and only secondarily affects the bone, the clinical findings would aid in the differential diagnosis. There are many clinical features that suggest a malignancy, including a rapidly growing soft tissue mass; indurated or rolled margins; ulcer, with or without pain; alteration in surface appearance of the tissue (whiteness, redness, mixture of red and white); dysgeusia, dysphonia, dysphagia; lymphadenopathy; sensory deficits; lack of healing after oral surgery; unintended weight loss and general feeling of unwellness.

Radiologic features of malignant lesions include a generally irregular radiolucent appearance (although some sarcomas and metastatic carcinomas can produce bone or other hard tissue) with an ill-defined border, without cortication or any sign of encapsulation (Figure 3.17A, Figure 3.17B, and Figure 3.17C). Frequently there are fingerlike projections into the surrounding bone. The lesion may totally destroy bone and cause the teeth to appear to float due to the complete loss of bony structure around them. They may destroy bony margins, such as the floor of the maxillary sinus, the buccal and lingual cortex, the walls of the inferior alveolar canal, and the lamina dura. They may also grow in the periodontal ligament space, causing it to appear wider than normal throughout and not just at the apex like periapical inflammation caused by pulpal disease.

Malignant lesions can be divided into four major types based on their origin: carcinomas (epithelial origin), metastatic tumors (from distant sites,

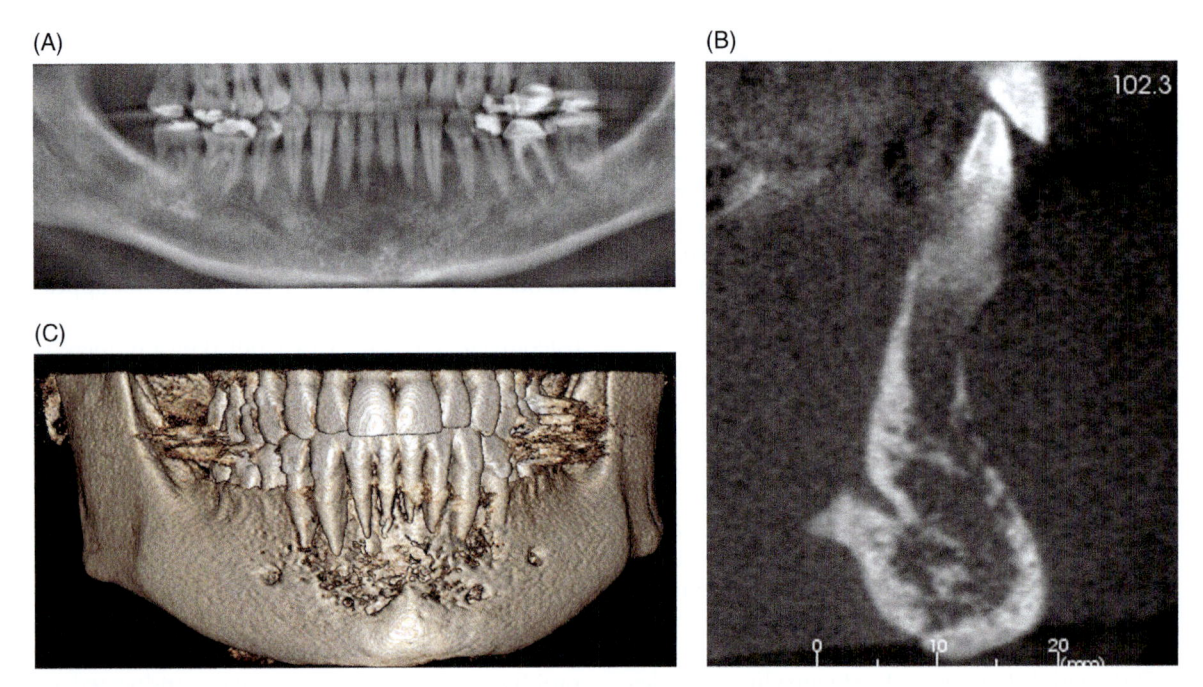

Figure 3.17A, B, and C Non-Hodgkin lymphoma in the anterior mandible: panoramic (A), sagittal (B), and 3D volumetric reconstruction (C) views. Note the ill-defined margins of the diffuse radiolucency, with loss of normal trabecular bone pattern and erosion of the buccal cortex. The 3D volumetric reconstruction (C) demonstrates the loss of buccal cortical bone. (Courtesy of Dr. David C. Hatcher, Sacramento, CA)

usually carcinomas), sarcomas (mesenchymal origin), and hematopoietic malignancies.

Most of the carcinomas that occur in the maxillofacial region arise in the soft tissues, such as the tongue, floor of mouth, soft palate, tonsils, and gingiva. Unless they invade bone as they grow, they will not be detected on radiologic examinations, including CBCT. Evaluation of the oral cavity by careful clinical examination should be done on all patients, including children. While most carcinomas occur in persons over the age of 50, malignancies can and do occur in young individuals.

If a malignant tumor is suspected from the findings of a clinical examination, generally other types of imaging examinations besides CBCT would be used to determine the full extent of the lesion in order to plan treatment, although CBCT could be helpful to evaluate for bone invasion by the tumor.

Epithelial malignancies can arise de novo in bone, without a soft tissue component, from epithelial cells remnant in the bone, but these are rare. Central carcinoma arising within bone occurs in the tooth-bearing areas, usually posterior mandible, and is similar to other carcinomas except that it has no connection with the soft tissue of the oral cavity.

Central mucoepidermoid carcinomas also occur typically in the posterior mandible. They frequently are less aggressive tumors and may resemble benign tumors with a multilocular appearance.

Secondary malignancies (metastatic tumors) in the jaws arise usually as a result of hematogenous spread from the primary tumor, which may arise from a number of different organs, including breast, prostate, lung, and kidney. Frequently the primary site is already known when a metastatic tumor is detected, but occasionally the metastasis may be the first sign of a malignancy. Most metastatic tumors occur in the posterior mandible, although the TMJ and the maxilla are also potential sites. Most metastatic tumors are radiolucent and have irregular margins, but tumors from the breast and prostate can also induce bone formation, giving the metastatic area a more radiopaque, frequently granular appearance.

Mesenchymal malignancies include osteosarcoma, chondrosarcoma, fibrosarcoma, and Ewing's sarcoma. All of these are rare in the jaws, occurring more often in other bones, particularly long bones. Osteosarcomas typically occur in the posterior mandible and may be radiolucent with an ill-defined margin, radiopaque, or mixed, depending on the amount of osteoid produced. If the tumor involves the periosteum, new bone may be produced at right angles to the surface, forming "sun-ray" or "hair-on-end" trabeculae. The normal bone pattern is lost, being replaced by tumoral bone of variable organization. Alteration of the width of the periodontal ligament space and distinctness of maxillary sinus floor and mandibular canal borders is not uncommon.

Most chondrosarcomas are of mixed density, with a flocculent appearance of new cartilage surrounded by calcification. Chondrosarcomas tend to be slower growing than other malignancies and may have a relatively well-defined margin compared to osteosarcomas. Fibrosarcomas contain collagen and elastin, made by malignant fibroblasts, and thus are radiolucent in appearance. They tend to infiltrate through the bone and thus may be larger than their radiographic appearance would suggest.

Ewing's sarcoma tends to occur in a younger age group but is rare in the jaws. It typically appears as a radiolucent lesion with ragged borders and may cause pathologic fracture.

Differential diagnosis of all of the sarcomas can be difficult because they can all look similar, depending on the amount of calcification occurring in them, and they may mimic osteomyelitis and other malignancies such as carcinomas.

The last group of jaw malignancies occurs in the hematopoietic system. Multiple myeloma is a neoplasm of malignant plasma cells and typically presents with multiple radiolucent lesions that appear "punched out," that is, well defined but with no cortical border or any type of bony reaction. While the jaws and skull can be affected, multiple myeloma is a systemic neoplasm that affects other areas more frequently.

Non-Hodgkin's lymphoma is a malignancy of cells of the lymphatic system. While it occurs most often within lymph nodes, it can occur in other locations, including the maxillary sinus, palate, tonsillar area, and bone, either as a primary tumor or secondary extension from a tumor in the lymph nodes. Differential diagnosis includes the other malignancies, as well as inflammatory lesions when the lymphoma occurs near the apex of a tooth.

If a primary or secondary malignancy is detected or suspected, rapid referral for further evaluation and management is needed. This may be to an oral surgeon for biopsy or to the patient's oncologist for a suspected metastatic lesion.

The dentist's role

To summarize the dentist's role with respect to the detection, diagnosis, and management of pathology observed on CBCT scans, there are two basic scenarios. In one, the scan is made specifically to evaluate some abnormal condition of the patient, detected originally either through history (patient complains of pain or swelling), clinical examination (facial asymmetry is observed), or other radiograph (a radiolucent or radiopaque lesion is noted on a panoramic or intraoral radiograph). In the second scenario, the scan is made for some purpose (implant, orthodontics) and an unexpected condition is observed on the scan.

Even though the basic goal is the same—to determine the nature of the condition and the type of management needed—the steps the dentist takes will be slightly different. In the first case, where an abnormality is expected, *before* the scan is made the clinician should do a *thorough* history and clinical examination: when did the symptoms first begin, what has the time course of symptoms been, what has the patient done to try to relieve the symptoms; what are the clinical findings with respect to teeth, bone, soft tissue; what are the results of intraoral and/or panoramic radiographs; what are the results of pulp testing? What is the provisional diagnosis based on all the information collected? What additional information, if any, is needed to make a diagnosis? What is the best method to get the additional information? Is CBCT really the best or would conventional CT or MRI be better?

In the second scenario, where an unexpected lesion is found on the CBCT, the clinician must go back to the patient and try to obtain the same information described above, but this time after the lesion is observed. That may mean that the questions and clinical examination and tests may be more focused to try to determine the nature of the condition.

Since the ultimate goal is the preservation and enhancement of the patient's health and well-being, it is critical that all abnormalities be detected and the nature of these abnormalities be determined. In many, probably most, cases the clinician using the CBCT in the dental office will be the one to make the diagnosis and plan the management, which frequently is simple observation without treatment. However, if there is any doubt about the diagnosis, or if the management of the condition is beyond the clinician's professional expertise, referral for further evaluation is appropriate.

Additional reading

Koenig, L.J., Tamimi, D., Harnsberger, H.R., Benson, B.W., Hatcher, D., Petrikowski, C.G., et al. (2012) Diagnostic Imaging, Oral and Maxillofacial. Salt Lake City, UT: Amirsys.

Neville, B.W., Damm, D.D., Allen, C.M., and Bouquot, J.E. (2002) Oral and Maxillofacial Pathology, 2nd ed. Philadelphia: WB Saunders.

White, S.C., and Pharoah, M.J., eds. (2009) Oral radiology, principles and interpretation, 6th ed. St. Louis: Mosby-Elsevier.

4 Diagnosis of Sinus Pathologies Using Cone Beam Computed Tomography

Aaron Miracle and Christian Güldner

This chapter will focus predominantly on the paranasal sinuses and temporal bone, regions of the extracranial head and neck relatively well suited to cone beam computed tomography (CBCT) imaging owing to complex bony anatomic detail and a relative paucity of soft tissue structures. Research establishing the clinical utility of CBCT in these regions is still preliminary, however, and there are many limitations to use in a diagnostic setting (Gupta et al., 2008; Miracle and Mukherji, 2009a, b). Poor low-contrast detectability is the overwhelming limitation with CBCT imaging, as many aggressive processes centered at the skull base within the extracranial head and neck involve soft tissue structures that are poorly visualized. When interpreting CBCT imaging in these regions (or any other for that matter), any aggressive lesions with bony destruction and most mass lesions warrant evaluation with MRI or contrast-enhanced CT (CECT) to better characterize the soft tissue composition and to delineate the extent of surrounding soft tissue involvement.

For practitioners trained in conventional multidetector CT (MDCT) interpretation, it is tempting to equate CBCT images with MDCT images processed with bone algorithms, and while there are distinct similarities, the differences in acquisition geometry, dose, image quality, and other technical parameters should be kept in mind. One notable difference between CBCT and MDCT is related to patient positioning. With CBCT imaging, the patient is often sitting up, and therefore dependent fluid and air–fluid levels will be oriented in the axial plane, making coronal and sagittal reformatted images ideal for identification. This becomes important in the setting of trauma, atraumatic sinus fluid (as in sinusitis), and middle ear effusions, among other disease processes.

Paranasal sinuses

The complex high-contrast anatomy of the paranasal sinuses and anterior skull base are attractive targets for CBCT (Balbach et al., 2011), where excellent spatial resolution and isotropic voxel acquisition generate quality images that can be reconstructed in multiple viewing planes. This section will briefly review the anatomy of the anterior skull base, pertinent anatomic variants that should be identified in the setting of sinus surgery, and paranasal sinus pathology that practitioners should be familiar with when interpreting CBCT images covering this anatomic region.

Cone Beam Computed Tomography: Oral and Maxillofacial Diagnosis and Applications, First Edition. Edited by David Sarment.
© 2014 John Wiley & Sons, Inc. Published 2014 by John Wiley & Sons, Inc.

Diagnostic sinus imaging

Despite being well suited for depicting fine detail of complex osseous structures such as those in the paranasal sinuses and anterior skull base, the role of CBCT in diagnostic sinus and skull base imaging is very limited. Paranasal sinus pathology covers a wide range of diverse disease processes, many of which are mucosal in origin and require discriminating contrast resolution for adequate evaluation (Yousem, 1993; Momeni et al., 2007). A variety of benign and malignant neoplasms, inflammatory soft tissue masses, postoperative complications, and infectious processes can present with similar symptoms, requiring selection of an imaging modality suited to identify the underlying disease process and guide further imaging. In most cases this will still be MDCT processed with both bone and soft tissue algorithms; however, MRI may be better suited as an initial imaging study in select situations. CBCT is not endorsed by the American College of Radiology (Mukherji et al., 2006; Rumboldt et al., 2009) for diagnostic sinus imaging, where evaluation of soft tissue windows is recommended.

Despite these limitations, paranasal sinus pathology will still be encountered incidentally in CBCT imaging performed for other indications (Maillet et al., 2011; Ritter et al., 2011), and therefore knowledge of important bony and soft tissue pathology is vital for practitioners interpreting CBCT images.

Sinusitis

Sinusitis is a common clinical affliction, most often encountered in the setting of antecedent viral upper respiratory tract infection. Most cases of sinusitis do not require imaging evaluation, and in the rare case where diagnostic imaging is indicated, MDCT is the appropriate initial diagnostic modality (Branstetter and Weissman, 2005; Brook, 2006; Eggesbo, 2006).

Acute

Acute sinusitis manifests as air fluid levels in one or more paranasal sinuses on CT imaging, often with a bubbly or frothy appearance (Figure 4.1). Viral pathogens are typically implicated; however, bacteria in so-called pyogenic sinusitis are also common. Top differential considerations include a posttraumatic blood level (often with associated maxillofacial fractures), noninfected postobstructive secretions, and pseudo fluid levels. Pseudo fluid levels represent flaccid mucous retention cysts, and upon careful inspection should demonstrate a rounded edge at the junction with adjacent bony partitions.

Chronic

Chronic sinusitis is characterized by mucoperiosteal thickening, occasionally with high-attenuation dessicated secretions or concretions in opacified sinus cavities that can be seen on soft tissue windowing of MDCT images but may not be as easily recognized on CBCT (Cymerman et al., 2011). Impaired mucociliary clearance of pathogenic sinonasal bacteria is implicated in the pathogenesis of chronic sinusitis, as will be discussed in a later section.

Fungal

Fungal sinusitis can be allergic, chronic, or invasive, the latter of which is a highly aggressive angioinvasive process and warrants immediate surgical evaluation. Invasive fungal sinusitis occurs in immunocompromised and diabetic patients and is characterized by a rapidly progressive course with invasion through the mucosa into bone, adjacent vessels, and soft tissue, with eventual extension to the orbits and intracranial structures. Invasive fungal sinusitis should be considered in any immunocompromised patient with findings suggestive of sinusitis with any concomitant bony erosion. Soft tissue infiltration with fat stranding is also a feature and cannot be adequately evaluated with CBCT. Intracranial and orbital extension in invasive fungal sinusitis is another feature that is incompletely evaluated with CBCT. MDCT and MRI are indicated for further evaluation if sinusitis with focal bone erosion is observed.

Chronic fungal sinusitis may be suspected if dense secretions are noted on MDCT, but this is unlikely to be recognized on CBCT imaging. Allergic fungal sinusitis or mycetoma should be entertained as possible diagnoses if a soft tissue mass with a matrix of calcifications is observed, especially if mucoperiosteal thickening from chronic sinusitis is seen.

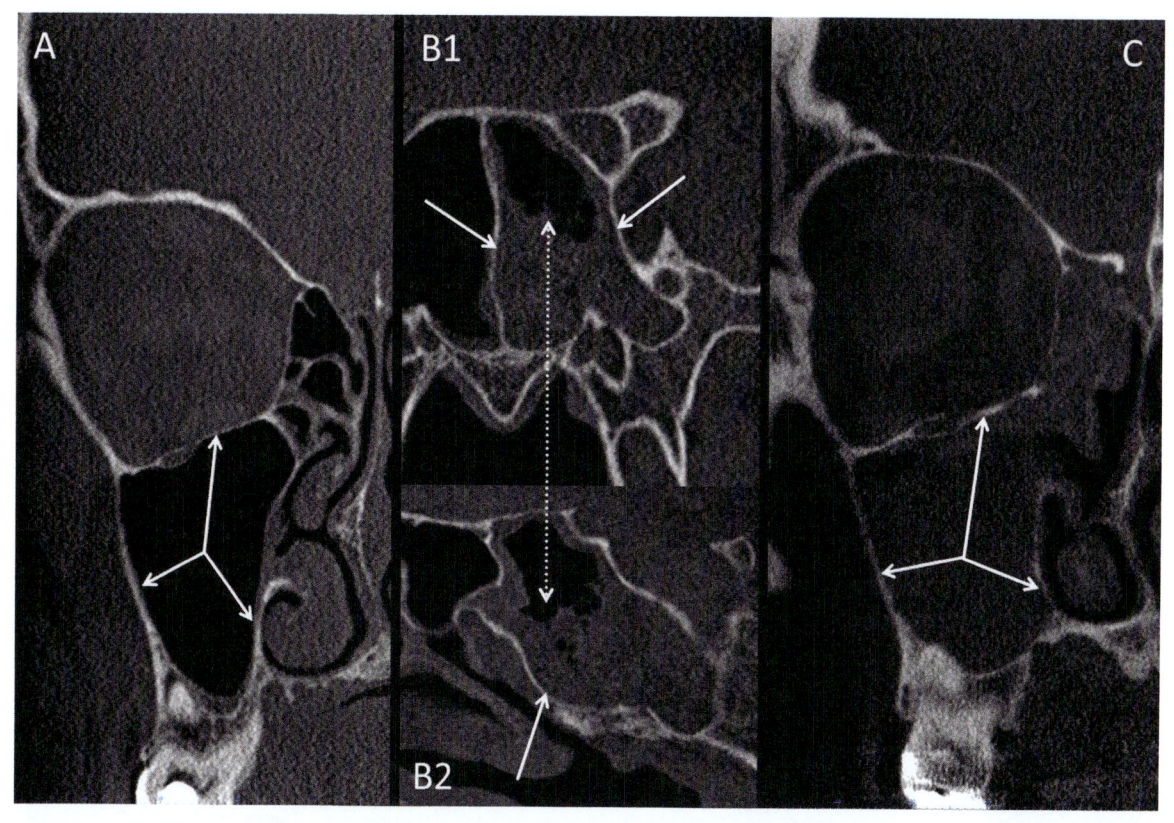

Figure 4.1 Sinusitis. A normal sinus (A) as well as acute sphenoid sinusitis (B1, B2) and chronic maxillary and ethmoid sinusitis (C) are shown. The sharply bounded right maxillary sinus (arrows) without mucosal thickening or secretions in A should be contrasted with coronal (B1) and sagittal (B2) images of a left sphenoid air fluid level with mucosal thickening and a frothy/bubbly appearance (dotted arrows), in this case of acute sphenoid sinusitis. Mucoperiosteal thickening involving the right ethmoid and maxillary sinus walls (arrows) in the coronal image in C is typical of chronic sinusitis.

Complications

Common complications of sinusitis include formation of inflammatory polyps, mucous retention cysts, and mucoceles, which will be addressed in subsequent sections. Several important complications of sinusitis cannot be sufficiently evaluated by CBCT imaging and warrant a brief discussion. Cavernous sinus thrombosis requires evaluation in soft tissue windows and is incompletely evaluated even with MDCT. Asymmetry of the cavernous sinuses in the setting of sinusitis should be further evaluated with CECT or MRI with gadolinium. Periorbital complications include preseptal cellulitis or abscess, optic neuritis and subperiosteal abscess. Subperiosteal abscesses appear as lentiform fluid collections arising from the lamina papyracea medial to the medial rectus muscle effacing extraconal fat. These should be evaluated with CECT. Intracranial complications are best assessed with gadolinium-enhanced MRI and include meningitis, epidural abscess, subdural empyema, cerebritis, and brain abscess. Superficial soft tissue complications such as subgaleal abscess and soft tissue changes from osteomyelitis are best evaluated with MRI or CECT.

Inflammatory polyps, mucoceles, and mucous retention cysts

Inflammatory polyps, mucoceles, and mucous retention cysts occur as complications of sinonasal inflammation, appear as uniform soft-tissue density lesions arising within sinus cavities, and can often be differentiated based on morphologic characteristics (Table 4.1). Mucous retention cysts are very common and result from mucous gland obstruction in the mucosa (Figure 4.2). Sinonasal polyps are pedunculated inflammatory mucosal lesions that can grow to obstruct sinus outflow. *Antrochoanal polyp* refers to the specific case of an inflammatory polyp arising from the maxillary antrum and prolapsing through the maxillary ostium into the nasal cavity and on occasion into the nasopharynx. Mucoceles occur most often in the frontal and ethmoid sinuses and can become infected (mucopyocele). Mucopyoceles require CECT or MRI for diagnosis.

Table 4.1 Common complications of sinonasal inflammation.

	Characteristic Findings
Inflammatory polyp	Polypoid soft tissue mass; ± visualized stalk; if prolapsing through sinus ostia, can appear dumbbell-shaped
Mucocele	Complete soft tissue opacification of sinus; ± bony remodeling/expansion
Mucous retention cyst	Round or dome-shaped soft tissue lesion; air still seen in the sinus

Silent sinus syndrome

Chronic obstruction of the maxillary infundibulum can result in maxillary atelectasis, with downward bowing of the maxillary roof/orbital floor and enophthalmos. The maxillary sinus is typically near-completely opacified with lateralization of the uncinate process toward the inferomedial orbital wall and consequent expansion of the middle meatus.

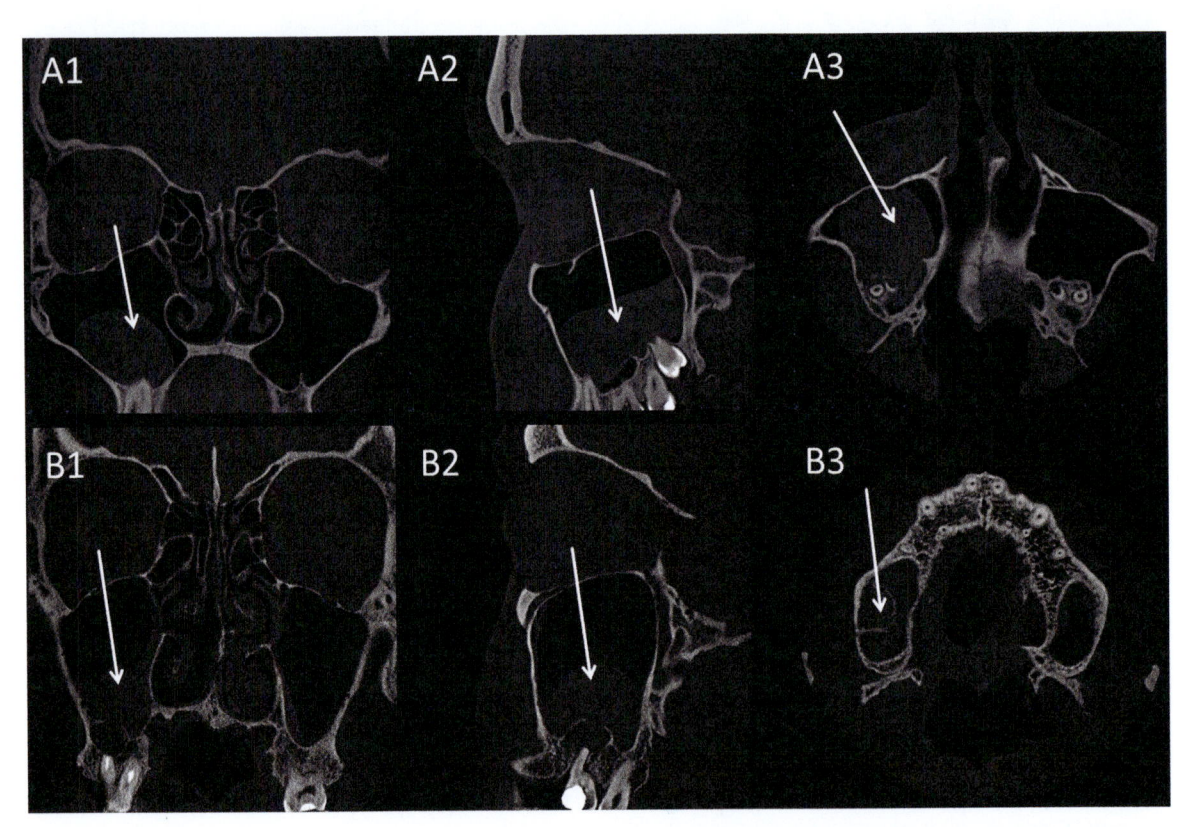

Figure 4.2 Mucous retention cysts. Coronal (A1, B1), sagittal (A2, B2), and axial (A3, B3) images demonstrate right maxillary mucous retention cysts, which are frequent findings in paranasal sinus imaging. They are rarely symptomatic and most often do not require therapy.

Fibro-osseous lesions

Although MDCT is the preferred modality for evaluating fibro-osseous lesions of the paranasal sinuses and skull base (Bolger et al., 1991), this group of lesions is likely to demonstrate a similar appearance on CBCT imaging and may be encountered incidentally. The pathologic potential of these lesions is typically related to mass effect; however, chondrosarcoma occasionally needs to be excluded in aggressive-appearing lesions.

Sinonasal osteomas

These lesions are benign and most often encountered in the frontal sinuses. They arise from the sinus wall and protrude into the sinus lumen with well-demarcated margins (Figure 4.3). They can be either cortical (uniformly cortical density) or fibrous (irregular internal matrix with a rim of cortical-density calcification).

Ossifying fibromas

These benign lesions are also well demarcated and expansile, invading the bone of origin. They can exhibit a ground-glass or mottled appearance of mixed bony and soft tissue density and can be confused with fibrous dysplasia. A characteristic finding is central calcified radiations with a dense rim, an appearance that is not typical of fibrous dysplasia.

Fibrous dysplasia

Fibrous dyplasia is a benign, ill-defined, heterogeneous expansile lesion of the medullary cavity. It can be classified as predominantly ground-glass, cystic (well-defined lytic lesions), pagetoid (inhomogeneous bony thickening), or a combination of these appearances.

Neoplasms and noninflammatory soft tissue pathology

The spectrum of noninflammatory soft tissue pathology in the paranasal sinuses is broad, and the vast majority of these lesions will be incompletely characterized by CBCT due to lack of intravenous contrast and poor low-contrast differentiation. Nevertheless, practitioners interpreting CBCT should be familiar with relevant pathology such that appropriate referral for CECT and/or MRI can be arranged. Noninflammatory soft tissue pathology will primarily appear as uniform soft-tissue-density space-occupying lesions on CBCT images and cannot be further evaluated. Many lesions, however, have characteristic locations, growth patterns, and patient characteristics that can guide the differential diagnosis before further evaluation with CECT and/or MRI.

Nonmalignant soft tissue masses include inverting papilloma, juvenile nasopharyngeal angiofibroma, frontoethmoid encephalocele, and benign mixed tumor. An inverting papilloma is a neoplastic

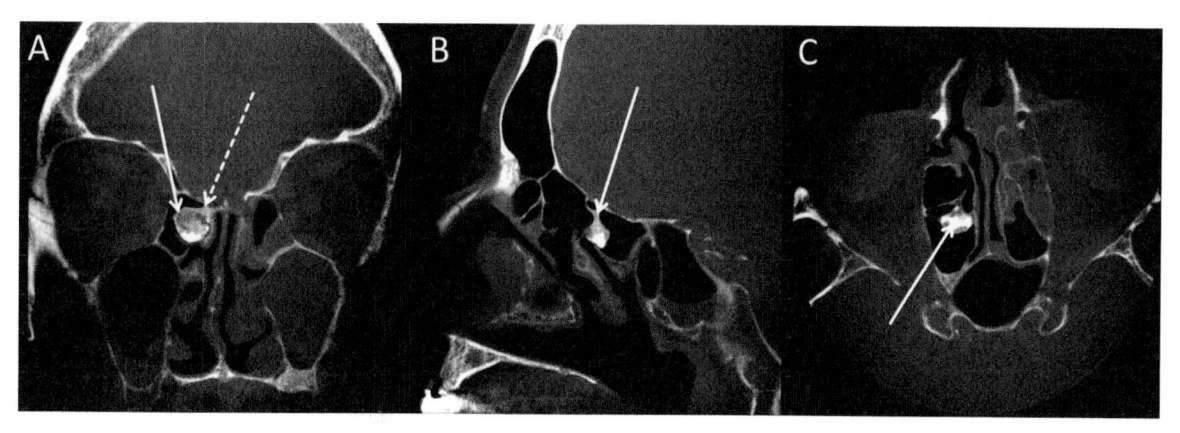

Figure 4.3 Sinonasal osteoma. Coronal (A), sagittal (B), and axial (C) images demonstrate a solid, mixed-density osseous lesion (white arrow) arising in a posterior ethmoid air cell consistent with an osteoma. Direct contact with the lateral lamella of the olfactory fossa (dotted arrow) makes decisions regarding therapy difficult in this patient.

growth directed into the mucosa and characteristically occurs on the lateral nasal wall centered on the hiatus semilunaris. There is an association with squamous cell carcinoma, and these lesions should be resected. Juvenile nasopharyngeal angiofibromas occur in male adolescents, arising from the nasal wall adjacent to the sphenopalatine foramen in the pterygopalatine fossa and can be locally aggressive but have no malignant potential. Frontoethmoid encephaloceles can occur congenitally or postraumatically but can also result from prior surgery. Soft tissue extruding from the anterior cranial fossa into the frontal or ethmoid sinuses suggests this diagnosis, but MRI is required for definitive determination. Benign mixed tumors, or pleomorphic adenomas, arise from rests of salivary glandular tissue and occasionally occur outside the major salivary glands. They appear as solitary expansile lesions of the nasal septum with bony remodeling. Contrast-enhanced imaging is necessary for appropriate characterization.

Malignant sinonasal tumors include squamous cell carcinoma—which accounts for 80% to 90% of malignant tumors in this region—as well as undifferentiated carcinoma (aggressive with extensive bony destruction), lymphoma, and minor salivary gland tumors. Primary sinonasal melanoma is rare. These lesions mainly present as soft tissue masses or opacification with bony destruction. All should be evaluated with gadolinium-enhanced MRI. The characteristic growth pattern of enthesioneuroblastoma, a highly aggressive and locally destructive tumor of the neurosensory receptor cells in the olfactory mucosa, deserves particular mention. These tumors exhibit extensive bony destruction and occur anywhere from the anterior skull base to the nasal turbinates. They classically involve the cribiform plate with extension into the anterior cranial fossa.

Wegener's granulomatosis

Wegener's granulomatosis is a noninfectious necrotizing vasculitis affecting the kidneys as well as the upper and lower respiratory tract (Benoudiba et al., 2003). Sinonasal involvement is typically characterized by inflammatory changes in the nasal cavity with occasional extension to the maxillary and ethmoid sinuses. Involvement of the other sinuses and extrasinonasal involvement is more rare. Characteristic imaging findings include nasal septal perforation, destruction of the turbinates and/or medial maxillary sinus wall, and nodular soft tissue masses distributed in the nasal cavity. MRI with gadolinium is the preferred imaging modality when there is expected extension beyond the sinuses.

Rhinolith

Chronic inflammatory response to a foreign body in the nasal cavity causes calcification and inflammatory soft tissue changes. The resulting rhinolith will appear as calcified material in the nasal cavity independent of the turbinates and bony septum. Common niduses for calcification include ectopic teeth, foreign bodies, and chronic blood clot.

Perioperative FESS

An emerging application for CBCT in the head and neck is perioperative imaging in the setting of functional endoscopic sinus surgery (FESS). FESS is predicated on the concept that mucociliary clearance in the paranasal sinuses occurs via predictable anatomic pathways converging on either (1) the osteomeatal complex (OMC), which constitutes the final drainage pathway of the maxillary, frontal, and anterior ethmoid air cells; or (2) the sphenoethmoidal recess, which is the final drainage pathway for the posterior ethmoid air cells and sphenoid sinuses (Daly et al., 2006; Bachar et al., 2007; Tam et al., 2010). The OMC comprises the maxillary sinus ostium, infundibulum, and middle meatus collectively. Posterior ethmoid air cells typically drain via the superior meatus or other ostia emptying beneath the superior turbinate, eventually reaching the sphenoethmoidal recess. Sphenoid sinuses typically drain into the sphenoethmoidal recess via the sphenoid ostia medial to the superior turbinates. These stereotypical drainage patterns are inconstant, and many important anatomic variants alter normal drainage pathways and can create points of anatomic narrowing. FESS is a minimally invasive mucosal-sparing technique aimed at restoring competent mucociliary clearance and sinus ventilation by targeting sites of drainage obstruction (Huang et al., 2009).

Preoperative evaluation before FESS should include MDCT imaging (Hoang et al., 2010), as underlying sinonasal mass lesions can present with symptomatology similar to chronic benign sinusitis. Important mimics and complications of chronic sinusitis that CBCT cannot reliably exclude or evaluate include, but are not limited to, tumor, encephalocele, subperiosteal abscess, epidural abscess, meningitis, and inflammatory involvement of the orbits. Preoperative imaging before FESS should also evaluate the optic nerves and optic contents, perimaxillary and extraconal fat, internal carotid arteries, preseptal and periorbital soft tissues, and if possible, the trigeminal nerve. Identifying variant anterior ethmoid arteries coursing below the skull base is also important.

Imaging should be delayed 4–6 weeks after initiation of medical therapy and should not be performed during symptoms of acute upper respiratory infection. Once the disease process has been characterized and after mass lesions have been excluded, attention should be turned to pertinent anatomic variants that may impact the surgical approach. The location of mucosal disease should also be assessed, as certain stereotyped patterns of disease implicate pathology in particular drainage pathways.

Multiplanar reformatted images are important when evaluating the paranasal sinuses, and particular viewing planes can be especially helpful when visualizing specific anatomic locations. One particularly attractive feature of CBCT imaging in the paranasal sinuses is the ability to reconstruct images in any viewing plane with high fidelity to the source data, a relatively unique feature of CBCT that is related to isotropic voxel acquisition technique.

The coronal plane allows optimal visualization of the OMC and also provides a relatively familiar viewing plane for surgeons accustomed to endoscopic surgery in the sinuses. Axial images provide the most advantageous views of the basal lamella dividing the anterior and posterior ethmoid air cells, as well as the sphenoethmoidal recess and sphenoidal ostia. The sphenoethmoidal recess is well visualized in the sagittal plane as well, which allows visualization of the posterior ethmoidal drainage pathway. Additionally, the frontal sinus, frontal sinus outflow tract, and anterior ethmoid drainage pathway into the middle meatus are often viewed in the sagittal plane.

Pertinent anatomic variants

Concha bullosa

Pneumatization of a nasal turbinate is referred to as concha bullosa (Figure 4.4) and in severe cases can cause obstruction of the OMC by mass effect, predisposing to sinus disease (Balbach et al., 2011).

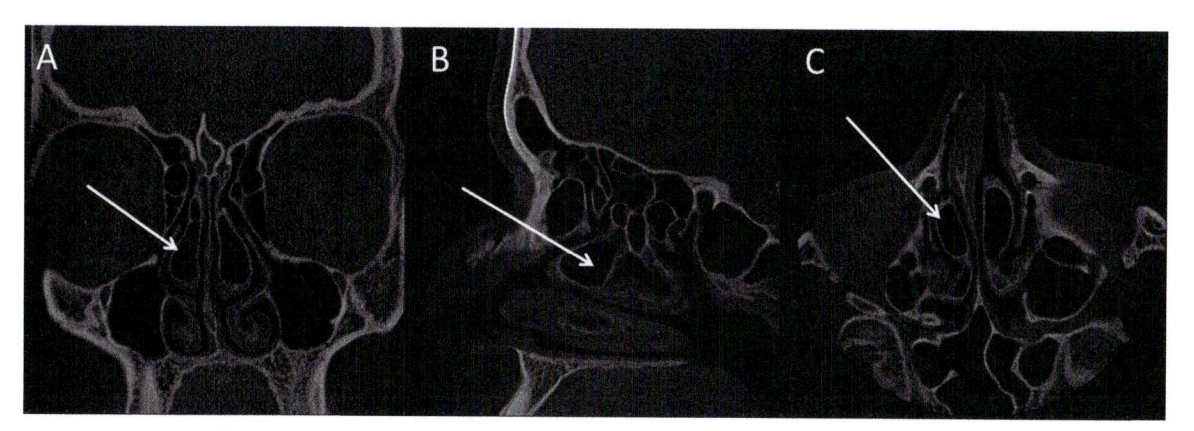

Figure 4.4 Middle turbinate pneumatization. Coronal (A), sagittal (B), and axial (C) images demonstrate extensive pneumatization of the middle turbinate (arrow), or concha bullosa mediana. Concha bullosa can cause obstruction of the infundibulum and is often associated with deviations of the nasal septum. Functional endoscopic sinus surgery (FESS) targeting the anterior ethmoid cells or infundibulum frequently involves reduction of the concha bullosa, typically the lateral wall.

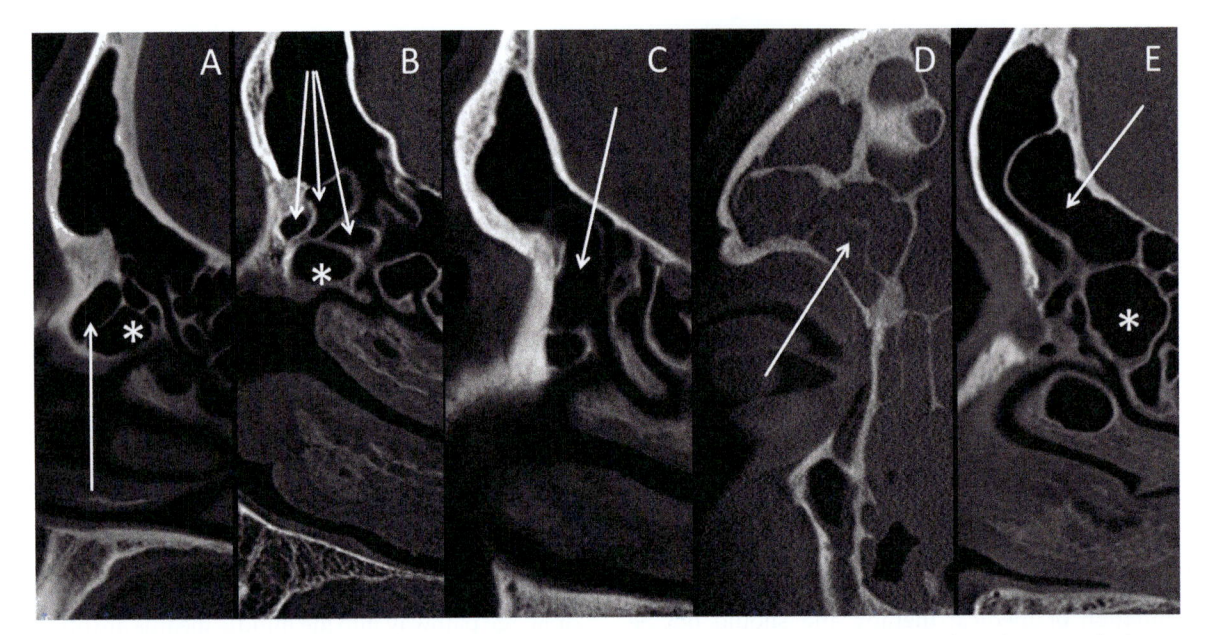

Figure 4.5 Frontal recess variants. Sagittal (A–C, E) and coronal (D) CBCT images demonstrate variant frontal recess cells that can lead to obstruction of frontal sinus outflow. Agger nasi cells are demonstrated in A and B (asterisks). In addition to the agger nasi cell, the anterior group of frontal recess cells includes frontal cells described by the Kuhn classification. A Kuhn 1 cell is depicted in A (arrow). A trio of Kuhn 2 cells are present in B (arrows). The Kuhn 3 cell in C (arrow) extends into the frontal sinus forming the anterior wall of the frontal sinus infundibulum. Kuhn 4 cells are single cells that pneumatize within the frontal sinus anteriorly and do not share a wall with the agger nasi cell (D, arrow). Within the posterior group of frontal recess cells, the frontal bullar cell (E) pneumatizes into the frontal sinus and projects above the ostium. Its posterior wall is the anterior skull base. An anterior ethmoidal bulla is marked by an asterisk in E.

Concha bullosa can be bulbous (involving the inferior bulbous portion of the turbinate), lamellar (pneumatized lamellar cells), or extensive (pneumatized bulbous turbinate and lamella).

Agger nasi pneumatization

Agger nasi cells are the most anterior of the anterior ethmoid cells (Figure 4.5) and with progressive pneumatization can expand to be bounded anteriorly by the frontal process of the maxilla, superiorly by the floor of the frontal sinus, inferomedially by the uncinate process, and inferolaterally by the lacrimal bone. Expanded agger nasi cells can obstruct drainage at the frontal recess and cause frontal sinusitis.

Uncinate process

The uncinate process forms the medial boundary of the infundibulum and as such is intimately related to the OMC and sinus outflow. Pneumatization of the uncinate bulla can cause obstruction of the OMC from mass effect. Lateral deviation of the uncinate process is also an important variant, as it can place the medial orbital wall at risk during instrumentation.

Haller's cells

Pneumatized cells inferolateral to the ethmoid bulla between the roof of the maxillary sinus and the floor of the orbit are termed Haller's cells (Figure 4.6) and can form the lateral wall of the infundibulm, causing OMC obstruction and maxillary sinusitis when enlarged.

Onodi cells

Expanded posterior ethmoid air cells (Figure 4.7) extending posteriorly into the sphenoid bone, occasionally as far posterior as the anterior clinoid process, are referred to as Onodi cells. Failure to recognize Onodi cells places the optic nerves at risk during FESS in the frontal recess.

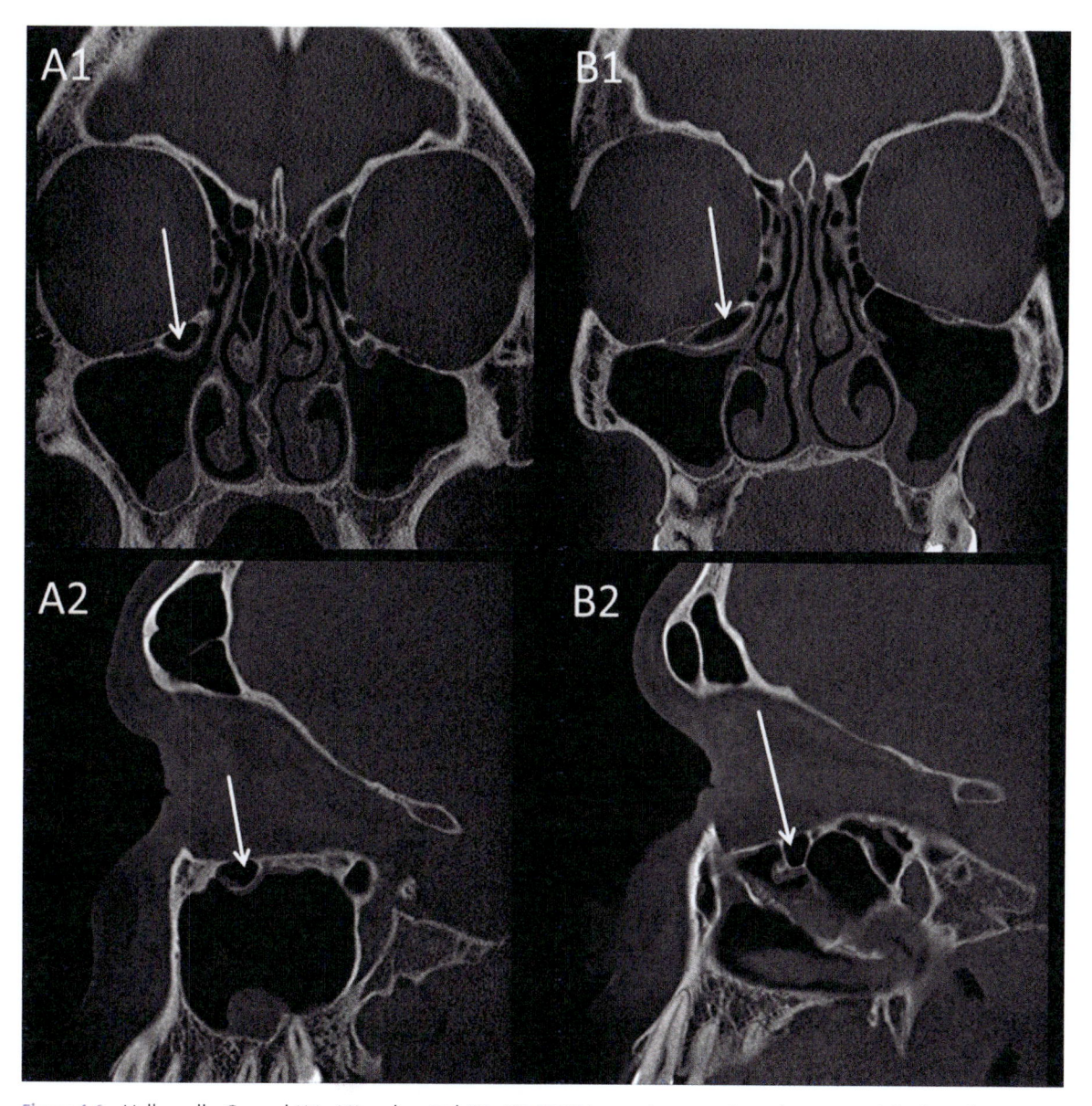

Figure 4.6 Haller cells. Coronal (A1, A2) and sagittal (B1, B2) CBCT images in two patients demonstrate inferolaterally pneumatized ethmoidal air cells, or Haller cells (arrows), which often form the lateral wall of the infundibulum and can contribute to infundibular obstruction. The patient in A has a small mucous retention cyst in the right maxillary sinus.

Nasal septum

Recognition of septal deflections and spurring can help determine the need for septoplasty during FESS procedures, depending on the extent and pattern of disease.

Olfactory fossa

The olfactory fossa is typically formed by the crista galli medially, the medial lamella inferiorly, and the lateral lamella laterally, with the fovea ethmoidalis marking the superolateral margin. Olfactory

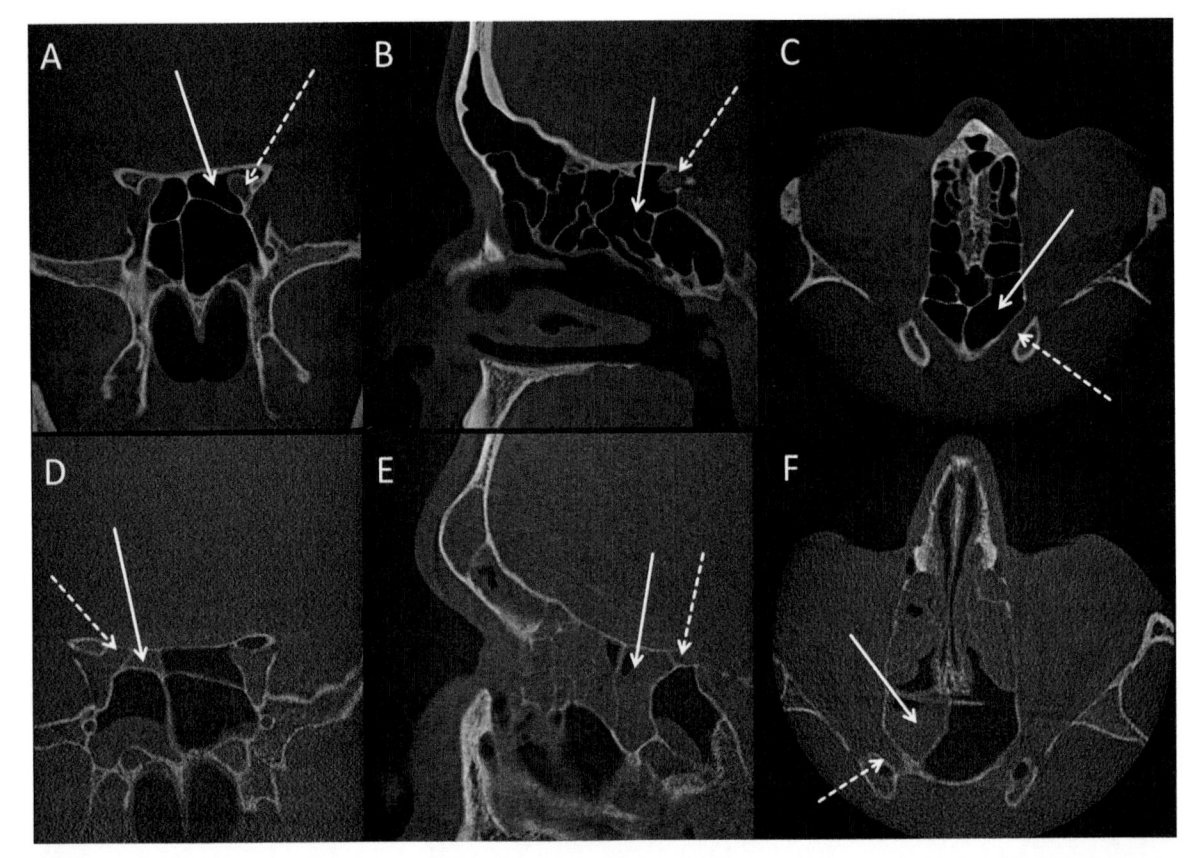

Figure 4.7 Onodi cells. Coronal (A, D), sagittal (B, E), and axial (C, F) CBCT images in two patients (A–C and D–F) demonstrate posterior ethmoidal air cells (white arrows) pneumatizing into the sphenoid bone immediately subjacent to the optic nerve in the optic canal (dotted arrows). FESS involving the ethmoid and sphenoid sinuses places the optic nerve at risk with this configuration. There is inflammatory mucosal thickening and secretions involving the ethmoid, frontal, and right sphenoid sinuses of the patient in D–F.

Table 4.2 Keros classification.

Keros Classification	Depth of Olfactory Fossa
I	<3 mm
II	3–7 mm
III	>7 mm

fossa variants can place the lateral lamella, the thinnest portion of the cribiform plate, at risk during endoscopic surgeries at the anterior skull base. The depth of the olfactory fossa can be graded based on the Keros classification (Table 4.2, Figure 4.8), measuring the distance between the fovea ethmoidalis and the medial lamella (Savvateeva et al., 2010). Keros type II anatomy is most common (Güldner, Diogo, et al., 2011; Saraiya and Aygun, 2009).

Lamina papyracea

Congenital or posttrauamatic dehiscence of the lamina papyracea can be identified prior to FESS, alerting the surgeon to the risk of damage to orbital contents in this area (Figure 4.9).

Frontal recess

The frontal infundibulum, frontal ostium, and frontal recess constitute the frontal sinus outflow tract, one of the narrowest anatomic apertures and a frequent site of drainage obstruction. Most commonly,

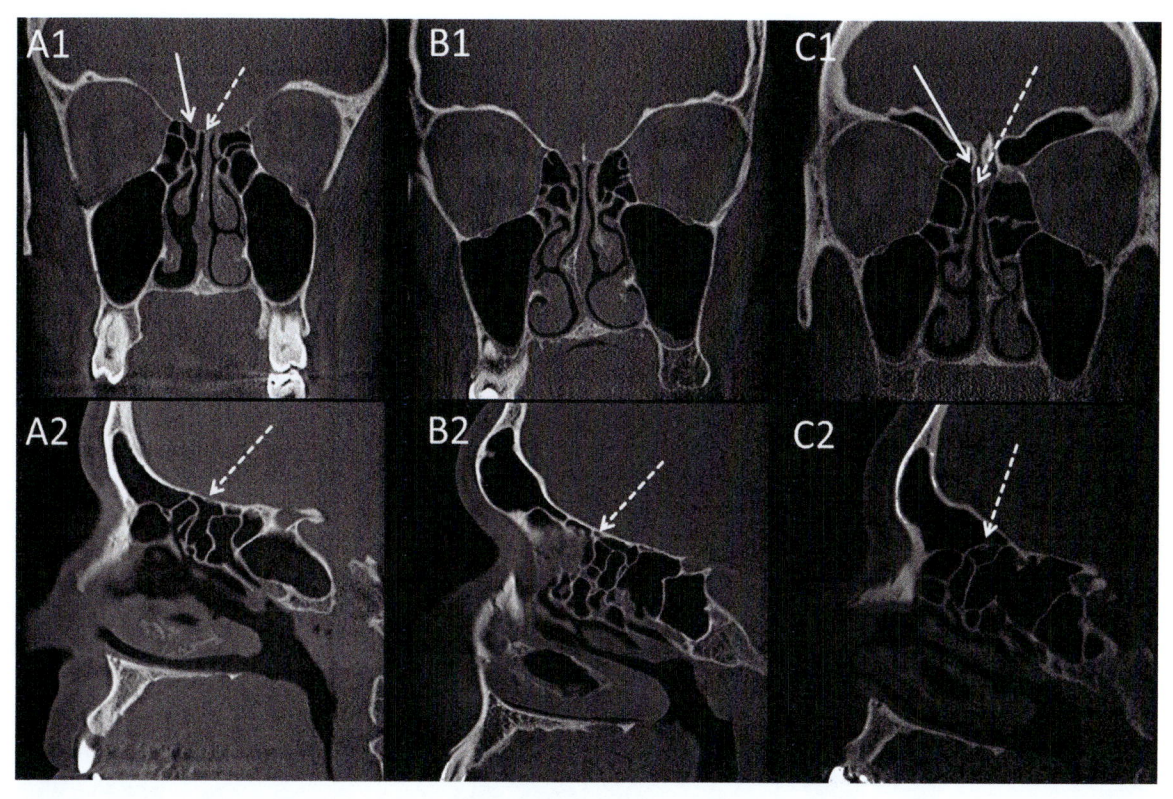

Figure 4.8 Olfactory fossa anatomy. The depth of the olfactory fossa can be described according to the Keros classification (A—Keros I; B—Keros II; C—Keros III). The relationship between the cribiform plate (dotted arrows) and lateral lamella is well demonstrated by coronal CBCT images (A1, B1, C1). Keros type I anatomy is typically associated with a course of the anterior ethmoid artery on the anterior skull base (A2, dotted arrow), whereas in Keros type III configuration the anterior ethmoid artery can run free through the ethmoidal cells (C2, dotted arrow).

the frontal recess is bordered anteriorly by the agger nasi cell, laterally by the lamina papyracea, and medially by the middle turbinate. The posterior border is formed by the ethmoid bulla, bulla lamella, and variably, the suprabullar cell. Anatomic variations in the frontal recess are particularly important, as it is one of the most difficult regions to treat endoscopically and one of the most common sites implicated in refractory sinusitis and in the need for revision FESS.

Frontal recess cells

Anterior ethmoid cells that pneumatize to form margins of the frontal sinus outflow tract are referred to collectively as frontal recess cells (Figure 4.5). The most constant of these is the agger nasi cell, which pneumatizes posteriorly to form the anterior border of the frontal recess. In addition to the agger nasi cell, several other variably pneumatized frontal recess cells can be important in the pathophysiology of frontal sinusitis and are discussed below.

The Kuhn classification (Table 4.3) describes four types of cells that, when present, pneumatize superiorly above the agger nasi cell to variably form the anterior wall of the frontal sinus, frontal infundibulum, or frontal recess. Along with agger nasi cells, these cells make up the anterior group of frontal recess cells.

The posterior group of frontal recess cells includes supraorbital ethmoid cells, frontal bullar cells, and suprabullar cells. Supraorbital ethmoid cells are located posterior to the frontal sinus and frontal recess and pneumatize from the orbital plate superolaterally over the orbit. These cells also drain into

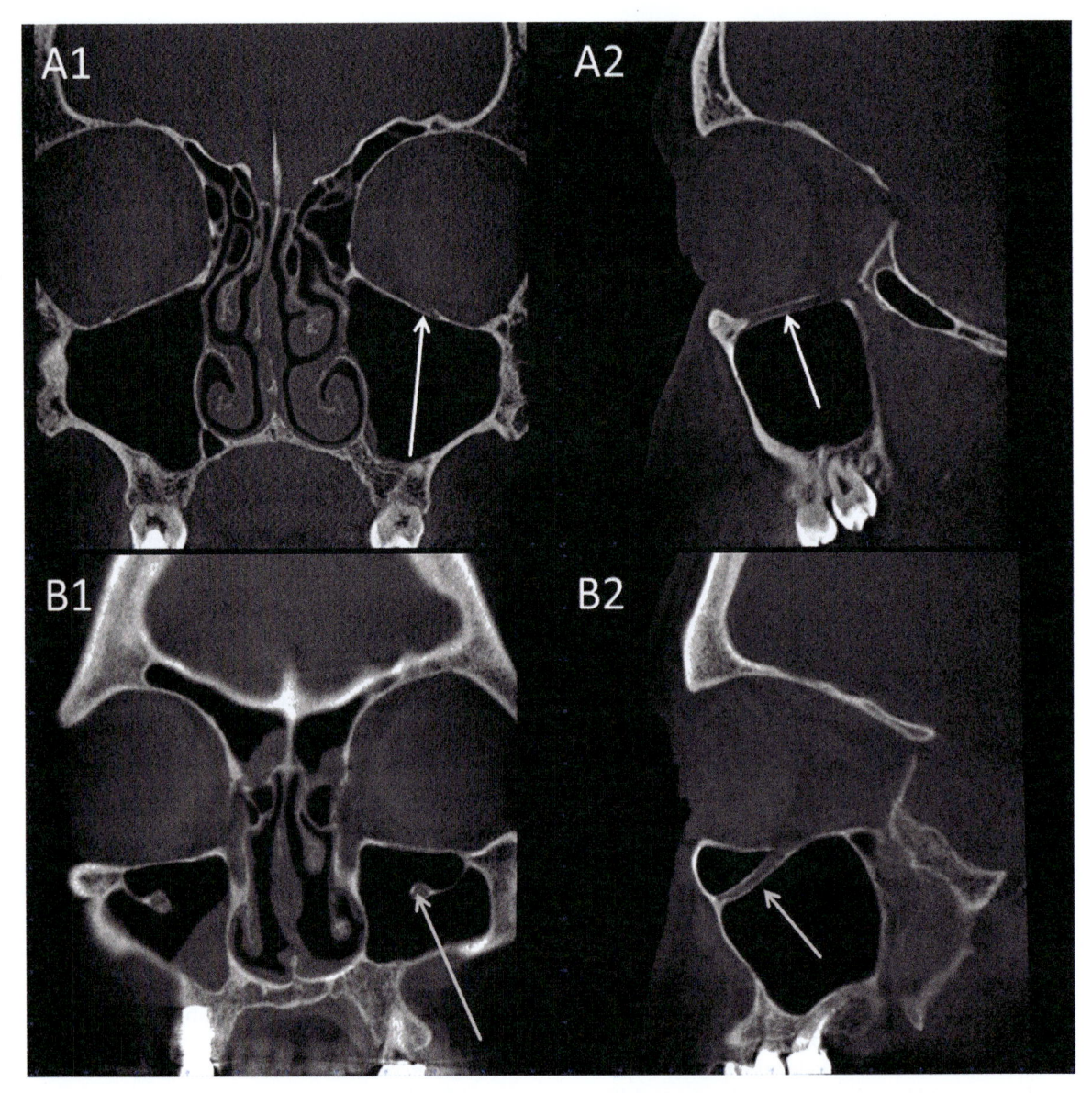

Figure 4.9 Infraorbital nerve. The course of the infraorbital nerve in the infraorbital canal is important in surgery within the maxillary sinus. Coronal (A1) and sagittal (A2) images demonstrate a closed course along the floor of the orbit (arrow). CBCT images in a second patient (B1, B2) depict a free course (arrow) within the maxillary sinus.

the frontal recess and can obstruct sinus outflow. Their ostia can also be mistaken for the frontal ostium endoscopically.

Suprabullar cells, a second variety of posterior frontal recess cells, are pneumatizations of the anterior skull base originating posterior to the frontal recess and extending anterosuperiorly only as far as the level of the frontal sinus ostium. They form the posterior border of the frontal recess when present.

Frontal bullar cells are similar in position to suprabullar cells, but they project superiorly into

Table 4.3 Kuhn classification.

Type	Description
1	Single cell without extension into the frontal sinus, not extending above the frontal ostium
2	Tier of 2 or more cells without extension into the frontal sinus, not extending above the frontal ostium
3	Single cell extending superiorly into the frontal sinus, forming the anterior wall of the infundibulum
4	Single cell pneumatized posteriorly into the frontal sinus, not abutting the agger nasi inferiorly

Box 4.1 Findings associated with recurrent symptoms after FESS.

Postoperative scarring
Residual outflow tract obstruction
 − remnant frontal recess cells
 − lateralization of the middle turbinate
 − retained uncinate
Osteoneogenesis
Inflammatory mucosal thickening
Recurrent polyposis
Previously undetected lesions
 − mucoceles
 − mucous retention cysts
 − neoplasms
 − fibro-osseous lesions

the frontal sinus above the ostium. Both frontal bullar cells and suprabullar cells can be mistaken for the anterior skull base when viewed endoscopically.

A final variety of frontal recess cells is the interfrontal sinus septal cell, which refers to pneumatization of the interfrontal sinus septum. These cells can extend posteriorly into the crista galli, a variant referred to as bulla galli.

Follow-up imaging after FESS

Postoperative complications following FESS can be divided into those that occur immediately postoperatively and those that manifest weeks to months later. In the immediate postoperative period, hemorrhage (especially from the anterior ethmoidal artery), orbital complications, and less frequently, violation of the anterior skull base with cerebrospinal fluid leak and/or damage to intracranial structures can be encountered. Appropriate imaging in these circumstances is always CECT and/or MRI with gadolinium, as CBCT lacks the ability to resolve important soft tissue structures in the orbits and anterior cranial fossa.

Recurrent symptoms after FESS

Outside the immediate postoperative period, patients may present with recurrent symptoms of sinusitis (Huang et al., 2009), in which case imaging evaluation can be indicated to determine the cause of continued symptoms. The most common causes of recurrent symptoms are postoperative scarring and unaddressed outflow tract obstruction. Less commonly, remnant frontal recess cells, retained uncinate process, lateralization of the middle turbinate, and osteoneogenesis are implicated as the source of recurrent symptoms. Inflammatory mucosal thickening and recurrent polyposis—in addition to scarring—are soft tissue findings on imaging that can be associated with sinusitis symptoms after FESS. Statistically, up to 23% of patients undergoing FESS for chronic sinusitis will require revision surgery for continued symptoms. Of this 23%, almost half require revision surgery for symptoms localized to the frontal sinuses. As such, close attention should be paid to the frontal sinus outflow tract on follow-up imaging, as revision FESS procedures are often directed to this anatomic area.

There are several findings on follow-up imaging after FESS that may predispose to recurrent symptoms (Box 4.1). Insufficient resection of agger nasi and other frontal recess cells can lead to residual obstruction or can serve as the substrate for scar formation postoperatively. Lateralization of the middle turbinate can also lead to obstruction and can result from turbinate manipulation or partial resection during initial FESS. Postoperative scarring and mucosal thickening are often implicated as causes of recurrent symptoms and cannot be differentiated based on nonenhanced CT features.

Patients who have a retained superior uncinate at its insertion can, in the setting of certain anatomic configurations, have a propensity for restenosis of the frontal recess outflow tract. In patients for whom the uncinate process inserts on the lamina papyracea or agger nasi, frontal sinus outflow proceeds directly medially into the middle meatus and the uncinate forms the lateral border of the frontal recess. For patients whose uncinate process inserts superiorly on the middle turbinate or skull base, frontal sinus outflow is directed into the ethmoid infundibulum, with the uncinate forming the medial wall of the frontal recess. In the aforementioned scenario of lateral uncinate insertion on the lamina papyracea or agger nasi, the ethmoid infundibulum ends blindly in the recessus terminalis, a recess that can remodel and expand outward with chronic sinusitis, medializing the uncinate and contributing to outflow obstruction. Retention of the superior uncinate insertion after FESS is not uncommon and should be excluded in cases of recurrent symptoms postoperatively.

Osteoneogensis, also referred to as hyperostosis, can be the result of chronic inflammation, previous trauma, or surgical manipulation with mucosal defects or mucosal stripping following FESS. Expanding osteoneogenesis postoperatively can restenose outflow tracts and cause recurrent symptoms.

Temporal bone

CBCT is an emerging technique for select imaging tasks in temporal bone imaging, and preliminary investigations are exploring roles in middle and inner ear implant imaging (Güldner, Wiegand, et al., 2011), surgical navigation (Kamran et al., 2010), and in defining particularly small high-contrast structures such as the middle ear ossicles and reuniting duct (Dalchow et al., 2006; Penninger et al., 2011). Use in general diagnostic imaging is still limited by lack of soft tissue contrast. Any practitioners interpreting CBCT images that include the lateral skull base in the field of view should be familiar with anatomy and pathology in this region, as it will be well delineated in many instances (Gupta et al., 2004).

Imaging evaluation in selected imaging tasks such as postoperative middle and inner ear reconstruction are beyond the scope of this chapter. Suffice it to say that middle and inner ear prostheses are generally well visualized with CBCT with relatively minimal streak artifact compared to MDCT (Majdani et al., 2009).

Inner ear

The inner ear refers to the structures internal to the oval and round windows and includes the cochlea, semicircular canals, and vestibule (collectively, the bony labyrinth) as well as the membranous labyrinth contained therein (Figure 4.10). The membranous labyrinth includes the utricle and saccule in the vestibule, the semicircular ducts, the scala media of the cochlea, and the endolymphatic duct and sac within the vestibular aqueduct. The perilymphatic space is also contained in the bony labyrinth and is composed of the space surrounding the utricle and saccule in the vestibule, the scala tympani and vestibuli in the cochlea, and the space in the semicircular canals surrounding the semicircular ducts. The perilymphatic space communicates with the subarachnoid space via the cochlear aqueduct (Yamane et al., 2011).

Congenital abnormalities

A normally developed inner ear consists of 2.5 turns of the cochlea, a separate vestibule, and normal size and configuration of the semicircular canals as well as cochlear and vestibular aqueducts (Figure 4.11). Multiple congenital abnormalities with characteristic imaging findings have been described but are beyond the scope of this chapter and are most likely to be encountered in the imaging workup of sensorineural hearing loss in a pediatric patient, a specialized area of clinical practice (Krombach et al., 2008; Kosling et al., 2009; Yiin et al., 2011).

Acquired inner ear lesions

Labyrinthitis

Labyrinthitis refers to inflammation involving the membranous labyrinth and is typically infectious, although autoimmune etiologies are also possible.

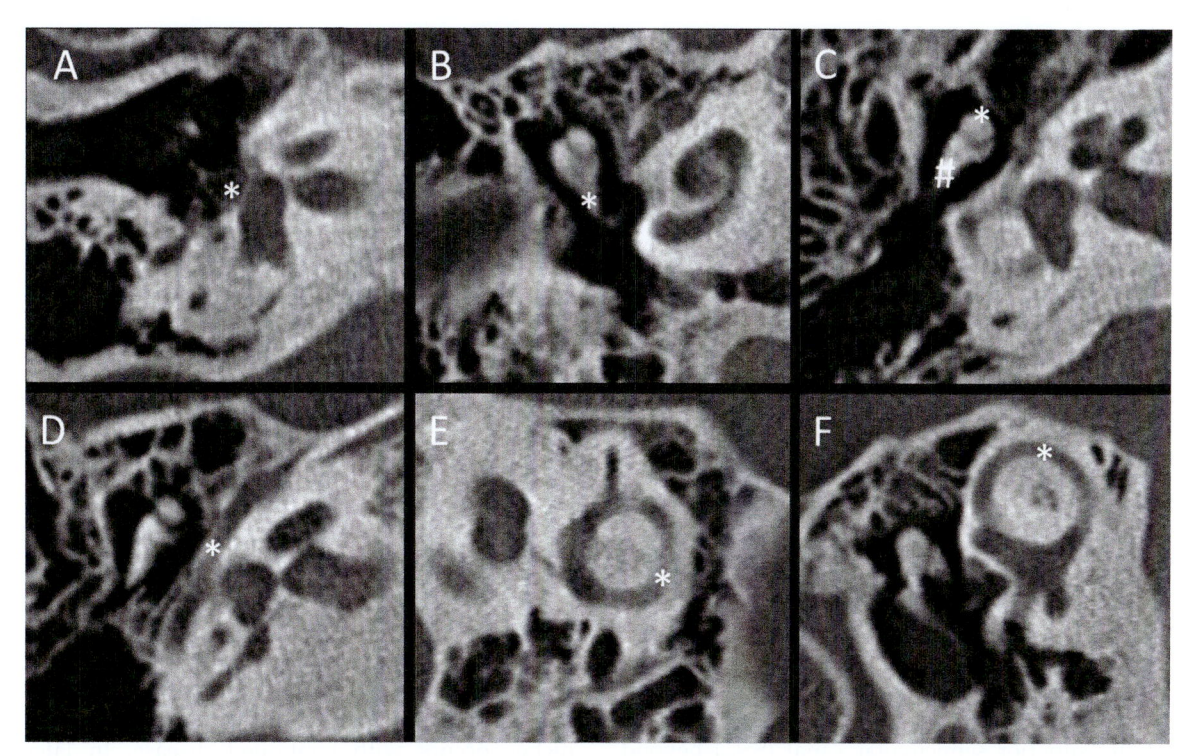

Figure 4.10 Normal temporal bone anatomy. Axial (A, C, D), coronal (B), and oblique (E, F) CBCT images depict the normal anatomy of the middle and inner ears. Both crura of the stapes (*) and the endplate can be seen articulating with the oval window in the oval window niche (A). The incudomalleolar joint (B and C) is seen in two different planes, demonstrating the head of the malleus (* in C) articulating with the body of the incus (#). The long limb of the incus is seen in B (*). In most patients, the bony coverage of the facial nerve in its tympanic segment can be visualized (D, *), demarcating the medial border of the mesotympanum. Oblique reformats demonstrating the posterior (E, *) and superior (F, *) semicircular canals can be constructed with high fidelity to the source data given the isotropic voxel acquisition afforded by CBCT imaging.

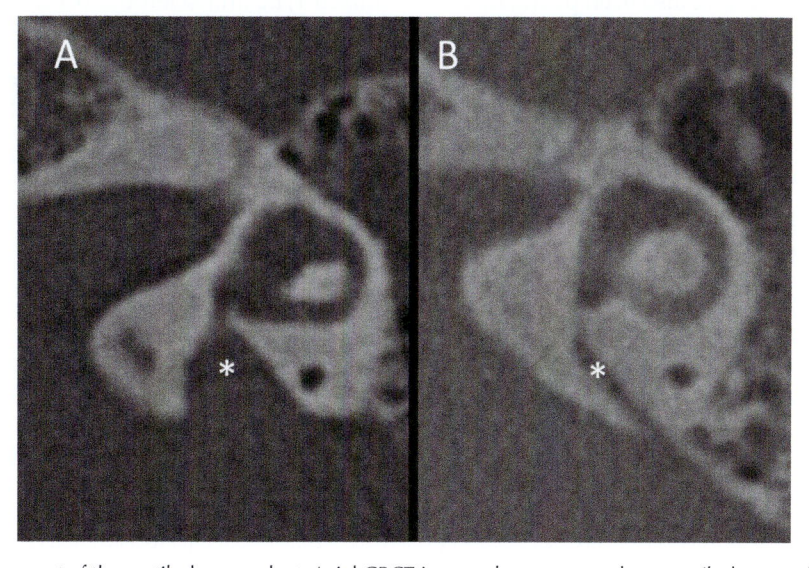

Figure 4.11 Enlargement of the vestibular aqueduct. Axial CBCT images demonstrate a large vestibular aqueduct (A). A normal vestibular aqueduct posterior and in-plane to the horizontal semicircular canal is provided for comparison (B). This congenital anomaly can cause varying degrees of sensorineural hearing loss and/or dizziness.

In infectious labyrinthitis, the causative agent is most commonly viral, although bacterial pathogens are also possible and represent more aggressive disease. Syphilitic labyrinthitis is more rare. The pathophysiology can be related to antecedent middle ear infection(s), meningitis, or hematogenous spread of viral infection. Posttraumatic etiologies and iatrogenic labyrinthitis after inner ear surgery are also possible. In the early phase of infection, CT imaging findings may not be present; but with progressive disease, ossification of the membranous labyrinth identified as osseous deposition within the bony labyrinth can be seen. Early manifestations of labyrinthitis before the onset of CT changes are better demonstrated with MRI (Maroldi et al., 2001).

Superior semicircular canal dehiscence

Frank dehiscence or extreme thinning of the roof of the superior semicircular canal (SSC) beyond the resolution of CBCT appears as an interruption or absence of the bony partition between the SCC and the middle cranial fossa. Identification of SSC dehiscence is important clinically, as it is a treatable cause of vestibular dysfunction. SSC dehiscence is typically idiopathic, possibly a developmental abnormality, but barotrauma and other posttraumatic causes have also been postulated.

Otosclerosis

Otoslcerosis is caused by a disruption in bone metabolism and consists of both a hypervascular spongiotic phase and a later sclerotic phase. Similar but pathophysiologically distinct from Paget's disease, it only affects the bony labyrinth of the inner ear and is typically bilateral. It occurs sporadically and is more common in men. Progressive disease can result in fixation of the stapedial footplate and conductive hearing loss.

Two forms of otosclerosis can be distinguished: fenestral and retrofenestral (Minor et al., 1998; Mong et al., 1999). Fenestral otosclerosis is more common and affects the fissula ante fenestram, the bony prominence demarcating the middle from inner ear just anterior to the oval window. The earliest CT evidence of fenestral otosclerosis is a lytic lesion involving the fissula ante fenestram (Figure 4.12; Lee et al., 2009). Extension to the cochlear promontory and oval/round window niches occurs with continued disease. In later phases, lytic lesions become expansile and spongiform. The final sclerotic phase appears as dense calcification (Maillet et al., 2011).

Retrofenestral, or cochlear, otosclerosis primarily affects the otic capsule and is identified in the early stages as pericochlear lucencies that can coalesce to form a lytic "halo." Progressive phases appear as mixed lytic and sclerotic foci that may ultimately

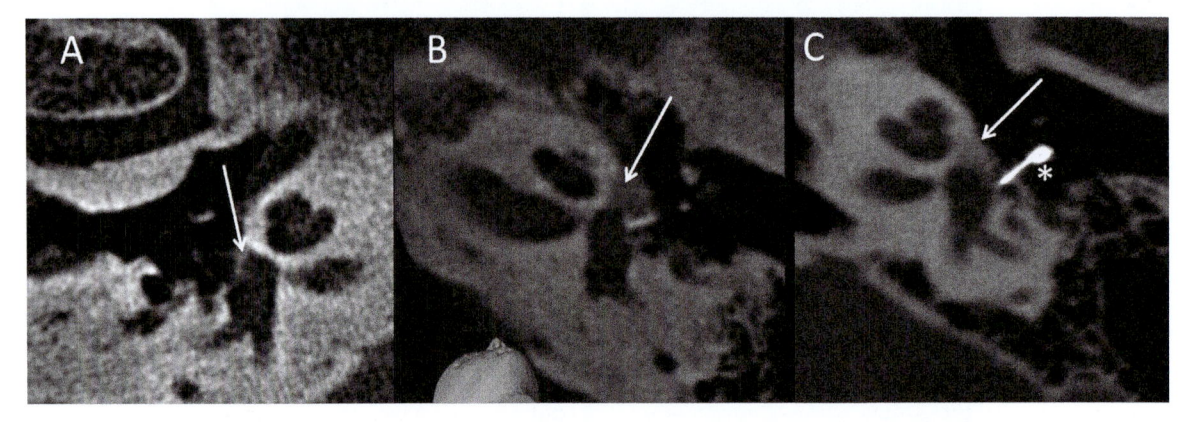

Figure 4.12 Otosclerosis. Coronal CBCT images at the level of the oval window niche and vestibule in three patients depict lucent lesions (arrows) involving the fissula ante fenestram (A) progressing retrofenestrally to involve the cochlea (B and C). Grade 1 otosclerosis is confined to the fissula ante fenestram and stapes footplate and is termed fenestral (A). Grade 2 otosclerosis subtotally involves the cochlea to varying degrees (B and C) with or without fenestral involvement. Grade 3 otosclerosis refers to diffuse and confluent involvement of the cochlea (not shown). Stapedectomy with placement of a stapes prosthesis is the therapy of choice (C).

appear predominantly sclerotic, although this can be difficult to identify in dense otic capsule bone. Retrofenestral otosclerosis often occurs with antecedent fenestral findings, so attention should be paid to the fissula ante fenestram when retrofenestral features are present.

Neoplasms

Evaluation of inner ear neoplasms is best performed with MRI, but CT can be useful in defining the extent of bony destruction. Incidental findings of inner ear tumors on CBCT can be inferred if soft tissue lesions arising within the inner ear spaces causing bony destruction are identified. Space-occupying soft tissue lesions in the inner ear include congential cholesteatomas, which can arise in the petrous apex and erode into the lanyrinth; metastases, which can be lytic, blastic, or both; lipoma; and endolymphatic sac tumors. Endolymphatic sac tumors are rare, and appear as retrolabyrinthine destructive soft tissue masses of the temporal bone, occasionally with elements of a calcified matrix.

Inner ear prosthesis

Cochlear implants are relatively well identified with CBCT and in some centers it is the modality of choice in their evaluation, as CBCT images typically afford lower levels of metallic streak artifact while maintaining high spatial resolution (Faccioli et al., 2009; Rafferty et al., 2006). The position of the inner ear prosthesis can sometimes be identified as within the scala tympani or scala vestibuli with CBCT and the electrode-modiolus relationship can be interrogated. A more complete discussion of inner ear implants is beyond the scope of this chapter (Marshall et al., 2005).

Middle ear

The middle ear can be segmented into the epitympanum, mesotympanum, and hypotympanum. The epitympanum is the superior-most space, separated from the mesotympanum by the tympanic isthmi at the level of the scutum and bounded superiorly by the tegmen tympani and aditus ad antrum into the mastoid sinus. The mesotympanum is bordered medially by the tympanic portion of the facial nerve, the cochlear promontory, and the fossae of the oval and round windows. Important structures in the posterior mesotympanum include the pyramidal eminence, sinus tympani, and facial nerve recess. The Eustachian canal arises from the anterior mesotympanum. The hypotympanum is the inferior-most recess in the tympanic cavity.

The middle ear houses the ossicles, whose anatomy can be well delineated with CBCT. The handle of the malleus is applied to the tympanic membrane, and the head articulates with the body of the incus. The lenticular process of the incus articulates with the head of the stapes, forming a complete ossicular chain from the tympanic membrane and handle of the malleus to the oval window via the stapes footplate (Stone et al., 2000; Monteiro et al., 2011).

Congenital abnormalities

Congenital abnormalities involving the middle ear include ossicular anomalies such as deformities, fixations, and absences, as well as hypoplasia of the middle ear cavity itself and underpneumatization of the mastoid. A detailed discussion of congenital and developmental abnormalities of the middle ear and their syndromic associations is beyond the scope of this chapter.

Otitis media

Acute

Predisposition to otitis media in the pediatric population is in part related to differences in orientation of the Eustachian tube and hypertrophy of lymphoid tissue. Acute cases are often encountered in this population, and imaging is usually not a necessary part of the diagnostic algorithm. Acute otitis media (AOM) can occur in adults as well, although it is less common, and appears as opacification of the middle ear cavity with or without an air fluid level and concomitant mastoid opacification. In an uncomplicated case of AOM, the ossicular chain is typically preserved. Mucoperiosteal inflammation can occur and eventually leads to osteomyelitis in severe cases, which presents as destructive erosion of cortical bone and trabeculae.

Advanced AOM can lead to coalescent mastoiditis, which refers to osteomyelitis of the mastoid. The imaging appearance is one of resorption of the trabeculae within the mastoid compared to the contralateral side, with eventual erosion into surrounding cortical bone and possible subperiosteal abscess formation. A subperiosteal abscess will most likely be occult on CBCT, and contrast-enhanced MDCT or MRI should be considered in the appropriate clinical setting. Inferior dehiscence of cortical bone adjacent to the insertion of the posterior digastric muscle suggests the diagnosis of Bezold's abscess, an aggressive soft tissue infection tracking along the path of the sternocleidomastoid muscle in the suprahyoid neck, eventually spreading within fascial planes into the mediastinum. MRI or CECT is necessary to assess the extent of spread in these cases, as lack of soft tissue resolution with CBCT precludes adequate evaluation of soft tissue involvement. Other complications of AOM include medial extension to the petrous apex, which will appear as opacification, resorption of traebeculae, and cortical erosion/destruction; epidural abscess; subdural abscess; and sigmoid sinus thrombosis. Needless to say, evaluation of suspected complications with CBCT is incomplete and further imaging should be immediately pursued (Lemmerling et al., 2008).

Chronic

Chronic otitis media (COM) refers to persistent inflammatory changes in the middle ear, the earliest imaging features of which are effusion and granulation tissue in the middle ear cavity. CBCT may demonstrate partial or complete opacification of the middle ear or adherent soft tissue in the absence of effusion. When both are present, lack of soft tissue discrimination will limit reliable evaluation. Clinical manifestations of COM include recurrent OM, hearing loss, and otalgia.

There is a spectrum of pathology related to chronic inflammation of the middle ear, and it can often be difficult to determine to what extent middle ear pathology is the result of recurrent or chronic inflammation/infection and to what extent pathology in the middle ear causes chronic inflammation and recurrent infections. In some instances the middle ear is predisposed to chronic otitis media and its sequellae due to obstruction of middle ear drainage, either from Eustachian tube obstruction or narrowing/obstruction of the tympanic isthmi separating the epitympanum (attic) from the mesotympanum. Narrowing can be congenital/developmental or related to acquired pathology as will be discussed below.

Related pathology in the middle ear includes tympanic membrane perforation or retraction, tympanosclerosis, and the spectrum of postinflammatory ossicular fixation, acquired cholesteatoma, and cholesterol granuloma. Underpneumatization of the ipsilateral mastoid is also associated with COM. Myringitis refers to inflammation of the tympanic membrane (Figure 4.13) and can occur with or without concomitant middle ear infection.

Postinflammatory ossicular fixation

Postinflammatory ossicular fixation occurs as a complication of AOM or COM and can lead to conductive hearing loss due to ossicular disruption. Three forms are typically described, chronic adhesive, tympanosclerosis, and fibro-osseous sclerosis. Chronic adhesive postinflammatory ossicular fixation refers to fixation of the ossicles with fibrous tissue and appears as soft tissue debris adjacent to the ossicles, most often around the stapes (causing stapedial fixation). Lack of middle ear effusion or erosions with a history of COM can suggest this diagnosis, but ultimately the appearance is nonspecific on CT and cannot be reliably differentiated from cholesteatoma and other soft tissue pathology.

Tympanosclerosis is distinguished pathologically by hyalinized collagen deposition and manifests radiologically as multifocal or discrete calcified densities within the middle ear cavity, often on the tympanic membrane or intimate to the ossicular chain. Fibro-osseous sclerosis is rare and can be differentiated from tympanosclerosis by the presence of lamellar new bone deposition.

Cholesteatoma

Cholesteatomas are one of the most common middle ear lesions, with an annual incidence of 9.2 per 100,000 in the adult population. They are distinguished histopathologically as nonneoplastic cysts of squamous cells which produce keratin lamellas

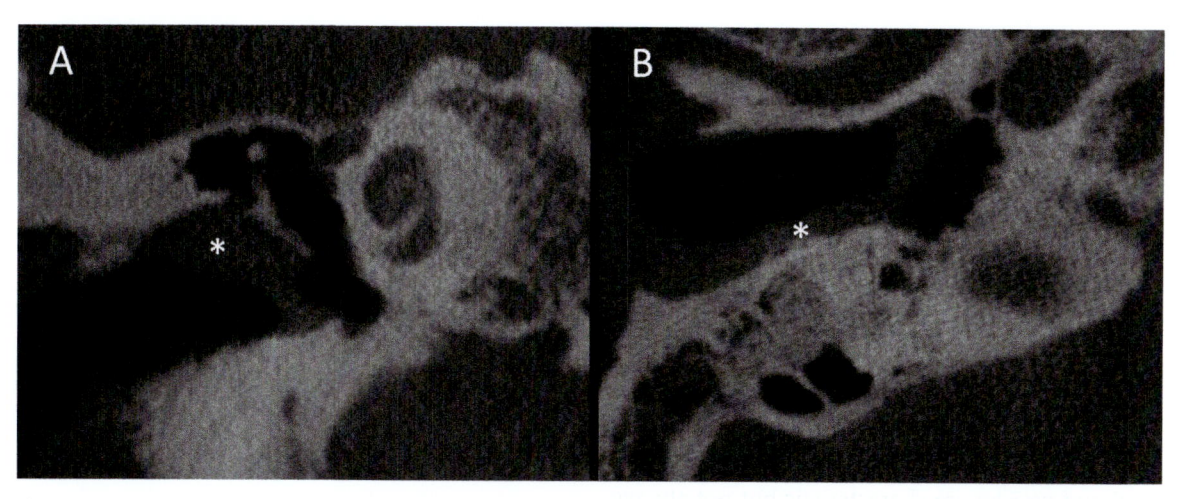

Figure 4.13 Chronic myringitis. Coronal (A) and axial (B) CBCT images demonstrating thickening of the tympanic membrane (A, *) with thickening of the dermis in the posterior external auditory canal (B, *). Normal mastoid pneumatization and a nonopacified middle ear cavity are typical in uncomplicated chronic myringitis.

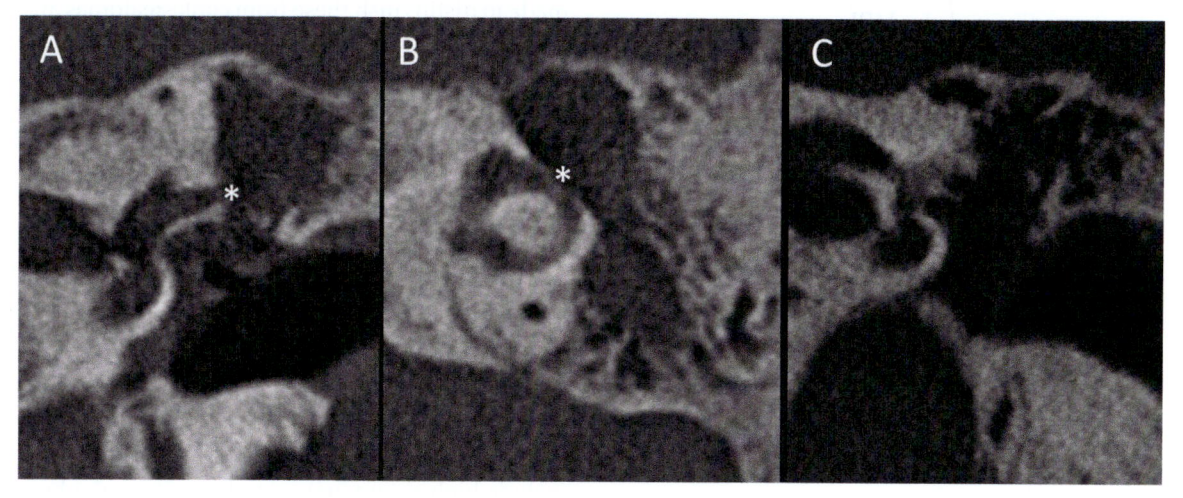

Figure 4.14 Pars flaccida cholesteatoma. Coronal (A, C) and axial (B) images demonstrate soft tissue centered in the epitympanum and extending into the mesotympanum and aditus ad antrum, with bony erosion causing dehiscense of the horizontal semicircular canal (* in A and B) and complete erosion of the ossicles, which are not seen within the epi- and mesotympanum (C). This lesion is centered in Prussak's space within the lateral epitympanum. The characteristic location and presence of bony erosions is compatible with cholesteatoma.

that then invaginate into the cyst. The external component is composed of mixed inflammatory cells and granulation tissue, occasionally with bony fragments.

The majority of cholesteatomas are acquired, but 2% may be congenital, in which case they can occur anywhere in the temporal bone and are histologically identical to epidermoid cysts encountered intracranially. Acquired cholesteatomas typically develop internal to the tympanic membrane (TM) and can be classified as either pars flaccida (arising from the pars flaccida of the TM) or pars tensa (developing through a perforation in the pars tensa of the TM). Pars flaccida cholesteatomas (Figure 4.14) are more common and are thought to be related to some combination of chronic infection and pressure differentials between the middle and external ear. Cholesteatomas can also develop in the posttraumatic and postsurgical settings.

Pars flaccida cholesteatomas are centered in Prussak's space, the epitympanic space lateral to the ossicles. Pars tensa cholesteatomas arise medial to the ossicles in the mesotympanum and can be secondarily acquired (through perforations in the TM) or congenital.

The typical CT appearance of a cholesteatoma is a uniform-density nondependent soft tissue mass that is sharply demarcated and expansile, centered in a characteristic location (Barath et al., 2011). Associated TM retraction and extension through the aditus ad antrum can be seen. Early erosion of the scutum as well as erosions of the tegmen tympani and ossicles are characteristic but not always present. Unfortunately, these imaging features are nonspecific on CT, as granulation tissue, secretions, cholesterol granulomas, and neoplasms can all exhibit a similar appearance (Table 4.4). Diagnosis is more readily made by MRI.

The most common complication of cholesteatoma is labyrinthine fistula, which can be inferred from dehiscence of the lateral semicircular canal. Facial nerve injury (erosion through the tympanic segment of the facial canal), extension into the internal auditory canal, and erosion of the mastoid trabeculations causing eventual automastoidectomy can also be seen. Dehiscence of the tegmen tympani or anterior epitympanic wall can suggest encephalocele or extension into the middle cranial fossa and warrants further evaluation with MRI. Erosion through the sigmoid sinus plate raises the possibility of sigmoid sinus thrombosis and is an indication for contrast-enhanced imaging.

Cholesterol granuloma

Cholesterol granulomas can be the sequela of chronic middle ear inflammation and are thought to result from chronic microhemorrhage and the formation of granulation tissue. Attempts can be made to distinguish these from cholesteatomas and hemorrhagic OM, but ultimately MRI is needed for more definitive distinction. The CT appearance is one of a smooth, expansile soft tissue mass in the middle ear, typically without ossicular erosions.

Vascular lesions

Important vascular lesions to recognize in the middle ear include aberrant internal carotid arteries and jugular bulb anomalies. An aberrant internal carotid artery will appear as a soft tissue mass coursing through the middle ear cavity that is continuous anteromedially with the petrous portion of the internal carotid artery. Jugular bulb anomalies include high-riding jugular bulbs and jugular bulb diverticuli. A high-riding bulb abuts the floor of the internal auditory canal and may protrude into the posteroinferior middle ear cavity if the sigmoid plate is dehiscent. Jugular bulb diverticuli, which are focal outpouchings from the jugular bulb, can also extend into the middle ear through a dehiscent sigmoid plate.

Neoplasms

Both primary and metastatic neoplasms of the middle ear are rare. Of the primary neoplasms, paragangliomas (glomus tumors) and schwannomas

Table 4.4 Evaluating the opacified middle ear.

Finding	Disease
Ossicular erosions	Cholesteatoma, glomus jugulare
Ossicular displacement	Cholesterol granuloma, schwannoma, glomus tympanicum
Nasopharyngeal soft tissue assymetry	Obstructing nasopharyngeal carcinoma
Dehiscence of facial nerve canal	Cholesteatoma
Tegmen tympani dehiscense	Cholesteatoma, encephalocele
Dehiscent lateral semicircular canal	Cholesteatoma
Calcified densities in the middle ear	Tympanosclerosis with COM
Lamellar new bone deposition	Fibro-osseous sclerosis with COM
Dehiscent sigmoid plate	Jugular bulb anomaly, cholesteatoma
Lucent fracture line	Temporal bone fracture

Note: COM = chronic otitis media.

are the most common. Rhabdomyosarcoma is a rare, highly aggressive tumor in children. The CT finding of a middle ear soft tissue mass with or without bony destruction is ultimately nonspecific, as cholesteatoma and other soft tissue lesions of the middle ear can have a similar appearance. Evaluation with MRI is mandatory in any suspected middle ear neoplasm.

Middle ear schwannomas can arise from the facial nerve or, less commonly, from Jacobson's nerve, the chorda tympani, or secondarily from CN VIII-XI extending into the middle ear. A soft tissue mass associated with the facial nerve canal or arising from the round window niche (Jacobson's nerve) is suspicious for schwannoma, but nonenhanced CT findings are nonspecific.

Middle ear glomus tumors arise from paraganglia associated with either Jacobson's nerve on the cochlear promontory (glomus tympanicum) or the internal jugular vein around the jugular foramen (glomus jugulare). Both present as soft tissue masses within the middle ear. Glomus tympanicum tumors appear to arise from the promontory, displace rather than destroy the ossicles, and are contained within the middle ear cavity. Glomus jugulare tumors arise from the jugular foramen and are more aggressive, exhibiting bony remodeling and ossicular destruction.

External auditory canal

Several pathologic processes in the temporal bone are particular to the external auditory canal (EAC) and deserve specific mention. Foremost among the nonneoplastic entities is malignant otitis externa, which will be discussed below. Other pathology which should be entertained in a differential of EAC disease includes cholesteatoma and squamous cell carcinoma. Both can appear as soft tissue lesions arising in the EAC with adjacent bony erosions, findings which make these entities difficult to distinguish from malignant otitis externa on imaging findings alone. Otoscopic findings as well as the clinical scenario should be considered.

In contrast, keratosis obturans is an idiopathic inflammatory lesion of the EAC causing fibrosis in the medial canal. It can be identified as soft tissue plugging extending up to the TM with mild bony enlargement of the EAC and no appreciable erosions. Bony lesions of the outer ear include osteoma, a densely corticated osseous lesion with either a bony stalk or broad base of attachment to the EAC; and EAC exostoses, which appears as bilateral circumferential bony narrowing of the canals, classically seen in chronic exposure to cold water.

Malignant otitis externa

Malignant (also known as necrotic) otitis externa is an invasive infectious process (classically pseudomonas) involving the EAC with risk of extension into the skull base toward the mastoid and petrous apex. Rarely, intracranial involvement can be seen. Advanced age and diabetes mellitus are risk factors. CT findings include soft tissue in the EAC with erosions involving adjacent EAC walls and middle ear structures. Erosions extending to the petrous apex and mastoid are present in more advanced disease (Sudhoff et al., 2008). MRI is indicated for evaluation of soft tissue extension into neck spaces inferiorly.

Trauma

Initial imaging in the setting of head trauma will be MDCT with or without CTA, as discriminating soft tissue resolution is needed to detect intracranial hemorrhage, cerebral edema, and vascular injuries, among other things. Despite CBCT's ability to detect bony skull base and maxillofacial fractures, the importance of identifying accompanying soft tissue and vascular pathology precludes the use of CBCT as the initial imaging modality. Dedicated temporal bone imaging with MDCT is often obtained if there is concern for laterobasal skull fracture, and multiplanar reconstructions are used to evaluate lucent fracture lines that may travel parallel to the imaging plane on axial slices (Schuknecht and Graetz, 2005; Saraiya and Aygun, 2009; Zayas et al., 2011).

Although CBCT has not been well evaluated in the setting of temporal bone trauma, CBCT images obtained secondarily for pre- or intraoperative navigation in the skull base and/or maxillodental regions may identify temporal bone fractures.

Maxillofacial trauma will be discussed separately. Upper cervical spine as well as condylar, clival, and transphenoidal skull base fractures are also serious injuries that are beyond the scope of this discussion.

Temporal bone trauma can have serious repercussions, including hearing loss (conductive or sensorineural), vestibular dysfunction, cerebrospinal fluid leak, and facial nerve paralysis, among other things. An opacified middle ear and/or soft tissue density in the mastoid air cells is highly suspicious of temporal bone fracture in the setting of trauma. Other secondary signs include air-fluid levels in the sphenoid sinuses, adjacent pneumocephalus, and air in the glenoid fossa of the TMJ. Intracranial extra-axial fluid collections and evidence of adjacent brain parenchymal injury are unlikely to be identified by CBCT.

Fractures are identified as linear lucencies that are distinguishable from normal cranial suture lines. The margins will often not be as well corticated as is seen with vascular channels and normal sutures. In the temporal bone, fractures are ideally classified as otic capsule-sparing or otic capsule-violating, depending on whether the fracture line extends to involve the bony labyrinth of the inner ear. The distinction is important clinically, as otic capsule-violating fractures are more commonly associated with sensorineural hearing loss, cerebrospinal fluid otorrhea, and facial nerve injury. Fractures can also be classified as longitudinal or transverse based on their relationship to the long axis of the petrous temporal bone, in which case transverse fractures are more likely to involve the otic capsule compared to longitudinal and are therefore considered to represent a more serious injury.

Once identified, it is important to follow the entire extent of the lucent fracture line(s), evaluating involvement of key middle and inner ear structures (Table 4.5). Extension to the external auditory canal is also relevant, as untreated EAC fractures can lead to canal stenosis. Disruption of the ossicular chain is not uncommon in temporal bone trauma and can lead to conductive hearing loss. The long process of the incus and stapedial crura are the most common sites of ossicular fracture, and incudostapedial separation is the most common dislocation injury.

Table 4.5 Temporal bone fracture.

Structure Involved	Clinical Concern
Ossicles	Conductive hearing loss
Carotid canal	Carotid artery injury
Facial nerve canal	Facial nerve injury
Cochlea	Sensorineural hearing loss
Vestibule	Risk of developing benign paroxysmal positional vertigo
Semicircular canals	Vertigo

Skull base

The skull base can be divided into anterior, central, and posterior compartments, with the temporal bone composing the lateral skull base, as discussed previously. The anterior skull base forms the floor of the anterior cranial fossa and the roof of the nasal cavity, orbits, and ethmoid sinuses. It is composed of the cribiform plate and crista galli medially, the orbital plates of the frontal bone more laterally, and the planum sphenoidale and lesser sphenoid wings posteriorly. Important bony foramina include the anterior and posterior ethmoid foramina transmitting the anterior and posterior ethmoid arteries respectively, as well as the cribiform plate foramina transmitting nerve fibers from cranial nerve (CN) I.

The central skull base is composed of the sphenoid bone, its greater wings, and the petrous temporal bone anterior to the petrous ridge. It forms the floor of the middle cranial fossa and the roof of the sphenoid sinus and infratemporal fossae. Central skull base foramina include the optic canal and superior/inferior orbital fissures, the carotid canal, the vidian canal, and foraminas rotundum, ovale, spinosum, and lacerum. CN II–VI are transmitted through central skull base foramina as well as the internal carotid, ophthalmic, and middle meningeal arteries.

The posterior skull base is composed of the posterior temporal bones and occipital bone and forms the floor of the posterior cranial fossa, the foramen magnum, and the superior boundary of the more posterior soft tissue compartments of the neck. Within the posterior skull base, CN VII–VIII are transmitted through the internal auditory canal, and CN IX–XII and the medulla oblongata pass through the foramen magnum. The jugular foramen is also a landmark of the posterior skull base. The foramen magnum is bounded anteriorly by the basilar quadrilateral plate of the occipital bone, laterally by the occipital condyles, and posteriorly by the squamous portion of the occipital bone.

Skull base imaging is traditionally accomplished by both MDCT and contrast-enhanced MRI, as both precise bony detail and soft tissue contrast are required for adequate evaluation (Curtin et al., 1998). Evaluation of the skull base is often performed in the setting of trauma as well as infection or malignancy to assess local extension and perineural spread of tumor, in which case CBCT is of limited value. Incidental skull base disease, however, can be encountered in CBCT scans ordered for other indications (Bremke et al., 2009).

Fibro-osseous lesions

Fibro-osseous pathology involving the skull base will appear similar to that encountered in other bony structures of the body. Paget's disease can involve the skull base, in which case it manifests as patchy or diffuse cortical thickening, blurring of cortico-medullary differentiation, and areas of osteolysis/demineralization. Osteopetrosis is another disease of bone metabolism that can be inherited in an autosomal dominant (adult presentation) or autosomal recessive (childhood presentation) manner. Autosomal dominant osteopetrosis is typically less severe than childhood autosomal recessive disease and appears as relatively uniform dense sclerosis and expansion of the skull base which can encroach on neural foramina and narrow the dural sinuses. The middle and inner ears may also be involved, causing conductive or sensorineural hearing loss. Fibrous dysplasia occurs in the skull base and can exhibit variable morphology including sclerotic, pagetoid, or predominantly cystic patterns as described previously.

Tumor and infection

Aggressive infectious processes that originate in the soft tissues of the head and neck can extend to the skull base and cause osteomyelitis. Classically this can be seen with coalescent mastoiditis, malignant otitis externa, and aggressive sinonasal infections such as invasive fungal sinusitis, although any infection can theoretically extend to the skull base if left untreated. Bone erosions are the hallmark of osteomyelitis, and obliteration of normal fat planes is often seen on MDCT (Chong, 2003). On CBCT, bony erosions with concordant clinical history/findings should raise concern for skull base osteomyelitis. Appropriate imaging evaluation when there is suspicion for skull base osteomyelitis includes MDCT and MRI.

Tumors that involve the skull base include many that have been discussed in the context of sinonasal and temporal bone pathology, as these tumors often extend to and/or arise from the anterior and lateral skull base. In brief, schwannomas, glomus tumors, and endolymphatic sac tumors are classic temporal bone tumors that involve the skull base. The vast majority of schwannomas arise from cranial nerves and are most commonly associated with CN VIII, although schwannomas of other cranial nerves are also encountered. Squamous cell carcinoma, enthesioneuroblastoma, and sinonasal undifferentiated carcinoma can all involve the skull base and have been discussed previously. Metastases and lymphoma should also be on the differential for skull base lesions with imaging features concerning for malignancy.

In addition to the tumors already discussed, chondrosarcoma, plasmacytoma, chordomas, and meningiomas also deserve mention. Chondrosarcomas are aggressive chondroid malignancies that can arise from the skull base, often centered at the petro-occipital fissure. They appear as expansile calcified tumors of the skull base and should be evaluated with MDCT and MRI. Skull base plasmacytomas are monoclonal plasma cell tumors that appear either as a soft tissue mass extending to and involving the skull base (extramedullary), or as lytic lesions centered within the skull base without defined sclerotic margins. Chordomas are rare tumors that arise from remnant notochord elements. They are typically centered in the clivus with imaging features of expansile, multilobulated lytic mass lesions. Meningiomas are relatively common and can arise from any region of the skull base with intracranial exposure, presenting as circumscribed extra-axial soft tissue masses centered on the intracranial dura mater with variable degrees of calcification. All skull base soft tissue masses, especially those with bony erosion, should be further evaluated with MRI.

Finally, benign tumors and tumorlike lesions of the skull base include eosinophilic granuloma and giant cell tumors. Eosinophilic granuloma (or Langerhans cell histiocytosis) is a rare, idiopathic disease of monoclonal histiocyte proliferation with formation of granulomatous tissue. The CT appearance is that of destructive lytic bone lesions, often with soft tissue mass(es). The calvarium is more commonly involved than the skull base, and the lateral skull base is the most typical extracalvarial site of involvement. CECT or MRI are required for more complete evaluation. Skull base giant cell tumors are benign lytic bone lesions that present as expansile soft tissue masses with a thin cortical rim, often centered in the sphenoid or temporal bones.

References

Bachar, G., Siewerdsen, J.H., Daly, M.J., Jaffray, D.A., and Irish, J.C. (2007). Image quality and localization accuracy in C-arm tomosynthesis-guided head and neck surgery. *Medical Physics*, 34(12): 4664–77.

Balbach, L., Trinkel, V., Güldner, C., Bien, S., Teymoortash, A., Werner, J.A., and Bremke, M. (2011). Radiological examinations of the anatomy of the inferior turbinate using digital volume tomography (DVT). *Rhinology*, 49(2): 248–52.

Barath, K., Huber, A.M., Stampfli, P., Varga, Z., and Kollias, S. (2011). Neuroradiology of cholesteatomas. *American Journal of Neuroradiology*, 32(2): 221–9.

Benoudiba, F., Marsot-Dupuch, K., Rabia, M.H., Cabanne, J., Bobin, S., and Lasjaunias, P. (2003). Sinonasal Wegener's granulomatosis: CT characteristics. *Neuroradiology*, 45(2): 95–9.

Bolger, W.E., Butzin, C.A., and Parsons, D.S. (1991). Paranasal sinus bony anatomic variations and mucosal abnormalities: CT analysis for endoscopic sinus surgery. *The Laryngoscope*, 101(1 Pt 1): 56–64.

Branstetter, B.F., IV, and Weissman, J.L. (2005). Role of MR and CT in the paranasal sinuses. *Otolaryngologic Clinics of North America*, 38(6): 1279–99.

Bremke, M., Sesterhenn, A.M., Murthum, T., Al Hail, A., Bien, S., and Werner, J.A. (2009). Digital volume tomography (DVT) as a diagnostic modality of the anterior skull base. *Acta Oto-Laryngologica*, 129(10): 1106–14.

Brook, I. (2006). Sinusitis of odontogenic origin. *Otolaryngology—Head and Neck Surgery*, 135(3): 349–55.

Chong, V. (2003). The skull base in oncologic imaging. *Cancer Imaging*, 4(1): 5–6.

Curtin, H.D., and Chavali, R. (1998). Imaging of the skull base. *Radiologic Clinics of North America*, 36(5): 801–17.

Cymerman, J.J., Cymerman, D.H., and O'Dwyer, R.S. (2011). Evaluation of odontogenic maxillary sinusitis using cone-beam computed tomography: Three case reports. *Journal of Endodontics*, 37(10): 1465–9.

Dalchow, C.V., Weber, A.L., Yanagihara, N., Bien, S., and Werner, J.A. (2006). Digital volume tomography: Radiologic examinations of the temporal bone. *American Journal of Roentgenology*, 186(2): 416–23.

Daly, M.J., Siewerdsen, J.H., Moseley, D.J., Jaffray, D.A., and Irish, J.C. (2006). Intraoperative cone-beam CT for guidance of head and neck surgery: Assessment of dose and image quality using a C-arm prototype. *Medical Physics*, 33(10): 3767–80.

Eggesbo, H.B. (2006). Radiological imaging of inflammatory lesions in the nasal cavity and paranasal sinuses. *European Radiology*, 16(4): 872–88.

Faccioli, N., Barillari, M., Guariglia, S., Zivelonghi, E., Rizzotti, A., Cerini, R., and Mucelli, R.P. (2009). Radiation dose saving through the use of cone-beam CT in hearing-impaired patients. *La Radiologia Medica*, 114(8): 1308–18.

Güldner, C., Diogo, I., Windfuhr, J., Bien, S., Teymoortash, A., Werner, J.A., and Bremke, M. (2011). Analysis of the fossa olfactoria using cone beam tomography (CBT). *Acta Oto-Laryngologica*, 131(1): 72–8.

Güldner, C., Wiegand, S., Weiss, R., Bien, S., Sesterhenn, A., Teymoortash, A., and Diogo, I. (2011). Artifacts of the electrode in cochlea implantation and limits in analysis of deep insertion in cone beam tomography (CBT). *European Archives of Oto-Rhino-Laryngology*. Published online 30 July 2011.

Gupta, R., Bartling, S.H., Basu, S.K., Ross, W.R., Becker, H., Pfoh, A., et al. (2004). Experimental flat-panel high-spatial-resolution volume CT of the temporal bone. *American Journal of Neuroradiology*, 25(8): 1417–24.

Gupta, R., Cheung, A.C., Bartling, S.H., Lisauskas, J., Grasruck, M., Leidecker, C., et al. (2008). Flat-panel volume CT: Fundamental principles, technology, and applications. *Radiographics: A Review Publication of the Radiological Society of North America*, 28(7): 2009–22.

Hoang, J.K., Eastwood, J.D., Tebbit, C.L., and Glastonbury, C.M. (2010). Multiplanar sinus CT: A systematic approach to imaging before functional endoscopic sinus surgery. *American Journal of Roentgenology*, 194(6): W527-36.

Huang, B.Y., Lloyd, K.M., DelGaudio, J.M., Jablonowski, E., and Hudgins, P.A. (2009). Failed endoscopic sinus surgery: Spectrum of CT findings in the frontal recess. *Radiographics: A Review Publication of the Radiological Society of North America*, 29(1): 177–95.

Kamran, M., Nagaraja, S., and Byrne, J.V. (2010). C-arm flat detector computed tomography: The technique and its applications in interventional neuroradiology. *Neuroradiology*, 52(4): 319–27.

Kosling, S., Omenzetter, M., and Bartel-Friedrich, S. (2009). Congenital malformations of the external and middle ear. *European Journal of Radiology*, 69(2): 269–79.

Krombach, G.A., Honnef, D., Westhofen, M., Di Martino, E., and Gunther, R.W. (2008). Imaging of congenital anomalies and acquired lesions of the inner ear. *European Radiology*, 18(2): 319–30.

Lee, T.C., Aviv, R.I., Chen, J.M., Nedzelski, J.M., Fox, A.J., and Symons, S.P. (2009). CT grading of otosclerosis. *American Journal of Neuroradiology*, 30(7): 1435–9.

Lemmerling, M.M., De Foer, B., VandeVyver, V., Vercruysse, J.P., and Verstraete, K.L. (2008). Imaging of the opacified middle ear. *European Journal of Radiology*, 66(3): 363–71.

Maillet, M., Bowles, W.R., McClanahan, S.L., John, M.T., and Ahmad, M. (2011). Cone-beam computed tomography evaluation of maxillary sinusitis. *Journal of Endodontics*, 37(6): 753–7.

Majdani, O., Thews, K., Bartling, S., Leinung, M., Dalchow, C., Labadie, R., et al. (2009). Temporal bone imaging: Comparison of flat panel volume CT and multisection CT. *American Journal of Neuroradiology*, 30(7): 1419–24.

Maroldi, R., Farina, D., Palvarini, L., Marconi, A., Gadola, E., Menni, K., and Battaglia, G. (2001). Computed tomography and magnetic resonance imaging of pathologic conditions of the middle ear. *European Journal of Radiology*, 40(2): 78–93.

Marshall, A.H., Fanning, N., Symons, S., Shipp, D., Chen, J.M., and Nedzelski, J.M. (2005). Cochlear implantation in cochlear otosclerosis. *The Laryngoscope*, 115(10): 1728–33.

Minor, L.B., Solomon, D., Zinreich, J.S., and Zee, D.S. (1998). Sound- and/or pressure-induced vertigo due to bone dehiscence of the superior semicircular canal. *Archives of Otolaryngology—Head and Neck Surgery*, 124(3): 249–58.

Miracle, A.C., and Mukherji, S.K. (2009a). Conebeam CT of the head and neck, part 1: Physical principles. *American Journal of Neuroradiology*, 30(6): 1088–95.

Miracle, A.C., and Mukherji, S.K. (2009b). Conebeam CT of the head and neck, part 2: Clinical applications. *American Journal of Neuroradiology*, 30(7): 1285–92.

Momeni, A.K., Roberts, C.C., and Chew, F.S. (2007). Imaging of chronic and exotic sinonasal disease: Review. *American Journal of Roentgenology*, 189(6 Suppl): S35-45.

Mong, A., Loevner, L.A., Solomon, D., and Bigelow, D.C. (1999). Sound- and pressure-induced vertigo associated with dehiscence of the roof of the superior semicircular canal. *American Journal of Neuroradiology*, 20(10): 1973–5.

Monteiro, E., Das, P., Daly, M., Chan, H., Irish, J., and James, A. (2011). Usefulness of cone-beam computed tomography in determining the position of ossicular prostheses: A cadaveric model. *Otology & Neurotology*, 32(8): 1358–63.

Mukherji, S.K., Gujar, S., Jordan, J.E., et al. (2006). ACR practice guideline for the performance of computed tomography (CT) of the extracranial head and neck in adults and children. *ACR Practice Guideline 2006* (Res 12, 17, 35).

Penninger, R.T., Tavassolie, T.S., and Carey, J.P. (2011). Cone-beam volumetric tomography for applications in the temporal bone. *Otology & Neurotology*, 32(3): 453–60.

Rafferty, M.A., Siewerdsen, J.H., Chan, Y., Daly, M.J., Moseley, D.J., Jaffray, D.A., and Irish, J.C. (2006). Intraoperative cone-beam CT for guidance of temporal bone surgery. *Otolaryngology—Head and Neck Surgery*, 134(5): 801–8.

Ritter, L., Lutz, J., Neugebauer, J., Scheer, M., Dreiseidler, T., Zinser, M.J., et al. (2011). Prevalence of pathologic findings in the maxillary sinus in cone-beam computerized tomography. *Oral Surgery, Oral Medicine, Oral Pathology, Oral Radiology, and Endodontics*, 111(5): 634–40.

Rumboldt, Z., Huda, W., and All, J.W. (2009). Review of portable CT with assessment of a dedicated head CT scanner. *American Journal of Neuroradiology*, 30(9): 1630–6.

Saraiya, P.V., and Aygun, N. (2009). Temporal bone fractures. *Emergency Radiology*, 16(4): 255–65.

Savvateeva, D.M., Güldner, C., Murthum, T., Bien, S., Teymoortash, A., Werner, J.A., et al. (2010). Digital volume tomography (DVT) measurements of the olfactory cleft and olfactory fossa. *Acta Oto-Laryngologica*, 130(3): 398–404.

Schuknecht, B., and Graetz, K. (2005). Radiologic assessment of maxillofacial, mandibular, and skull base trauma. *European Radiology*, 15(3): 560–8.

Stone, J.A., Mukherji, S.K., Jewett, B.S., Carrasco, V.N., and Castillo, M. (2000). CT evaluation of prosthetic ossicular reconstruction procedures: What the otologist needs to know. *Radiographics*, 20(3): 593–605.

Sudhoff, H., Rajagopal, S., Mani, N., Moumoulidis, I., Axon, P.R., and Moffat, D. (2008). Usefulness of CT scans in malignant external otitis: Effective tool for the diagnosis, but of limited value in predicting outcome.

European Archives of Oto-Rhino-Laryngology, 265(1): 53–6.

Tam, A.L., Mohamed, A., Pfister, M., Chinndurai, P., Rohm, E., Hall, A.F., et al. (2010). C-arm cone beam computed tomography needle path overlay for fluoroscopic guided vertebroplasty. *Spine*, 35(10): 1095–9.

Yamane, H., Takayama, M., Sunami, K., Sakamoto, H., Imoto, T., and Anniko, M. (2011). Visualization and assessment of saccular duct and endolymphatic sinus. *Acta Oto-Laryngologica*, 131(5): 469–73.

Yiin, R.S., Tang, P.H., and Tan, T.Y. (2011). Review of congenital inner ear abnormalities on CT temporal bone. *The British Journal of Radiology*, 84(1005): 859–63.

Yousem, D.M. (1993). Imaging of sinonasal inflammatory disease. *Radiology*, 188(2): 303–14.

Zayas, J.O., Feliciano, Y.Z., Hadley, C.R., Gomez, A.A., and Vidal, J.A. (2011). Temporal bone trauma and the role of multidetector CT in the emergency department. *Radiographics*, 31(6): 1741–55.

5 Orthodontic and Orthognathic Planning Using Cone Beam Computed Tomography

Lucia H. S. Cevidanes, Martin Styner, Beatriz Paniagua, and João Roberto Gonçalves

Introduction

Technology development has led to scientific advances in diagnosis and treatment planning in orthodontics and oral maxillofacial surgery. Evidence-based dentistry seems to be a light at the end of a tunnel of benefits, costs, interests, and ethics that will potentially lead to improved quality of life for patients. Specifically, three-dimensional (3D) diagnostic assessment of facial morphology at baseline and overtime has the potential to allow more effective and rational clinical decision making for orthodontic and orthognathic surgery patients. With the availability of cone beam computed tomography (CBCT), the preparation of the surgical plan is shifting from using 2D radiographic images to 3D images and models. In the past ten years, a number of research centers and commercial companies have strived to provide software environments that allow preparation of the operative plan on 3D models of the skeletal structures extracted from the CBCT. As these planning systems begin to be used in clinical practice, it is important to validate the clinical application of these methods, critically assess the difficulty of transferring virtual plans into the operating room, and assess long-term treatment outcomes of surgery. Studies on the 3D bone remodeling and displacements with surgery have helped elucidate clinical questions on variability of outcomes of surgery (Cevidanes, Bailey, et al., 2005; Carvalho et al., 2010; Tucker et al., 2010). Accuracy and reliability of this tool, increased costs, and radiation exposure are some of the aspects to be discussed in this transition.

In this chapter we discuss applications of CBCT to diagnosis, treatment planning, and approaches to measure changes over time. The image analysis tools for 3D images, specifically color maps and 3D "closest point" quantification, have been adapted by us for use with cone beam CTs of the craniofacial complex and have brought significant contribution to clinical needs as they broaden the diagnosis and narrow the treatment targets. However, the closest point method measures displacement that occurs with orthognathic surgery as the smallest separation between the boundaries of the same structure, which may or may not be the appropriate directional distance between equivalent boundaries or landmarks on pre- and postsurgery images. The closest point method cannot be used to quantify longitudinal changes and fails to quantify rotational and large translational movements. Other 3D morphometric

---

Cone Beam Computed Tomography: Oral and Maxillofacial Diagnosis and Applications, First Edition. Edited by David Sarment.
© 2014 John Wiley & Sons, Inc. Published 2014 by John Wiley & Sons, Inc.

approaches under development will also be discussed in this chapter.

Applications of 3D CBCT imaging for diagnosis and treatment planning

Although some clinicians have used CBCT routinely in the orthodontic practice, there are questions on whether the diagnostic benefits justify the radiation dose and the routine use of CBCT. Current applications of 3D CBCT imaging in orthodontics include the following diagnosis and assessment of treatment for complex orthodontic conditions.

Alveolar bone and tooth morphology and relative position

CBCT allows evaluation of buccal and lingual plates of the alveolar bone, bone loss or formation, bone depth and height, presence or absence of unerupted teeth, tooth development, tooth morphology and position, amount of bone covering the tooth, proximity or resorption of adjacent teeth. For such application, the image acquisition can utilize a small or medium field of view that includes an arch quadrant or both upper and lower arches, depending on the clinical indication (Figure 5.1). Such findings in CBCT images may lead to modifications in the orthodontic treatment planning (such as avoid extraction, change plan of which tooth to extract, or placement of bone plates and mini-screws), reduced treatment duration, and improved control of additional root resorption in the ortho-surgical planning (Molen, 2010; Leung et al., 2010; Tai et al., 2010; Becker et al., 2010; Botticelli et al., 2010; Katheria et al., 2010; Leuzinger et al., 2010; Tamimi and ElSaid, 2010; Van Elslande et al., 2010; SHemesh et al., 2011; Sherrard et al., 2010; Treil et al., 2009).

Temporomandibular joint evaluation

For detecting TMJ bony changes, panoramic radiography and MRI have only poor to marginal sensitivity (Ahmad et al., 2009). For this reason, CBCT has recently replaced other imaging modalities as the modality of choice to study TMJ bony changes (Alexiou et al., 2009; Helenius et al., 2005; Koyama et al., 2007). The Research Diagnostic Criteria for Temporomandibular Disorders (RDC/TMD; Dworkin and LeResche, 1992) was revised recently to include image analysis criteria for various imaging modalities (Ahmad et al., 2009). The RDC/TMD validation project (Schiffman et al., 2010; Truelove et al., 2010; Schiffman et al., 2010) concluded that revised clinical criteria alone, without recourse to imaging, are inadequate for valid diagnosis of TMD and had previously underestimated the prevalence of bony changes in the TMJ. TMJ pathologies that result in alterations in the size, form, quality, and spatial relationships of the osseous joint components lead to skeletal and dental discrepancies in the three planes of space. In affected condyles, the perturbed growth and/or bone remodeling, resorption, and apposition can lead to progressive bite changes that are accompanied by compensations in the maxilla, "non-affected" side of the mandible, tooth position, occlusion and articular fossa, and unpredictable orthodontic outcomes (Kapila et al., 2011; Bryndahl et al., 2006).

Like any other joint, the temporomandibular joint (TMJ) is prone to a myriad of pathologies that could be didactically divided as "degenerative pathologies" and "proliferative pathologies" (also see chapter 3 for details). Such pathologies can dramatically affect other craniofacial structures and be easily recognized, or the TMJ pathology can be challenging to diagnose even to experts when its progression is subtle and limited, though still clinically relevant (Figure 5.2). In any situation,

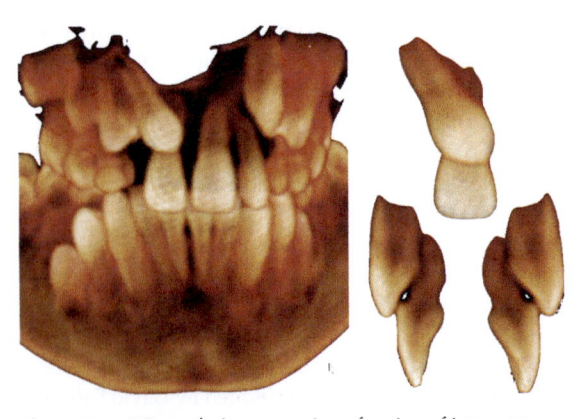

Figure 5.1 3D renderings cropping of region of interest to assess the position of the impacted canine.

longitudinal quantification of condylar changes has the potential to improve clinical decision making, by identifying the most appropriate and beneficial therapy.

The TMJ is unique in relation to the other joints in our body. Adult joint bone surfaces are composed of hyaline cartilage, but the TMJ's bone surfaces are composed of fibro cartilage, which allows a tremendous ability to adapt morphologically according to function. The threshold between functional physiologic stimulus with its positive biochemical effects on the TMJ and joint overloading that leads to degenerative changes is beyond current knowledge (Ishida et al., 2009; Blumberg et al., 2008; Burgin and Aspden, 2008; Roemhildt et al., 2010; Scott and Athanasiou, 2006; Verteramo and Seedhom, 2007). This threshold is influenced by a multitude of factors, including but not limited to the joint loading vectors and their magnitude (Gallo et al., 2008), and patient inherited or acquired (genetic and mostly epigenetic) factors including hormonal and autoimmune imbalances. Current methods to detect pathological conditions in a cross-sectional diagnostic assessment (bone scintigraphy and positron emission tomography) are highly sensitive; however, they do not have enough specificity, as there are no standard normal values for baseline assessments. Longitudinal 3D quantification using CBCTs offers a relative low-cost/low-radiation technology (compared to PET-CT and bone scintigraphy) and can make a significant difference on treatment planning as an additional biomarker or risk factor tool. The use of biomarkers to aid diagnosis in temporomandibular joint disorders is very promising, but it is not novel. Several biomarkers, including C-reactive protein, have previously been identified in blood and in synovial fluid biopsies of patients with TMJ condylar bone resorption and related to the pathological progress (Fredriksson, et al., 2006; Nordahl et al., 2001; Alstergren and Kopp, 2000). Such techniques, still currently restricted to academic environments and research centers, are certainly very promising and will complement CBCT three-dimensional techniques that are already a clinical tool protocol.

Airway assessment

Airway morphology (see chapter 9 for details) and changes overtime with surgery, growth, and its relationship to obstructive sleep apnea have been recently assessed in CBCTs (Abramson et al., 2011; Schendel et al., 2011; Iwasaki et al., 2011; Schendel and Hatcher, 2010; Conley, 2011; Lenza et al., 2010; El and Palomo, 2010). However, the boundaries of the nasopharynx superiorly with the maxillary and paranasal sinuses, and the boundaries of the oropharynx with the oral cavity anteriorly and inferiorly with the larynx, are not consistent among subjects. Additionally, image acquisitions and airway shape and volume will vary markedly with functional stage of the dynamic process of breathing and head posture. If head posture is not correctly reproduced in longitudinal studies, differences in head posture will lead to variability in airway dimensions. Longitudinal assessments of mandibular setback have not shown consistent reduction of airway space, nor have mandibular propulsion devices shown enlargement of the airway space

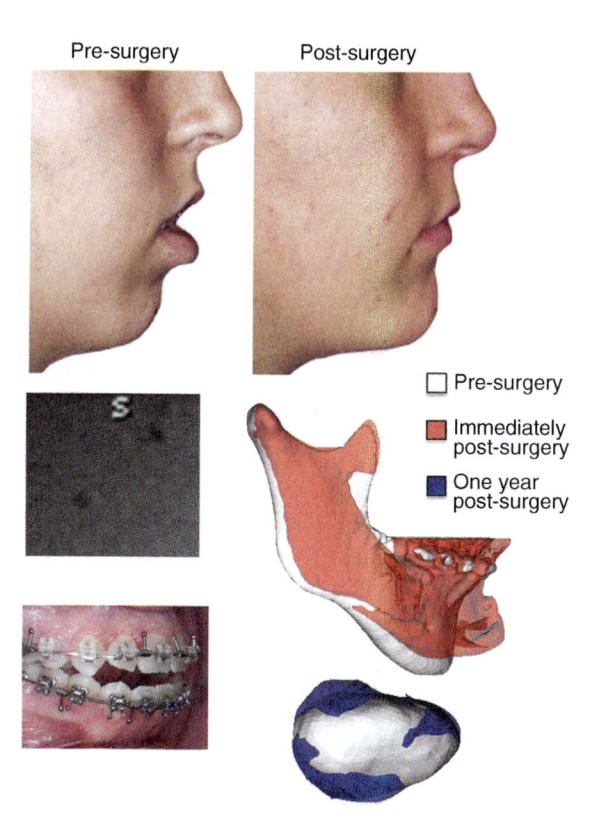

Figure 5.2 Two-jaw surgery where disc displacement without capture at open bite was diagnosed in MRI. Surgical correction included disc repositioning. Please note in blue the condylar remodeling 1 year post-surgery.

Pre-surgery — Splint removal — 1 year post-surgery

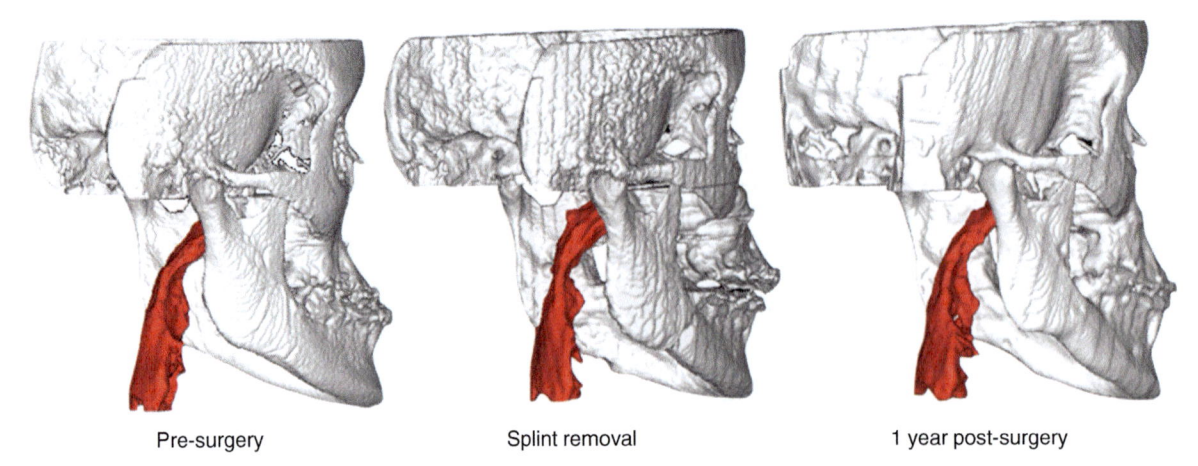

Figure 5.3 Longitudinal assessments of mandibular setback reveal reduction of airway space of the lower portion of the pharynx at splint removal. However, this airway space reduction is no longer observed at 1 year post-surgery.

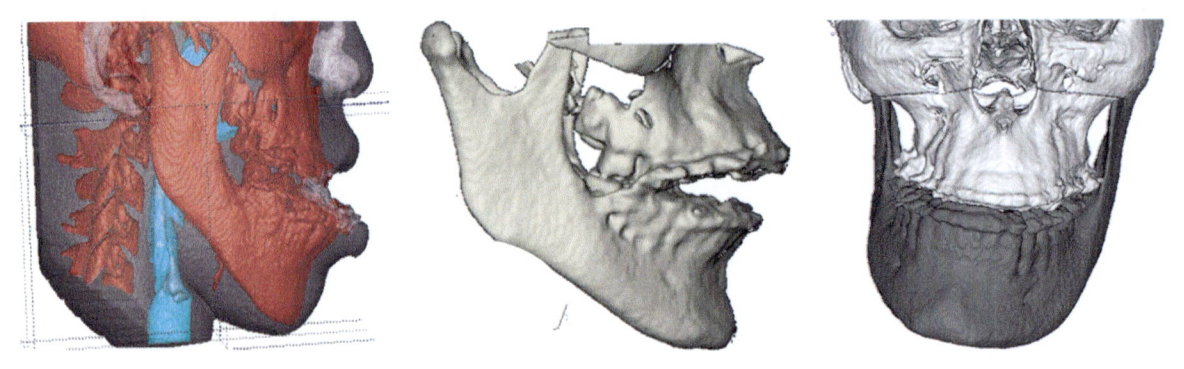

Figure 5.4 Skeletal antero-posterior, vertical, and transverse discrepancies shown in surface models.

that might be helpful for obstructive breathing conditions (Figure 5.3). Retroglossal airway changes after extraction of four bicuspids and retraction of lower anterior teeth or after significant surgical mandibular advancement or setback are prone to great variability and are still under scrutiny in studies.

Dentofacial deformities and craniofacial anomalies

CBCT imaging offers the ability to analyze facial asymmetry and antero-posterior, vertical, and transverse discrepancies (Figure 5.4). The virtual treatment simulations can be used for treatment planning in orthopedic corrections and orthognathic surgery and for printing surgical splints. Computer-aided jaw surgery is increasingly in use clinically due to the possibility of incorporating a high level of precision for accurately transferring virtual plans into the operating room. In complex cases, follow-up CBCT acquisitions, for growth observation, treatment progress, and posttreatment observations, may be helpful to assess stability of the correction overtime (Agarwal, 2011; Behnia et al., 2011; Dalessandri et al., 2011; Ebner et al., 2010; Edwards, 2010; Jayaratne, Zwahlen, Lo, and Cheung, 2010; Kim et al., 2011; Abou-Elfetouh et al., 2011; Lloyd et al., 2011; Gateno et al., 2011; Almeida et al., 2011; Cevidanes et al., 2010; Orentlicher et al., 2010; Jayaratne, Zwahlen, Lo, Tam, et al., 2010; Popat and Richmond, 2010; Schendel and Lane, 2009).

The methods for computer-aided systems in jaw surgery follow procedures from the image scanners to the operating room (Figure 5.5) and have

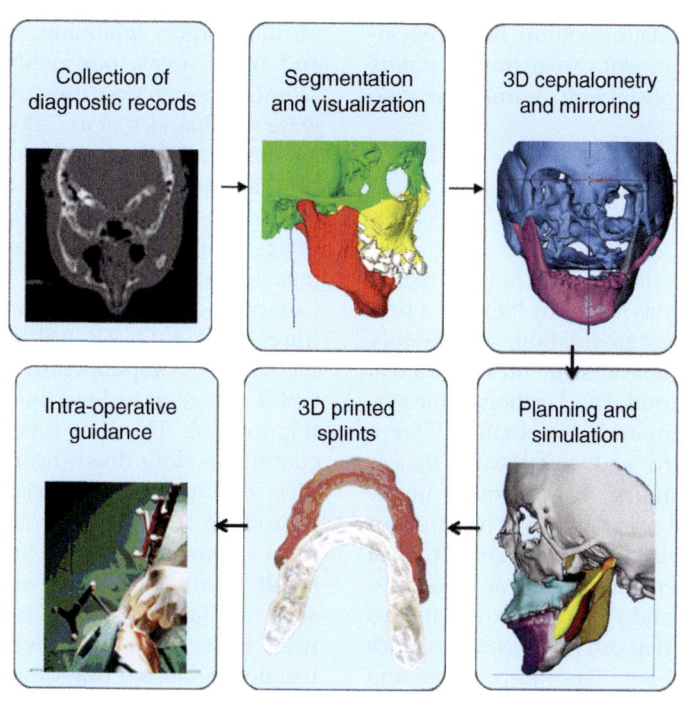

Figure 5.5 Steps in computer-assisted surgery.

included commercially a number of systems, such as Medical Modeling (Texas) and Maxilim (Medicim, Mechelen, Belgium). The advantages of those systems are that they do not require time or computer expertise for the surgeon, and for a service fee, the commercial companies construct surface models from CBCTs and impressions or digital dental casts registered to the CBCT, perform the virtual surgery, and print surgical splints. The computer-aided surgery steps include (1) data acquisition: collection of diagnostic data; (2) image segmentation: identification of anatomic structures of interest in the image data sets and visualization of 3D display of the anatomic structures; (3) diagnosis: extraction of clinical information from the 3D representations of the anatomy, for example, by using mirroring planes; (4) planning and simulation: preparation of an operative plan by using the virtual anatomy, and preparation of a simulation of the outcome; (5) 3D printed surgical guides or individually fabricated synthetic grafts or prosthetic repair; and (6) intraoperative guidance: assistance for intraoperative realization of the virtual plan.

(1) Collection of diagnostic records

Diagnosis of skeletal discrepancies is based on visual data coming from different sources: clinical examination, 3D photographic examination, CBCT, CT, MRI, and digital dental models. Computer-assisted systems must integrate different records in order to characterize the orthodontic diagnosis and formulate the treatment plan. Multimodality registration is available for a number of commercial software programs, such as 3DMDvultus (3DMD, Atlanta, GA), Maxilim (Medicim, Mechelen, Belgium), Dolphin Imaging (Dolphin Imaging & Management Solutions, Chatsworth, CA), InVivo-Dental (Anatomage, San Jose, CA), and SimPlant OMS (Materialise, Leuven, Belgium). The CMFApp software (developed under the funding of the Co-Me network; CMFApp software, 2012) and Slicer3 (3DSlicer software, 2012; National Alliance for Medical Image Computing, NIH Roadmap) provide uniform medical data handling preoperative grey level image (CBCT, CT, MRI), skeletal models, acquired dental occlusion, operative plans, diagnostic data (3D cephalometry, mirrored structures), planning data (osteotomy lines, repositioning plans), guidance data (registration points and transformations), postoperative image, and so forth.

(2) Segmentation and visualization of anatomic structures of interest

The acquired DICOM files can be imported into diverse 3D image analysis software. Next, in a process known as image segmentation, we identify and delineate the anatomical structures of interest in the image. In orthodontics and orthognathic surgery, the goal of segmentation is to obtain a 3D representation of the hard and soft tissues that is usable for virtual planning. Even though image segmentation has been a field of active research for many decades, it remains one of the hardest, most frequently required steps in image processing systems. There does not and cannot exist a standard segmentation method that can be expected to work equally well for all tasks. The morphology and position of the condyles, and the internal surface of the ramus and maxilla are critical for careful virtual surgery planning. To best capture these and other areas, our method of choice for the segmentation procedures utilizes ITK-SNAP software (Yushkevich et al., 2006), which has received continuous NIH support for further open-source software development. ITK-SNAP was developed, based on the NIH Visualization Tool Kit and Image Tool Kit (ITK), as part of the NIH Roadmap Initiative for National Centers of Biomedical Computing. The automatic segmentation procedures in ITK-SNAP utilize two active contour methods to compute feature images based on the CBCT image gray level intensity and boundaries (Figure 5.6). The first method causes the active contour to slow down near edges, or discontinuities, of intensity. The second causes the active contour to attract to boundaries of regions of uniform intensity. After obtaining the segmentation result, manual postprocessing is normally necessary. Artifacts resulting from metallic elements need to be removed. Lower and upper jaws are usually connected due to insufficient longitudinal image resolution and must be separated in the temporomandibular joint and on the occlusal surface

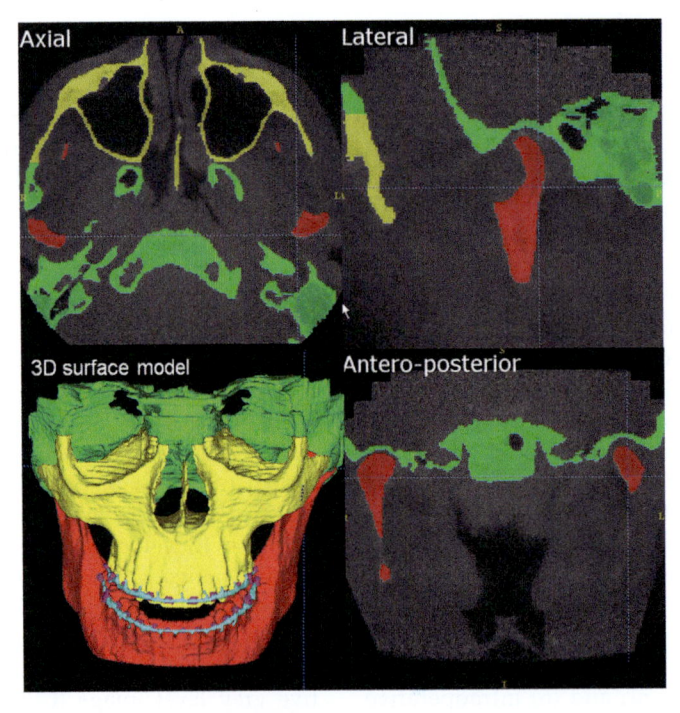

Figure 5.6 Construction of surface models using ITK-SNAP.

in particular. For this reason, it has been recommended that the CBCT be taken in centric occlusion with a stable and thin bite registration material (Swennen et al., 2009). On a laptop computer equipped with 1 GB of RAM, the initial mesh generation step typically takes about 15 minutes. Manual postprocessing usually takes longer, up to a couple of hours (separation of the jaws can be particularly tedious).

Two technological options are available to visualize these structures three dimensionally. The first is surface-based methods, which require the generation of an intermediate surface representation (triangular mesh) of the object to be displayed, providing very detailed shading of the facial surfaces at any zoom factor. The second is volume-based methods, which create a 3D view directly from the volume data (Pommert et al., 1996). The advantage of a surface-based method is the very detailed shading of the facial surfaces at any zoom factor. Also, any other three-dimensional structure that can be represented by a triangular mesh can be easily included in the anatomical view (e.g., implants imported from CAD implant databases). The majority of existing cranio-maxillofacial surgery planning software uses surface-based visualization. An obvious disadvantage of surface-based methods is the need for an intermediate surface representation. The advantage of a volumetric method is that volumetric operations are immediately visible in three dimensions, as well as in cross-sectional images. For example, virtual osteotomies can be applied on the original image dataset and seen in three dimensions (see chapter 7 for more details). The main limitation of this representation is the difficulty of establishing the boundaries between tissues and assigning the proper color/transparency values to obtain the desired display. Moreover, the image intensity for a given tissue can vary between patients and scanners (e.g., bone density varies with age and metabolic status; there are variations in scanner calibrations). Virtual cutting operations are much more difficult to simulate in voxel-wise representations. Further evolutions in software and graphics hardware that combine both surface- and volume-based visualization technologies have great potential as they offer complementary information and might expedite the process.

(3) Diagnosis using 3D cephalometry and mirroring techniques

Morphometrics is the branch of mathematics studying shapes and shape changes of geometric objects. Cephalometrics is a subset of morphometrics. Clinically, it is used to analyze a set of points, either of anatomical meaning or from an abstract definition (such as middle point between two other points), and understanding of facial morphology is described by angles and linear measurements (Figure 5.7). Surface and shape data available in 3D imaging provide new characterization schemes, based on higher order mathematical entities (e.g., spline curves and surfaces). For example, Cutting et al. (1996) and Subsol et al. (1998) introduced the concept of ridge curves for automatic cephalometric characterization. Ridge curves (also known as crest lines) of a surface are the loci of the maximal curvature, in the associated principal curvature directions. The ridge lines of a surface convey very rich and compact information, which tends to correspond to natural anatomic features. Lines of high curvature are typical reference features in the craniofacial skeleton. Future studies will establish new standards for 3D measurements in the craniofacial skeleton. New developments in this area might lead to comprehensive 3D morphometric systems, including surface-based and volume-based computed shape measurements (Figure 5.8).

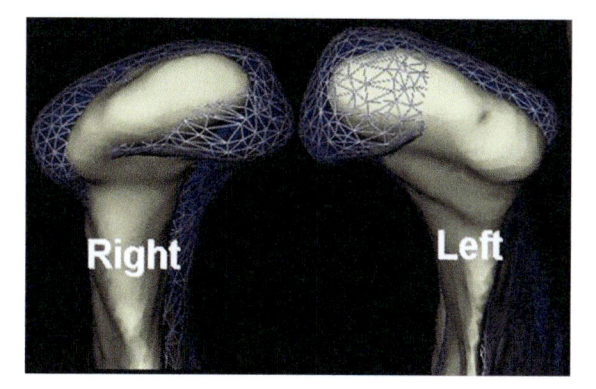

Figure 5.7 Overlay of pre-surgery (solid) and 1 year post-surgery (mesh) surface models of the mandibular condyles. The condylion landmarks in the pre-surgery and 1 year post-surgery could not be homologous points in the condyles, when marked bone changes have occurred.

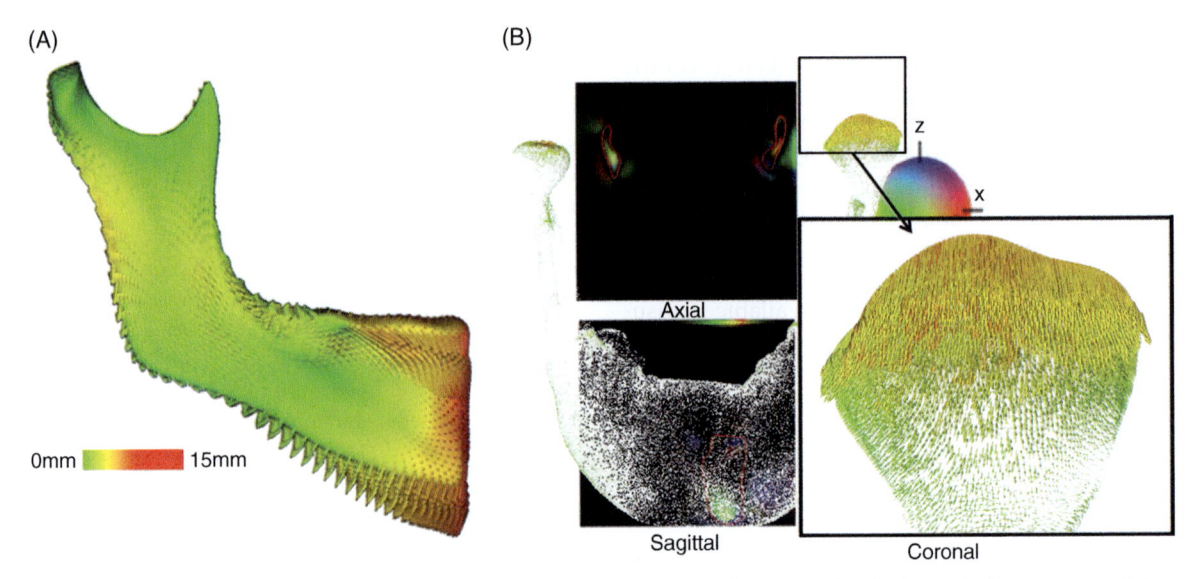

Figure 5.8 Correspondence shape analysis methods. (A) Vectors color maps of correspondent before and after surgery models using surface-based models that are parameterized into point-based models. (B) Color maps using tensor-based morphometry.

They could also lead to "four-dimensional" (4D) shape information, which integrates evolution over time in the analysis, an application of great relevance allowing early diagnosis of postintervention unexpected positional changes. Clinical decisions could therefore be influenced to avoid further complications.

(4) Surgical planning and simulation

After establishment of the diagnosis, the next step is to use the 3D representations of the anatomy to plan and simulate the surgical intervention. In orthognathic surgery, corrective interventions designate procedures that do not require an extrinsic graft, and reconstructive interventions are designated for situations in which a graft is used. In corrective procedures, it is important to determine the location of the surgical cuts, to plan the movements of the bony segments relative to one another, and to achieve the desired realignment intraoperatively. In reconstructive procedures, problems arise in determining the desired implant or graft shape. In the case of implants and prosthesis, the problems are to select the proper device and shape it, or to fabricate an individual device from a suitable biocompatible material. With a graft, the difficulties lie in choosing the harvesting site, shaping the graft, and placing the implant or graft in the appropriate location (Chapuis, 2006).

Virtual osteotomies allow for planning of cuts as well as position and size of fixation screws and plates, taking into account the intrinsically complex cranial anatomy. The surface model can also include regions of thin (or absent) bone, such as the maxillary sinus anterior wall, which can create sudden discontinuities in the mesh, as well as inner structures (e.g., mandibular nerve canal). After the virtual osteotomy, the virtual surgery with relocation of the bony segments can be performed with quantification of the planned surgical movements (Chapuis et al., 2007; De Momi et al., 2006; Krol et al., 2005; Chapuis, Langlotz, et al., 2005; Chapuis, Ryan, et al., 2005). Relocation of the anatomical segments with six degrees of freedom is tracked for each bone fragment. This allows for the correction of the skeletal discrepancy for a given patient and simultaneous tracking of measurements of X, Y, and Z translation and rotation around each of these axes. The rendering of the new position can be used as an initial suggestion to the surgeon, for discussions of the 3D orthodontic and surgical treatment goals, and/or for printing surgical splints if high-resolution scans of the dental structure are registered to the

CBCT and if the software tool presents an occlusion detection functionality.

Simulation of soft tissue changes
Methods that attempt to predict facial soft tissue changes resulting from skeletal reshaping utilize approximation models, since direct formulation and analytical resolution of the equations of continuum mechanics is not possible with such geometrical complexity. Different types of models have been proposed: displacements of soft tissue voxels are estimated with the movements of neighboring hard tissue voxels (Schutyser et al., 2000), bone displacement vectors are simply applied on the vertices of the soft tissue mesh (Xia et al., 2000), and multilayer mass-spring models (Teschner et al., 2001; Keeve et al., 1996; Mollemans, et al., 2007), finite element models (Westermark et al., 2005; Chabanas et al., 2003; Schendel and Montgomery, 2009), and mass tensor models (Keeve et al., 1998) assume biological properties of soft tissue response. In any case, thorough validation reports for all these methods are still lacking. Comparisons of the simulation with the postoperative facial surface have not yet been performed. Surgical planning functions generally do not fulfill the requirements enumerated above for the preparation of quantitative facial tissue simulation. Other functionalities that have been incorporated into different software systems include simulation of muscular function (Zachow et al., 2001), distraction osteogenesis planning (Gladilin et al., 2004), and 4D surgery planning (Gateno et al., 2003).

(5) Intraoperative surgical navigation

During surgical procedures, achieving the desired bone segment realignment freehand is difficult. Further, segments must often be moved with very limited visibility, for example, under the (swollen) soft tissues. Approaches used currently in surgery rely largely on the clinician's experience and intuition. In maxillary repositioning, for example, a combination of dental splints, compass, ruler, and intuition are used to determine the final position. It has been shown that in the vertical direction (in which the splint exerts no constraint), only limited control is achieved (Vandewalle et al., 2003). While the surgical splint guides the position of the maxilla relative to the mandible, in two-jaw surgeries the spatial position of the two jaws relative to the face is influenced by the splint precision and the trans-surgical vertical assessment. As splints are made over teeth while guiding bone changes away from those teeth, small splint inaccuracies may result in significant bone position inaccuracies. The predictability of precise osteotomies in the wide variety of patient morphologies and consequent controlled fractures such as in the pterigoyd plates, sagittal split osteotomies, or interdental cuts are still a concern. In reconstructive procedures, the problems of shaping and placing a graft or implant in the planned location also arises. Surgical navigation systems have been developed to help accurately transfer treatment plans to the operating room.

Tracking technology
Different tracking technologies (Langlotz, 2004; Kim et al., 2009) for the displacement of a mobilized fragment in the course of an osteotomy can be used with respective advantages and disadvantages:

1. *Ultrasound:* An array of three ultrasound emitters is mounted on the object to be tracked, but the speed of sound value can vary with temperature changes and the calibration procedure is very delicate.
2. *Electromagnetic tracking:* A homogeneous magnetic field is created by a generator coil. Ferromagnetic items such as implants, instruments, or the operation table can interfere strongly with these systems, distorting the measurements in an unpredictable way. Newer systems claim reduction of these effects and feature receivers the size of a needle head, possibly heralding a renewal of interest for electromagnetic tracking in surgical navigation (examples are the 3D guidance trackstar, Ascension, Burlington, VT; StealthStation AXIEM, Medtronic, Louisville, CO; and Aurora, Northern Digital Inc., Ontario, Canada).
3. *Infrared optical tracking devices:* These rely on pairs or triplets of charged coupled devices that detect positions of infrared markers. A free line of sight is required between the cameras and markers.

Longitudinal assessments using CBCT

Over the last decade we have utilized longitudinal CBCT images for assessment of treatment outcomes. Even with the availability of 3D images, there are critical barriers that must be overcome before longitudinal quantitative assessment of the craniofacial complex can be routinely performed. These are outlined below.

Radiation from CBCT acquisition

The use of 3D images for treatment planning and follow-up raises concerns regarding radiation dose, requiring guidelines for specific applications rather than indiscriminate use.

Construction of 3D surface models

Longitudinal quantitative assessment of growth, surgical correction, and stability of results requires construction of 3D surface models. Segmentation, the process of constructing 3D models by examining cross-sections of a volumetric data set to outline the shape of structures, remains a challenge (Adams and Bischof, 1994; Ma and Manjunath, 2000; Lie, 1995; Moon et al., 2002). Many standard automatic segmentation methods fail when applied to the complex anatomy of patients with facial deformity. The methods described by Gerig et al. (2003) address these technical difficulties and have been adapted by Cevidanes et al. (2005, 2006, 2010) in our laboratory to construct 3D craniofacial models.

Image registration

Image registration is a core technology for many imaging tasks. The two obstacles to widespread clinical use of nonrigid (elastic and deformable) registration are computational cost and quantification difficulties, as the 3D models are deformed (Christensen et al., 1996; Rueckert et al., 1999; Hajnal et al., 2001). Nonrigid registration is required to create a composite of several different jaw shapes preoperatively to guide the construction of 3D surface models (Thompson et al., 1997). However, to evaluate surgical displacements, rigid registration has advantages for longitudinal assessments (Maes et al., 1997). We have developed (Cevidanes, Bailey, et al., 2005; Cevidanes, Phillips, et al., 2005; Cevidanes et al., 2006) a novel sequence of fully automated voxel-wise rigid registration at the cranial base and superimposition (overlay) methods (Figure 5.9). The major strength of this method is that registration does not depend on the precision of the 3D surface models. The cranial base models are only used to mask anatomic structures that change with growth and treatment. The registration procedures actually compare voxel by voxel of gray-level CBCT images, containing only the cranial base, to calculate rotation and translation parameters between the two images.

Regional superimposition in the anterior cranial base does not completely define the movement of the mandible relative to the maxilla. Future studies are needed to investigate the use of different 3D regional superimposition areas. Currently, superimposition of 3D surface models is still too time consuming and computing intensive to apply these methods in routine clinical use. Our current focus is on developing a simplified analysis so that soon these methods can be used clinically.

Quantitative measurements

Precise quantitative measurement is required to assess the placement of bones in the desired position, the bone remodeling, and the position of surgical cuts and fixation screws and/or plates relative to risk structures. Current quantification methods include the following:

a. *Volume* changes (Thompson et al., 1997) reflect increase or decrease in size, but structural changes at specific locations are not sufficiently reflected in volume measurements; volume assessment does not reveal location and direction of proliferative or resorptive changes, which would be relevant for assessment clinical results.
b. *Landmark*-based measurements (Rohr, 2001) present errors related to landmark identification. Locating 3D landmarks on complex

(A)   (B)

☐ Pre-surgery
■ Immediately post-surgery (red)
■ One year post-surgery (blue)

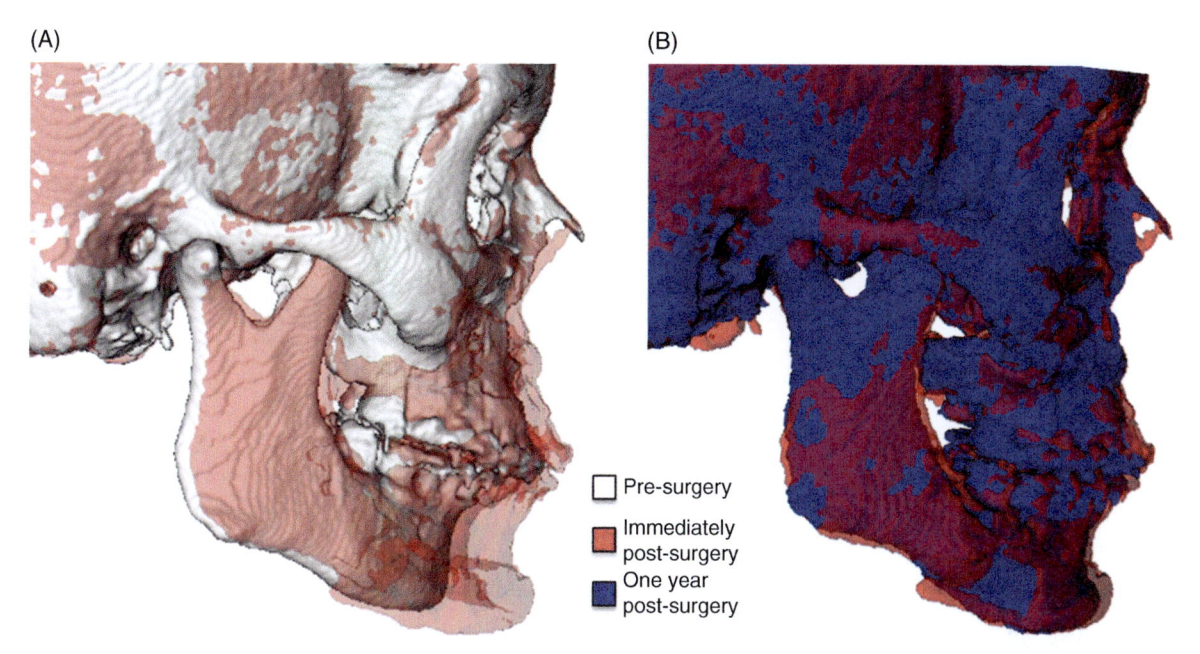

Figure 5.9 Longitudinal follow-up of treatment outcomes of surgery. Surface models of pre-surgery (white), immediately after surgery (red), and 1 year post-surgery (blue) were superimposed on the cranial base. (A) Overlay of pre-surgery and immediately after surgery. (B) Overlay of immediately after surgery and 1 year post-surgery.

curving structures is not a trivial problem for representation of components of the craniofacial form (Dean et al., 2000). As Bookstein (1991) noted, there is a lack of literature about suitable operational definitions for the landmarks in the three planes of space (coronal, sagittal, and axial). Gunz et al. (2004) and Andresen et al. (2000) proposed the use of semi-landmarks, that is, landmarks plus vectors and tangent planes that define their location, but information from the whole curves and surfaces must also be included. The studies of Subsol et al. (1998) and Andresen et al. (2000) provided clear advances toward studies of curves or surfaces in 3D, referring to tens of thousands of 3D points to define geometry.

c. *Closest point* measurements between the surfaces can display changes with color maps, as proposed by Gerig et al. (2001). However, the closest point method measures closest distances, not corresponding distances between anatomical points on two or more longitudinally obtained images (Figure 5.10). For this reason, the closest point measurements completely fail to quantify rotational and large translational movements, and this method cannot be used for longitudinal assessments of growth or treatment changes, nor the physiologic adaptations, such as bone remodeling that follows surgery.

d. *Shape correspondence:* The SPHARM-PDM framework (Styner et al., 2006; Gerig et al., 2001) was developed as part of the National Alliance of Medical Image Computing, (NAMIC, NIH Roadmap for Medical Research), and has been adapted for use with CBCTs of the craniofacial complex (Paniagua, Cevidanes, Walker, et al., 2010; Paniagu, Cevidanes, Zhu, et al., 2010). SPHARM-PDM is a tool that computes point-based models using a parametric boundary description for the computing of shape analysis. The 3D virtual surface models are converted into a corresponding spherical harmonic description (SPHARM), which is then sampled into a triangulated surface (SPHARM-PDM). This work presents an improvement in outcome measurement as compared to closest point

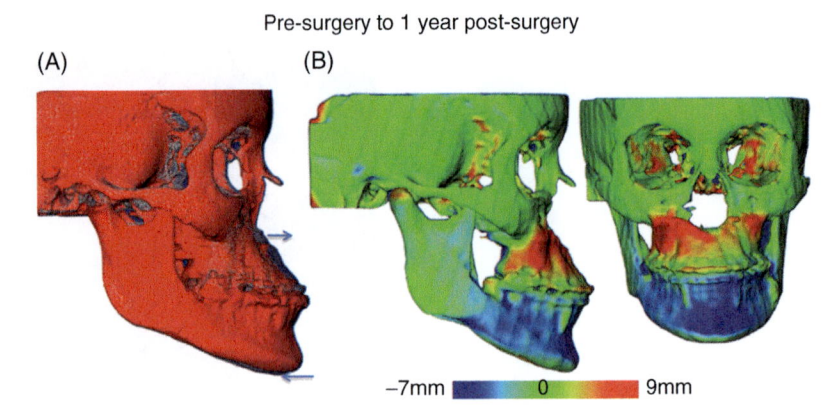

Figure 5.10 Lateral and frontal view of closest point distance color maps between pre-surgery and 1 year post-surgery. (A) Overlay of pre-surgery (red) and 1 year post-surgery (semi-transparent mesh) surface models where the arrows point to the direction of jaw displacements 1 year post-surgery. (B) The color maps are displayed in the 1 year post-surgery model and show the amount of maxillary advancement in red and mandibular setback in blue.

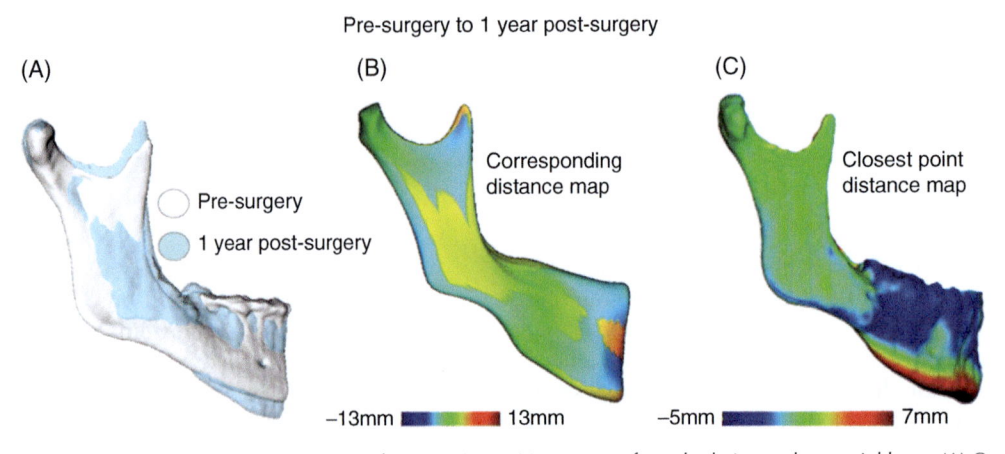

Figure 5.11 What do color maps measure? Note that superimposition was perfomed relative to the cranial base. (A) Overlay of pre-surgery (white) and 1 year post-surgery (blue) surface models. (B and C) Two different types of color maps displayed in the 1 year post-surgery model. (B) Correspondent point-based color maps that reflect the pattern of bone changes shown in A. (C) Closest point surface distance color maps. Note that because the remodeling of the ramus was marked, the pattern of the color map does not reflect the actual remodeling and minimizes the measured surface changes.

correspondence–based analysis. This standard analysis is currently used by most commercial and academic softwares but does not map corresponding surfaces based in anatomical geometry, and it usually underestimates rotational and large translational movements. Closest point color maps measure surgical jaw displacement as the smallest separation between boundaries of the same structure, which may not be the right anatomical corresponding boundaries on pre- and postsurgery anatomical structures (Figure 5.11).

References

3DSlicer software. http://www.slicer.org/. Accessed March 1, 2012.

Abou-Elfetouh, A., Barakat, A., and Abdel-Ghany, K. (2011). Computed-guided rapid-prototyped templates for segmental mandibular osteotomies: A preliminary report. *Int J Med Robot*, 7(2): 187–92.

Abramson, Z., Susarla, S.M., Lawler, M., Bouchard, C., Troulis, M., and Kaban, L.B. (2011). Three-dimensional computed tomographic airway analysis of patients with obstructive sleep apnea treated by maxillomandibular advancement. *J Oral Maxillofac Surg*, 69(3): 677–86.

Adams, R., and Bischof, L. (1994). Seeded region growing. *IEEE Trans Pattern Analysis and Machine Intelligence*, 16(6): 641–7.

Agarwal, R. (2011). Anthropometric evaluation of complete unilateral cleft lip nose with cone beam CT in early childhood. *J Plast Reconstr Aesthet Surg*, 64(7): e181–2.

Ahmad, M., Hollender, L., Anderson, Q., Kartha, K., Ohrbach, R.K., Truelove, E.L., John, M.T., and Schiffman, E.L. (2009). Research diagnostic criteria for temporomandibular disorders (RDC/TMD): Development of image analysis criteria and examiner reliability for image analysis. *Oral Surg Oral Med Oral Pathol Oral Radiol Endod*, 107(6): 844–60; NIHMS121369.

Alexiou, K., Stamatakis, H., and Tsiklakis, K. (2009). Evaluation of the severity of temporomandibular joint osteoarthritic changes related to age using cone beam computed tomography. *Dentomaxillofac Radiol*, 38(3): 141–7.

Almeida, R.C., Cevidanes, L.H., Carvalho, F.A., Motta, A.T., Almeida, M.A., Styner, M., et al. (2011). Soft tissue response to mandibular advancement using 3D CBCT scanning. *Int J Oral Maxillofac Surg*, 40(4): 353–9.

Alstergren, P., and Kopp, S. (2000). Prostaglandin E2 in temporomandibular joint synovial fluid and its relation to pain and inflammatory disorders. *J Oral Maxillofac Surg*, 58(2): 180–8.

Andresen, R., Bookstein, F.L., Conradsen, K., Ersboll, B.K., Marsh, J.L., and Kreiborg, S. (2000). Surface-bounded growth modeling applied to human mandibles. *IEEE Trans Med Imaging 2000*, 19: 1053–63.

Becker, A., Chaushu, C., and Casap-Caspi, N. (2010). Cone-beam computed tomography and the orthosurgical management of impacted teeth. *J Am Dent Assoc*, 141: 14S–18S.

Behnia, H., Khojasteh, A., Soleimani, M., Tehranchi, A., and Atashi, A. (2011). Repair of alveolar cleft defect with mesenchymal stem cells and platelet derived growth factors: A preliminary report. *J Craniomaxillofac Surg*. Epub 2011 March 21.

Blumberg, T.J., Natoli, R.M., and Athanasiou, K.A. (2008). Effects of doxycycline on articular cartilage GAG release and mechanical properties following impact. *Biotechnol Bioeng*, 100(3): 506–515. doi:10.1002/bit.21778.

Bookstein, F.L. (1991). *Morphometric tools for landmark data* (1st ed.). Cambridge, England: Cambridge University Press.

Botticelli, S., Verna, C., Cattaneo, P.M., Heidmann, J., and Melsen, B. (2010). Two- versus three-dimensional imaging in subjects with unerupted maxillary canines. *Eur J Orthod*, Epub 2010 December 3:1–6.

Bryndahl, F., Eriksson, L., Legrell, P.E., and Isberg, A. (2006). Bilateral TMJ disk displacement induces mandibular retrognathia. *J Dent Res*, 85: 1118–23.

Burgin, L.V., and Aspden, R.M. (2008). Impact testing to determine the mechanical properties of articular cartilage in isolation and on bone. *J Mater Sci Mater Med*, 19(2): 703–11. doi:10.1007/s10856-007-3187-2.

Carvalho, Fde. A., Cevidanes, L.H., da Motta, A.T., Almeida, M.A., and Phillips, C. (2010). Three-dimensional assessment of mandibular advancement 1 year after surgery. *Am J Orthod Dentofac Orthop*, 137(4Suppl): S53.e1-S53.e12.

Cevidanes, L.H.S., Bailey, L.T.J., Tucker Jr., G.R., Styner, M.A., Mol, A., Phillips, C.L., et al. (2005). Superimposition of 3D cone-beam CT models of orthognathic surgery patients. *Dentomaxillofacial Radiology*, 34(6): 369–75.

Cevidanes, L.H.S., Phillips, C.L., Tulloch, J.F.C., and Proffit, W.R. (2005). Superimposition of 3D cone-beam CT models of orthognathic surgery patients. In: J.A. McNamara, ed., *3D Imaging*. Moyers Symposium Series.

Cevidanes, L.H.S., Styner, M.A., and Proffit, W.R. (2006). Image analysis and superimposition of 3D cone-beam CT models. *Am J Orthod Dentofacial Orthop*, 129(5): 611–8.

Cevidanes, L.H.S., Tucker, S., Styner, M., Kim, H., Chapuis, J., Reyes, M., et al. (2010). Three-dimensional surgical simulation. *Am J Orthod Dentofac Orthop*, 138(3): 361–71.

Chabanas, M., Luboz, V., Payan, Y. (2003). Patient specific finite element model of the face soft tissues for computer-assisted maxillofacial surgery. *Med Image Anal*, 7(2): 131–51.

Chapuis, J. (2006). *Computer-aided cranio-maxillofacial surgery*. PhD thesis, University of Bern.

Chapuis, J., Langlotz, F., Blaeuer, M., Hallermann, W., Schramm, A., and Caversaccio, M. (2005). A novel approach for computer-aided corrective jaw surgery. 3rd International Conference on Computer-Aided Surgery around the Head, Berlin, Germany. 2005 August.

Chapuis, J., Ryan, P., Blaeuer, M., Langlotz, F., Hallermann, W., Schramm, A., et al. (2005). A new approach for 3D computer-assisted orthognathic surgery—first clinical case. Conference on Computer Assisted Radiology and Surgery, Berlin, Germany. 2005 June.

Chapuis, J., Schramm, A., Pappas, I., Hallermann, W., Schwenzer-Zimmerer, K., Langlotz, F., et al. (2007). A new system for computer-aided preoperative planning and intraoperative navigation during corrective jaw surgery. *IEEE Trans Inf Technol Biomed*, 11(3): 274–87.

Christensen, G.E., Rabbitt, R.D., Miller, M.I. (1996). Deformable templates using large deformation kinematics. *IEEE Trans Image Processing*, 5:1435–47.

CMFApp software. http://co-me.ch/. Accessed March 1, 2012.

Conley, R.S. (2011). Evidence for dental and dental specialty treatment of obstructive sleep apnoea. Part 1: the adult OSA patient and Part 2: the paediatric and adolescent patient. *J Oral Rehabil*, 38(2): 136–56.

Crum, W.R., Hartkens, T., and Hill, D.L. (2004). Non-rigid image registration: Theory and practice. *Br J Radiol*, 77(2): S140–53.

Cutting, C.B., Bookstein, F.L., Taylor, R.H. (1996). Applications of simulation, morphometrics, and robotics in craniofacial surgery. In: R. Taylor, S. Lavallee, G. Burdea, and R. Mosges, eds., *Computer Integrated Surgery* (pp. 641–62). Cambridge, MA: MIT Press.

Dalessandri, D., Laffranchi, L., Tonni, I., Zoti, F., Piancino, M.G., Paganelli, C., et al. (2011). Advantages of cone beam computed tomography (CBCT) in the orthodontic treatment planning of cleidocranial dysplasia patients: A case report. *Head Face Med*, 27: 7–6.

De Momi, E., Chapuis, J., Pappas, I., Ferrigno, G., Hallermann, W., Schramm, A., et al. (2006). Automatic extraction of the mid-facial plane for craniomaxillofacial surgery planning. *Int J Oral Maxillofac Surg*, 35(7): 636–42.

Dean, D., Hans, M.G., Bookstein, F.L., and Subramanyan, K., (2000). Three-dimensional Bolton-Brush Growth Study landmark data: Ontogeny and sexual dimorphism of the Bolton Standards cohort. *Cleft Palate Craniofac J*, 37: 145–55.

Ebner, F.H., Kürschner, V., Dietz, K., Bültmann, E., Nägele, T., and Honegger, J. (2010). Craniometric changes in patients with acromegaly from a surgical perspective. *Neurosurg Focus*, 29(4): E3.

Edwards, S.P. Computer-assisted craniomaxillofacial surgery. (2010). *Oral Maxillofac Surg Clin North Am*, 22(1): 117–34.

El, H., and Palomo, J.M. (2010). Measuring the airway in 3 dimensions: A reliability and accuracy study. *Am J Orthod Dentofacial Orthop*, 137(4 Suppl): S50.e1–9; discussion S50-2.

Fredriksson, L., Alstergren, P., and Kopp, S. (2006). Tumor necrosis factor-alpha in temporomandibular joint synovial fluid predicts treatment effects on pain by intraarticular glucocorticoid treatment. *Mediators Inflamm*, 2006(6): 59425.

Gallo, L.M., Gössi, D.B., Colombo, V., and Palla, S. (2008). Relationship between kinematic center and TMJ anatomy and function. *J Dent Res*, 87(8): 726–30.

Gateno, J., Teichgraeber, J.F., and Xia, J.J. (2003). Three-dimensional surgical planning for maxillary and midface distraction osteogenesis. *J Craniofac Surg*, 14(6): 833–9.

Gateno, J., Xia, J.J., and Teichgraeber, J.F. (2011). New 3-dimensional cephalometric analysis for orthognathic surgery. *J Oral Maxillofac Surg*, 69(3): 606–22.

Gerig, G., Jomier, M., and Chakos, M. (2001). Valmet: A new validation tool for assessing and improving 3D object segmentation. In: W. Niessen and M. Viergever, eds, *MICCAI 2001: Proceedings of the International Society and Conference Series on Medical Image Computing and Computer-Assisted Intervention* (pp. 516–28); 2001 Oct 14–17; Utrecht, Netherlands. Berlin: Springer.

Gerig, G., Prastawa, M., Lin, W., and Gilmore, J. (2003). Assessing early brain development in neonates by segmentation of high-resolution 3T MRI [Short Paper, Lecture Notes in Computer Science LNCS #2879], pp. 979–80.

Gerig, G., Styner, M., Jones, D., Weinberger, D., and Lieberman, J. (2001). Shape analysis of brain ventricles using SPHARM. *MMBIA Proceedings*. IEEE 2001: 171–8.

Gladilin, E., Zachow, S., Deuflhard, P., Hege, H.C. (2004). Anatomy- and physics-based facial animation for craniofacial surgery simulations. *Med Biol Eng Comput*, 42(2): 167–70.

Gunz, P., Mitteroecker, P., Bookstein, F.L. (2004). Semilandmarks in three dimensions. In: D.L. Slice, editor. Modern morphometrics in physical anthropology. New York: Kluwer Academic.

Hajnal, J.V., Hill, D.L.G., Hawkes, D.J., eds. (2001). *Medical image registration*. Boca Raton: CRC Press.

Helenius, L.M., Hallikainen, D., Helenius, I., Meurman, J.H., Könönen, M., Leirisalo-Repo, M., Lindqvist, C. (2005). Clinical and radiographic findings of the temporomandibular joint in patients with various rheumatic diseases: A case control study. *Oral Surg Oral Med Oral Pathol Oral Radiol Endod*. 99: 455–63.

Ishida, T., Yabushita, T., and Soma, K. (2009). Effects of a liquid diet on temporomandibular joint mechanoreceptors. *J Dent Res*, 88(2): 187–91.

Iwasaki, T., Saitoh, I., Takemoto, Y., Inada, E., Kanomi, R., Hayasaki, H., et al. (2011). Evaluation of upper airway obstruction in Class II children with fluid-mechanical simulation. *Am J Orthod Dentofacial Orthop*, 139(2): e135–45.

Jayaratne, Y.S., Zwahlen, R.A., Lo, J., and Cheung, L.K. (2010). Three-dimensional color maps: A novel tool for assessing craniofacial changes. *Surg Innov*, 17: 198.

Jayaratne, Y.S., Zwahlen, R.A., Lo, J., and Tam, S.C., Cheung, L.K. (2010). Computer-aided maxillofacial surgery: An update. *Surg Innov*, 17(3): 217–25.

Kapila, S., Conley, R.S., and Harrell Jr., W.E. (2011). The current status of cone beam computed tomography imaging in orthodontics. *Dentomaxillofacial Radiology*, 40: 24–34.

Katheria, B.C, Kau, C.H., Tate, R., Chen, J.-W., English, J., and Bouquot, J. (2010). Effectiveness of impacted and supernumerary tooth diagnosis from traditional radiography versus cone beam computed tomography. *Ped Dent*, 32(4): 304–9.

Keeve, E., Girod, B., and Girod, S. (1996). Computer-aided craniofacial surgery. H.U. Lemke, editor, *Computer Assisted Radiology*. Paris, France.

Keeve, E., Girod, S., Kikinis, R., and Girod, B. (1998). Deformable modeling of facial tissue for craniofacial surgery simulation. *Comput Aided Surg*, 3(5): 228–38.

Kim, H., Jurgen, P., Krol, Z., Caversaccio, M., Nolte, L.P., Zeilhofer, H.F., Gonzales, M.A. (2009). Clinical applications of computer-aided planning and navigation system for cranio-maxillofacial surgery. CAS-H 2009. Leipzig, Germany, Book of Abstracts.

Kim, Y.-I., Park, S.-B., Son, W.-S., and Hwang, D.-S. (2011). Midfacial soft-tissue changes after advancement of maxilla with Le Fort I osteotomy and mandibular setback surgery: Comparison of conventional and high Le Fort osteotomies by superimposition of cone-beam computed tomography volumes. *J Oral Maxillofac Surg*, 2011 April 14.

Koyama, J., Nishiyama, H., and Hayashi, T. (2007). Follow-up study of condylar bony changes using helical computed tomography in patients with temporomandibular disorder. *Dentomaxillofac Radiol*, 36: 472–7.

Krol, Z., Chapuis, J., Schwenzer-Zimmerer, K., Langlotz, F., and Zeilhofer, H.F. (2005). Preoperative planning and intraoperative navigation in the reconstructive craniofacial surgery. *J Med Inform Tech*, 9: 83–9.

Langlotz, F. (2004). Localizers and trackers for computer assisted freehand navigation. In: F. Picard, L.-P. Nolte, A.M. Digiola, B. Jamaraz, eds., *Hip and Knee Surgery—Navigation, Robotics, and Computer Assisted Surgical Tools* (pp. 51–3). Oxford University Press.

Lenza, M.G., Lenza, M.M., Dalstra, M., Melsen, B., Cattaneo, P.M. (2010). An analysis of different approaches to the assessment of upper airway morphology: a CBCT study. *Orthod Craniofac Res*, 13(2): 96–105.

Leung, C.C., Palomo, L., Griffith, R., and Hans, M.G. (2010). Accuracy and reliability of cone-beam computed tomography for measuring alveolar bone height and detecting bony dehiscences and fenestrations. *Am J Orthod Dentofac Orthop*, 137(4 Suppl): S109–19.

Leuzinger, M., Dudic, A., Giannopoulou, C., and Killaridis, S. (2010). Root-contact evaluation by panoramic radiography and cone-beam computed tomography of super-high resolution. *Am J Orthod Dentofac Orthop*, 137(3): 389–92.

Lie, W.N. (1995). Automatic target segmentation by locally adaptive image thresholding, *IEEE Trans. Image Processing*, 4(7): 1036–41.

Lloyd, T.E., Drage, N.A., and Cronin, A.J. (2011). The role of cone beam computed tomography in the management of unfavourable fractures following sagittal split mandibular osteotomy. *J Orthod*, 38(1): 48–54.

Ma, W.Y., and Manjunath, B.S. (2000). Edge flow: A technique for boundary detection and image segmentation. *IEEE Trans. Image Processing*, 9(8): 1375–88.

Maes, F., Collignon, A., Vandermeulen, D., Marchal, G., Suetens, P. (1997). Multimodality image registration by maximization of mutual information. *IEEE Trans Med Imaging*, 16: 187–98.

Molen, A.D. (2010). Considerations in the use of cone-beam computed tomography for buccal bone measurements. *Am J Orthod Dentofac Orthop*, 137(4 Suppl): S130-5.

Mollemans, W., Schutyser, F., Nadjmi, N., Maes, F., and Suetens, P. (2007). Predicting soft tissue deformations for a maxillofacial surgery planning system: From computational strategies to a complete clinical validation. *Med Image Anal*, 11(3): 282–301.

Moon, N., Bullitt, E., Leemput, K., and Gerig G. (2002). Model-based brain and tumor segmentation. *Proc. 16th Int Conf on Pattern Recognition ICPR 2002* (pp. 528–531), editors: R. Kasturi, D. Laurendeau, C. Suen, IEEE Computer Society.

Nordahl, S., Alstergren, P., Eliasson, S., and Kopp, S. (2001). Radiographic signs of bone destruction in the arthritic temporomandibular joint with special reference to markers of disease activity: A longitudinal study. *Rheumatology (Oxford)*, 40(6): 691–4.

Orentlicher, G., Goldsmith, D., and Horowitz, A. (2010). Applications of 3-dimensional virtual computerized tomography technology in oral and maxillofacial surgery: Current therapy. *J Oral Maxillofac Surg*, 68(8): 1993–59.

Paniagua, B., Cevidanes, L., Walker, D., Zhu, H., Guo, R., and Styner, M. (2010). Clinical application of SPHARM-PDM to quantify temporomandibular joint arthritis. *Comput Med Imaging Graph*, December 23.

Paniagua, B., Cevidanes, L., Zhu, H., and Styner, M. (2010). Outcome quantification using SPHARM-PDM toolbox in orthognathic surgery. *Int J Comput Assist Radiol Surg*, December 16.

Pommert, A., Riemer, M., Schiemann, T., Schubert, R., Tiede, U., Hohne, K.H. (1996). Three-dimensional imaging in medicine: Methods and applications. In: R. Taylor, S. Lavallee, G. Burdea, and R. Mosges, eds., *Computer Integrated Surgery* (pp. 155–74). Cambridge, MA: MIT Press.

Popat, H., and Richmond, S. (2010). New developments in three-dimensional planning for orthognathic surgery. *J Orthod*, 37(1): 62–71.

Roemhildt, M.L., Coughlin, K.M., Peura, G.D., Badger, G.J., Churchill, D., Fleming, B.C., et al. (2010). Effects of increased chronic loading on articular cartilage material properties in the lapine tibio-femoral joint. *J Biomech*, 43(12): 2301–8.

Rohr, K. (2001). Landmark-based image analysis: Using geometric and intensity models. *Computational Imaging and Vision Series*, Vol. 21. London: Kluwer Academic.

Rueckert, D., Sonoda, L.I., Hayes, C., Hill, D.L.G., Leach, M.O., and Hawkes, D.J. (1999). Nonrigid registration using free-form deformations: Application to breast MR images. *IEEE Trans Med Imaging*, 18: 712–21.

Dworkin, S.F., and LeResche, L. (1992). Research diagnostic criteria for temporomandibular disorders: Review, criteria, examinations, and specifications, critique. *J Craniomandib Disord*, 6: 301–55.

Schendel, S., Powell, N., and Jacobson, R. (2011). Maxillary, mandibular, and chin advancement: Treatment planning based on airway anatomy in obstructive sleep apnea. *J Oral Maxillofac Surg*, 69(3): 663–76.

Schendel, S.A., and Hatcher, D. (2010). Automated 3-dimensional airway analysis from cone-beam computed tomography data. *J Oral Maxillofac Surg*, 68(3): 696–701.

Schendel, S.A., and Lane, C. (2009). 3D orthognathic surgery simulation using image fusion. *Semin Orthod*, 15: 48–56.

Schendel, S.A., and Montgomery, K. (2009). A web-based, integrated simulation system for craniofacial surgical planning. *Plast Reconstr Surg*, 123(3): 1009–106.

Schiffman, E.L., Ohrbach, R., Truelove, E.L., Tai, F., Anderson, G.C., Pan, W., et al. (2010). The Research Diagnostic Criteria for Temporomandibular Disorders. V: Methods used to establish and validate revised Axis I diagnostic algorithms. *J Orofac Pain*, 24(1): 63–78.

Schiffman, E.L., Truelove, E.L., Ohrbach, R., Anderson, G.C., John, M.T., List, T., et al. (2010). The Research Diagnostic Criteria for Temporomandibular Disorders. I: Overview and methodology for assessment of validity. *J Orofac Pain*, 24(1): 7–24.

Schutyser, F., Van Cleynenbreugel, J., Ferrant, M., Schoenaers, J., Suetens, P. (2000). Image-based 3D planning of maxillofacial distraction procedures including soft tissue implications. *Medical Image Computing and Computer-Assisted Intervention*. 1935: 999–1007.

Scott, C.C., and Athanasiou, K.A. (2006). Mechanical impact and articular cartilage. *Crit Rev Biomed Eng*, 34(5): 347–78.

Shemesh, H., Cristescu, R.C., Wesslink, P.R., and Wu, M.-K. (2011). The use of cone-beam computed tomography and digital periapical radiographs to diagnose root perforations. *JOE*, 37(4): 513–16.

Sherrard, J.F., Rossouw, P.E., Benson, B.W., Carrillo, R., and Buschang, P.H. (2010). Accuracy and reliability of tooth and root lengths measured on cone-beam computed tomographs. *Am J Orthod Dentofac Orthop*, 137(4 Suppl): S100-8.

Styner, M., Oguz, I., Xu, S., Brechbuhler, C., Pantazis, D., Levitt, J., et al. (2006). Framework for the statistical shape analysis of brain structures using Spharm-PDM. Special edition open science workshop at MICCAI. *Insight J*, pp. 1–7. Available at http://hdl.handle.net/1926/215.

Subsol, G., Thirion, J.P., and Ayache, N. (1998). A scheme for automatically building three-dimensional morphometric anatomical atlases: Application to a skull atlas. *Med Image Anal*, 2(1): 37–60.

Swennen, G.R., Mollemans, W., De Clercq, C., Abeloos, J., Lamoral, P., Lippens, F., et al. (2009). A cone-beam computed tomography triple scan procedure to obtain a three-dimensional augmented virtual skull model appropriate for orthognathic surgery planning. *J Craniofac Surg*, 20(2): 297–307.

Tai, K., Hotokezak, H., Park, J.H., Tai, H., Miyajima, K., Choi, M., et al. (2010). Preliminary cone-beam computed tomography study evaluating dental and skeletal changes after treatment with a mandibular Schwarz appliance. *Am J Orthod Dentofac Orthop*, 138(3): 262.e1-262.e11.

Tamimi, D., and ElSaid, K. (2009). Cone beam computed tomography in the assessment of dental impactions. *Semin Orthod*, 15: 57–62.

Teschner, M., Girod, S., and Girod, B. (2001). 3-D simulation of craniofacial surgical procedures. *Stud Health Technol Inform*, 81: 502–8.

Thompson, P.M., MacDonald, D., Mega, M.S., Holmes, C.J., Evans, A.C., Toga, A.W. (1997). Detection and mapping of abnormal brain structure with a probabilistic atlas of cortical surfaces. *J Comput Assist Tomogr*, 21: 567–81.

Treil, J., Braga, J., Loubes, J.-M., Maza, E., Inglese, J.-M., Casteigt, J., et al. (2009). 3D tooth modeling for orthodontic assessment. *Semin Orthod*, 15: 42–7.

Truelove, E., Pan, W., Look, J.O., Mancl, L.A., Ohrbach, R.K., Velly, A.M., et al. (2010). The Research Diagnostic Criteria for Temporomandibular Disorders. III: Validity of Axis I diagnoses. *J Orofac Pain*, 24(1): 35–47.

Tucker, S., Cevidanes, L.H.S., Styner, M., Kim, H., Reyes, M., Proffit, W., et al. (2010). Comparison of actual surgical outcomes and 3-dimensional surgical simulations. *J Oral Maxillofac Surg*, 68(10): 2412–21.

Van Elslande, D., Heo, G., Flores-Mir, C., Carey, J., and Major, P.W. (2010). Accuracy of mesiodistal root angulation projected by cone-beam computed tomographic panoramic-like images. *Am J Orthod Dentofac Orthop*, 137(4 Suppl): S94-S99.

Vandewalle, P., Schutyser, F., Van Cleynenbreugel, J., and Suetens, P. (2003). Modeling of facial soft tissue growth for maxillofacial surgery planning environments. *IS4TH*, 2003: 27–37.

Verteramo, A., and Seedhom, B.B. (2007). Effect of a single impact loading on the structure and mechanical properties of articular cartilage. *J Biomech*, 40(16): 3580–9.

Westermark, A., Zachow, S., and Eppley, B.L. (2005). Three-dimensional osteotomy planning in maxillofacial surgery including soft tissue prediction. *J Craniofac Surg*, 16(1): 100–4.

Xia, J., Samman, N., Yeung, R.W., Shen, S.G., Wang, D., Ip, H.H., et al. (2000). Three-dimensional virtual reality surgical planning and simulation workbench for orthognathic surgery. *Int J Adult Orthod Orthognath Surg*, 15(4): 265–82.

Yushkevich, P.A., Piven, J., Hazlett, H.C., Smith, R.G., Ho, S., Gee, J.C., et al. User-guided 3D active contour segmentation of anatomical structures: Significantly improved efficiency and reliability. *Neuroimage*, 31(3): 1116–28.

Zachow, S., Gladilin, E., Zeilhofer, H.F., and Sader, R. (2001). Improved 3D osteotomy planning in craniomaxillofacial surgery. Medical Image Computing and Computer-Assisted Intervention: 4th International Conference, Ultrecht, The Netherlands; October 2001.

6 Three-Dimensional Planning in Maxillofacial Reconstruction of Large Defects Using Cone Beam Computed Tomography

Rutger Schepers, Gerry M. Raghoebar, Lars U. Lahoda, Harry Reintsema, Arjan Vissink, and Max J. Witjes

Introduction

Large maxillofacial bone defects have been a reconstructive challenge throughout time. In case of small bony defects, bridging can be performed using free iliac crest grafts. When defects are too big or lack sufficient soft tissue to support the graft, free vascularized osseous flaps are usually necessary to close the defects. However, bony reconstruction of such defects does not always restore function. Masticatory function, especially, often remains unfavorable because of problems with retention and stabilization of the prosthesis after reconstruction with vascularized grafts. This problem can be solved by placing dental implants in these osseous flaps to retain a denture, thus improving mastication and speech (Schmelzeisen et al., 1996). When dental implants are considered part of the treatment plan, correct positioning of the osseous component of the free flap is eminent to allow for implant placement at the preferred anatomical locations from a prosthodontic perspective. When the bone transplant is incorrectly positioned, impants often have to be placed in a suboptimal position for prosthodontic rehabilitation. As a result, the postoperative function and esthetics of the implant-retained mandibular prosthesis are often impaired, thereby negatively affecting the patient's quality of life (Zlotolow et al., 1992). Therefore, when implant placement is desired in osseous free flaps, a precise preoperative plan is essential (Albert et al., 2010; de Almeida et al., 2010). For this type of reconstruction, imaging of the defect should provide sufficient data to reliably perform the planning. In the preoperative phase of such reconstructions, a computed tomogram (CT) has been the standard imaging modality for several decades. However, with the introduction of the cone beam CT, a versatile tool has been introduced which has replaced the standard CT in planning craniofacial defect reconstructions.

In the past years cone beam CT (CBCT) has become increasingly popular because it combines good image quality with a relatively low radiation dose. Its versatility is enhanced now that software has become available that allows virtual treatment planning in implantology and maxillofacial surgery.

This chapter shows the complete CBCT-based virtual workflow of fully digitally planned primary and secondary reconstructions of maxillofacial

---

Cone Beam Computed Tomography: Oral and Maxillofacial Diagnosis and Applications, First Edition. Edited by David Sarment.
© 2014 John Wiley & Sons, Inc. Published 2014 by John Wiley & Sons, Inc.

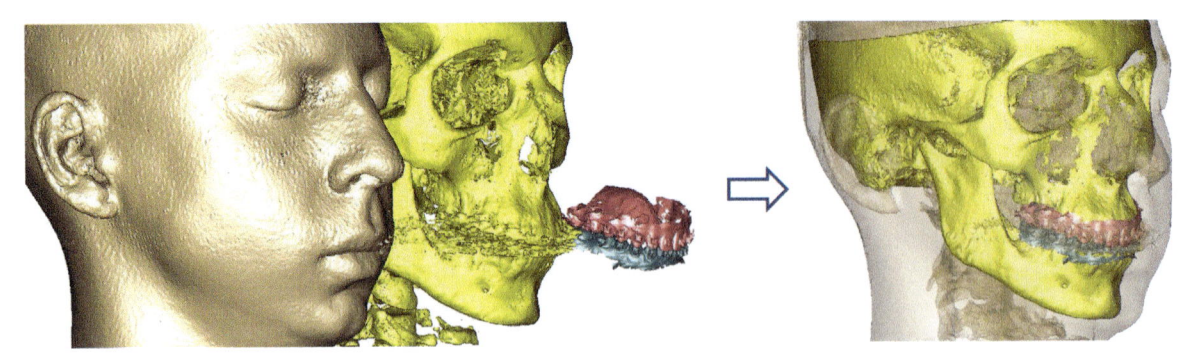

Figure 6.1 Fusion of the 3D models of the face (CBCT), bony structures (CBCT), and dentition (Lava Chairside Oral Scan) produces a 3D augmented model of the face.

defects with osseous flaps and implant-retained prosthetic reconstructions.

3D augmented virtual model

To start the digital workflow, a detailed 3D model is needed from the patient's face, bony structures, and dentition (3D augmented model). Computer software packages, such as Simplant (Materialize Dental, Leuven, Belgium) or ProPlan CMF (Synthes, Solothurn, Switzerland and Materialise, Leuven, Belgium) can reconstruct a detailed 3D volume out of CBCT DICOM (Digital Imaging and Communications in Medicine) data by software volume rendering. The volumes are constructed of voxel-based data, requiring the input of a threshold of a grey value of the specific voxel corresponding with the skin or bone of the patient. For skin and bone this usually results in a detailed 3D model of high quality from CBCT data. For conventional CT as well as CBCT it is still not possible to accurately display the dentition. Metal used in most fillings and crowns produce scattering artifacts in the CBCT scan; therefore, a detailed 3D model of the dentition has to be obtained in another way. This can be implied easiest by scanning an impression or a dental cast with a CBCT out of which a detailed 3D model can be derived. Now 3D optical intraoral scanners such as the Lava Chairside Oral Scanner C.O.S. (3M ESPE, St. Paul, USA) have become available. These scanners are highly accurate and can produce a 3D surface model of the dentition. This produces a more detailed 3D model compared to the impression or cast scan. A 3D augmented virtual model of the maxillofacial region is thus created by importing the 3D optically obtained dentition model into the 3D model of the bone and skin in the correct anatomical location (Figure 6.1).

CBCT-based virtual planning of resection and reconstruction

Planning and surgery of primary reconstruction immediately after tumor ablative surgery

Reconstruction of large maxillofacial defects with free vascularized grafts directly after tumor ablation has become a standard treatment modality and is widely accepted and used (Taylor et al., 1975). Direct reconstruction provides jaw stability and tissue support for favorable esthetic reconstruction of the face and adequate filling of the defect. The resection of a bone tumor or bone-invading tumor can be planned virtually from CBCT data. The shape of the graft can also be planned virtually. Virtual shaping of the graft at the donor site helps to adequately fill the defect created by tumor resection. In case of a large hemi maxillary defect, a deep circumflex iliac artery flap can be used to reconstruct the defect. The required shape of the iliac crest is often complex due to the complex facial bone geometry of the midface. The starting point is the virtual resection of the tumor, which is planned on a CBCT of the head and virtually simulated in ProPlan CMF (Figure 6.2A). The CBCT scan serves as a base for importing other data into the software. In this case, a CT scan of the iliac crest is then made and a 3D virtual bone model is created and positioned in the defect, creating a virtual reconstruction of the defect (Figure 6.2B). A resection guide can be designed and printed by additive manufacturing. This guide is used to exactly shape the iliac crest graft while the vascular blood supply is still intact. The planned outcome of the shape of the iliac crest graft can be printed (Materialize, Leuven, Belgium) in resin. This printed model can be used after the resection of the tumor to ensure that the graft fits well in the defect before harvesting the graft. As has been pointed out before, restoring masticatory function is highly important for a patient. To adequately restore function, implants are needed. In primary reconstructive planning, implants can be planned and guided into the bone graft. It is possible to insert implants either while the graft is still at the donor site or after the graft is fixed in the recipient jaw and blood circulation is reestablished. An important advantage of inserting implants in the graft at the donor site is that these implants can then be used to guide the placement of the graft in the jaw defect. A positioning guide can be screwed on the implants to guide intraoral fixation of the graft in the proper position. After consolidation of the graft, a superstructure can be produced to start the prosthetic phase.

Preoperative virtual planning

Resection margins of bone tumors or tumors that invade bone can be determined on (CB)CT scans. Normally these margins are translated to the operating room by measuring the distance of anatomical landmarks to the tumor margins on a CT scan of the target area. These are used in the operating room to determine the resection plane clinically. Planning of the resection margins and planes on CBCT scans can be adequately visualized in ProPlan CMF. Resection planes can be planned on a 3D model to virtually resect the tumor (Figure 6.3A). These planes can be visualized in 3D and in axial, sagittal, and coronal planes in the CT slices (Figure 6.3B). The anatomical information in the planes is used to precisely plan the resection cuts. Bone-supported cutting guides can be designed and printed by additive manufacturing to guide tumor resection intraoperatively (Figure 6.4). CBCT information on the shape of the bone surface

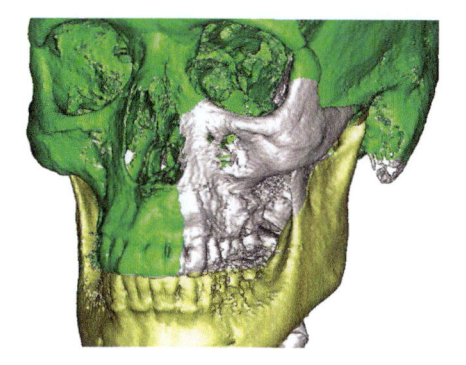

Figure 6.2A 3D bone model of a CBCT showing the tumor region on the left processus of the maxilla in the molar region. The resection area of the maxilla is shown (grey).

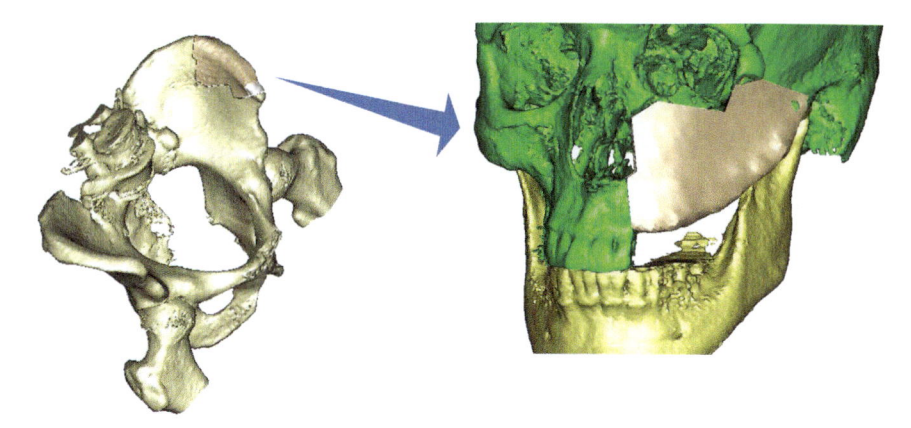

Figure 6.2B 3D bone model of a CT of the iliac crest (left) with the planned graft segment DCIA in the maxillary defect position (right).

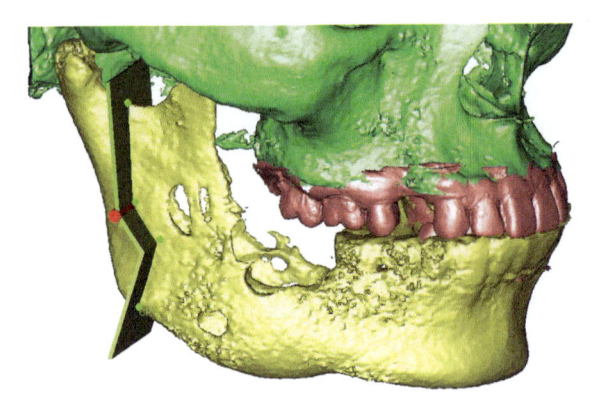

Figure 6.3A 3D model of a mandible with an ameloblastoma located in the right corpus. The resection plane is shown in green, representing the distal resection border of the tumor.

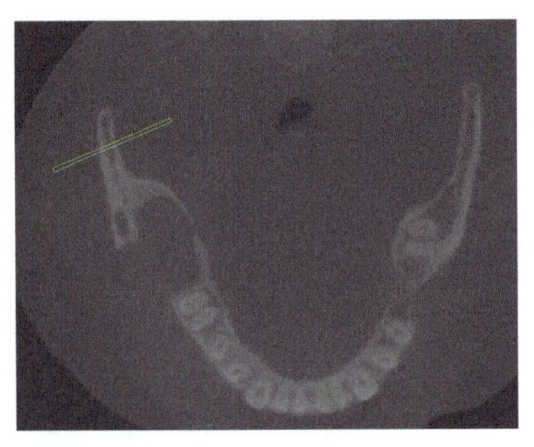

Figure 6.3B Axial slice of a mandible with an ameloblastoma located in the right corpus; the planned resection plane is shown in green, corresponding with the plane in Figure 6.3A.

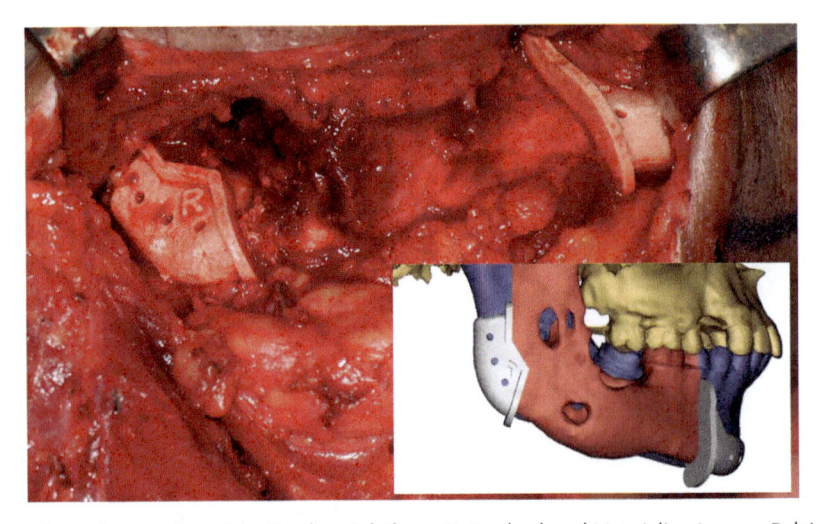

Figure 6.4 The insert shows the resection guides (Synthes, Solothurn, Switzerland; and Materialise, Leuven, Belgium) virtually planned to resect the tumor; this corresponds to the intraoperative situation showing the 3D printed resection guides on the mandible.

is very accurate, yielding cutting guides that exactly fit to the actual bone surface. Often the guides only fit in one position on the bone. This leads to an optimization of sparing the surrounding healthy bone due to the versatility of cutting planes without compromising the tumor-free margins (Figure 6.5). Primary reconstruction with a free vascularized bone graft can be performed in the same 3D plan as the tumor resection (Figure 6.6). This can include the planning of dental implants in the graft that can be used for dental rehabilitation after bone consolidation.

Planning and surgery of secondary reconstruction of pre-existing maxillofacial defects

Choice of free vascularized osseous flap

An essential step is selecting the type of free vascularized bone graft that adequately bridges the defect. Several choices are available in order to reconstruct a large defect of the upper and lower jaw. These mainly include the free fibula as the workhorse (Lopez et al., 2010), the iliac crest, and

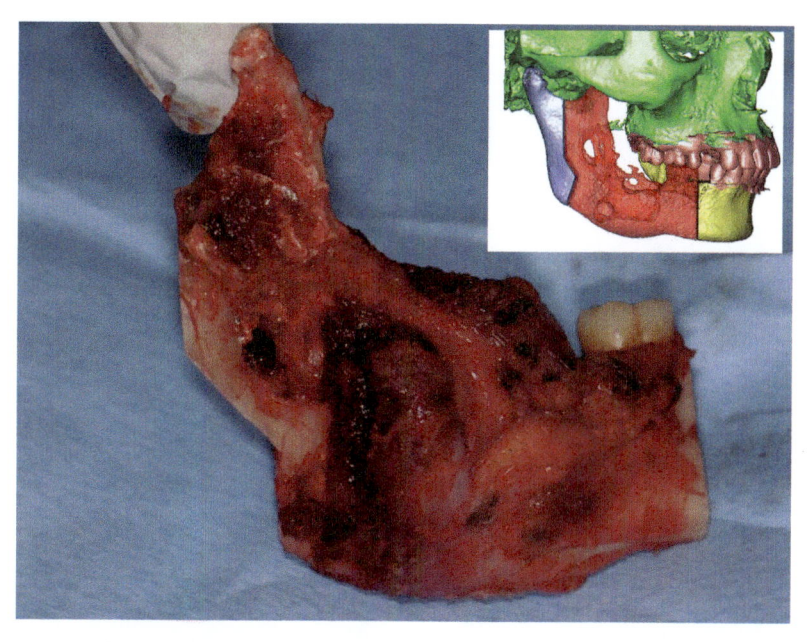

Figure 6.5 The tumor resected and guided out of the mandible; the insert shows the virtual plan of the resection.

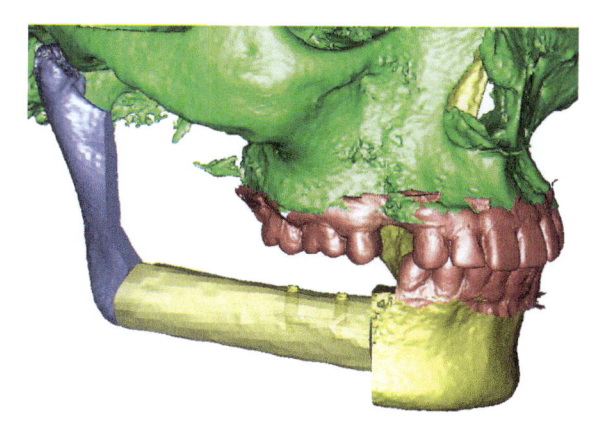

Figure 6.6 The defect created after virtual tumor resection is reconstructed with a fibula segment with two implants.

theoretically others, such as, for instance, the medial femoral condyle or the scapula. For each flap an example will be given to demonstrate how these flaps can be used in the treatment plan.

For large bone defects, the free fibula has many advantages and is therefore most widely used. The fibula is a long bone of the lower extremity. It has a tubular shape with a thick, dense cortical bone layer around the entire circumference that renders it one of the strongest and longest bones available for transfer. The length of the fibula graft can easily exceed 20 cm. During harvesting, it is necessary to leave approximately 6 cm of bone distally and proximal, in order to maintain stability of the knee and ankle joint. Furthermore, implant survival in a vascularized fibula is known to be high, which might be due to the presence of dense cortical bone contributing to adequate initial implant stability (Chiapasco et al., 2006; Gbara et al., 2007).

The deep circumflex iliac artery (DCIA) free flap is more challenging to dissect, and the length and diameter of the vascular pedicle to the iliac crest is less predictable (Cordeiro et al., 1999). In addition, a certain amount of muscle needs to be harvested as well, making this flap less pliable and more difficult to shape. However, if large combined soft tissue and bone defects need to be reconstructed, for instance the maxilla with a substantial palatal defect, the DCIA flap has been advocated as the flap of choice. The cortical layer of the bone is thinner compared to the fibula, which makes it less favorable for implant placement due to less initial stability.

Due to the unique anatomic location of the scapula, with its option to be harvested as a chimerical flap, indications to be used as a replacement

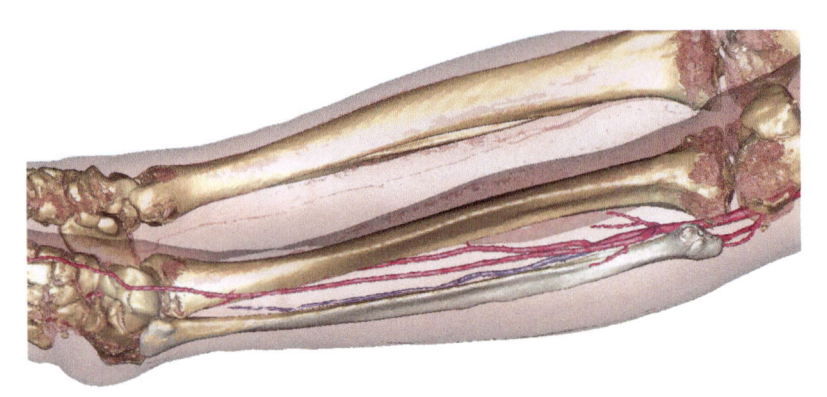

Figure 6.7A 3D model of a CT angiogram of the lower legs, showing the bones, arterial vascular supply of the left lower leg (pink-blue), and the skin (transparent).

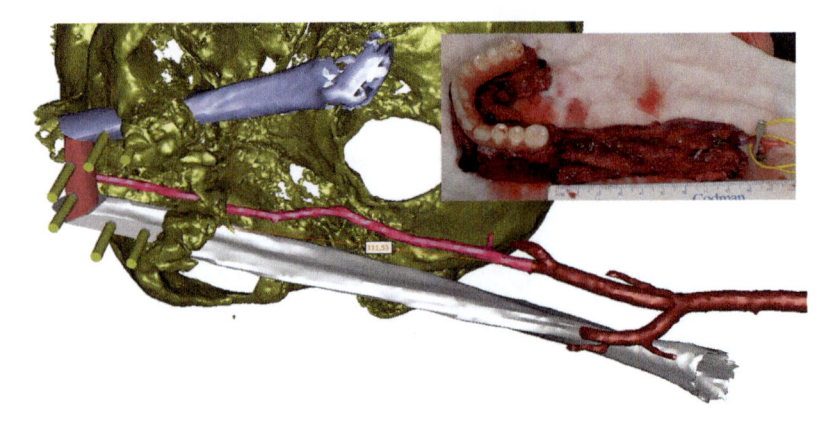

Figure 6.7B 3D model of the skull of a patient with a large bony defect of nearly the entire maxilla. A fibula reconstructive plan is shown with three segments of the fibula combined with the arterial blood vessels. The fibular artery is shown in purple; this artery is subsequently harvested as a part of the graft to use for the recirculation of the graft on the recipient side. The insert on the upper right shows the fibula graft with an implant-supported prosthesis fixated on the graft. The arteriovenous vessel pedicle is shown with a length of 11 cm, corresponding to the length of the fibular artery in the plan.

of maxillofacial bone are limited. The donor site, which is also a drawback of the DCIA flap compared to the fibula, is very unfavorable in the scapula when it comes to osseous free flaps. All of the above-mentioned flaps currently cannot be imaged with a CBCT. Therefore, a combination of craniofacial imaging with CBCT and flap imaging with conventional CT is still necessary.

3D virtual model of the bone and vessels

For the planning of the reconstruction, the anatomy of the donor bone as well as its vascular support are essential in determining the possibilities and limits of the reconstruction. For virtual planning of some flaps it is possible to obtain information on the bone and the 3D spatial orientation of its vessels (Eckardt and Swennen, 2005). Both can be visualized in a CT angiogram with intravenous contrast in some flaps (Figure 6.7A, Figure 6.7B). Voxel-based threshold volume rendering can visualize a 3D model of the bone, including the arteriovenous blood vessels of the donor bone segment. In the planning of the graft segmentation, the vessels are relocated together with the bone graft to reconstruct the defect. Sufficient vessel length of the donor segment is needed to reach the vessels in the neck for recirculation of the blood

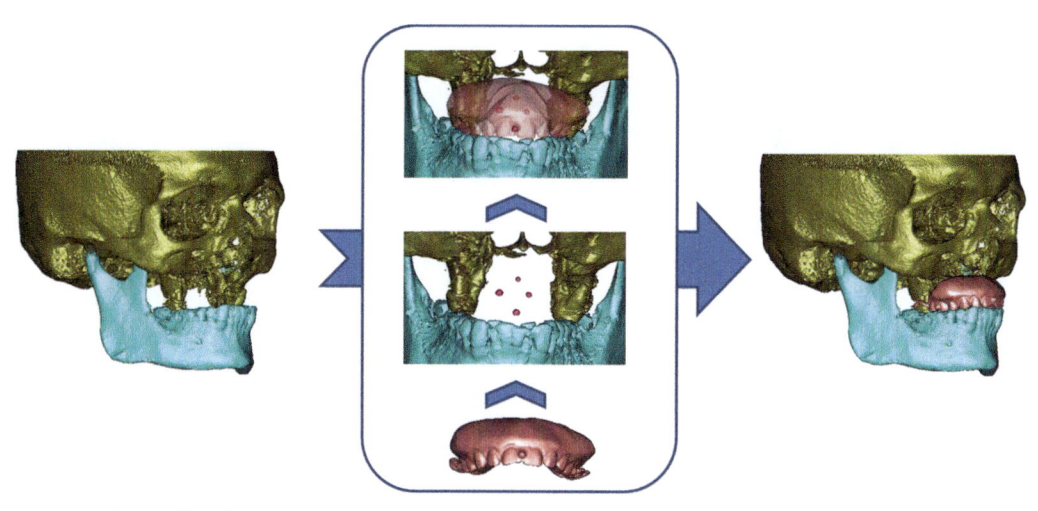

Figure 6.8A Matching of the denture and the 3D bone models can be performed in a double scan procedure. The patient is scanned with a CBCT wearing the denture (with glass particles on it, shown by the red dots); after this, the denture is scanned separately. Both scans are matched on glass particle geometry into a fusion model.

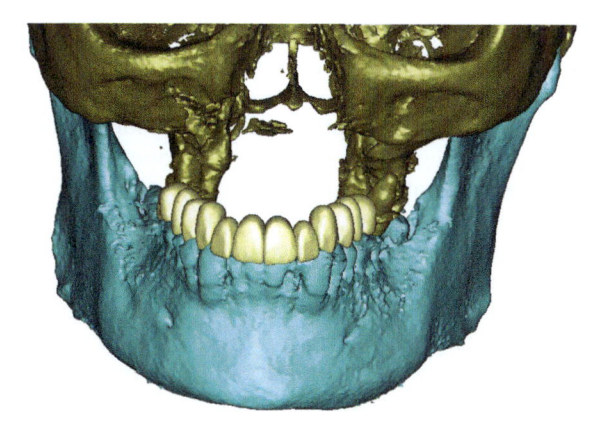

Figure 6.8B 3D augmented virtual model of a patient with a large bony defect of the left maxilla. A reconstruction plan is shown with a double barrel fibula graft, three implants, and a virtual teeth set-up.

supply, especially when considering reconstruction of the maxilla.

3D virtual setup of the dentition

Irrespective of the type of reconstruction and free flap, the planning starts from the occlusion of the dentition. An ideal dental setup is needed to determine the optimal position of the elements in the defect. In edentulous or partial dentulous patients the prosthesis or wax-up can be virtualized. In this case a CBCT scan has to be made of the patient's head with the full or partial denture in occlusion. Because the density of the denture (voxel value) is too close to the density of soft tissue, the denture has to be scanned separately (double scan procedure) in the CBCT. Matching of the denture with the patient scan is usually done by fixing several glass particles to the denture; the CBCT scan of the patient and the separate scans of the dentures can then be matched on particle geometry (Figure 6.8A). In patients with a maxillofacial defect, the defect size and anatomy are clearly visualized in the augmented model. The 3D augmented model with the defect clearly visualized is the starting point of reconstructive planning.

In Simplant there is also the possibility to create a virtual setup of teeth (Figure 6.8B). It is very important for this dental setup to be accurate, because the planning of the bone graft and the implants are deducted from this. This planning should be performed from a prosthodontist point of view to ensure that the setup is functional. In the planning phase a combination of several decisions have to be made. The first decision is the type of dental rehabilitation to aim at. In edentulous patients this can be an implant-supported bar, retained denture, or a hybrid structure. In dentulous patients an implant-supported bridge or implant-supported crowns are more desirable.

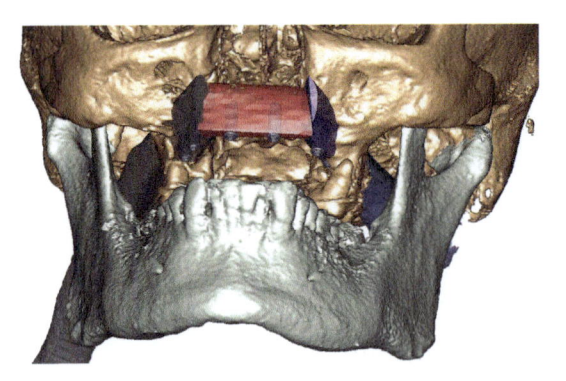

Figure 6.9A Plan of implants in a segmented fibula to reconstruct the bone defect of nearly the entire maxilla. The molars showed severe loss of periodontium and periradicular bone; removal of the molars was therefore inevitable. The reconstructive planning was made taking this into account.

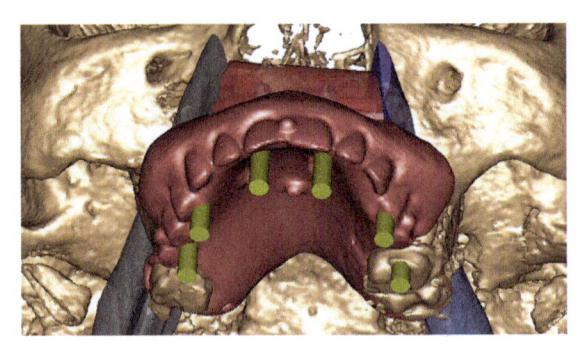

Figure 6.9B The position of the implants and the fibula segments were planned according to the desired position of the prosthesis to optimally support the prosthesis. In green the implant restorative spaces are shown, located in the centerline of the implants.

3D virtual planning of the bone graft and the implants

Once the setup of the missing dentition is determined, the planning continues with the selection of the type of donor graft. The choice of the graft usually has several aspects. First, the graft has to anatomically fill the defect and provide sufficient support to the implant-supported dental structure. Next, the blood supply of the graft has to be sufficient, with sufficient vessel length for recirculation attachment. The distance of the graft to the acceptor vessels of the neck can be large, especially when the reconstruction concerns a defect in the maxilla. The combination of the angiography and the CT is perfect for 3D planning because the configuration of the vessels and the bone can be visualized together.

The CT-angiography has to be added to the 3D virtual augmented model in ProPlan CMF. This is done by importing the CT-angiography DICOM data into the software plan of the patient. The 3D volume of the selected bone graft and the arteries can be created by selecting the proper voxel threshold of bone and the intravenous contrast. The bone graft can be situated in the preferred anatomical location in the bone defect of the maxilla or mandible that has to be reconstructed. The shape of the bone graft usually doesn't exactly match with the shape of the bone in the missing jaw segment. Especially in larger defects, the shape of the maxillary or mandibular segment that has to be reconstructed differs from the graft shape. The donor graft can therefore be segmented to follow the shape of the defect. One has to bear in mind that the blood supply of the segments decreases with diminishing segment size, increasing the risk of graft necrosis in small segments. Virtual bone cuts can be created in the 3D model of the bone graft, segmenting the graft to properly match the defect anatomy and meanwhile aiming at a functional position of the implant-supported structure. The definitive position of the bone graft has to reach both goals. Planning of the graft and the implants is done simultaneously to achieve the best position of both (Figure 6.9A, Figure 6.9B). The geometrical arterial vessel position to the bone graft is monitored closely in the planning process. The vessel length that can be used is anatomically identified and the position of the vessel to the bone is taken into account in planning the bone graft. For instance, if the left and right fibulas are both suitable as a transplant, the vessel geometry often determines the choice of side to reach the best location of the vessels to be connected to the recipient vessels of the neck.

Once the optimal position of the implants is determined in the graft, the implant position can be locked to the graft segments. The segments can then be relocated to their original position before segmentation, giving the implant position in the original bone graft. The drilling guide is designed on the periosteum of the original bone graft, and in the case of a fibula graft, skin is supported on the lateral malleolus to prohibit axial sliding. The

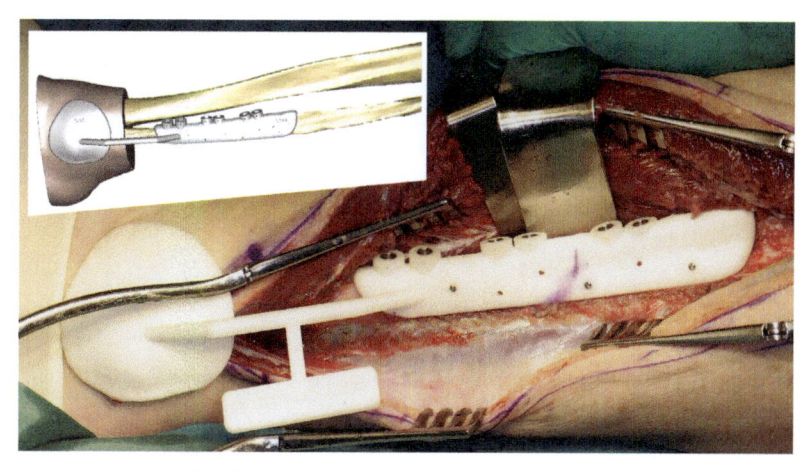

Figure 6.10 The insert shows the virtual drilling guide (ProPlan CMF). The drilling guide is situated on the periosteum of the fibula graft and is skin supported on the lateral maleolus to prohibit axial sliding. The guide is printed through selective laser sintering and sterilized using gamma irradiation. The guide is fixated with three miniscrews (KLS Martin Group, Tuttlingen, Germany).

guide is printed with a 3D printer and sterilized using gamma irradiation (Figure 6.10).

Prefabrication of the bone graft

In secondary reconstruction of maxillofacial defects, it is preferable to use prefabricated grafts since it will provide an accurate plan of the reconstruction as well as the possibility of soft tissue lining around the dental implants. Rohner et al. (2003) described a method to prefabricate a free vascularized fibula to obtain optimal support of the superstructure and to create a stable peri-implant soft tissue layer. The prefabrication includes preoperative planning of implant insertion, osteotomies of the fibula, and planning of a skin graft on the fibula for a thin lined soft tissue reconstruction. The analysis of the craniofacial defect and the reconstruction in this technique is performed on printed stereolithograpic models. Here we describe the 3D virtual planning of the technique of prefabrication.

The first surgical phase includes placement of the dental implants in the bone graft, registration of the exact location of the implants in the graft, and covering the bone with a split thickness skin graft. In the first step, the dissection is only carried out to the interosseous membrane, exposing the anterior margin of the fibula to receive the dental implants. The drilling guide should be placed precisely and fixed to the bone with miniscrews (Figure 6.10). Guided implant drilling, in the case of dense bone guided tapping and guided implant insertion, are subsequently performed. After placement of the implants, the guide is removed. Even with guided implant placement, small deviations will occur in the implant position compared to the planned position. An intraoperative optical scan of the implants with scan abutments (E.S. Healthcare, Dentsply International, Inc.; Figure 6.11) is made to register the deviation. Here the Lava Oral Scanner was used to register the exact position and angulations of the implants (Figure 6.12A). Hereafter, the fibula is covered with a split thickness skin graft taken from the ipsilateral thigh of standard thickness (Figure 6.12B) and a Gore-Tex patch (W.L. Gore and Associates, Flagstaff, USA). The wound is closed primarily with a drain left in place for 1 to 2 days, and the implants and split skin are left to heal for approximately 6 weeks.

Virtual planning of the suprastructure and the cutting guide preceding the second surgical step

The optical scan can be imported in the ProPlan CMF software as an STL file (STereoLithography file) format matched with the scan caps, resulting in the position of the scan caps and implant position

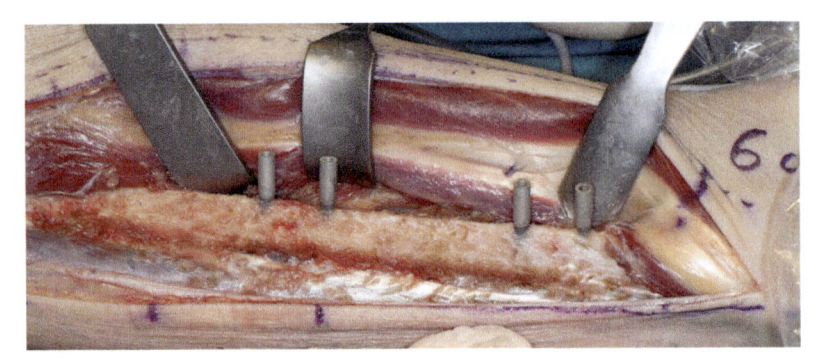

Figure 6.11 The fibula of the right lower leg after insertion of four implants. Scan caps are fixed on the fibula for registration of the implant position in the fibula.

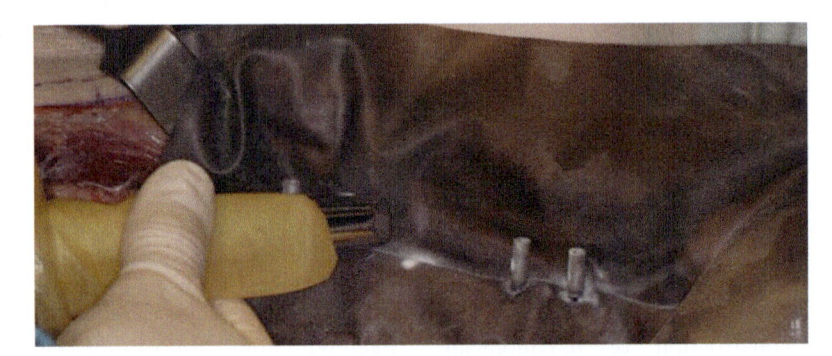

Figure 6.12A The fibula is covered with a rubber dam with punched holes for the scan caps. A thin dusting with titanium dioxide powder was applied and the Lava COS was used to register the position of the scan caps and thus the position of the implants.

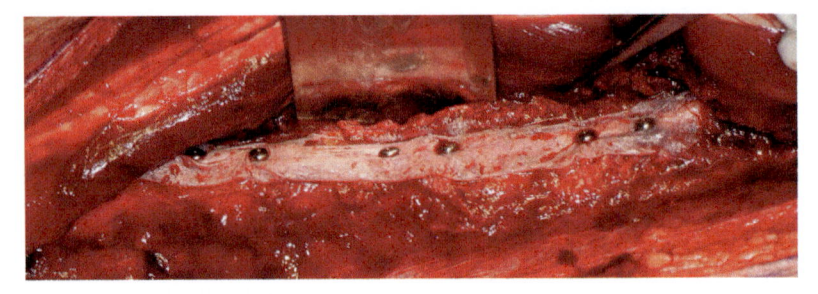

Figure 6.12B The peri implant fibula is covered with a split thickness skin graft of a standard thickness; the implants are covered with cover screws.

in the graft. The optical scan is compared with the planned position of the implants and matched to this ideal position. The superimposed fusion model with the accurate position of the implants is uploaded In ProPlan. The data are then sent to a specialized CAD-CAM (computer-aided design and computer-aided milling) company for design and fabrication of the suprastructure out of titanium (E.S. Healthcare, Dentsply International, Inc.; Figure 6.13). The suprastructure design is imported in ProPlan and checked for its shape. To position the implant suprastructure–supported fibula in the correct dimension to the antagonist dentition, an intermediate occlusal guide was

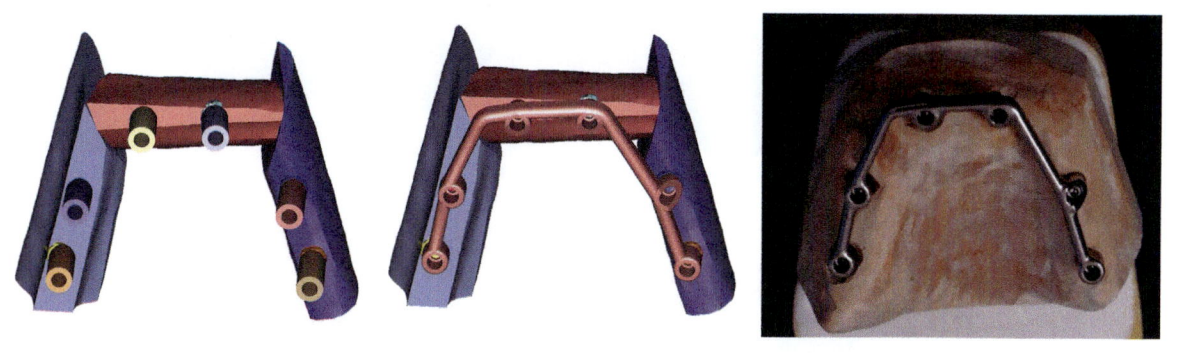

Figure 6.13 The digitized position of the scan caps and implants are matched with the planned implant position (left). The suprastructure is designed digitally on the scan cap positions (middle) and milled out of titanium (E.S. Healthcare, Dentsply International, Inc.; right). On this model a prosthesis can be designed.

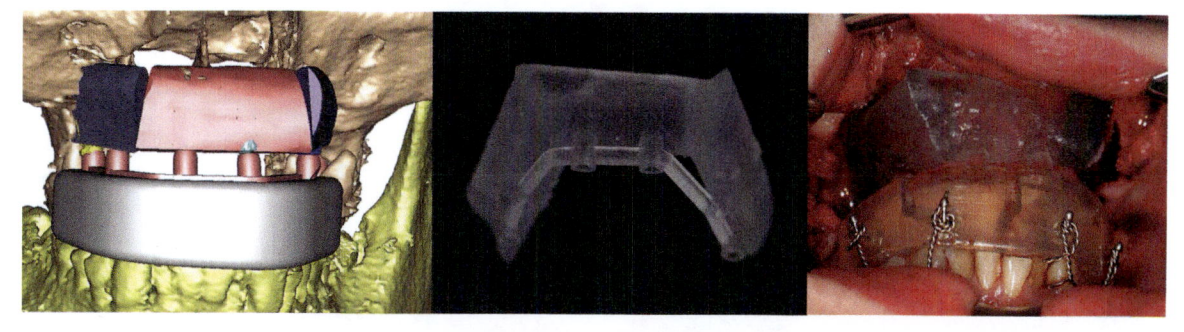

Figure 6.14 3D model of the upper jaw reconstruction (left; see also Figure 6.11). A 3D print of the surgical outcome, including the implants and the virtual designed bar can be made (middle). This 3D print can be used together with the occlusal guide (see also Figure 6.11) intraorally to resect the defect edges until they properly match the graft dimensions (right).

virtually planned in ProPlan and printed with a 3D printer into a model. The occlusal guide functions as an antagonist dental cast positioner in the articulator to plan and finish the prosthesis or bridge. In case of a bar-retained prosthesis, this occlusal guide can also function as a positioner of the bar-supported fibula during reconstruction. To transfer the virtual plan of the segmentation of the graft to the actual surgery, a cutting guide is designed. Fixation of the guide is planned on the implants in the graft. The guide is printed with a 3D printer and sterilized using gamma irradiation.

Preparation of the recipient jaw area

In most large maxillofacial defects the bone needs to be shaped to fit the graft properly without compromising the blood supply of the graft. This includes the shaping of the bony borders of the defect and the local soft tissue. There are generally two ways to prepare the defect. One possibility is to design a cutting guide, either bone or dentition supported, to perform the shaping of the defect. The planned graft will fit into the planned resection. Another possibility is to print the 3D planned suprastructure and the connected bone graft in a 3D stereolithographic model. This 3D model resembles the transplant exactly and can be used intraorally in the defect to prepare the defect (Figure 6.14). Once the model fits the defect, the transplant will fit as well (Figure 6.15). A meticulous preparation of the recipient area is mandatory: the graft and especially the attached vessels are delicate and thereby easily damaged during positioning in the defect. This positioning should therefore be minimized to avoid trauma to the graft. Also, ischemia time is known to be a significant factor in flap survival. The use of a 3D stereolithograpic model mimicking the bony graft, the implants, and the suprastructure will

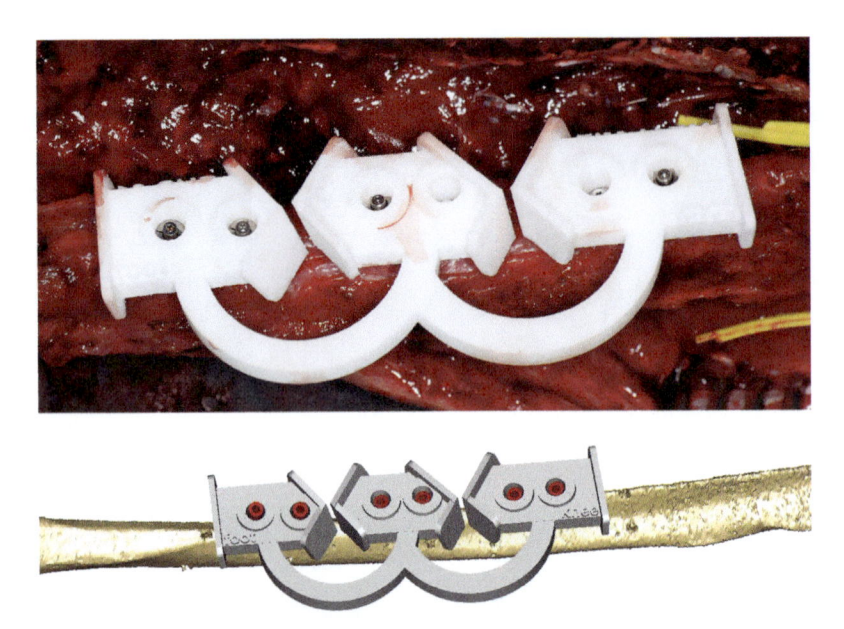

Figure 6.15 Selective laser sintering model of the cutting guide (Synthes, Solothurn, Switzerland; and Materialise, Leuven, Belgium) fixed on the implants with Nobel guide fixation screws in the left fibula (above). The virtual cutting guide shown on the fibula (ProPlan CMF; below).

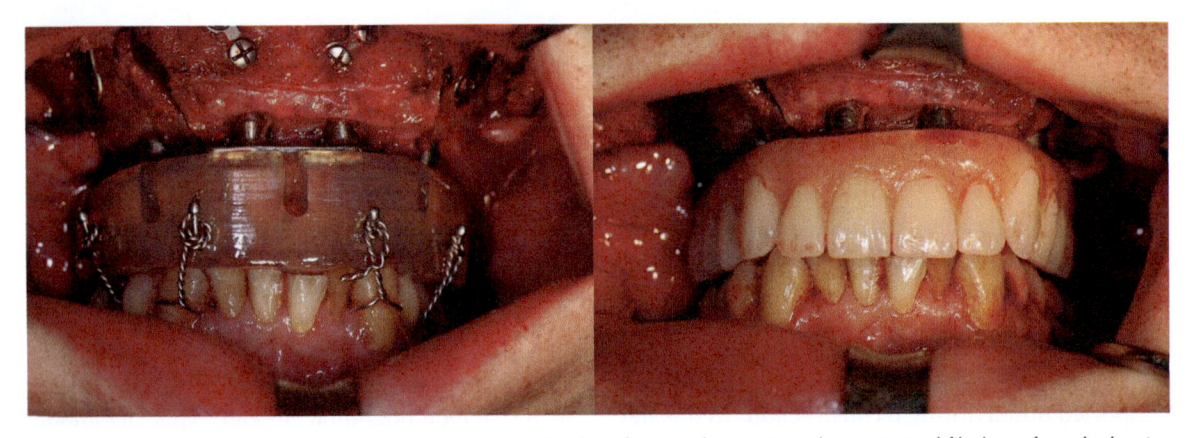

Figure 6.16 After preparation of the defect edges, the occlusal guide is used to position the segmented fibula graft on the bar in the maxillary defect (left). The fibula graft is fixated on the zygomatic bone and on the infraorbital bone using 1.5-mm titanium plates (Synthes, Solothurn, Switzerland). The prosthesis in the proper occlusion intraorally (right).

reduce "fondling" with the graft and significantly shorten ischemia time.

Reconstructive surgery of the jaw

The second surgical step, usually 6 weeks after the prefabrication to allow the implants sufficient time for osteointegration, includes harvesting of the implant-bearing transplant. While the vascular support of the graft stays intact (the fibula remains in situ), osteotomies are performed using the implant-supported cutting guide (Figure 6.15) to shape the transplant to the correct size and form. Thereafter, the suprastructure connecting the implants is placed. The prefabricated bone graft with the suprastructure in place is cut from its blood supply and transferred to the intraoral recipient site. Here, the intermediate occlusal guide is used (Figure 6.16). In the case of a bridge or hybrid structure, a positioning wafer is made to

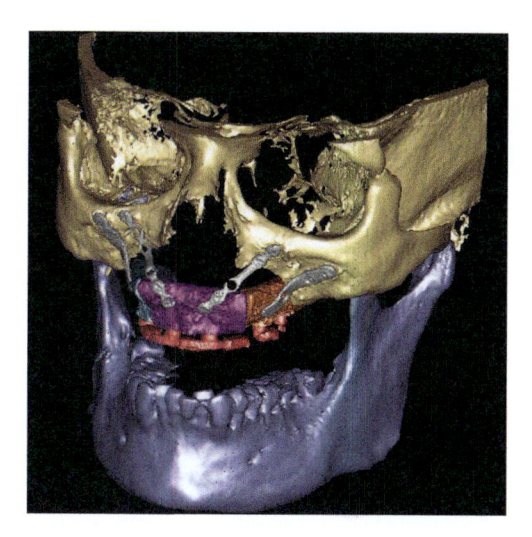

Figure 6.17A 3D segmented model of a postoperative CBCT scan after reconstruction of the maxilla with a three-segment fibula bone and a bar on implants.

guide the graft and suprastructure into the desired occlusion. The skin graft, which represents the neo-mucosa at this point, is sutured to the oral mucosa (Chang et al., 1999).

Evaluation of the surgery

CBCT scans provide the possibility of postoperative analysis for evaluation of the outcome of the surgery. The CBCT scan shows all dimensions of the reconstruction outcome (Figure 6.17A). The DICOM files from the scan can be imported into ProPlan; these can then be superimposed on the original reconstruction plan (Figure 6.17B). It is now easy to visualize how well reconstructive segments match the plan (Roser et al., 2010). Postoperative CBCT scans can also be used to evaluate consolidation of the graft bone segments to the defect edges (Figure 6.17C).

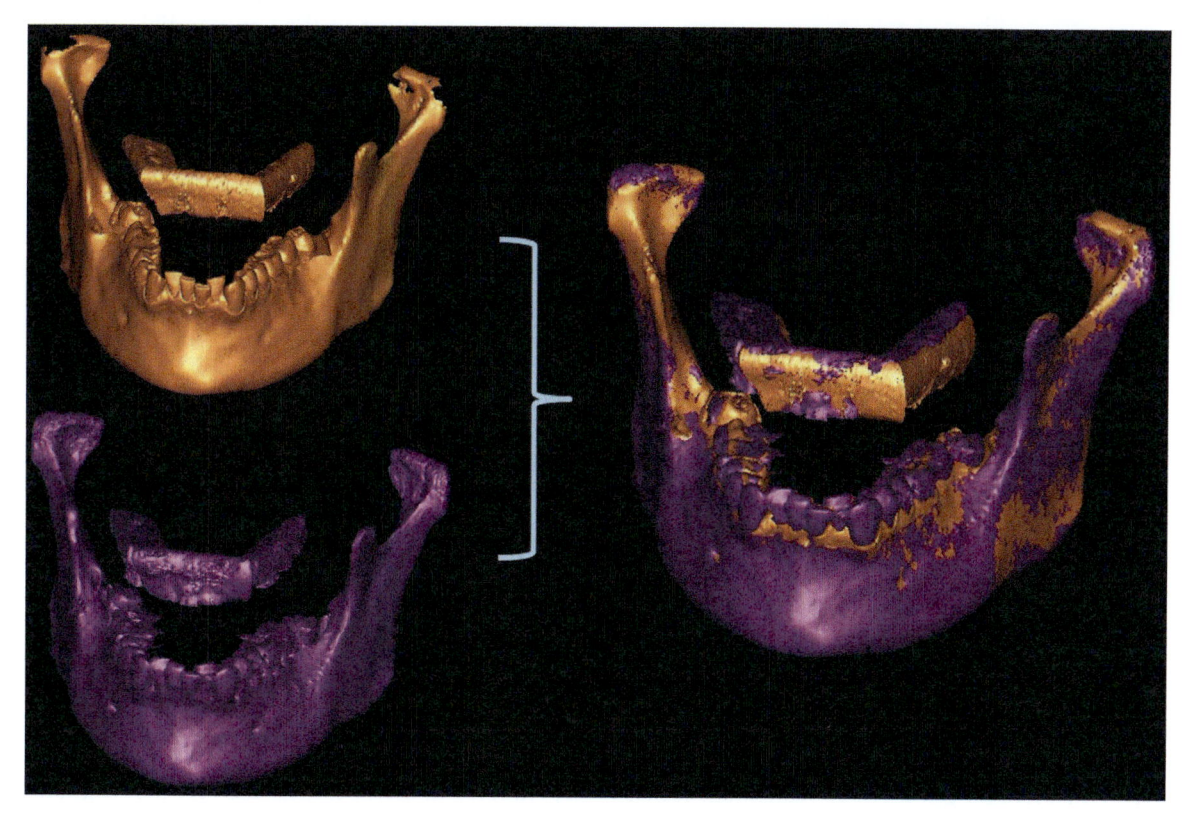

Figure 6.17B 3D model of the fibula parts and the lower jaw of the plan (orange) and the 3D model of fibula parts and the mandible extracted out of the postoperative CBCT scan (purple). The superimposition fusion model was aligned on the mandible, showing a high similarity between the planned position of the fibula parts and the surgical outcome.

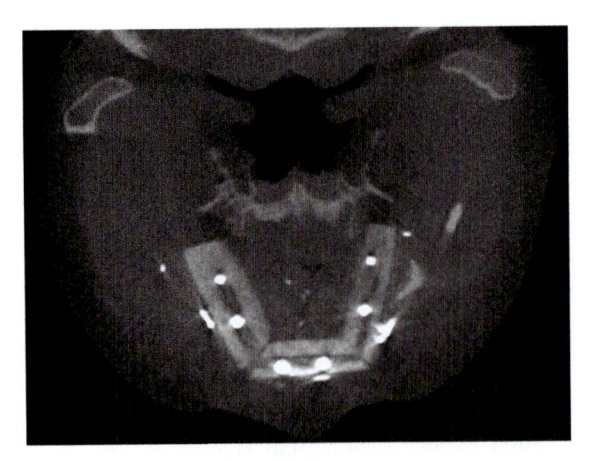

Figure 6.17C Postoperative axial CBCT slide showing the beginning phase of consolidation between the fibula segments. On conventional OPG this would not be visible in this precise manner.

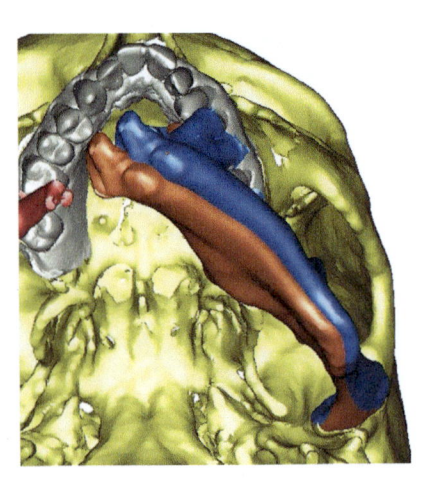

Figure 6.19 Lateral condylar rotation of the mandibular left corpus was performed (brown part, before rotation; blue part, after rotation).

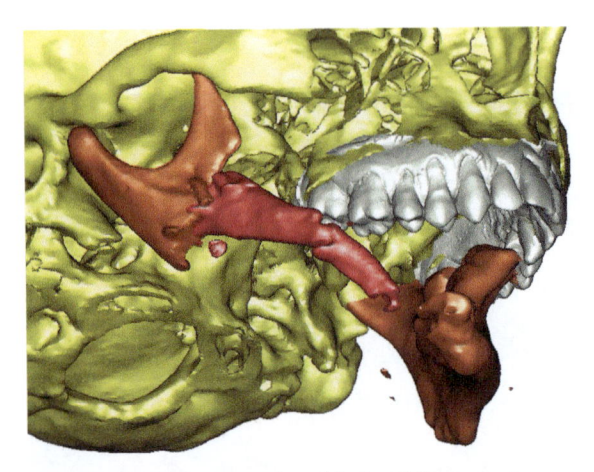

Figure 6.18 3D augmented model of a CBCT of a male patient 25 years after resection of the right corpus of the mandible and reconstruction with a rib graft. Resorption of the rib graft (red) can be clearly seen. Migration of the left mandible is shown with severe dental compensation.

Case report of a secondary reconstruction

At the age of 16 (1983), a male patient was diagnosed with an ameloblastoma of the right corpus of the mandible. A partial mandibula resection was performed, as well as immediate reconstruction with a free rib graft. Thirty years later, the rib graft was fractured and resorbed, leaving a mobile discontinuity of the mandible (Figure 6.18). The patient had a full dentition in the upper jaw and a remaining dentition in the left mandible. The left mandibular segment had migrated to the medial side over the years, showing dental compensation of the lower remaining premolars and molar. The patient was offered a reconstruction with a free fibula flap including an implant-based prosthesis, and removal of the remaining dentition in the lower jaw. Function of the temporomandibular joints was sufficient, and nearly normal condylar rotation and translation was possible. Lateral rotation of the left mandibular segment was possible to a certain extent. A 3D augmented model was obtained in ProPlan CMF with a CBCT and a scan of the dentition. The left corpus was virtually rotated to the left, preserving condylar seating to compensate for the medial migration. A more favorable position of this segment for reconstruction was thus realized (Figure 6.19). Reconstruction was planned with removal of the remaining rib graft and placement of a two-segment fibula with four implants, one of which was planned for the anterior mandibular left corpus. A bone-supported guide was planned for insertion of this implant. The remaining three implants were inserted in the fibula. All implants were placed during the first operation and their position was recorded digitally with the Lava Oral Scanner. The scan was superimposed on the plan using the remaining outer

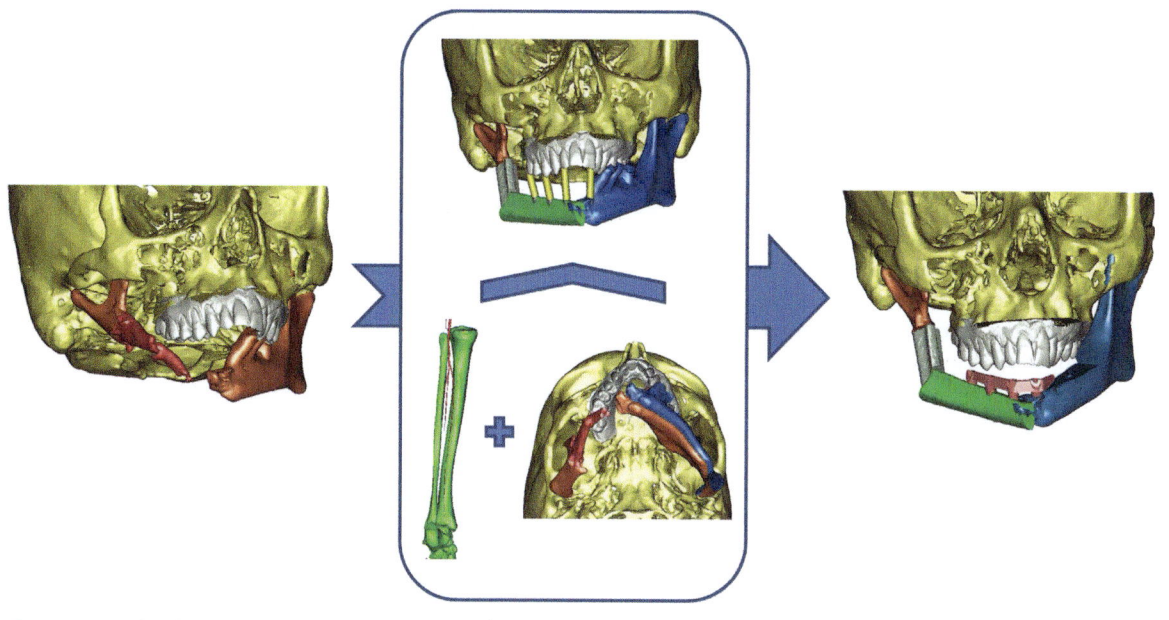

Figure 6.20 The planning of the reconstruction with two fibula segments is shown in several steps. A bar is designed on three implants in the fibula and one implant in the mandible. The teeth in the left mandibular corpus were extracted during the reconstruction surgery.

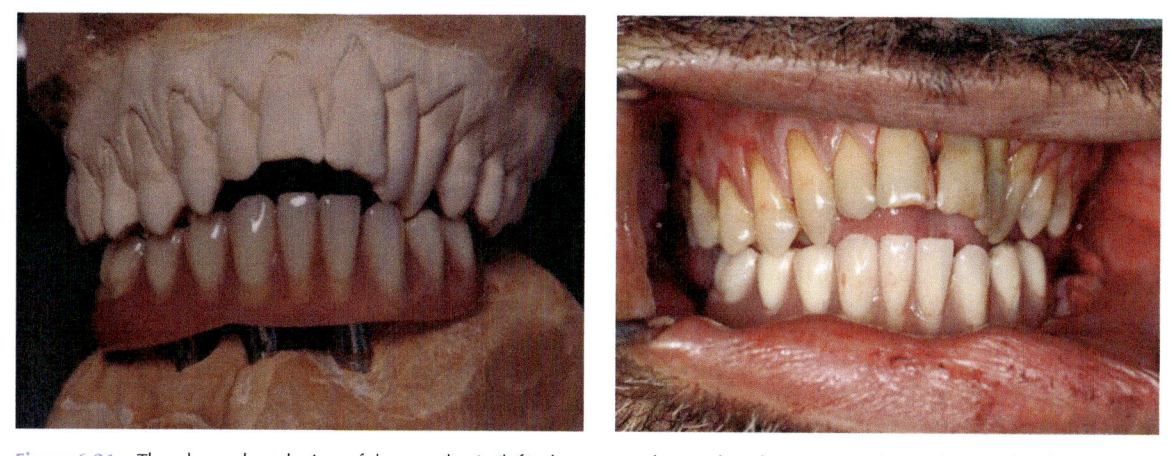

Figure 6.21 The planned occlusion of the prosthesis (left) almost exactly matches the postoperative occlusion after the reconstruction.

surface of the premolars and molar on the CBCT as a reference. A titanium bar and dental prosthesis were planned on the implants and fabricated. During the second surgical phase of the reconstructive surgery, the remaining mandibular molars were removed and the alveolar ridge was trimmed down to gain intermaxillary prosthetic height (Figure 6.20). Fixation of the fibula to the left corpus of the mandible was performed with the bar on implants and to prohibit rotation around the mandibular implant, with a 1.5-mm mini plate (Synthes, Solothurn, Switzerland). The bar and the prosthesis showed a favorable fit and occlusion (Figure 6.21). Healing was uneventful, showing a clinically and radiologically favorable consolidation. After 30 years the patient was able to eat steak.

Discussion

For complex reconstructions of maxillofacial defects, the CBCT scan provides an excellent basis for 3D virtual preoperative planning and postoperative evaluation. The CBCT apparatus is usually situated in the maxillofacial surgery department and is thus easily accessible. This is particularly important in reconstructive planning cases, because the patient has to be scanned in the right interrelation of the upper and lower jaw, which can then be checked by the surgeon or prosthodontist. Scanning the patient wearing a teeth setup can only be done this way.

In primary resection of tumors it is possible to plan the planes of the bone resection in software based on CBCT-derived data. Cutting guides can be produced to guide the resection exactly as planned. For primary and secondary reconstruction, drilling guides for guided implant insertion and cutting guides can be produced by 3D printing. As this chapter shows, the CBCT scan is the basis of these resection and reconstruction guides.

Secondary reconstruction of maxilla-mandibular defects using prefabricated bone grafts always implies that the patient must be willing to undergo at least two surgical procedures. There are three major benefits of using prefabricated bone grafts instead of bone grafts without preplanning of the graft position. First, by planning from the occlusion the prosthodontist is aiming for the optimal implant position in the bone flap, thereby trying to safeguard that implant placement and prosthetic rehabilitation are not impaired by wrong placement of implants and bone. Second, the skin graft provides an excellent thin covering around the implants of the fibula bone (Figure 6.12B; Chang et al., 1999), as in large maxillofacial defects there is usually not only a bony defect but also a lack of soft tissue. Third, ischemia time of the flap is kept to a minimum, because the shaping and cutting of the fibula as well as the fixation of the bridge onto the implants can be done with the fibula still in situ and perfused. This reduces the time needed to place the construct into the jaw defect, thus increasing the chances of successful free flap transplantation (Jokuszies et al., 2006). Even in cases of primary reconstruction of large defects during ablative surgery, virtual planning is very useful and can prevent incorrect positioning of the bone graft (as described in the primary reconstruction section).

3D printing of anatomical parts and guides is essential to allow for precise translation of the planning to the operating room. It saves operating time and therefore cost; also, it helps to reduce ischemia time. CBCT and 3D software are the basis for virtual planning technique, as described above. The fusion of optical 3D scan files and CT-angiography data extends the power of 3D surgical planning. 3D virtual planning provides an essential, powerful tool for complex reconstructions of maxillofacial defects. Computer-aided design can create all necessary guides, and additive manufacturing can print them (Hirsch et al., 2009). We foresee that for complex reconstructions, 3D virtual planning combined with 3D printing of surgical guides might evolve to become the standard approach and treatment.

References

Albert, S., Cristofari, J.P., Cox, A., Bensimon, J.L., Guedon, C., and Barry, B. (2010). Mandibular reconstruction with fibula free flap: Experience of virtual reconstruction using Osirix, a free and open source software for medical imagery. *Ann Chir Plast Esthet*, 56(6): 494–503.

Chang, Y.M., Chan, C.P., Shen, Y.F., and Wei, F.C. (1999). Soft tissue management using palatal mucosa around endosteal implants in vascularized composite grafts in the mandible. *Int J Oral Maxillofac Surg*, 28(5): 341–3.

Chiapasco, M., Biglioli, F., Autelitano, L., Romeo, E., and Brusati, R. (2006). Clinical outcome of dental implants placed in fibula-free flaps used for the reconstruction of maxillo-mandibular defects following ablation for tumors or osteoradionecrosis. *Clin Oral Implants Res*, 17(2): 220–8.

Cordeiro, P.G., Disa, J.J., Hidalgo, D.A., and Hu, Q.Y. (1999). Reconstruction of the mandible with osseous free flaps: A 10-year experience with 150 consecutive patients. *Plast Reconstr Surg*, 104(5): 1314–20.

de Almeida, E.O., Pellizzer, E.P., Goiatto, M.C., Margonar, R., Rocha, E.P., Freitas, A.C. Jr., et al. (2010). Computer-guided surgery in implantology: Review of basic concepts. *J Craniofac Surg*, 21(6): 1917–21.

Eckardt, A., and Swennen, G.R. (2005). Virtual planning of composite mandibular reconstruction with free fibula bone graft. *J Craniofac Surg*, 16(6): 1137–40.

Gbara, A., Darwich, K., Li, L., Schmelzle, R., and Blake, F. (2007). Long-term results of jaw reconstruction with microsurgical fibula grafts and dental implants. *J Oral Maxillofac Surg*, 65(5): 1005–9.

Hirsch, D.L., Garfein E.S., Christensen, A.M., Weimer, K.A., Saddeh, P.B., and Levine, J.P. (2009). Use of computer-aided design and computer-aided manufacturing to produce orthognathically ideal surgical outcomes: A paradigm shift in head and neck reconstruction. *J Oral Maxillofac Surg*, 67(10): 2115–22.

Jokuszies, A., Niederbichler, A., Meyer-Marcotty, M., Lahoda, L.U., Reimers, K., and Vogt, P.M. (2006). Influence of transendothelial mechanisms on microcirculation: Consequences for reperfusion injury after free flap transfer. Previous, current, and future aspects. *J Reconstr Microsurg*, 22(7): 513–8.

Lopez-Arcas, J.M., Arias, J., Castillo, J.L., Burgueno, M., Navarro, I., Moran, M.J., et al. (2010). The fibula osteomyocutaneous flap for mandible reconstruction: A 15-year experience. *J Oral Maxillofac Surg*, 68(10): 2377–84.

Rohner, D., Jaquiery, C., Kunz, C., Bucher, P., Maas, H., and Hammer, B. (2003). Maxillofacial reconstruction with prefabricated osseous free flaps: A 3-year experience with 24 patients. *Plast Reconstr Surg*, 112(3): 748–57.

Roser, S.M., Ramachandra, S., Blair, H., Grist, W., Carlson, G.W., Christensen, A.M., et al. (2010). The accuracy of virtual surgical planning in free fibula mandibular reconstruction: Comparison of planned and final results. *J Oral Maxillofac Surg*, 68(11): 2824–32.

Schmelzeisen, R., Neukam, F.W., Shirota, T., Specht, B., and Wichmann, M. (1996). Postoperative function after implant insertion in vascularized bone grafts in maxilla and mandible. *Plast Reconstr Surg*, 97(4): 719–25.

Taylor, G.I., Miller, G.D., and Ham, F.J. (1975). The free vascularized bone graft. A clinical extension of microvascular techniques. *Plast Reconstr Surg*, 55(5): 533–44.

Zlotolow, I.M., Huryn, J.M., Piro, J.D., Lenchewski, E., and Hidalgo, D.A. (1992). Osseointegrated implants and functional prosthetic rehabilitation in microvascular fibula free flap reconstructed mandibles. *Am J Surg*, 164(6): 677–81.

7 Implant Planning Using Cone Beam Computed Tomography

David Sarment

Introduction

Prior to surgically placing dental implants, a careful planning must be performed. Several factors are considered to ensure the successful placement of implants. The dimensions, locations, and positioning of implants should all be determined prior to surgery. Thus, it is necessary to evaluate osseous structures in detail and develop a vision of the prosthetic outcome, so that available bone volume and density, as well as anatomic limitations, are uncovered.

To this effect, there are several diagnostic tools, including radiography. Two-dimensional radiographs are a projection of the anatomy onto a film or detector. The two most commonly used methods are panoramic and periapical radiographs. Because of their ease of access, they are adequate techniques for screening, detection of obvious pathology, and initial measurements. However, they are subject to significant deformation inherent to the projection angles or centers of rotations. In a 1994 comparison of radiographic methods, Sonick et al. demonstrated that measurements performed on periapical and panoramic images could deviate 2–3 mm. They also reported a maximum deviation reaching 7.5 mm for panoramic images (Sonick et al., 1994).

Interestingly, not only these dimensions are significant, but it is not possible to know which image is most distorted. By contrast, in the same study, computed tomography (CT) distortion was 0.2 mm and would reach a maximum of 0.5 mm. Therefore, the examiner can consider all measurements to be accurate within 0.5 mm and be in the "safe zone" at all times. Interestingly, this study and others were conducted using conventional CT, with the expectation that better results would be found using cone beam computed tomography (CBCT). In 2000, the American Academy of Oral and Maxillofacial Radiology published a position statement, based on a thorough review of the literature available at the time, and recommended some type of cross-sectional imaging for implant planning (Tyndall and Brooks, 2000). Again, if the original studies were repeated at the present time, using CBCT in place of conventional CT, the three-dimensional modality would be expected to improve. However, a similar distortion would likely occur with two-dimensional radiographs because it is mostly due to factors extrinsic to image acquisition itself.

Although three-dimensional radiography has superior diagnostic value than two-dimensional images, this information alone is often insufficient

---

Cone Beam Computed Tomography: Oral and Maxillofacial Diagnosis and Applications, First Edition. Edited by David Sarment.
© 2014 John Wiley & Sons, Inc. Published 2014 by John Wiley & Sons, Inc.

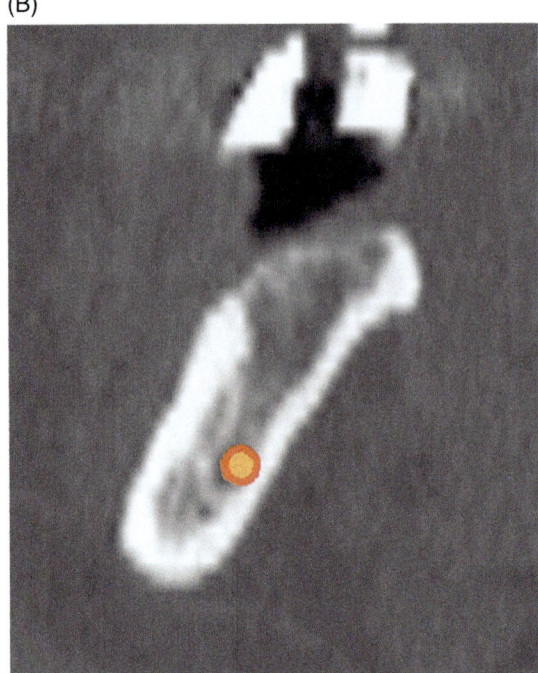

Figure 7.1 (A) This hopeless premolar can be removed and an implant immediately placed because bone is adequate and abundant where needed. (B) In the first mandibular edentulous location, a scannographic guide demonstrates that placement of an implant in the long axis of the future restoration would in fact bring the apex of an implant towards the lingual concavity. The decision can be made prior to surgery to angle the implant, place a shorter fixture, or avoid this site.

to place implants in ideal or adequate locations for restorative purposes. This is because, even in the presence of bone, the prosthetic demand might require an implant position that would be outside of the osseous envelope (Figure 7.1). Consequently, it is often necessary to project the restorative expectation onto the radiographic image, using a radiographic guide, in order to visualize bone and future restorations simultaneously. To this effect, the availability of in-office three-dimensional radiography creates the flexibility of positioning a radiographic guide in the presence of the clinician. This is in contrast to referring a patient to a center or hospital, where the technician might not be aware of the positioning of a dental guide, and the patient supine position together with the difficulties of scanning might compromise the outcome.

There are other practical advantages of using in-office scanning. For example, when using a small field of view, it is possible to rescan an area of interest after treatment has been rendered to document healing or evaluate a bone graft. The ability to quickly diagnose and plan for treatment is a significant advantage when care must be rendered in a timely fashion due to patient discomfort or pain. Combined with surgical guides, the use of CBCT and implant planning software allows for a predictable surgery (Nickenig and Eitner, 2007). However, there are limitations to CBCT. Image contrast is limited, and the presence of dental restorations significantly deteriorates image quality. Furthermore, radiation levels are significant and imaging can only be used reasonably.

Image quality and implant planning

The quality of CBCT, as discussed in chapter 1, significantly impacts diagnosis. Voxel size, contrast, and artifacts are important factors to consider when viewing and planning implants. To optimize the use of the machine, the least amount of radiation yielding accurate measurements should be utilized (Dawood et al., 2012). Three-dimensional renderings are utilized during the diagnosis treatment

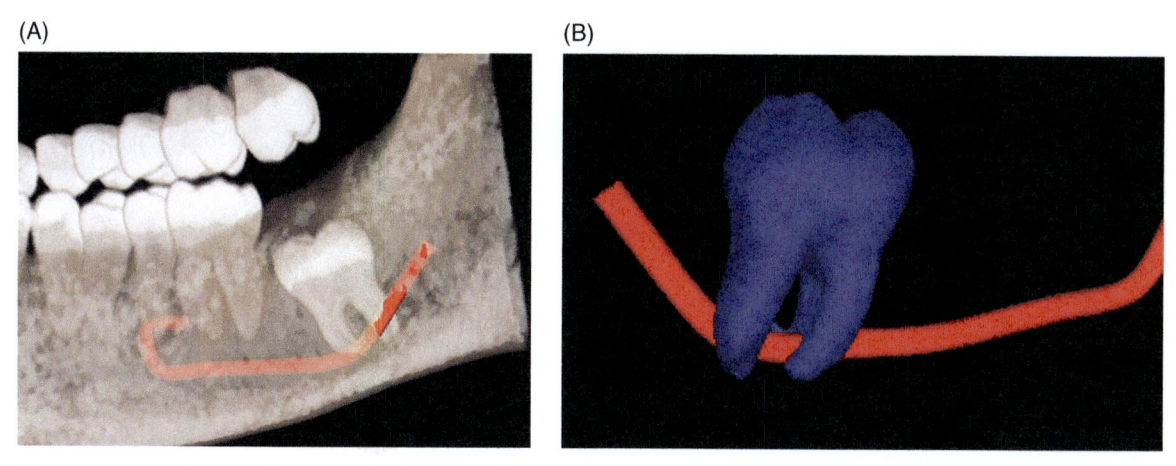

Figure 7.2 (A) Volume rendering is difficult to utilize for discerning the relationship between the roots and the mandibular nerve. With surface rendering, specific anatomy can be assigned various colors with threshold methods. (B) Because objects are now separated, they can be removed from the rendering, providing a view of specific areas. In this case, the roots and their relationship to the nerve can be viewed precisely.

phase and must be accurate to provide a true representation of bone. Unfortunately, it is common to find a discrepancy between the expected anatomy and the actual topography discovered during surgery. Although several factors affect image quality (Ritter et al., 2009), viewing is most affected by image rendering method and three-dimensional calculation thresholds.

Image rendering can be performed in two ways: volume rendering and surface rendering. Volume rendering is a three-dimensional display mostly available on cone beam and spiral CTs standard software. It is best understood as a cloud of pixels with some level of transparency. By contrast, surface rendering is obtained using conversion software to calculate the surface of the image and show it with small triangles.

The example in Figure 7.2 illustrates the use of surface rendering versus volume rendering. Figure 7.2A shows volume rendering of a second molar in close proximity with the mandibular nerve. Software (Uniguide, France) is then utilized to import DICOM files and prepare a surface rendering of the anatomy. In contrast to volume rendering, surface rendering uses thresholds to discern anatomic features. Since each voxel is assigned a certain Hounsfield unit that represents a gray value, it is possible to instruct the computer to eliminate voxels that are outside of a window of gray values. For examples, if an object such as a tooth, denser than adjacent bone, is believed to be extractable using a window of units ranging from 1000 to 1500, then surrounding voxels of smaller values are assigned to a different object (in this case, bone). Once rendered, each object can be displayed together or separately. Figure 7.3 also illustrates the use of this technique, called segmentation, for treatment planning. In this case, orthodontic implants are desired. Virtual implants are introduced to the rendering while separating anatomical features, and future osteotomies can be planned carefully. Surface rendering is therefore a superior method for viewing CBCT anatomy and planning implants. In addition, software can perform calculations such as Boolean operations that consist of detecting common areas overlaid by two objects, or subtracting unnecessary anatomy. However, because the approach is dependent upon threshold values, this arbitrary decision can also affect the outcome since true anatomy can slightly differ. In Figure 7.4, bone is represented at two different thresholds, demonstrating how changes in values can significantly affect the rendering.

Once a three-dimensional image has been rendered on a computer screen, it can also be exported for three-dimensional printing. Although CAD/CAM is most often used for fabrication of a surgical guide, it is also possible to produce CAD/CAM medical models and utilize these for implant planning (Rasmussen, 2000). In Figure 7.5, a stereolithographic medical model was ordered and planning was performed on the transparent model.

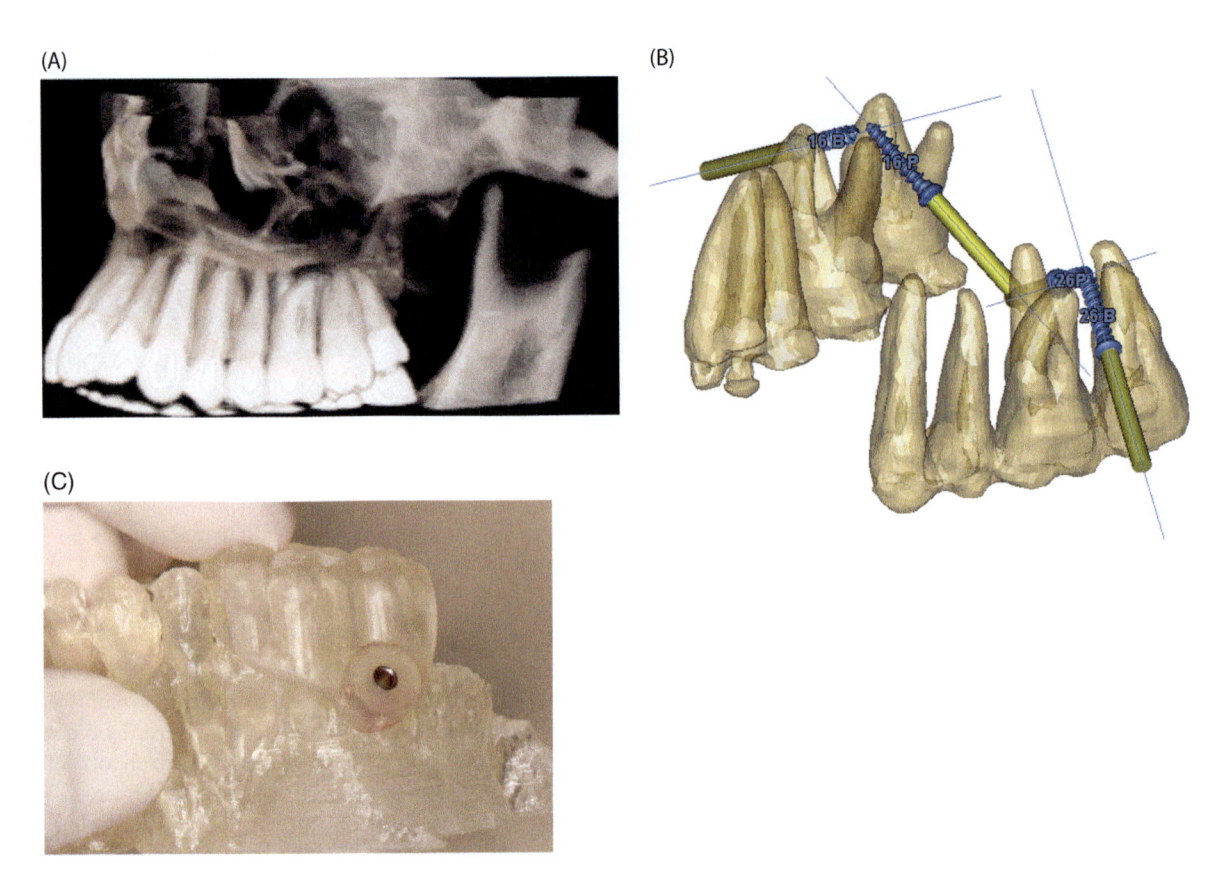

Figure 7.3 (A) Four orthodontic interradicular implants are planned, but volume rendering is difficult to utilize to depict the precise anatomy. (B) Using software (Uniguide, France), segmentation of anatomic features is performed and bone is eliminated from the rendering, allowing for the depiction of virtual implants and their accurate relationship to adjacent roots. (C) A CAD/CAM surgical guide (see chapter 8) is then fabricated. Implants are placed accurately.

A surgery on the plastic was conducted while visualizing the anatomy. A surgical guide was then fabricated in the laboratory, using acrylic and traditional methods. Again, bone surface found on the model is only as good as software segmentation and rendering. If the surface is misinterpreted because of limited contrast, the model may not be a true representation of bone. This is particularly true if bone grafting was first performed.

Anatomic evaluation

Prior to placing a dental implant, it is necessary to evaluate the anatomy in order to prevent intrusion to undesirable areas, prepare for bone augmentation, and optimize implant stability and position. Furthermore, implant therapeutic options have become more sophisticated in recent years, and more delicate evaluations are often necessary. This includes prosthetic demands, surgical techniques, and intricate treatment planning with other specialties such as orthodontics. Other chapters focus on several aspects of surgical methods. This chapter focuses on practical anatomic considerations as applied to the daily practice of dental implants.

Bone density

Density of bone is an important factor for implant placement, and there are several critical elements with regard to density. First, thickness of cortical bone can be evaluated to anticipate the ability to stabilize the implant when minimal bone height is otherwise available. High resolution available with

(A) (B)

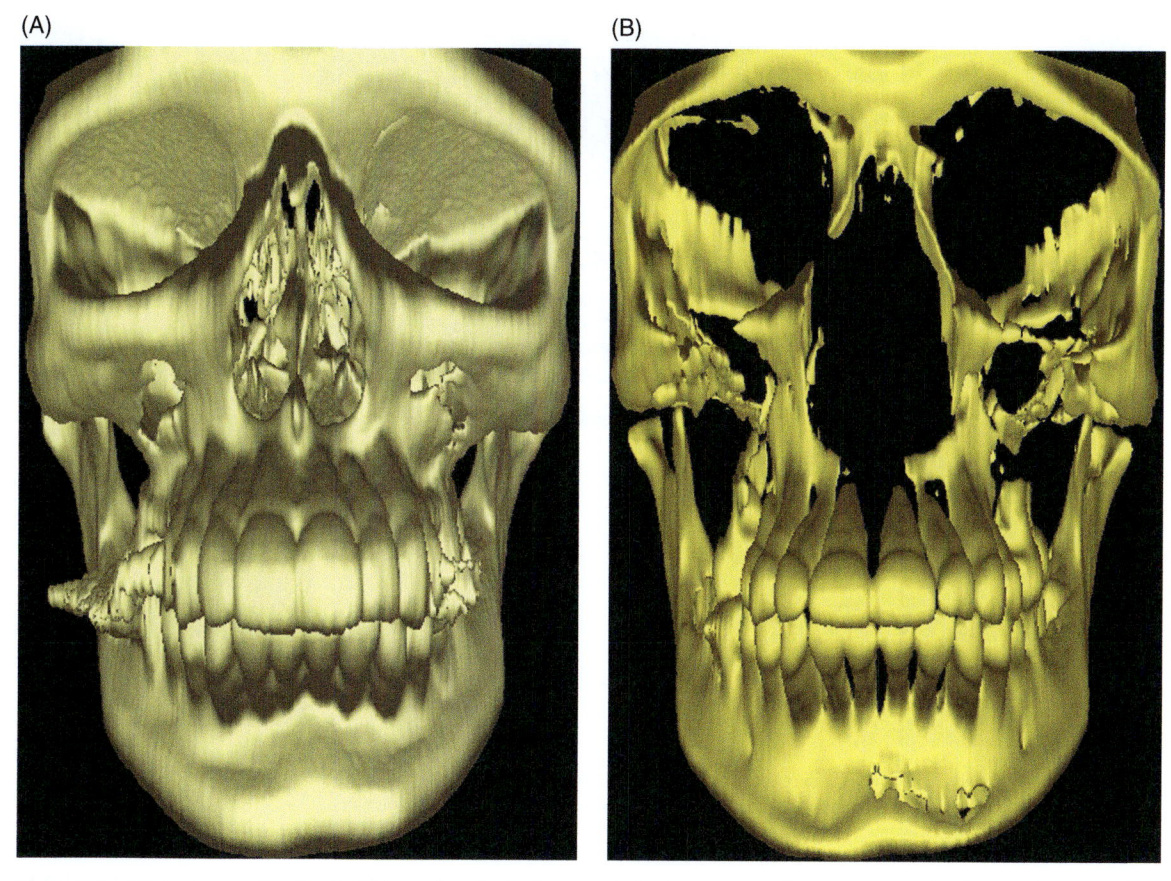

Figure 7.4 (A) A conservative threshold is used to depict bone and eliminate surrounding tissues. (B) The threshold is modified to increase the window and some bone of lesser density is no longer visible.

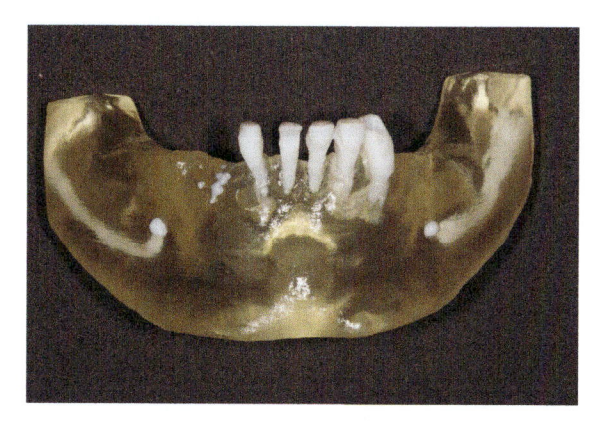

Figure 7.5 A medical CAD/CAM model was ordered using the office CBCT. The model shows bone surface and hopeless teeth. A rehearsal of surgery can be performed on the model, including extractions and bone reduction.

CBCT provides an adequate measurement of cortical bone thickness. Second, medullar bone density can be evaluated as well: a visual appreciation of density is possible, which allows for anticipation of the clinical scenario. Knowing that poor density will be found at surgery influences the implant protocol, perhaps leading to the decision to undersize the osteotomy. In contrast, high density might require further osseous preparation, such as pre-tapping of the osteotomy site.

It is important to remember that CBCT is less reliable than conventional CT with regard to precise density measurements. Compared to conventional machines, which are calibrated within a few Hounsfield units, cone beam machines are not so precise, and discrepancies exist from patient to patient as well as within a single scan. Yet there is

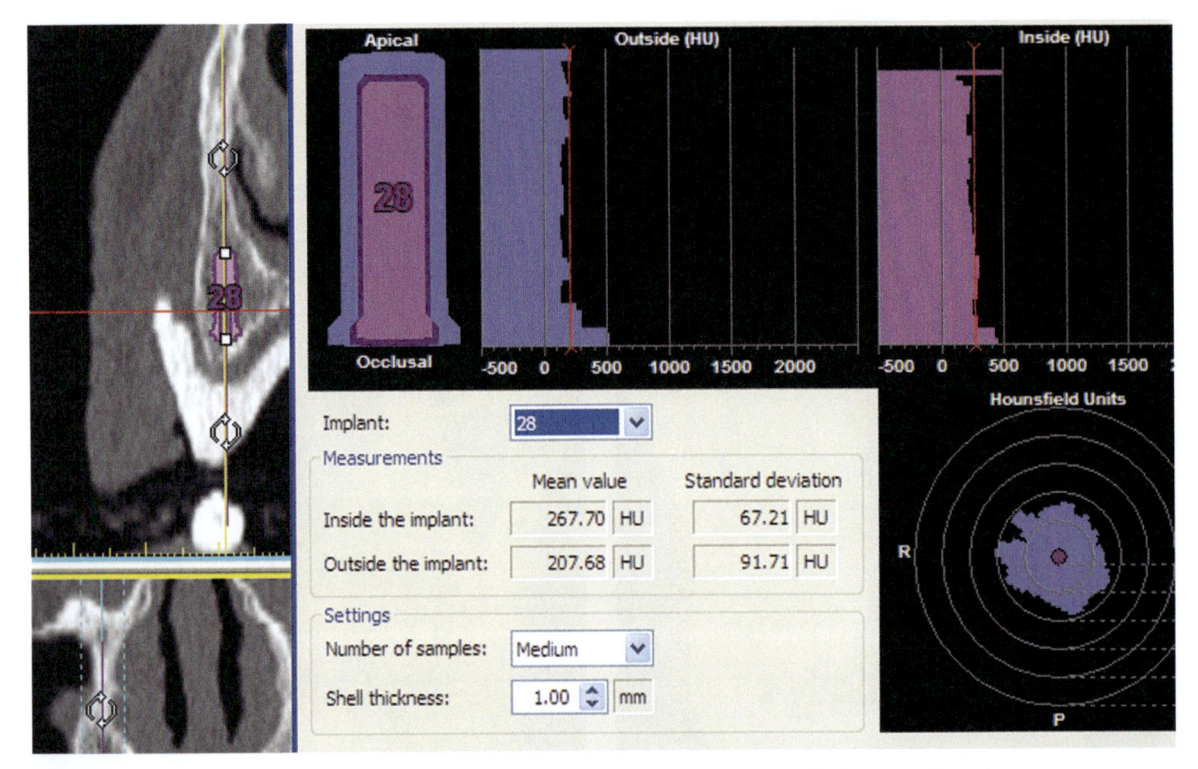

Figure 7.6 A third party software is utilized to investigate bone density in the vicinity of a future implant. The computer can analyze surrounding Hounsfield units and render graphs to approximate bone density.

some evidence that a correlation is generally present (Norton and Gamble, 2001; Song et al., 2009; Naitoh, Aimiya, et al., 2010). As a result, implant planning software often provides calculation tools that render a representation of density in the vicinity of a virtual implant: a potential implant location is selected by overlaying the drawing of an implant onto the CT image using a dedicated software tool. Software gathers Hounsfield levels within voxels surrounding the potential implant. A rendering is then produced, usually utilizing color schemes and figures to represent the expected density (Figure 7.6).

Considerations for maxillary sinus augmentations

When planning for an implant at the posterior maxilla, the anatomy of the maxillary sinus must be understood. The first consideration is bone height: if insufficient, bone grafting may be necessary. The ability to precisely measure bone height below the maxillary sinus allows for the selection of a surgical method. If available bone is sufficient to obtain primary stability, then it is conceivable to use an osteotomy technique, or a simultaneous placement and Caldwell-Luc sinus grafting technique. If this distance is insufficient to expect primary stability, a sinus augmentation alone is planned.

Osteotomy techniques

When using an augmentation through the osteotomy approach, a precise measurement can be performed using CBCT. In addition, the local anatomy can be precisely evaluated, at times allowing for a flapless approach (Fornell et al., 2012). Because the image can be manipulated, local measurements can be positioned in the expected axis of the future osteotomy. As a result, the distance from the crestal bone to the floor of the sinus is known prior to surgery. In techniques where 2 mm

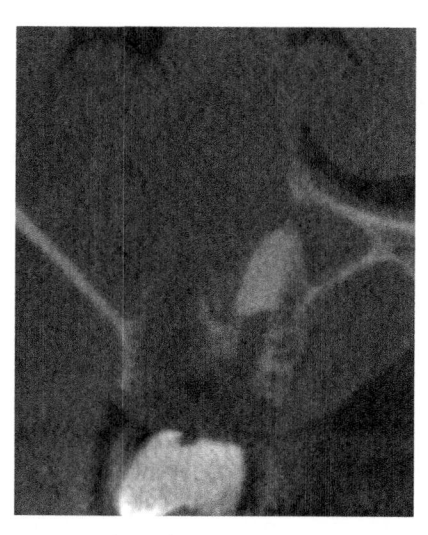

Figure 7.7 A single tooth implant site shows sinus pathology, lack of vertical bone, proximity of the maxillary sinus, a communication, and a root remnant. A periapical radiograph would be insufficient to anticipate these issues.

are first subtracted prior to fracturing the cortical bone towards the sinus, an adequate estimate is available. In fact, it can be argued that a periapical radiograph taken during surgery might not be necessary since a true visualization would not be obtained.

In the example of Figure 7.7, an extraction had been recently performed and the placement of a dental implant was expected. A root remnant was to be removed, but more importantly, a soft tissue communication with the maxillary sinus was evident. In evaluating the area for bone augmentation, it was found that the bucco-lingual dimension was flat. Interestingly, although the initial preference to approach the area surgically was to utilize a window, it was determined that the extraction socket would give better access to the area of interest for several reasons. First, the window would have been at a significant buccal distance to the future implant location, and good access and visualization would have been difficult. Second, elevation of the maxillary soft tissue in the area of the extraction socket would have been difficult, with possible tear due to the fresh extraction. Furthermore, elevation to the medial wall would have been delicate, with the likelihood to graft the buccal portion of the sinus only. Finally, bone graft would have had to be placed in sufficient volume to reach the window and packing would have been difficult. As a result, it was decided to utilize the extraction socket to approach the area and graft the site.

Another example where a CBCT is useful is the single premolar site. In a typical case, the sinus floor above the area of interest would be somewhat flat and regular. Yet, it is possible to find a significant slant and, at times, a bucco-lingual septum interrupting the floor, therefore forcing the surgeon to modify the surgical approach. Unique nuances of the local anatomy are best studied using CBCT and would be more difficult to depict without it.

Caldwell-Luc approaches

When choosing a Caldwell-Luc sinus augmentation approach, CBCT enhances the surgical preparation and execution. First, the presence of soft tissue pathology can be ruled out, or addressed appropriately. Because CBCT is present in the office and radiation doses are reduced when compared to conventional CT, updating the anatomy with a new examination after treatment of sinus pathology is reasonable (Figure 7.8). Furthermore, specific dimensions of the sinus in the area of interest can be studied, and might influence the surgical approach. Typically, the sinus width and shape are important dimensions to visualize prior to entering the area. Once known, a good localization and size of the window is easily identified while the depth of the graft can be predicted. In fact, a measurement can be recorded and utilized during surgery to ascertain that the sinus membrane has been elevated to the medial wall, in situations where direct visualization is difficult.

Another important anatomic limitation when preparing for a maxillary sinus surgery is the presence of septi, which might interfere with the localization of the window. In the presence of a septum, the clinician can easily and accurately locate it, and then determine if the window can be displaced mesially or distally. When necessary, two windows can be created. Furthermore, elevation of the sinus membrane can purposely be performed against the septum: the clinician, knowing to look for the bony interference, will reflect the membrane using a modified angle of the surgical instrument while continuing to maintain bone contact.

In other instances, unusual sinus anatomy can be depicted, revealing mesio-distal walls or complete separations within the maxillary sinus. A two-dimensional radiograph such as a panoramic or a periapical film would not reveal compartments, leaving the element of surprise at the time of surgery. For instance, in Figure 7.9, two separate sinuses are present, one a medial and one a buccal compartment. CBCT was performed for the purpose of preparing for a sinus elevation and later implant placement. In view of the anatomic structures, it would have been possible to take the unusual approach of accessing the most medial sinus with a secondary window. Yet, because the outcome was unpredictable and out of the routine practice, it was decided to avoid grafting all together. As a result, the surgical treatment plan and prosthetic plan were affected and modified to accommodate this new limitation. It is interesting to note that the initial treatment plan was established using a panoramic radiograph and, if a CBCT had not been requested, it is likely that grafting of the most buccal sinus only would have been performed as it would have been impossible, at the time of surgery, to detect the mesio-distal wall. Consequently, the area could not have been implanted.

Considerations at the mandible

Mandibular anatomy

At the mandible, several anatomic considerations are better understood using three-dimensional radiography. For example, the localization of the mandibular nerve is more precisely measured in three dimensions, and more importantly, unusual

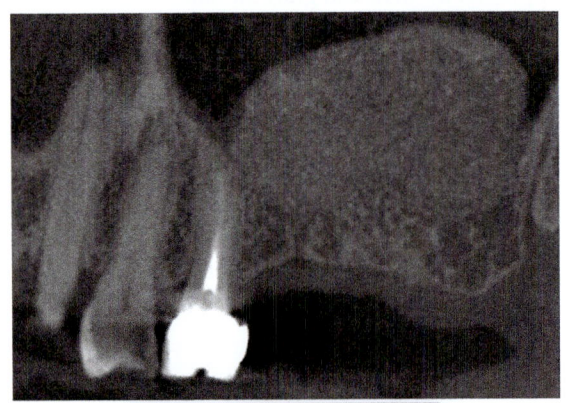

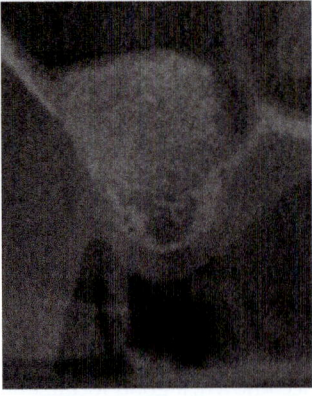

Figure 7.8 A maxillary sinus is evaluated after grafting. This second scan is useful to ascertain grafting success and prepare the implant surgery.

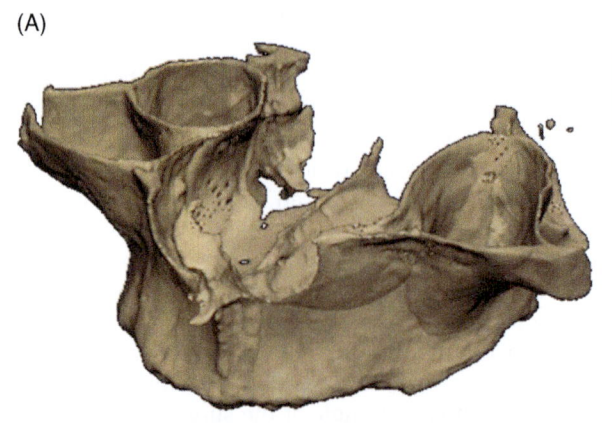

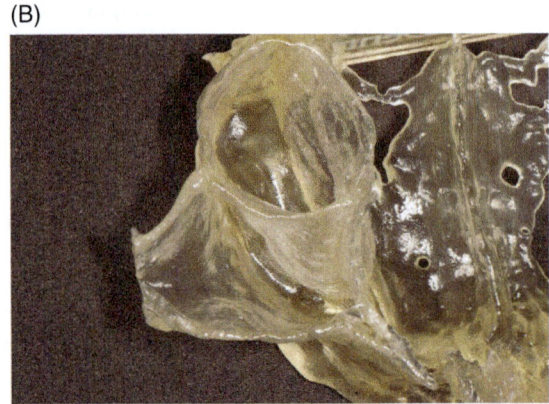

Figure 7.9 The three-dimensional rendering (A) of a maxilla shows a right sinus divided in a buccal and palatal compartments. (B) The biomodel is easier to view. Its manipulation is convenient for treatment planning.

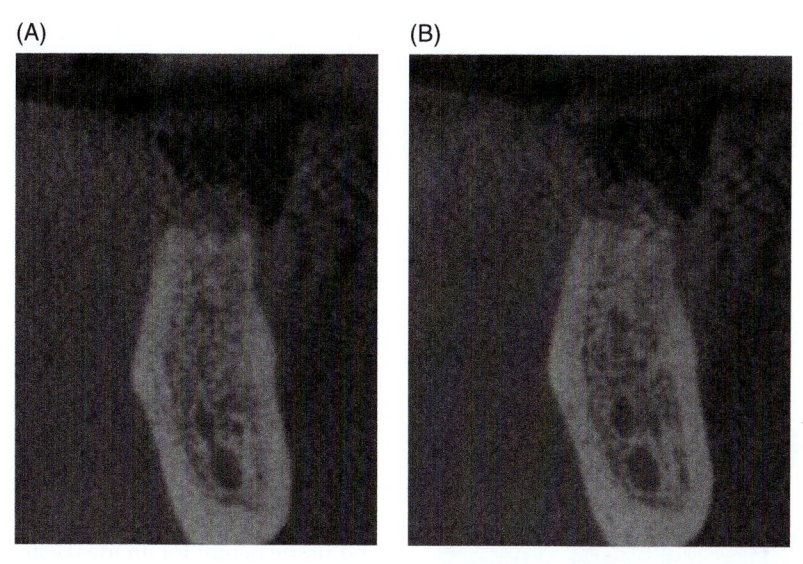

Figure 7.10 The mandibular nerve is bifid, and a significant branch continues mesial to the mental foramen. (A) This cross-section is located in the second premolar area, and shows the beginning of the nerve division. (B) This cross-section is located about 2 mm mesial to the first section, once the two branches are distinguishable.

anatomy such as bifid canals can and should be safely identified. The ability to scroll through fine images also allows for a good visualization of the mental foramen as well as anatomic variations in this area. In the case presented in Figure 7.10 the nerve splits in two large branches distal to the mental foramen. As a result, if placement of an implant in the vicinity of the mental foramen is considered, it might be more reasonable to maintain a greater distance than usual for the osteotomy, or to place an implant coronal to the secondary mesial branch. In fact, the presence of such a branch past the mesial aspect of the mental foramen is common and more easily identifiable on a CBCT (Orhan et al., 2011). Because contrast is inferior using CBCT, it is in fact possible that detection of the cortical bone defining the mandibular canal could be more difficult than traditional CT. Other considerations at the mandible include the presence of bone canals in the interforaminal area. According to Tepper et al. it is always present. Its identification might prevent its perforation and possibly prevent bleeding (Tepper et al., 2001). Similar to implant site evaluation, it is also possible to radiograph the block donor site when such a method is necessary. The symphyses of the mental area are easily radiographed and measurements easily obtained to assess the position and size of the block.

Diagnosis

Endodontic treatment versus implantation

The presence of a CBCT in the office allows for imaging of a tooth with a guarded prognosis. When the decision to extract a tooth is questionable, it is often because endodontic treatment is a reasonable approach. Often, further treatment such as a crown elongation is also necessary and the survival of the tooth is debatable. There is ample research evaluating the long-term success of endodontic treatment and demonstrating outcomes equivalent to implant success rates. In addition, CBCT helps enhance endodontic treatment and retreatment (see chapter 10). Yet the precise third dimension provided by CBCT might assist in the decision making, not only in evaluating the difficulty of treating the tooth but also in recognizing the possible obstacles in implant placement. In the example of Figure 7.11, a periapical radiograph of a tooth with a guarded prognosis is representative of such a situation. Once a CBCT has been performed, the decision to remove the tooth is more easily made: the extent of the lesion is significant enough to choose extraction and later replacement of this second molar. Figure 7.12 illustrates a case considered for root coverage. Once a

CBCT is taken, the lack of cuspid bone support becomes evident and an extraction with implant placement is preferred.

In Figure 7.13, it is possible to appreciate the positions of fractures endured during a sport accident on this lateral incisor. Two bucco-lingual fractures are identifiable, showing their relationship to the pulp and adjacent bone support. Upon identification of the fracture lines, the decision to remove the tooth and place an implant is easily made, although endodontic treatment was first considered: a significant crown elongation and possible orthodontic forced-eruption would be necessary prior to restoring the tooth, leaving a short root and an esthetic defect. In contrast, bone is present for an immediate implant placement after extraction, maintaining the buccal bone with minimal grafting and tissue height for an ideal esthetic outcome.

Extraction

When the extraction is performed, the maintenance of remaining supporting osseous material is critical to subsequent implant treatment, bone grafting, or implant placement. In particular, the buccal bone plate can be difficult to preserve because of its thickness. For instance, in the esthetic zone, such as in Figures 7.13 and 7.14, this structure is particularly susceptible to surgical trauma. In some instances, a fenestration or dehiscence might be visible using CBCT. Only a radiographic method capable of detecting fine areas can serve the clinician in analyzing a thin buccal bone plate. Once detected, the clinician can better prepare for the surgical act by allocating more time to expand the alveole and perhaps by modifying techniques to limit buccal pressures.

Similarly, interradicular bone for posterior teeth is another delicate structure to manage during tooth removal. Once identified, the clinician can also modify the surgery to preserve this precious bone structure. For instance, the decision to section roots prior to attempting an elevation can be taken for the purpose of avoiding buccal tension on the interradicular structure. Because of the ability to travel through occluso-apical sections and modify angles, it is also possible to note if roots possess angles or apical fusion which might interfere with its mobilization. In fact, once a root form is understood anatomically, its path of extraction can also be anticipated. CBCT is a method of choice for such fine analysis

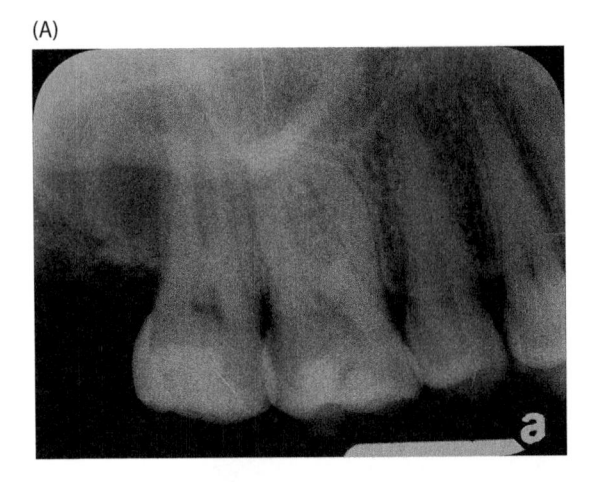

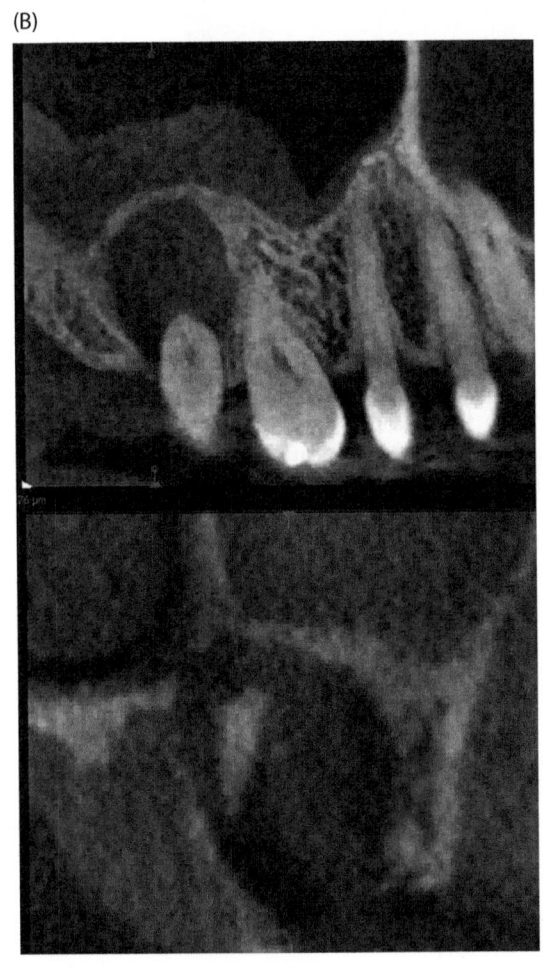

Figure 7.11 (A) A periapical radiograph shows a lesion distal to the second molar. Probing is significant and watched for about 12 months. (B) A CBCT demonstrates the extent of the lesion, including communication to the sinus and nasal cavity.

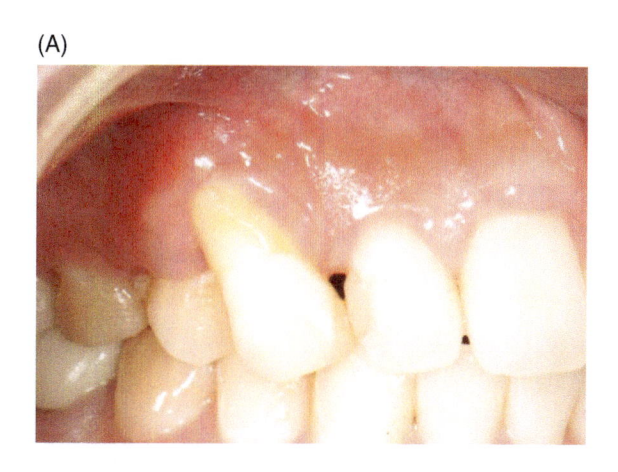

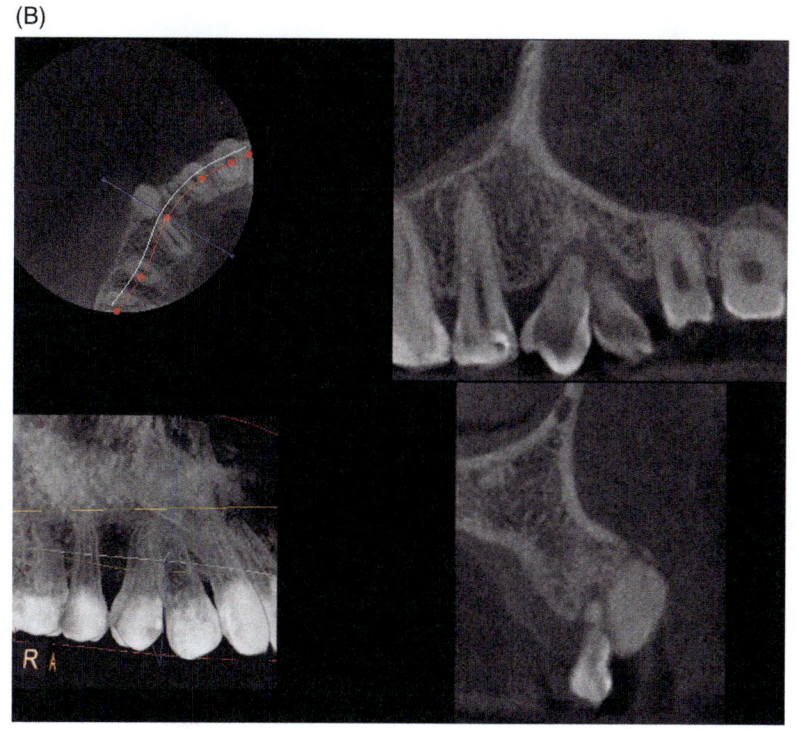

Figure 7.12 (A) A cuspid is considered for root coverage, but (B) inadequate bone support instead suggests an extraction and implant placement.

because of the practical access to the machine, fine imaging, and relatively reasonable radiation.

Orthodontic evaluation

Another indication for CBCT is in the analysis of an implant site while orthodontic movement is anticipated or in progress. A typical example is a patient with missing lateral incisors. When possible, it is preferable to analyze the surgical anatomy before or prior to completion of tooth movement. It is not uncommon to find that adjacent roots converge apically, resulting in a lack of mesio-distal distance at mid-root or more apically. The use of CBCT can confirm if adequate space is present, and when insufficient, it is possible to request a torque movement. Again, when patients are of age to

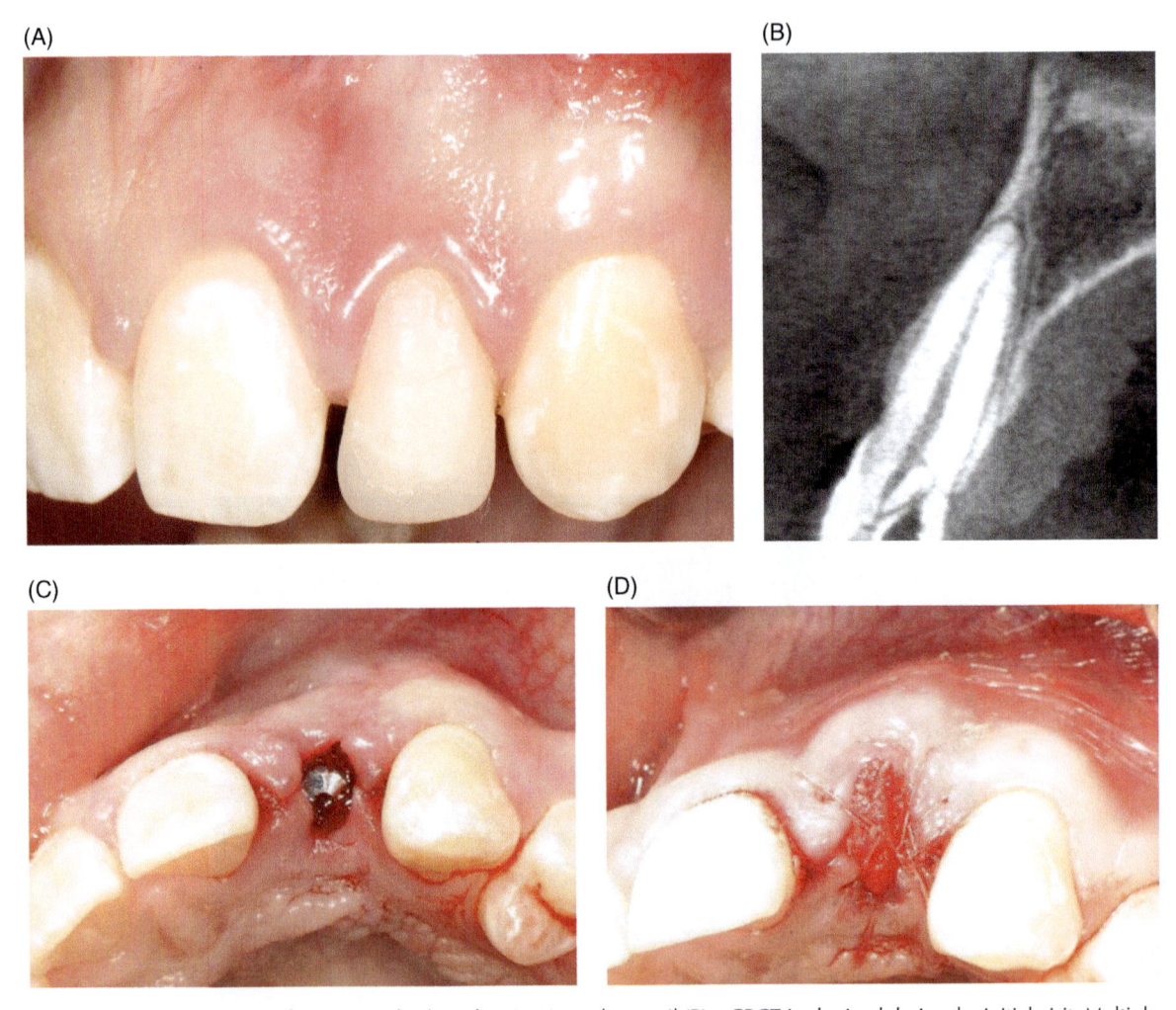

Figure 7.13 (A) The extent of trauma on this lateral incisor is unclear until (B) a CBCT is obtained during the initial visit. Multiple fractures are evident, leading to a replacement with an implant. (C) The tooth is carefully removed while maintaining the buccal plate, and an implant is immediately inserted. (D) A bone graft is also packed prior to placement of a collagen membrane.

receive CBCT, it is also conceivable to perform a second local CBCT to confirm that space has been established. In Figure 7.15, the orthodontist was about to complete treatment. A panoramic radiograph was insufficient to note that the mesio-distal distance at mid-root level was reduced due to root convergence. Once tooth movement was modified, the area was radiographed a second time to confirm that a narrow diameter implant had now become an option.

Furthermore, mini-implants as anchoring devices for orthodontic applications can take advantage of CBCT to evaluate interradicular space and bone thickness. Once implant planning has been performed, the osteotomy must accurately be placed between roots. Recently, while the use of CAD/CAM surgical guides is more commonly used for definitive implants, their application to mini-implants has also been explored (Kim et al., 2008).

Immediate implantation

When immediate implantation is a consideration, the ability to confirm that adequate bone is available for primary stability is a concern. CBCT is an

(A)

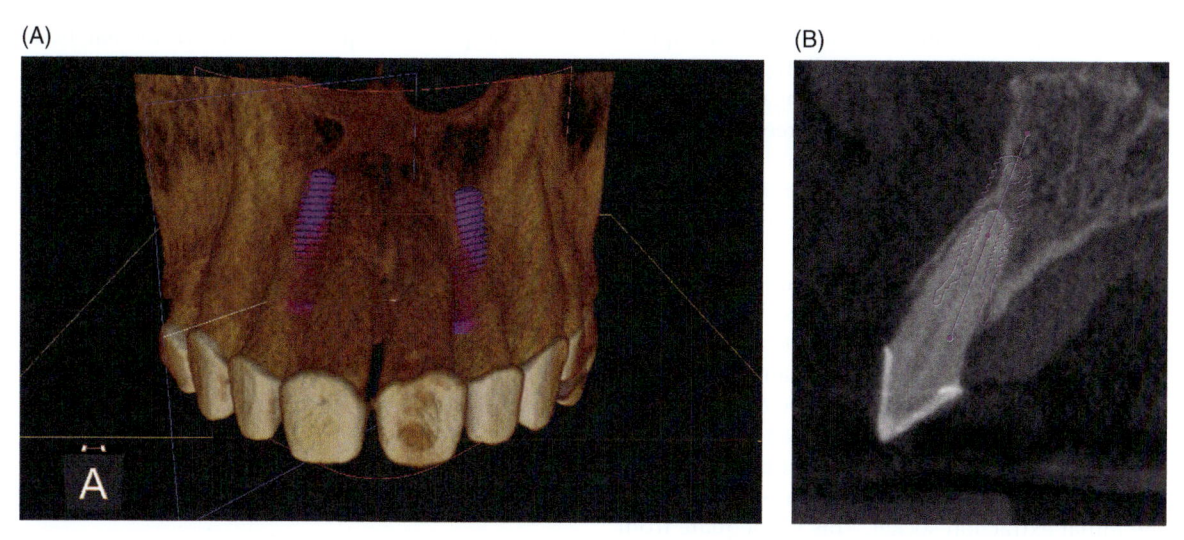

(B)

Figure 7.14 (A) The rendering shows virtual implant apices coming through the buccal plates. (B) The thin buccal plate is more evident on this cross-section.

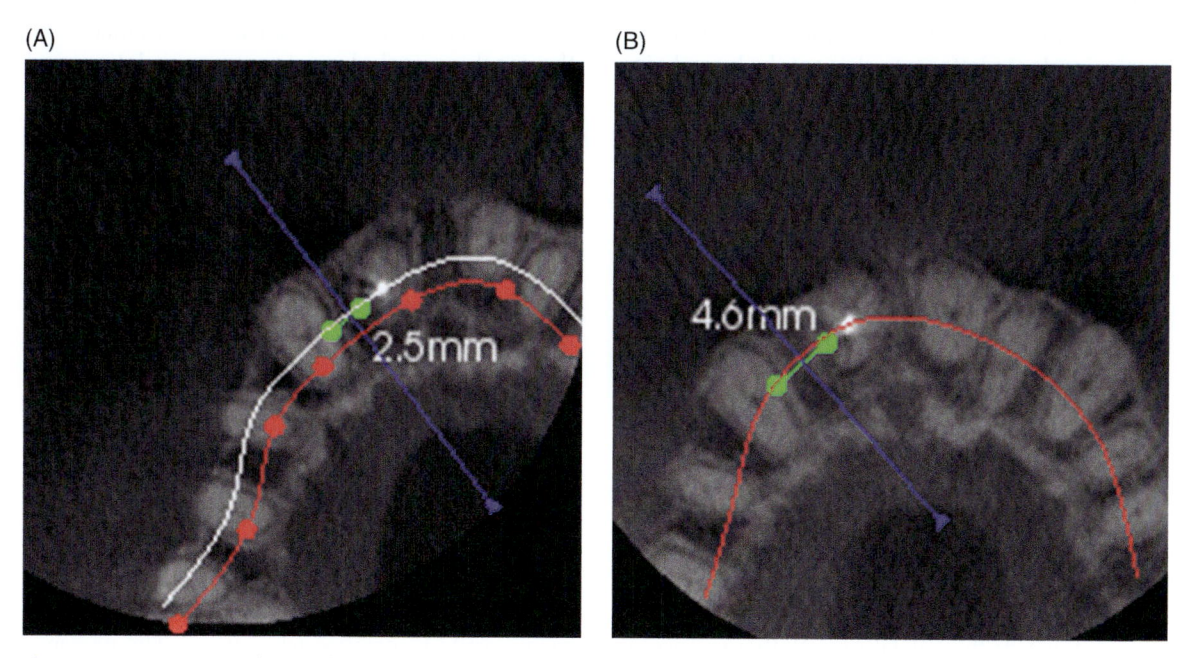

(A)

(B)

Figure 7.15 (A) A preimplant evaluation is performed during orthodontic treatment. A future lateral incisor implant is desired, but the space is insufficient in the apical region. (B) Orthodontic movement is modified with further divergence of the roots and the CBCT update now shows adequate space.

option to validate the presence of apical or interradicular bone. It is then possible to appreciate how much bone-implant contact is expected, and what area of the future implant would remain in the alveole. Furthermore, it is also possible to anticipate where the implant can be located to gain stability. Using a three-dimensional fine radiograph, the clinician can predetermine the available bone and be more confident that primary stability can be achieved. The localization of the implant may or may not be centered on the extraction socket, apical bone might be available for anchorage, and selection of a wide enough implant to engage the socket walls can be performed using three-dimensional evaluation.

At the maxillary anterior quadrant, the implant will engage the palatal wall of bone while knowledge of the buccal bone wall is critical (Braut et al., 2011). A CBCT image can provide adequate measurements of these two areas. More importantly, an implant emulation can be performed at this stage to ensure that the implant localization and angulation does not have to be compromised while searching for anchorage (Kan et al., 2011). Indeed, it is common to find implants placed with a significant buccal angulation because they follow the initial extraction socket. This is adequate from the surgical aspect, but the restoration is more difficult to achieve because the abutment is significantly angulated. Furthermore, in highly esthetic cases with thin buccal tissues, there is a high risk for the implant platform to show at the buccal gingival margin. In an effort to avoid this issue, the careful clinician would prepare the osteotomy more palatally and with the desire to direct the long axis of the implant towards the tooth cingulum (Figure 7.13C, Figure 7.13D). Therefore, the presence of a palatal wall and apical bone are critical to an ideal immediate implant placement. CBCT, again, is a useful tool to carefully study these specific dimensions. Figure 7.14 illustrates how a prosthetically driven implant placement causes the apical portion of implants to perforate the buccal plate.

In the maxillary premolar area, tooth anatomy significantly impacts the localization of an immediate implant at the time of extraction. For example, a single-rooted tooth can easily provide guidance for an osteotomy. In contrast, when two divergent roots are present, the implant osteotomy might digress towards the palatal root. With a periapical radiograph, it is more difficult to decipher the tooth anatomy, whereas a CBCT shows root anatomy and bone morphology. At the mandible, tooth anatomy is usually less significant to an immediate implant placement. However, localization of the mental foramen is critical because the osteotomy might be apical to the socket in order to obtain primary stability, thus approaching this important anatomic limitation.

In the posterior quadrants, interradicular bone is often utilized to anchor an immediate implant. Again, a two-dimensional radiograph provides a limited view of this anatomy. Another consideration is the presence of the maxillary sinus, which can at times follow the anatomy of the molar roots. Once the tooth is removed, little bone height remains to prepare an osteotomy and bone density can be low. If an internal sinus elevation is to be performed, it is preferable to anticipate the procedure using proper diagnosis. At the mandible, the availability of bone is also limited by the possible presence of the mandibular nerve.

Small implant restorations

For a single tooth implant, bone morphology is studied precisely on CBCT. The mesio-distal dimension can be measured, using a virtual ruler, on the axial view: typically, software provided with the machine includes image manipulation and initial measurements such as rulers. The user can scroll axial views and select a level at which the measurement is most useful. It is important to note that axial views are cross-sections of the scanned volume. Consequently, head position impacts this view: axial view should ideally be perpendicular to the plane of occlusion, but if the patient was "head down" or "head up" during scanning, the axial cut might intersect the anatomy at a different angle: the mesio-distal measurement is impacted because it is artificially greater than it should be. Notably, some software can help the user correcting for this error by providing a function to rotate the patient's head on a separate scout-type view. This is only available on CBCT units with large fields of view. When a small area has been imaged, it is difficult to view and appreciate the plan of occlusion, and therefore the mesio-distal measurements could be erroneously trusted. The presence of adjacent teeth usually provides reliable anatomic landmarks such as cemento-enamel junctions from which measurements can be made. Once an arch has been traced on an axial view, a thin artificial "panoramic" image is created on which mesio-distal measurements can also be performed.

The bucco-lingual evaluation, although precise, is also dependent upon angles. This time, the cross-section is a reconstructed view perpendicular

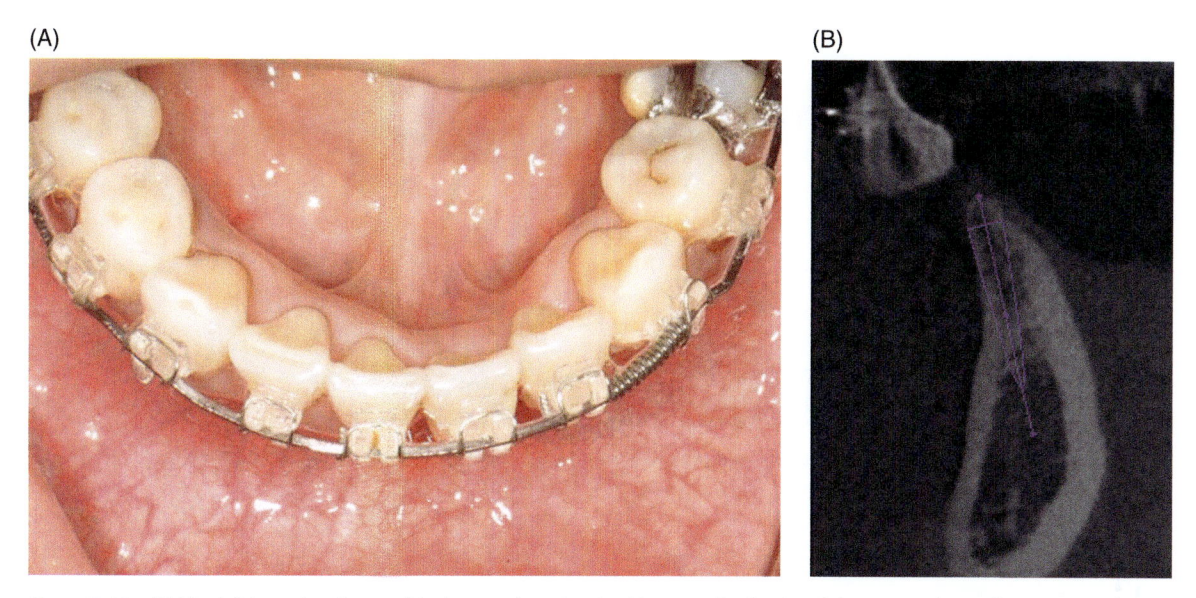

Figure 7.16 (A) The left lateral and central incisor are hopeless in this postorthodontic adult patient. The teeth are removed, roots sectioned, and crowns reattached to the wire. (B) A CBCT is then taken and shows that buccal bone is missing significantly if an ideal implant placement is to be achieved. This dimension cannot be seen on a two-dimensional radiograph.

to the occlusal tracing. This line is user defined and easily modified. Yet it is important to keep in mind that a cross-section relies upon this tracing because dimensions can also be significantly impacted. Similarly, bone height is viewed on the same cross-sectional image and is influenced by left-right patient head tilt. Again, some software provides correction tools, and small field of view images are more difficult to correct. But in this particular direction, a measurement can be made at an angle.

Notably, the presence of adequate bone is insufficient for an ideal implant placement. The ridge might be located more lingually than desired (Figure 7.16), or at an angle that prevents a prosthetically driven implant placement. The use of a scannographic guide is then essential to project the restorative plan onto the anatomy (Sarment et al., 2003). For a single tooth implant, adjacent teeth can also help guide the implant position: when looking at the cross-section, it is possible to modify its thickness to create an artificial projection of adjacent teeth towards the area of interest. For segmental cases, it is not possible to use this method and a scannographic guide, containing barium sulfate or another radio-opaque material, is necessary to identify the location of the future restoration (Figure 7.17).

Regardless of the scanning method used, the use of a surgical guide is recommended to transfer planning to surgery, so as to achieve a better accuracy of placement (Behneke et al., 2012).

Evaluation of the edentulous arch

With small field of views, multiple scanning might be necessary. Some manufacturers provide software methods to stitch images together: areas that overlay are recognized as identical on multiple data sets, and algorithm is written to reconcile these series of images into one file. It is important to recognize that image quality is usually slightly decreased for large scanning, because the amount of data would otherwise be overwhelming. Therefore, the pitch between sections is decreased several-fold. The clinical impact is minimal, but the clinician should understand the consequence of utilizing the appropriate protocol to optimize it to the clinical purpose.

Evaluation of the edentulous arch using CBCT also requires a scannographic guide to better anticipate the restorative outcome. Typically, the lack of plane of occlusion should be addressed prior to scanning so that planning can be performed

(A) (B)

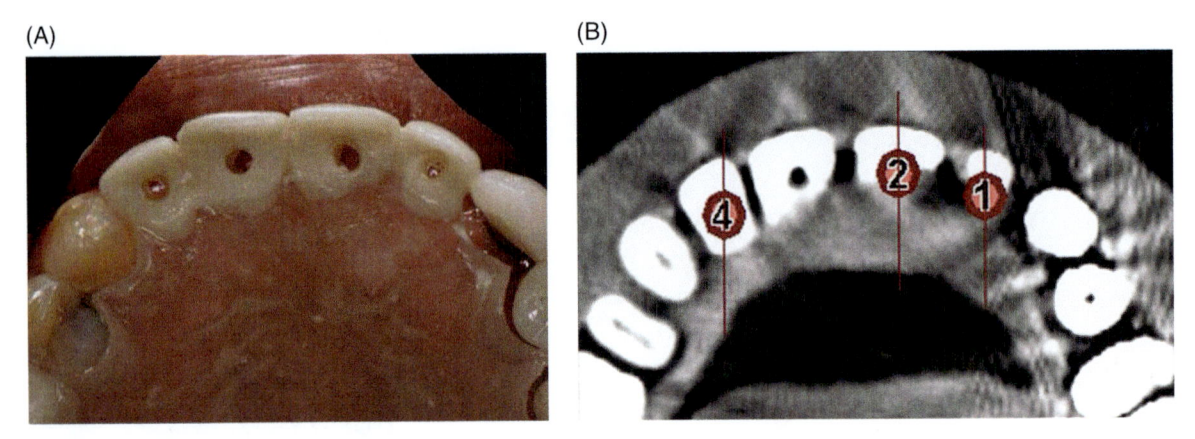

Figure 7.17 (A) A scannographic guide is prepared prior to scanning. (B) Once images are acquired, future restorative teeth are visualized.

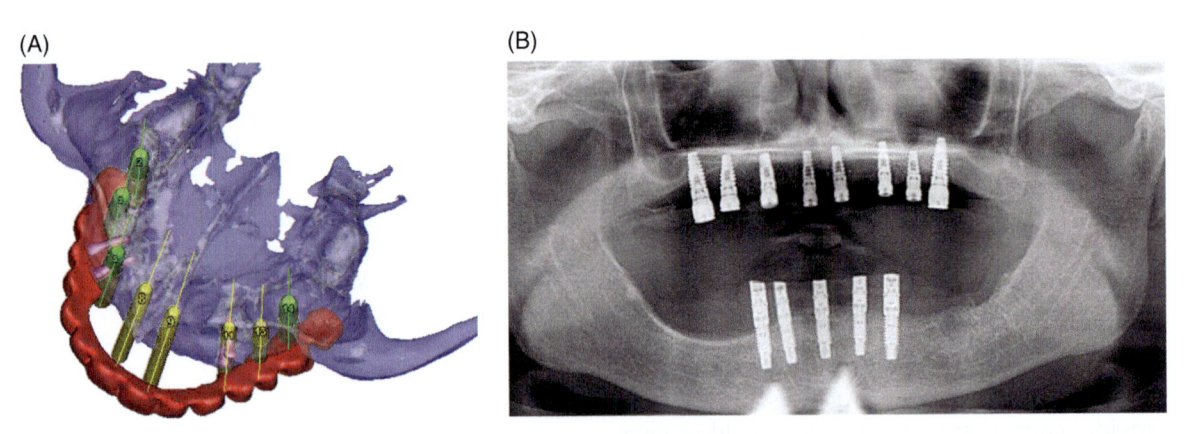

(A) (B)

Figure 7.18 (A) Various densities are segmented and assigned separate colors on the screen. (B) The panoramic radiograph has limited value to appreciate the prosthetic challenge.

accordingly. The best method to visualize the future occlusal plane is to fabricate a scannographic guide that imitates the final restoration. The guide should contain radio-opaque material in sufficient concentration to yield a contour on the screen, yet without causing image distortion seen with very dense objects (i.e., streak artifacts or beam hardening). Barium sulfate is usually mixed with acrylic. The guide can contain various concentrations of barium sulfate, which produces distinct densities (Sarment and Misch, 2002). When later exported to an implant-planning software, these various shades of gray can be segmented, assigned a color, and artificially removed on the screen for better viewing of other parts of images, such as the anatomy alone (Figure 7.18). Furthermore, when a soft tissue–supported surgical guide is expected, it is necessary to provide a duplicated denture with a radio-opaque base in order to identify soft tissue contours. In this instance, a double scanning protocol can be requested by the guide manufacturer. This second acquisition can also be performed on the CBCT unit, and will later help with segmentation and fabrication of the CAD/CAM surgical guide.

Scanning update

Because the level of radiation is somewhat reasonable, in particular when using small field of views CBCT, it is possible to scan an area of interest a second time. The decision must be carefully made in view of the use of additional radiation. However, the clinical benefit can be significant enough in

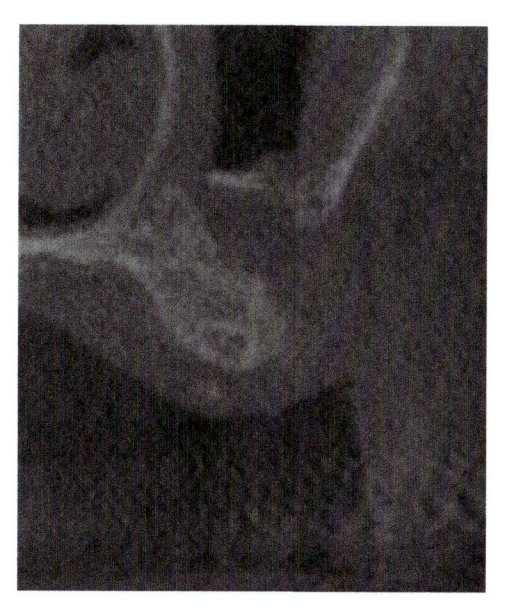

Figure 7.19 This maxillary sinus augmentation has healed poorly and the window area is invaded with soft tissue only. On a two-dimensional radiograph, bone augmentation appears adequate.

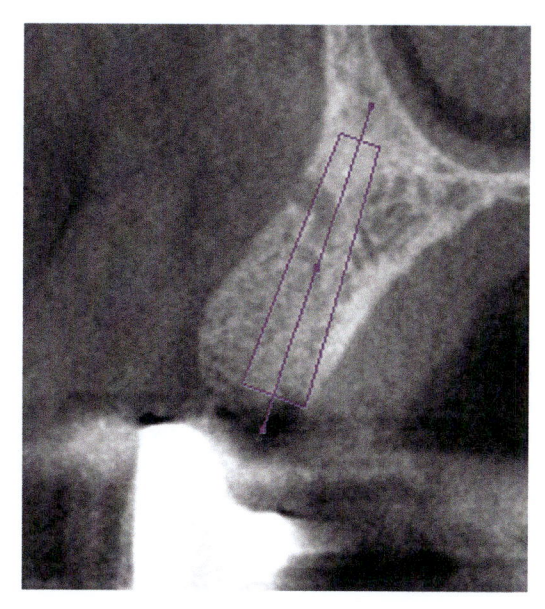

Figure 7.20 A ridge preservation graft was placed after extraction of a maxillary cuspid. CBCT scanning prior to implant surgery shows a void at the apical end of the alveole. Virtual implant planning shows that an ideally located implant would mostly traverse the graft while its apex would be in soft tissue.

specific situations. As is often the case, there are few published guidelines for rescanning, and the clinician should use good judgment.

In the evaluation of the maxillary sinus, it is common to find pathology. If transient, soft tissue appearance might vary significantly within days. More importantly, once the patient has been referred to an otorhinolaryngologist and treated successfully, a decision must be made to use the original images or rescan the area. The medical specialist might have used other means to evaluate the results, such as direct vision and patient interview. Therefore, the exact state of the sinus to be entered for bone grafting is unknown. Furthermore, many months might have passed since the initial visit. In addition, there is value in rescanning a grafted maxillary sinus because the presence of new bone is essential to implant placement. When relying on the initial images, it is difficult to anticipate the success of the bone graft, and a two-dimensional radiograph, just like the initial evaluation, is insufficient to provide an accurate visualization of new bone (Figure 7.19, Figure 7.20). CBCT scanning can evaluate the new volume, localization, and density of bone. Within the graft, areas of lesser density can be anticipated as well. Although the clinical signifi-cance of these variations within the graft remains unclear at this time, the clinician can modify the surgical protocol in two different ways. First, a longer implant length might be preferred in order to engage sufficient stabilizing bone. Second, the osteotomy might be undersized, in areas of lower density, so that greater compression is gained in low-density areas, in a manner similar to that of poor native bone quality.

It is questionable whether scanning after implant placement is of use (Corpas et al., 2011), in particular because the presence of titanium produces significant artifacts (Schulze et al., 2010). For research purposes, Peleg et al. followed up implant placement with scanning in order to evaluate anatomy parameters (Peleg et al., 1999). These and other authors (Murakami et al., 1999) found that healing was good but that a significant percentage of implants were not in contact with bone, in spite of their clinical success. When a flapless approach is utilized, postsurgical scanning might be of greater interest to ensure the penetration of implants into bone (Van Assche et al., 2010). In a more recent study, Naitoh et al. reported on bone to implant contact assessment after successful implantation, and claimed that such evaluation is possible using CBCT (Naitoh, Nabeshima, et al., 2010).

Similarly, large bone augmentations such as block grafts can be imaged in preparation of implantation. The success of the graft and possible areas of graft resorption can be anticipated. The surgical approach may also be affected, in particular when regrafting might be necessary. For instance, a small approach could be preferred if the graft appears intact. In contrast, if an apical area needs to be accessed for further grafting, then a larger initial incision is preferable. The knowledge gained during rescanning is used for better incisions and a more effective surgery. A similar decision making can be applied to all grafting, including smaller areas.

Conclusion

There are limitations to the use of CBCT when preparing for the placement of implants. The presence of adjacent metallic restorations such as crowns or endodontic posts is a common problem. Image artifacts are significant enough to render the image unusable to diagnosis. In contrast, a standard radiograph has better value in these situations. This situation arises often in evaluating a potential crack, typically in the area of an endodontically treated tooth and in the presence of a post. For the same reason, the possible crack is masked by artifacts.

This is also true when an implant has been placed in the vicinity. It is also important to remember that postimplantation evaluation of peri-implant bone is very limited. Beam hardening and artifacts are simply misinterpreted for a lack of bone. Therefore, in cases of ailing or failing implants, CBCT is usually not the image of choice.

The presence of a CBCT in a dental office has a significant impact on the workflow. Obviously, the initial consultation should include, when appropriate, the use of scanning. In order to best utilize the technology, it is recommended to develop an internal protocol to clarify the decision tree to all members of the team. A well-informed staff will be trained to accommodate the schedule for scanning and will be prepared to acquire the radiograph when a patient is first seen for dental implantation.

Furthermore, the clinician should decide to take the time to read the radiograph while the patient is present, or to schedule a second visit for treatment planning. More importantly, it is possible to obtain an over-read by a dental and maxillofacial radiologist (see chapter 3) to rule out pathology.

Over the last few years, CBCT machines have become more refined, often offering the option of a small field of view scanning to minimize radiation (Farman, 2009). While guidelines are being developed by dental specialties, the clinician must rely on the reasonable use of the technology in order to utilize it when the benefit outweighs the possible risk. The issue at hand is that benefit and risk are loosely defined. Yet, with regard to dental implants and associated grafting, the clinical benefit is obvious because accurate implant planning is now available.

References

Behneke, A., Burwinkel, M., and Behneke, N. (2012). *Clinical Oral Implants Research*, 23: 416–23.

Braut, V., Bornstein, M. M., Belser, U., and Buser, D. (2011). *International Journal of Periodontics & Restorative Dentistry*, 31: 125–31.

Corpas Ldos, S., Jacobs, R., Quirynen, M., Huang, Y., Naert, I., and Duyck, J. (2011). *Clinical Oral Implants Research*, 22: 492–9.

Dawood, A., Brown, J., Sauret-Jackson, V., and Purkayastha, S. (2012). *DentoMaxilloFacial Radiology*, 41: 70–4.

Farman, A.G. (2009). *Oral Surgery Oral Medicine Oral Pathology Oral Radiology & Endodontics*, 108: 477–8.

Fornell, J., Johansson, L.A., Bolin, A., Isaksson, S., and Sennerby, L. (2012). *Clinical Oral Implants Research*, 23: 28–34.

Kan, J.Y., Roe, P., Rungcharassaeng, K., Patel, R.D., Waki, T., Lozada, J.L., and Zimmerman, G. (2011). *International Journal of Oral & Maxillofacial Implants*, 26: 873–6.

Kim, S.H., Kang, J.M., Choi, B., and Nelson, G. (2008). *World Journal of Orthodontics*, 9: 371–82.

Murakami, K., Itoh, T., Watanabe, S., Naito, T., and Yokota, M. (1999). *J Periodontol*, 70: 1254–9.

Naitoh, M., Aimiya, H., Hirukawa, A., and Ariji, E. (2010a). *International Journal of Oral & Maxillofacial Implants*, 25: 1093–8.

Naitoh, M., Nabeshima, H., Hayashi, H., Nakayama, T., Kurita, K., and Ariji, E. (2010b). *Journal of Oral Implantology*, 36: 377–84.

Nickenig, H.J., and Eitner, S. (2007). *Journal of Cranio Maxillo Facial Surgery*, 35: 207–11.

Norton, M.R., and Gamble, C. (2001). *Clin Oral Implants Res*, 12: 79–84.

Orhan, K., Aksoy, S., Bilecenoglu, B., Sakul, B.U., and Paksoy, C.S. (2011). *Surgical & Radiologic Anatomy*, 33: 501–7.

Peleg, M., Chaushu, G., Mazor, Z., Ardekian, L., and Bakoon, M. (1999). *J Periodontol*, 70: 1564–73.

Rasmussen, O.C. (2000). In *Phidias Rapid Prototyping in Medicine*, Vol. 4 Materialise, Inc., pp. 10–12.

Ritter, L., Mischkowski, R.A., Neugebauer, J., Dreiseidler, T., Scheer, M., Keeve, E., et al. (2009). *Oral Surgery Oral Medicine Oral Pathology Oral Radiology & Endodontics*, 108.

Sarment, D.P., Al-Shammari, K., and Kazor, C.E. (2003). *Int J Period Rest Dent*, 23: 287–95.

Sarment, D.P., and Misch, C.E. (2002). *Int Mag Oral Implantol*, 3: 16–22.

Schulze, R.K., Berndt, D., and d'Hoedt, B. (2010). *Clinical Oral Implants Research*, 21: 100–7.

Song, Y.D., Jun, S.H., and Kwon, J.J. (2009). *International Journal of Oral & Maxillofacial Implants*, 24: 59–64.

Sonick, M., Abrahams, J., and Faiella, R.A. (1994). A comparison of the accuracy of periapical, panoramic, and computerized tomographic radiographs in locating the mandibular canal. *Int Oral Maxillofac Implants*, 9: 455–60.

Tepper, G., Hofschneider, U.B., Gahleitner, A., and Ulm, C. (2001). *Int J Oral Maxillofac Implants*, 16: 68–72.

Tyndall, A.A., and Brooks, S.L. (2000). Selection criteria for dental implant site imaging: A position paper of the American Academy of Oral and Maxillofacial Radiology. *Oral Surg Oral Med Oral Pathol Oral Radiol Endod*, 89: 630–7.

Van Assche, N., van Steenberghe, D., Quirynen, M., and Jacobs, R. (2010). *Journal of Clinical Periodontology*, 37: 398–403.

8 CAD/CAM Surgical Guidance Using Cone Beam Computed Tomography

George A. Mandelaris and Alan L. Rosenfeld

Introduction

Management of diagnostic and clinical information utilizing patient-specific 3D volumetric data and computer software is transforming oral health care. This paradigm shift, the result of technology advances and improved access to 3D imaging, benefits patients and clinicians most when an accurate diagnosis can be made that enhances the delivery of therapy.

Implant placement has been and continues to be intuitive for most clinicians throughout the world. Research over the past decade has demonstrated that this approach to osteotomy site preparation carries the greatest magnitude of error compared to approaches where computer-generated stereolithographic surgical guides are utilized (Sarment, Sukovic, et al., 2003; Jung et al., 2009). While less than optimal implant placement may appear to be rather trivial at the time of operation, the prosthetic reconciliation required to compensate can lead to a less than satisfactory prosthetic outcome and complicate patient care (Spielman, 1996; Beckers, 2003).

Since 1999, advances in implant surgical guide development through computer-aided design/computer-aided manufacturing (CAD/CAM) have allowed for osteotomy site preparation to occur alone (partial guidance) or in combination with the delivery of an endosseous osseointegrated dental implant through a single guide (total guidance). The shared qualities between all CAD/CAM generated surgical guides include the following: (1) They are designed to reflect consideration of patient-specific anatomy that has been acquired through computed tomography, either mutislice spiral CT (MSCT) or cone beam CT (CBCT). (2) They are based on a presurgical prosthetically directed plan that is determined after clinical examination to understand patient-specific regional anatomy and vital structure orientation prior to surgery. (3) They are generated through computer software applications that are utilized to analyze regional anatomy and simulate planned surgical and prosthetic therapy (Vrielinck et al., 2003; Schneider et al., 2009).

The process involved in CAD/CAM implant surgical guide design and utilization is a prosthetically driven approach to implant therapy that usually benefits from the use of a scanning appliance. A scanning appliance is critical for predictable prosthetic outcomes because it allows the prosthetic parameters to be transferred to the CT dataset for coordinated interdisciplinary planning in the preoperative phase of therapy (Israelson et al., 1992; Basten and Kois, 1996; Mecall and

---

Cone Beam Computed Tomography: Oral and Maxillofacial Diagnosis and Applications, First Edition. Edited by David Sarment.
© 2014 John Wiley & Sons, Inc. Published 2014 by John Wiley & Sons, Inc.

Rosenfeld, 1992; Mecall and Rosenfeld, 1996). This type of appliance is arguably the most critical aspect of the computer-guided implantology process. They are often misunderstood, incorrectly designed, and not utilized to their full potential.

The opportunity to utilize stereolithographic medical modeling coupled with three-dimensional patient-specific CT information creates a variety of guide support strategies. These strategies include fabrication of bone, tooth, tooth-mucosa, or exclusively mucosal-supported surgical drilling guides (with or without implant delivery) that can facilitate the delivery of implant therapy in a more precise and efficient manner with less patient discomfort when compared to the conventional methods (Rosenfeld et al., 2006a, 2006b, 2006c; Mandelaris and Rosenfeld, 2008; Mandelaris et al., 2010). The purpose of this chapter is to give an overview of CAD/CAM surgical guidance using CBCT imaging. The authors have published extensively on the details of computer-guided implantology (Rosenfeld et al., 2006a, 2006b, 2006c; Mandelaris and Rosenfeld, 2008; Mandelaris et al., 2009; Mandelaris and Rosenfeld, 2009a, 2009b; Mandelaris et al., 2010).

While several companies make CAD/CAM-generated surgical guides and multiple software manufacturers exist in the marketplace, the computer software planning system and CAD/CAM-generated surgical guides utilized and described in this chapter are SimPlant and the SurgiGuide family from Materialise Dental (Leuven, Belgium). In addition, while many cone beam computed tomography (CBCT) companies exist, the images and 3D volumes demonstrated in this chapter will be from the Carestream Dental 9300 CBCT unit.

Rapid prototyping and medical modeling

Rapid prototyping is a method of producing solid physical hardcopies of human anatomy from three-dimensional computer data (Popat, 1998). All rapid prototyping techniques are based on the same principle of constructing a 3D structure in layers. The most direct benefits to the dental implant patient include (1) a greater understanding of the treatment requirements and commitment needed for successful therapy; (2) a significant reduction in surgical time and proportional decrease in postsurgical pain, discomfort, and swelling; and (3) the ability to review the risks and benefits with the patient for a better understanding of anticipated outcomes as well as alternative types of treatment.

Medical modeling has several principal uses (Swaelens, 1999; Erickson et al., 1999; Webb, 2000). The first is to enable visualization of anatomical features such as tumor size and location, bone morphology, and orientation of vital structures. The second is to facilitate communication between interdisciplinary team members involved in patient treatment. The third is to enable the rehearsal of surgical procedures such as osteotomy preparation, implant positioning, abutment selection, and implant provisionalization. Complex surgical intervention can be performed prior to patient intervention.

Stereolithography

Stereolithography is the most well known and used rapid prototyping technique. It is also the technique most commonly used for the generation of medical models and computer-generated drilling guides used during the progressive drilling sequence in dental implant surgery (Erickson et al., 1999). Accuracy and reliability are two of the distinguishing characteristics of the stereolithographic process (Barker et al., 1994). In addition, stereolithography allows for medical models to be generated that are transparent, constructed in a timely manner, cost effective, and allow for selective colorization of regions of visual interest (Wouters, 2001; Figure 8.1,

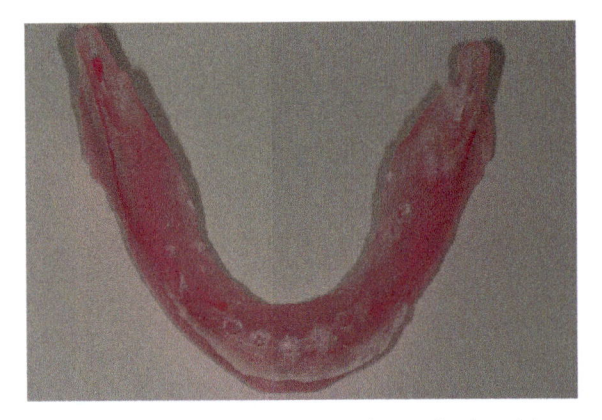

Figure 8.1 A mucosal stereolithographic medical model with five interforamina osteotomy site preparations as a part of the presurgical workup. Note the colorization of the inferior alveolar nerve and mental foramen.

Figure 8.2). The dimensional accuracy of anatomical skull replicas derived from three-dimensional CT imaging using the rapid prototyping technique of stereolithography has been shown to be less than one millimeter, another important quality of this technology (Cheng and Wee, 1999; Campbell et al., 2002; Gopakumar, 2004).

Pretreatment analysis

Determining surgical and dental anatomy requirements for the patient seeking dental implant rehabilitation are key factors leading to an esthetic, functional, and biologically acceptable tooth replacement solution. Case type patterns representing various forms of edentulism have been described in previous publications (Mecall, 2009). These case type patterns allow for classification of residual ridge resorption, changes in overall volume of bone and soft tissue, and prosthetic requirements to restore form and function. Table 8.1 describes the five case type patterns and typical corresponding treatment. The success of prosthetic outcomes is dependent upon multiple variables, including proper dental space appropriation, which directly influences the reconstructive requirements of both hard and soft tissue. This

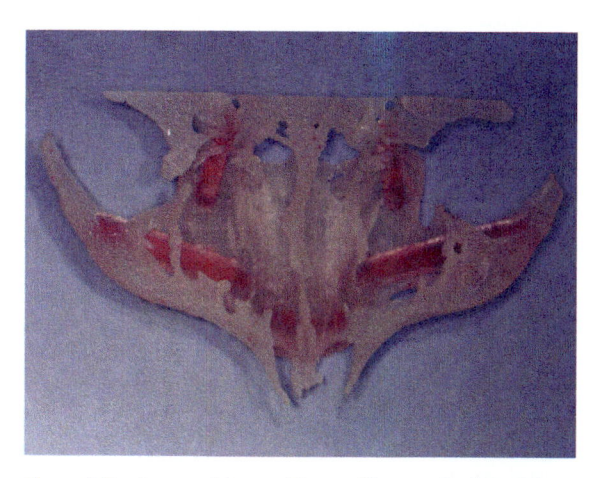

Figure 8.2 A stereolithographic maxillary medical model with selective colorization of planned trans-sinusal implants (pterygoid and zygoma). Courtesy of Dr. Philippe Tardieu (Dubai, UAE).

Table 8.1 Computer-guided implantology treatment planning based on case type patterns.

Case type	Scanning Appliance	Type of Wax-up Indicated	Corresponding Anatomy
I	Tooth-form	Tooth-form	Dental and surgical anatomy within normal limits
II, III, and IV	Full-contour	Full-contour	Dental anatomy may or may not be within normal limits; determination of the volume of hard and soft tissue augmentation for optimal final tooth position required. Surgical anatomy requires augmentation; volume and/or position of tissue need to be determined.
IV and V	Partial or complete denture	Trial tooth setup	Complete edentalism; dental and possibly surgical anatomy require modification
IV and V	Provisional restoration	Tooth-form	Dental anatomy only requires modification
IV or V	Patient's existing prosthesis	None, but the existing prosthesis must meet all acceptable prosthodontic criteria	Complete edentalism; dental and possibly surgical anatomy require modification. Fiduciary markers required.

Source: Mecall, 2009.

assessment improves the likelihood that an implant replacement solution will be successful from a biologic, esthetic, phonetic, and functional perspective. These determinants are assessed through a diagnostic wax-up and the selection of the most appropriate scanning appliance. A properly positioned and stabilized scanning appliance worn during CT/CBCT imaging transfers meaningful prosthetic information into the imaging dataset. This enables the surgical treatment plan to be as effective as possible. Prosthetically directed and collaboratively based treatment planning leads to predictable patient outcomes that can be planned before surgical intervention occurs. This process is referred to as restorative leadership. Restorative leadership allows the interdisciplinary team members to embrace a computer-guided implantology framework called collaborative accountability, which ultimately focuses on the patient outcome (Rosenfeld et al., 2006a, 2006b, 2006c; Mandelaris and Rosenfeld, 2008). This creates an atmosphere of disclosure and interactive discussion that allows the patient to become an active participant in the treatment planning process. The restorative leadership process and collaborative accountability framework (a codiscovery process) is described below for each case type pattern leading to dental implant tooth replacement therapy.

The restorative leadership process: Case type pattern identification and patient-specific diagnostic wax-ups

Case type pattern identification helps to identify patient characteristics and categorize dental and surgical requirements for treatment. In addition, identifying case type patterns allows the implant team to estimate the costs and duration of treatment as a part of the preoperative workup. The restorative leadership process usually begins with the prosthetic dentist and consists of appropriate dental radiographs and securing mounted diagnostic study models. The mounted study models should reflect the patient in a reproducible articulated position. Rehabilitation of partial or complete edentulism consists of a diagnostic wax-up that is either tooth form, full contour, or a trial tooth setup (whereby anatomically correct denture teeth are used). This leads to the fabrication of an accurate scanning appliance in preparation for prosthetically meaningful volumetric imaging (CT/CBCT). Identification of case type patterns are based on the individual requirements of dental and surgical anatomy. The patient-specific tooth position and bone/soft tissue volume required to satisfy outcome goals of the final prosthesis must be established during the diagnostic phase. The utilization of case type patterns allows the prosthetic outcome goals to set surgical performance standards required to support the prosthetic outcome. This is a distinct paradigm shift compared to the historic nature of implant therapy.

Case type pattern I

A case type pattern I identifies the patient and requirements limited to dental anatomy since the residual ridge (i.e., surgical anatomy–soft and hard tissue volume/position) does not require modification to enable an optimal prosthetic outcome (Figure 8.3A and B, Figure 8.4A). Essentially, the dental anatomy is either missing or intact (i.e., tooth is present), but the surgical anatomy is sufficient for optimal tooth replacement. This case type pattern may be applied to a patient who has lost a natural tooth but had a socket preservation procedure and the resulting surgical anatomy is intact, so only the dental anatomy requires workup. Alternatively, this case type pattern could apply to a patient who has not lost a natural tooth but has suffered a nonrestorable fracture or a resorptive process where tooth replacement is required and an immediate implant is an option (Figure 8.4 A and B). In this situation, when the dental and surgical anatomy have not been altered by tooth loss, no scanning appliance is needed (i.e., the natural tooth will serve as the optimal final tooth position). 3D masks can be created to separate the tooth from adjacent neighboring anatomy to optimize planning and fixture positioning during computer-guided implant surgery (Figure 8.5A through F).

Case type patterns II and III

In case type patterns II and III, appropriating dental space/anatomy is given high priority. The dental anatomy may or may not be within normal limits. The surgical anatomy, however, will require modification to enable an optimal regional anatomy/volume to be realized in the final prosthetic outcome. In other words, the bone and/or

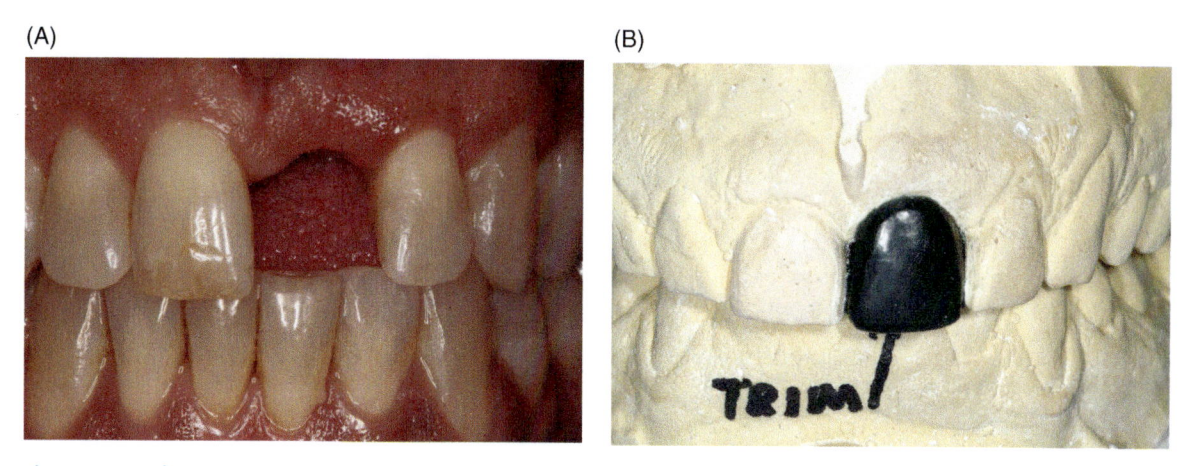

Figure 8.3A and B Case type pattern I clinical features of a patient with missing maxillary right central incisor #8. Dental anatomy only requires workup; surgical anatomy does not require modification.

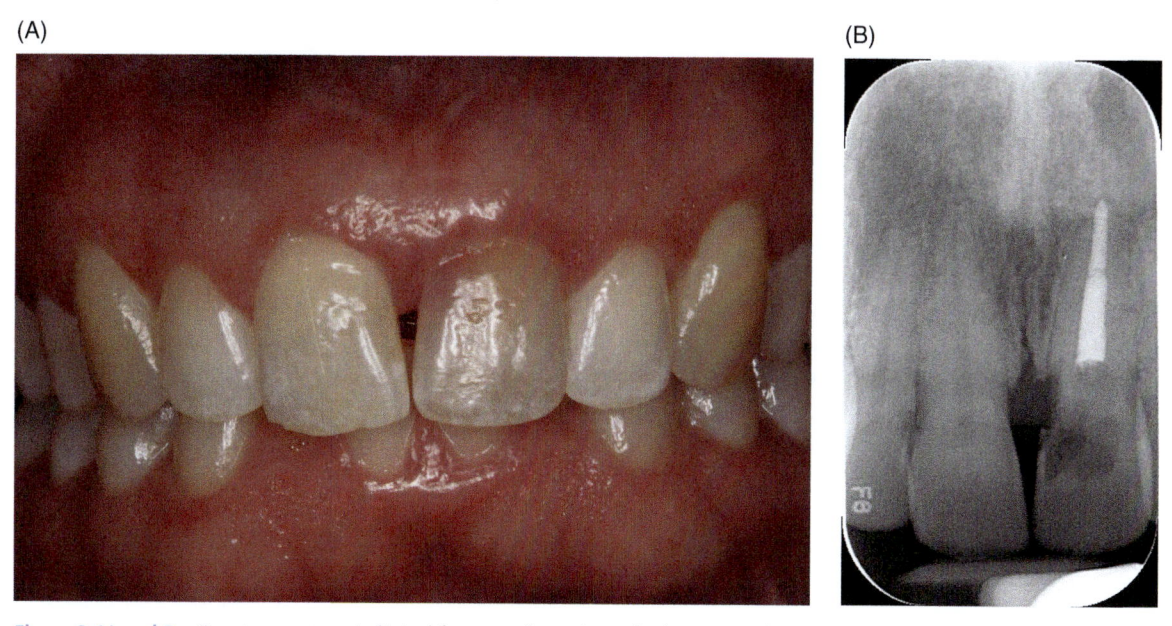

Figure 8.4A and B Case type pattern I clinical features of a patient who has not yet lost maxillary left central incisor (#9). Dental anatomy only requires workup; surgical anatomy does not require modification. Figure 8.4B demonstrates the radiograph resorption defect, substantiating a hopeless prognosis.

soft tissue volume requires some form of augmentation, but the dental anatomy can simply be developed through a wax-up. A full-contour diagnostic wax-up is performed to establish optimal tooth position and proportion as well as an optimal surrounding bone/soft tissue environment within the established prosthetic outcome goals.

Case type pattern II situations include gingival asymmetry or color alterations, early facial bone loss, mucogingival abnormalities, or thin periodontal biotypes or may involve occlusal instability (Figure 8.6A and B).

This case type pattern is usually limited to one or two teeth and may require orthodontic forced

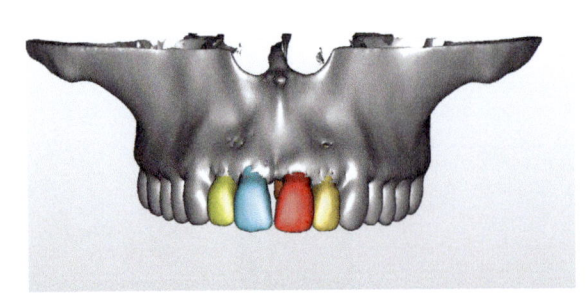

Figure 8.5A 3D construction of maxillary CBCT volume. Masks created include maxilla and individual teeth #7–#10.

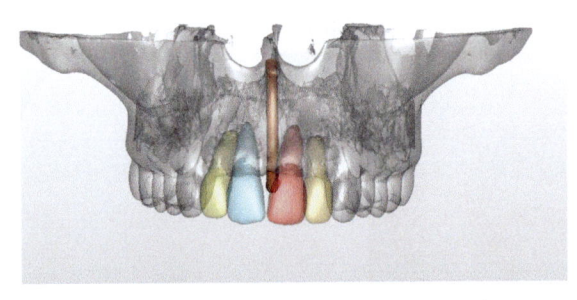

Figure 8.5B 3D construction of maxillary CBCT volume. Masks created include maxilla and individual teeth #7–#10. Transparency toggle tool turned on for root anatomy visualization in 3D.

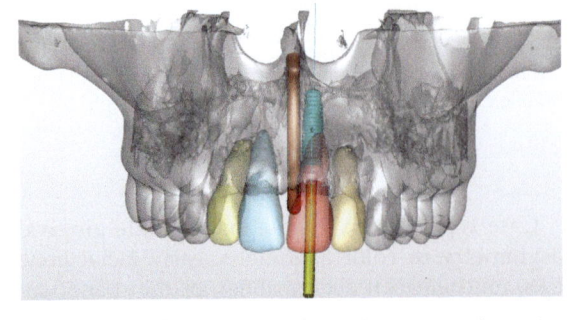

Figure 8.5C 3D construction of maxillary CBCT volume. Masks created include maxilla and individual teeth #7–#10. Virtual implant placement at the #9 position. Transparency toggle tool turned on for root anatomy visualization in 3D.

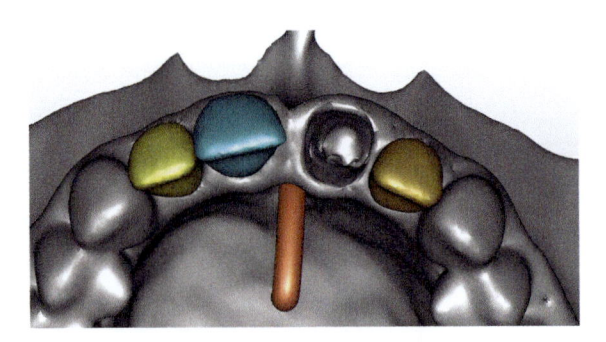

Figure 8.5D Occlusal view of anterior maxilla of 3D reconstruction. Mask of tooth #9 toggled off to simulate extraction.

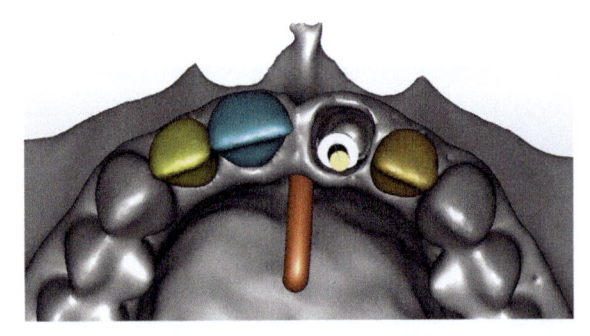

Figure 8.5E Occlusal view of anterior maxilla of 3D reconstruction. Mask of tooth #9 toggled off to simulate extraction and immediate implant. Note the implant:alveolus discrepancy, which will require management.

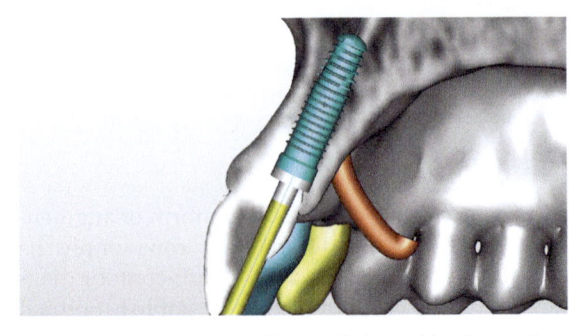

Figure 8.5F Cross-sectional view of planned implant at the #9 position with clip art rendering engaged (3D cross-section simulated onto 2D-cross section).

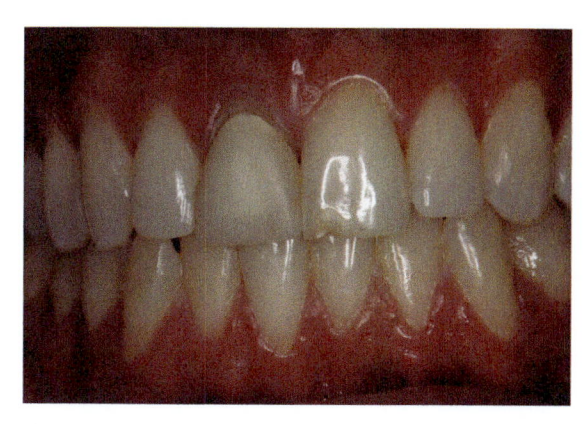

Figure 8.6A Case type pattern II clinical features of a patient with a nonrestorable and endodontically failing maxillary right central incisor #8. Dental anatomy is within normal limits, but surgical anatomy requires augmentation (note the thin periodontium).

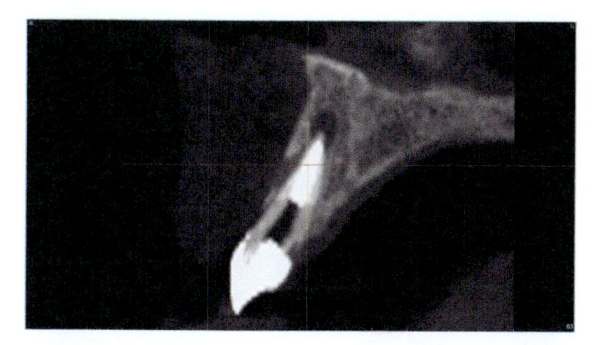

Figure 8.6B CBCT imaging and cross-sectional view of #8.

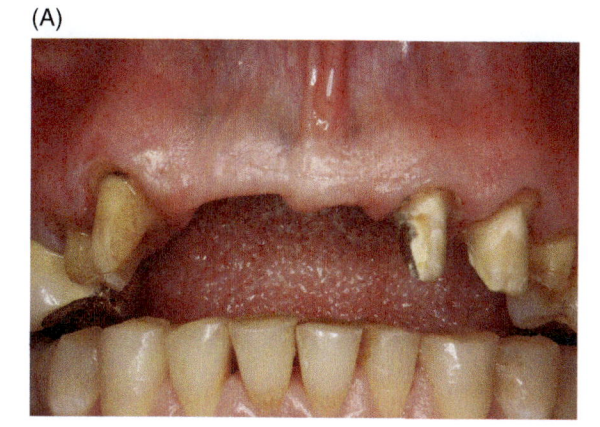

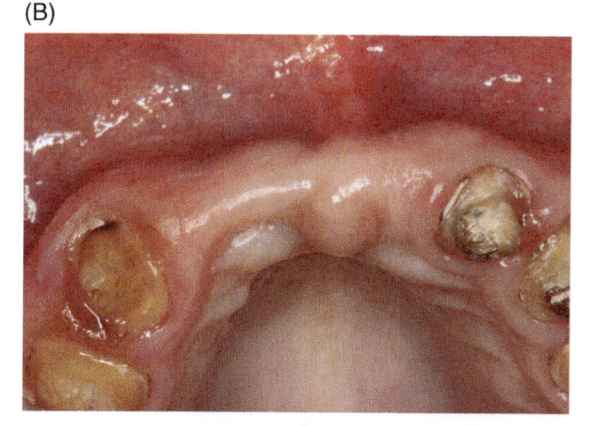

Figure 8.7A and B Case type pattern III clinical features of a patient with partial edentulism #7–#10. Dental anatomy is mostly within normal limits, but surgical anatomy requires augmentation and volume/position of tissue needs to be determined. Predominantly horizontal with some vertical bone loss.

eruption or connective tissue grafting to gain sufficient soft tissue volume such that the dental anatomy has a resulting normal proportion.

Case type pattern III cases are defined predominantly by horizontal bone loss (with some degree of vertical bone loss as a result of the postextraction resorption phenomenon; Figure 8.7A and B). These cases generally demonstrate a dental space appropriation anatomy considered to be of normal proportion. However, surgical anatomy is deficient and the required volume of tissue needs to be determined in order to establish an optimal surgical environment. The full-contour diagnostic wax-up creates a simulation of the dental anatomy and volume of bone/soft tissue which is transferred into a scanning appliance. This facilitates prosthetically relevant CBCT imaging and surgical planning to support the principles of restorative leadership and collaborative accountability (Figure 8.8).

Case type pattern IV

Case type pattern IV cases are defined predominantly by vertical bone loss (Figure 8.9) but demonstrate some level of horizontal resorption secondary to the postextraction resorption. These cases may demonstrate altered occlusal vertical dimension, reduced mesiodistal spacing, and some occlusal instability. Both surgical and dental anatomy require modification to establish optimal

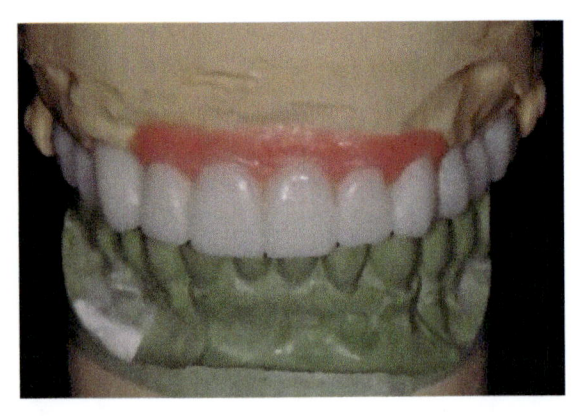

Figure 8.8 Full-contour diagnostic wax-up. Reprinted with permission from Mecall, 2009.

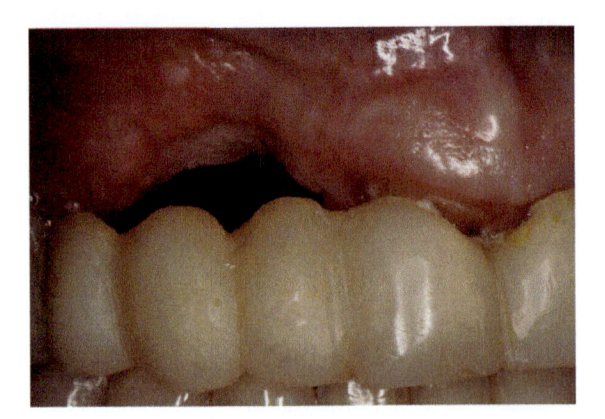

Figure 8.9 Case type pattern IV clinical features of a patient with partial edentulism. Dental and surgical anatomy require modification. Predominantly vertical with some horizontal bone loss.

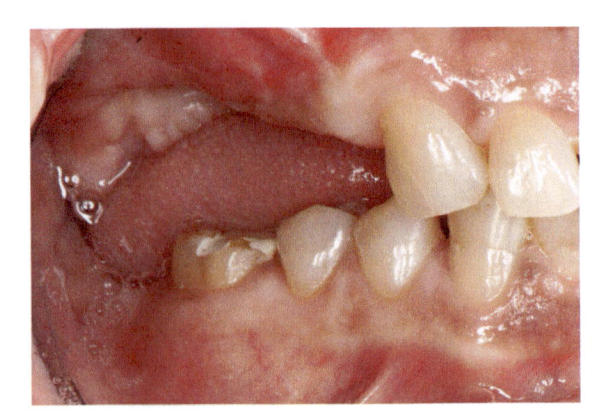

Figure 8.10A Case type pattern IV clinical features of a patient with partial edentulism #2–#5. Dental and surgical anatomy require modification. Predominantly vertical with some horizontal bone loss.

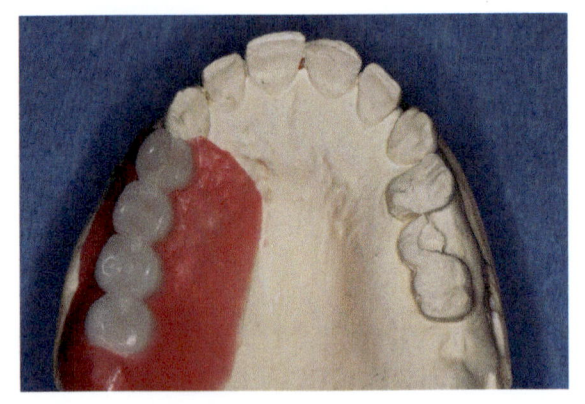

Figure 8.10B Full-contour diagnostic wax-up for case type pattern IV clinical features of a patient with partial edentulism of the maxillary right posterior.

dental proportion/position and hard/soft tissue volume. This can be determined in the form of a full-contour diagnostic wax-up for those situations involving limited tooth loss or in the form of a trial tooth setup for more extensive tooth loss using anatomically correct denture teeth (Figure 8.10A and B).

Case type pattern V

Case type pattern V cases are characterized by advanced horizontal and vertical bone loss (Figure 8.11). They are situations of complete edentulism where advanced residual ridge resorption has usually occurred. Concomitantly, there is loss of perioral musculature support and occlusal instability. These cases require a trial tooth setup using anatomically correct denture teeth to establish an optimal dental anatomy and a favorable hard/soft tissue volume (Figure 8.12). Anatomically correct denture teeth are mandatory because they more appropriately reflect natural tooth dimensions representative of realistic prosthetic outcome dimensions for implant-supported prosthodontics. In these situations, the surgical (bone and soft tissue) and dental anatomy is generally altered such that both environments require modification.

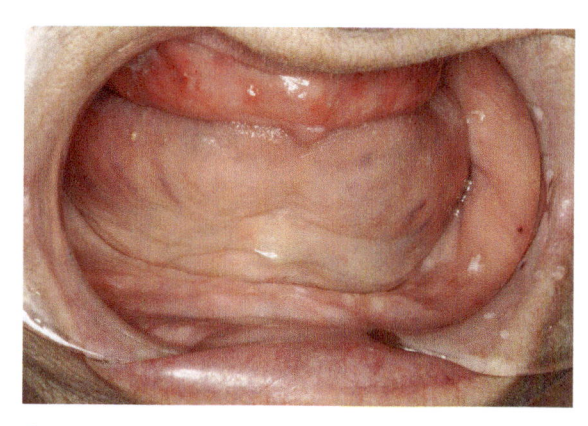

Figure 8.11 Case type pattern V clinical features of a patient with complete edentulism. Dental and surgical anatomy require modification. Significant vertical and horizontal bone loss.

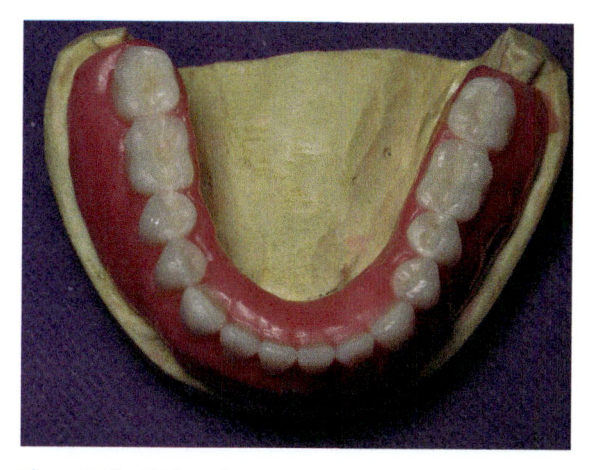

Figure 8.12 Trial tooth setup.

This requires that surgical and prosthetic landmarks be established, which allows for optimal esthetics, phonetics, and function to be realized in the prosthetic diagnostic phase.

Once the tooth form, full-contour wax-up, or trial tooth setup are completed, representing "optimal" dental and regional anatomy, a scanning appliance is fabricated. The appliance must reflect that which was created in the diagnostic wax-up or trial tooth setup.

Scanning appliances

Scanning appliances were traditionally used to reflect the optimal final prosthetic tooth position in an edentulous space within the regional anatomy under investigation (Basten and Kois, 1996). The earliest type of appliance was a simple tooth silhouette outline created by painting a thin barium sulfate coating on a vacuform resin sheet (Mecall and Rosenfeld, 1992). This enabled the identification of tooth form to be evaluated against existing regional anatomy viewed in the CT dataset. Its earliest use was limited to plain film analog CT images. This format was awkward and not user friendly. With the evolution in computer software and CT-guided implant technology, four types of scanning appliances have emerged (Mecall, 2009). The choice reflects the extent of edentulism and disruption of regional anatomy. The four types are outlined below.

1. Tooth form

This type of scanning appliance is typical for a patient who has dental and surgical anatomy within normal limits–in essence, a case type pattern I or II situation. The optimal, final tooth position is represented by a solid 30% barium sulfate (by weight) tooth and should contain a negative image center representing the center of the tooth or screw access hole emergence. The barium tooth can reside within a 0.040-inch vacuform wafer which covers sufficient teeth in the arch so that the appliance is stable. Ideally, inspection windows should be created at three different cusp tip points so that a triangulated plane is created and seating verification can be confirmed through visual inspection. The 30% barium sulfate standard can be substituted with other acceptable radiodense materials. The density of these materials should not compete with regional anatomic images or create artifacts that would negatively influence radiographic interpretation. A radiolucent interocclusal bite registration is also useful to ensure that the appliance is fully seated in a reproducible and accurate manner at an open vertical dimension during CBCT imaging. In some cases, the pontic or receptor site might need to be developed in the soft tissue (i.e., surgical anatomy) to allow complete seating of the scanning appliance reflecting optimal tooth form (Figure 8.13).

2. Full contour

A full-contour scanning appliance may be used for case type pattern II cases and is always used for case type patterns III and IV situations. They consist of a barium sulfate gradient differential. The dental anatomy should be represented as a solid tooth using 30% barium sulfate by weight while the

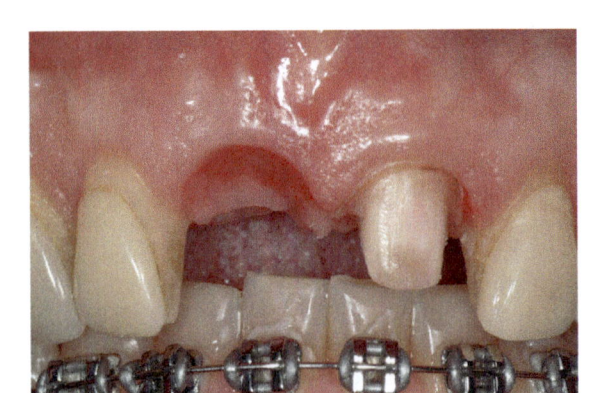

Figure 8.13 Pontic/receptor site development performed in preparation for CBCT diagnostics. Tooth form provisional/scan appliance utilized. Development of receptor site allows complete seating of the appliance, reflecting optimal tooth position and proportion.

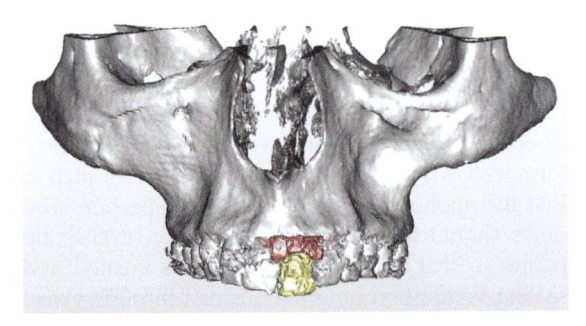

Figure 8.14A 3D reconstruction of CT diagnostics for the maxilla. #9 is a planned implant site. Masks included reflect bone + additional teeth, scanning appliance/dental anatomy for #9, and surgical anatomy/soft tissue position/volume for #9.

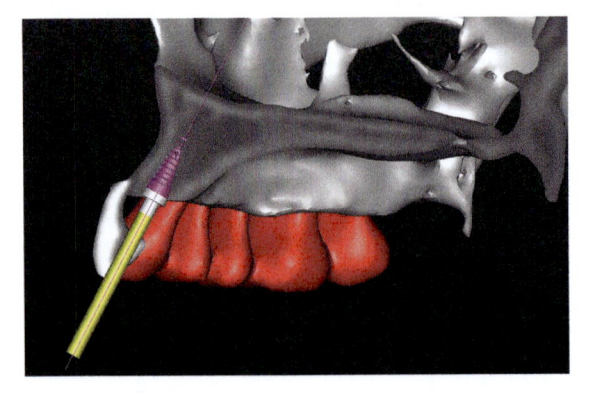

Figure 8.14B 3D reconstruction of CT diagnostics for the maxilla with cross-sectional view. Clip art rendering tool engaged. 2D cross-section is imposed on 3D reconstruction.

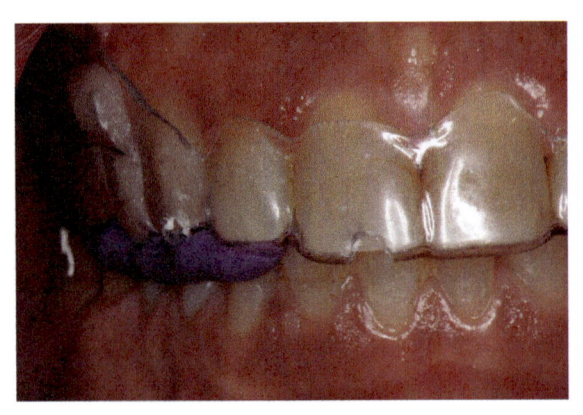

Figure 8.15A Full-contour scanning appliance in place. Radiolucent interocclusal bite registration used to ensure complete seating.

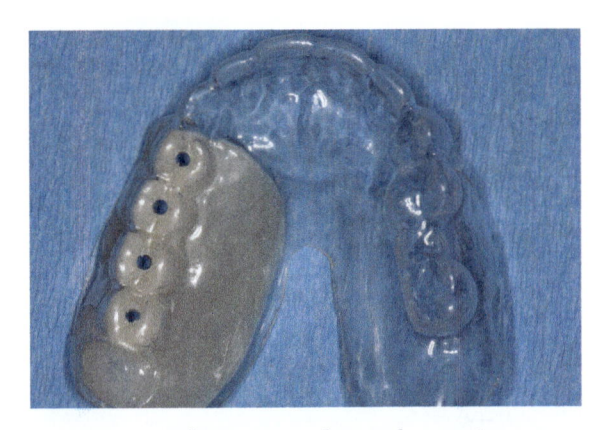

Figure 8.15B Full-contour vacuform wafer scanning appliance. Dental anatomy is 30% barium with negative image centers. Surgical anatomy (soft tissue volume/position) is represented in 10% barium.

modified bone/soft tissue representation is 10% barium sulfate by weight. This barium gradient differential allows the dental anatomy to be segmented from the proposed bone/soft tissue requirements as viewed in the dataset images. This allows all existing and proposed anatomy to be viewed interactively as independent masks through computer software (Figure 8.14A and B, Figure 8.15A–C). As in the tooth-form scanning appliance, negative image holes should be positioned in the prosthetic center of the teeth or proposed screw access holes. The barium tooth/teeth and soft tissue can reside within a 0.040-inch vacuform wafer. The wafer must incorporate enough teeth in the arch so that the

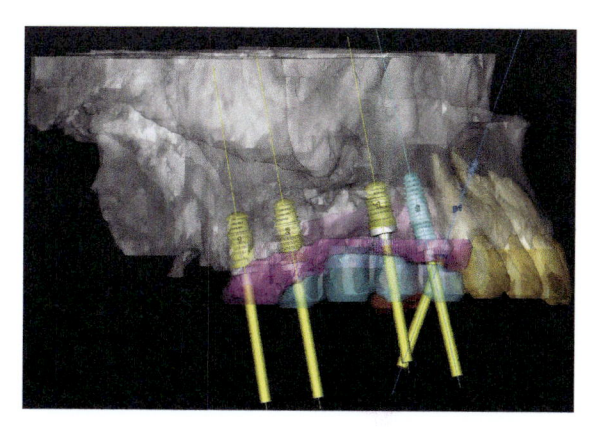

Figure 8.15C 3D reconstruction with multiple masks for prosthetically directed implant planning. Masks include natural teeth, maxilla, scan appliance dental anatomy/teeth, scan appliance surgical anatomy/soft tissue position/volume.

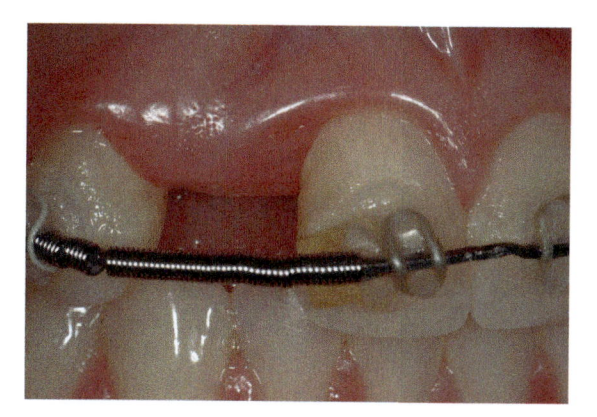

Figure 8.16A Case type pattern II patient clinical presentation. Implant treatment planning to ensue for #7. Note the mild soft tissue volume loss requiring full-contour wax-up. Edentulous site requires pontic/receptor site modification/development if the proper tooth proportion is to be able to seat properly.

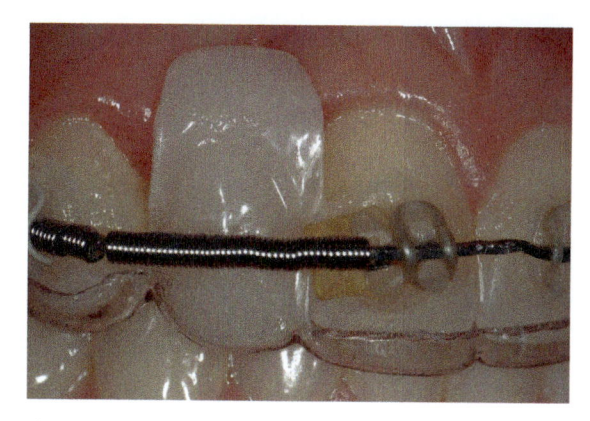

Figure 8.16B Case type pattern II patient clinical presentation. Ridge-lapped full-contour scanning appliance in place. Ridge-lapped scan appliance used to allow for full proportion of tooth #7 to be visualized because the receptor/pontic site was not developed preoperatively.

appliance is stable when seated. This appliance will generally involve more surface area in direct contact with residual ridge soft tissue. In cases such as a congenitally missing lateral incisor where the vertical soft tissue position is optimal but deficient in horizontal volume, the edentulous ridge may not allow seating of a full-contour appliance. The pontic receptor site soft tissue might need to be modified to enable complete seating of the scanning appliance. If not addressed, this situation often results in a ridge-lapped scanning appliance, which can complicate implant planning if a totally guided approach is used (Figure 8.16A and B). As for all vacuform-based scanning appliances, inspection windows should be made at three different cusp tips so that a triangulated plane is created and seating verification can be confirmed through visual inspection. A radiolucent interocclusal bite registration is also useful to ensure that the appliance is fully seated at an open vertical dimension for CBCT imaging.

3. Denture scannoguide

In the situation where a patient's existing partial or complete denture meets all the fundamental prosthodontic criteria of success, requiring no further modifications or setup, the prosthesis itself can be used as the scanning appliance, utilizing the dual scan protocol (see section on CBCT imaging protocols). The Tardieu scanning appliance is a separate laboratory processed barium gradient differential scanning appliance and has been previously published (Tardieu, 2009). It consists of a partial denture or complete denture consisting of anatomically correct denture teeth. The teeth are 30% barium sulfate and the base is 10%. This scanning appliance is fabricated either after a trial tooth setup has been performed when a new denture is needed, or by duplicating an existing acceptable denture (Figure 8.17A and B). This establishes the proper phonetic, functional, and physiologic requirements that will be

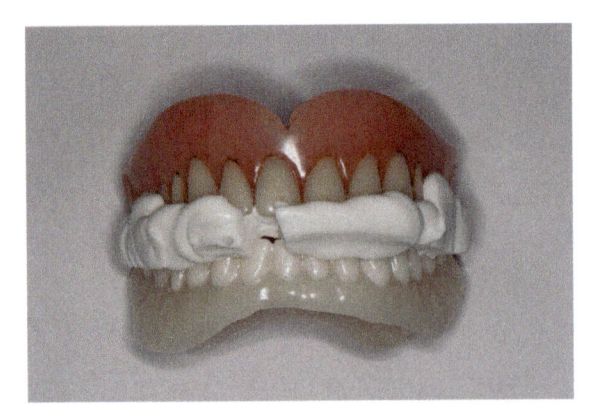

Figure 8.17A Denture scannoguide created for the completely edentulous mandible. The patient's maxillary denture is shown with bite registration created to ensure complete seating and to verify accurate positioning.

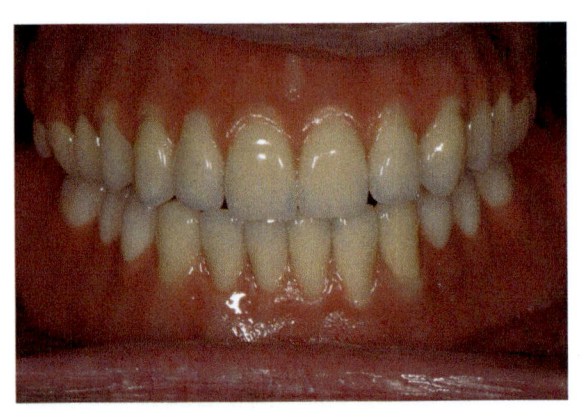

Figure 8.18 Accurate complete dentures for a patient seeking implant rehabilitation. Dentures are correct in all prosthodontic criteria. Scanning appliance creation is not needed. Patient will utilize existing dentures as the scanning appliances. Fiduciary markers are required and dual scan CBCT protocol will be used.

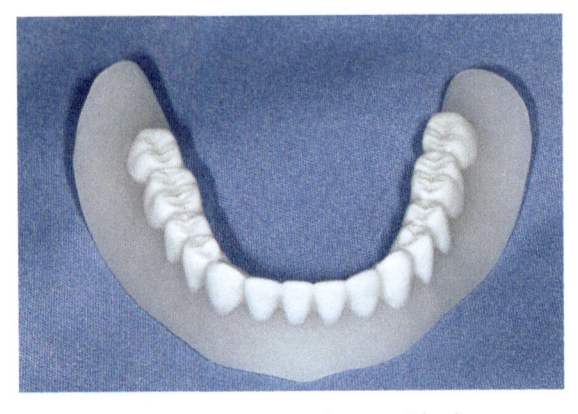

Figure 8.17B Denture scannoguide created for the completely edentulous mandible. Dental anatomy (teeth) is 30% barium and surgical anatomy (soft tissue volume/denture base) is 10% barium.

incorporated in the scanning appliance. If a trial tooth setup is not required and the existing prosthesis meets all satisfactory prosthodontic requirements, it can be utilized as a scannoguide for imaging purposes (using a dual scan protocol; Figure 8.18). An interocclusal bite registration should be created so that complete seating of the scanning appliance can be verified. The bite registration is critical in these cases since it allows for accurate cross-mounting of the scanning appliance, virtual rapid prototype duplicate of the denture/scan appliance, and CAD/CAM surgical guide generated from the CBCT dataset and stereolithographic process. In situations involving immediate delivery of interim implant-supported teeth, cross-referencing ensures a more accurate prosthesis occlusion.

4. Provisional restoration or natural tooth

In the case of a provisional restoration, 30% barium sulfate may be used for the missing tooth. However, if a provisional restoration spans more than the future implant site, corresponding abutment teeth should include significantly less barium sulfate. Using a concentration of more than 10% barium sulfate by weight for neighboring abutment tooth preparations may make it difficult, if not impossible, to decipher between scanning appliance and natural tooth structure. The competition between teeth and scanning appliance should be limited or reduced as much as possible. This will help ensure an accurate registration of the optically scanned stone model with the surgical planning software when the CAD/CAM guide is fabricated. In the case of a natural tooth that is to be lost due to a fracture, a resorptive process, or from another cause, the dental anatomy is already present and considered optimal. In these cases, the natural tooth serves as the scanning appliance for which optimal tooth position can be evaluated against regional anatomy and from which surgical planning can meaningfully commence (Figure 8.4A and B, Figure 8.5A–F).

CBCT imaging protocols

There are two scanning appliance protocols that can be used to transfer prosthetically relevant information to the CBCT dataset. They are described below:

1. *Single scan protocol.* This protocol implies that the patient is imaged with a fully seated scanning appliance. It is the traditional method for importing prosthetically meaningful data to the CT dataset (Figure 8.19A–C).
2. *Dual scan protocol.* This protocol is used when a differential barium gradient scanning appliance is not required. Either the patient's existing prosthesis meets acceptable criteria or one has been fabricated. Multiple fiduciary markers are attached to the appliance in strategic positions (Figure 8.20A–D). The fiduciary markers allow spatial orientation, which facilitates registration of the radiolucent acrylic denture with the CBCT dataset (SimPlant; Materialise Dental, Glen Burnie, MD, USA). Again, a radiolucent interocclusal bite registration ensures that the patient is imaged with the appliance firmly compressing the supporting soft tissues, avoiding black air-pocket artifact indicative of a poorly positioned appliance. Then, the appliance itself is imaged using a protocol recommended by the CT/CBCT manufacturer to image acrylic. Acrylic requires much lower radiation exposure for imaging when compared to bony structures. Registration of the two scans can be accomplished with commercially available proprietary imaging software. This registration process embeds the scanning appliance within the imaging dataset. The major benefit of the dual scan protocol is that a separate scanning appliance is not needed. This saves time and reduces the cost of diagnostics. However, it does not marginalize the need to ensure that the scanning appliance is an accurate prosthodontic prosthesis. The imaging technology used in computer-guided implantology is only effective when the correct diagnostic information is incorporated in the CT/CBCT study.

Collaborative accountability

The concept of collaborative accountability is preceded by the prosthetic leadership process. The restorative leadership process and case type pattern identification leading to proper scanning appliances has been previously described in this chapter. The surgical planning can be incorporated into stereolithographic drilling guides that can be used for accurate osteotomy preparations and implant delivery using a variety of guide support platforms.

The ability to incorporate the parameters of a successful prosthetic outcome into a CT dataset marks a collaborative breakthrough for the implant team (surgeon, prosthetic doctor, laboratory technologist, and patient). This paradigm shift is the fundamental basis for the current concept of collaborative accountability (Rosenfeld et al., 2006a, 2006b, 2006c; Mandelaris and Rosenfeld, 2008). This context allows the presurgical roles and responsibilities of the implant team to be determined. There are five aspects that describe the collaborative accountability context:

1. The prosthetic dentist assumes a leadership role in interdisciplinary collaboration by setting the treatment performance standards for those participating in patient care.
2. Prosthetic outcome determines surgical performance requirements, and becomes the responsibility of the implant surgeon.
3. Preoperative, not intraoperative, planning drives the treatment.
4. Stereolithographic medical modeling can reduce the so-called surgical talent gap. In other words, the placement of dental implants no longer relies on traditional "mental navigation" but rather on precise computer-guided implant positioning that is planned presurgically.
5. The very nature of a collaborative process focuses on the patient's outcome. This preoperatively defines treatment limitations, expectation, and costs in an atmosphere of disclosure.

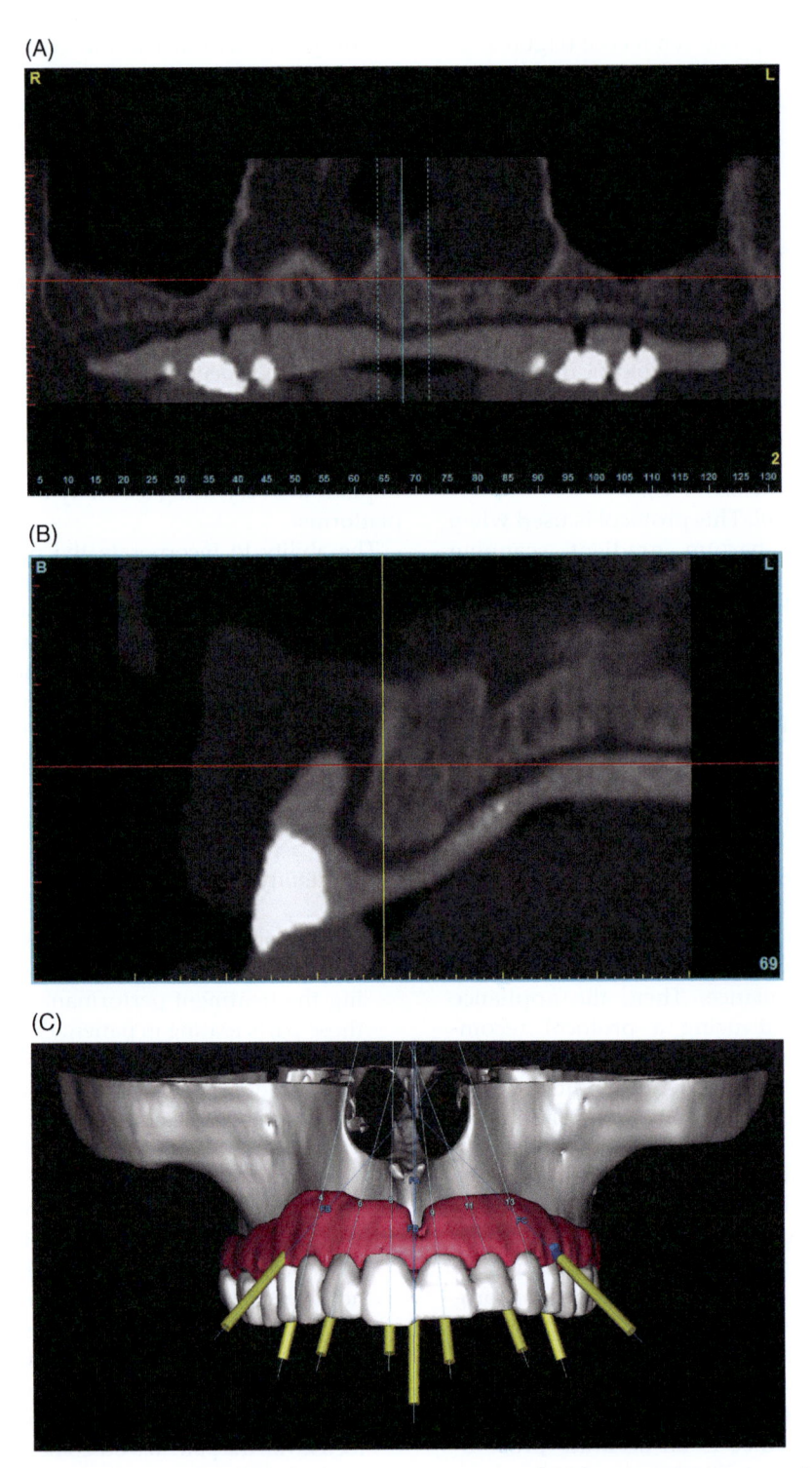

Figure 8.19A–C Panoramic, cross-sectional, and 3D reconstruction views of single scan CBCT imaging technique for a patient with complete edentulism in the maxilla. Denture scannoguide in place with radiolucent interocclusal bite registration.

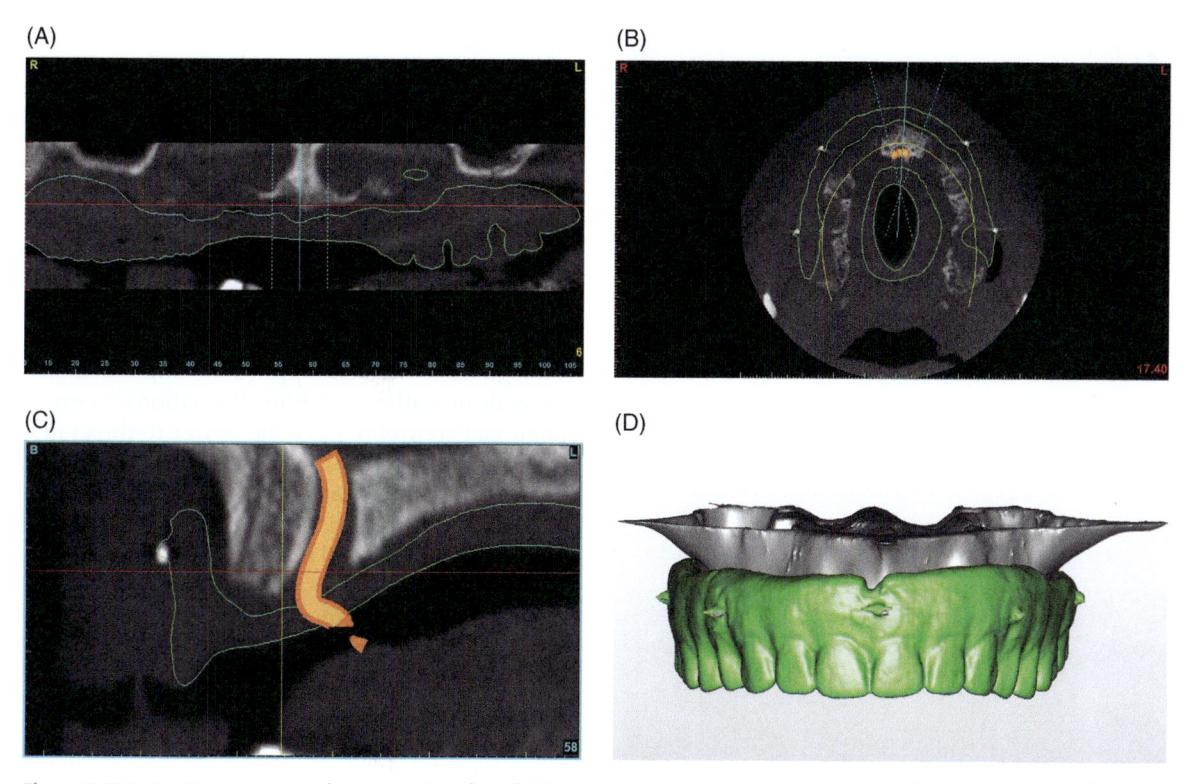

Figure 8.20A–D Panoramic, axial, cross-sectional, and 3D reconstruction views of dual scan CBCT imaging technique for a patient with complete edentulism in the maxilla. Patient's existing denture was used as the scanning appliance. Note multiple fiduciary markers in place at strategic positions.

CAD/CAM surgical guides

Introduction

Most diagnostic scans are obtained using cone beam computed tomography (CBCT) scanners. As previously discussed, scanning appliances are an important part of the imaging process. Surgical guides are designed and fabricated using CT/CBCT scans with meaningful diagnostic anatomical information embedded within the study. Viewing and surgical treatment planning software enables the clinician to extract and manipulate relevant data set information critical to the planning process. The fabrication of rapid prototype (RP) stereolithographic surgical guides is dependent upon pretreatment analysis and identification of case type patterns, appropriate scanning appliance imaging protocols that incorporate the principles of restorative leadership and collaborative accountability (Rosenfeld et al., 2006a, 2006b, 2006c). Guided surgical planning and guided surgical drilling is not a passing fad. Anticipated worldwide growth is substantial (Armheiter, 2006). Surgical guides can assist in the selection of the least traumatic surgery within the context of evidence-based information with maximum consideration for principles of wound healing and prosthetic biomechanics (de Almeida et al., 2010).

Definition and classification

The first aspect of guide definition and classification is that RP-generated surgical guides can accommodate and facilitate different surgical implant delivery methods that include either *partial* or *complete* CAD/CAM surgical guidance. (Figure 8.21A and B). Inherent to all CAD/CAM-generated surgical guides is the element of drilling tube prolongation (i.e., drilling tube elongation). Prolongation is a critical concept to determining feasibility,

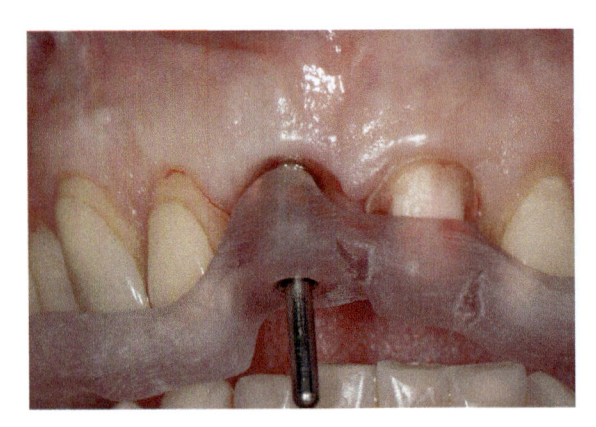

Figure 8.21A Example of tooth-supported, partially guided CAD/CAM surgical guide to facilitate osteotomy site preparation only for #8 without bone exposure. Implant placement will occur manually.

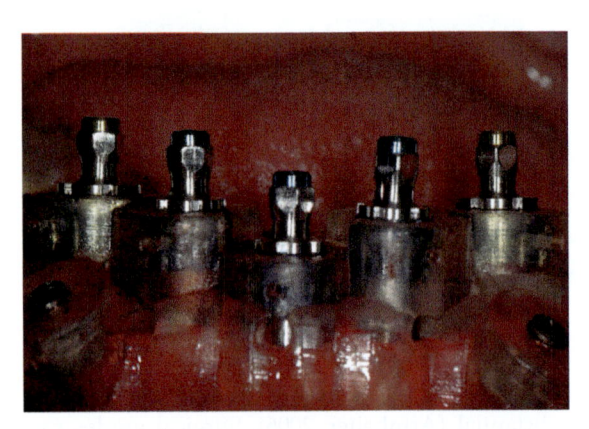

Figure 8.21B Example of bone-supported, totally guided CAD/CAM surgical guide with multiple stabilization screws in place. Five interforamina implants delivered. This guide type controls all three planes of ostetomy site preparation as well as the implant delivery.

guide development/fabrication, and realistic execution of vertical depth control in computer-guided implant surgery using CAD/CAM surgical guides. (Mandelaris et al., 2009). Figure 8.22, parts A through C, demonstrates the concept of prolongation.

Partial CAD/CAM surgical guidance implies assisted osteotomy preparation with or without depth control requiring manual implant installation. Partial guidance can be utilized in both fully and partially edentulous patients. Partial guidance can include successive guides representing increasing drill tube diameters or a single master tube with drill diameter reduction key inserts (Figure 8.23). The accuracy of partially guided implant placement has been documented by numerous authors (Sarment, Al-Shammari, et al., 2003; Sarment, Sukovic, et al., 2003; van Steenberghe et al., 2003; Vrielinck et al., 2003; Ganz, 2003; Di Giacomo et al., 2005; van Assche et al., 2007; Ganz, 2007). Total guidance implies axial (buccolingual and mesiodistal) and vertical depth control during osteotomy preparation and implant placement. Total guidance is also applied to implant delivery with or without additional rotational control. Rotational control to have the power to direct hex orientation is implant manufacturer dependent. Figure 8.24 demonstrates a totally guided implant system whereby rotational control of hex orientation is incorporated. All totally guided implant systems utilize a single surgical guide. These totally guided osteotomy and implant delivery systems are manufactured by specific implant companies to deliver their proprietary dental implants. It is important to remember that all totally guided implant delivery systems share similar characteristics. First, they are accurate. Second, they are sophisticatedly engineered. Third, they are efficient. Fourth, they are programmer dependent. Fifth and most important, they are all "brain dead." The patient-specific nature of any RP totally navigated implant delivery system is the result of the doctor's collaborative prosthetically directed treatment plan, which is developed by managing and manipulating information facilitated by using interactive planning software. The paradox nature of these systems allows the surgeon to deliver an accurate plan accurately or an inaccurate plan accurately. In other words, one can deliver a poorly conceived plan accurately. The delivery system does not know the difference. Figure 8.25 highlights the computer-guided implant treatment pathway process. Figure 8.26 and Figure 8.27 demonstrate the decision making and CAD/CAM guide application algorithms for partial and complete CAD/CAM guide usage in the partially and completely edentulous patient, respectively.

The second aspect of guide definition and classification is the guide support options. The case type pattern identification facilitates the selection of the most appropriate scanning appliance. The scanning appliance not only represents the surgical and

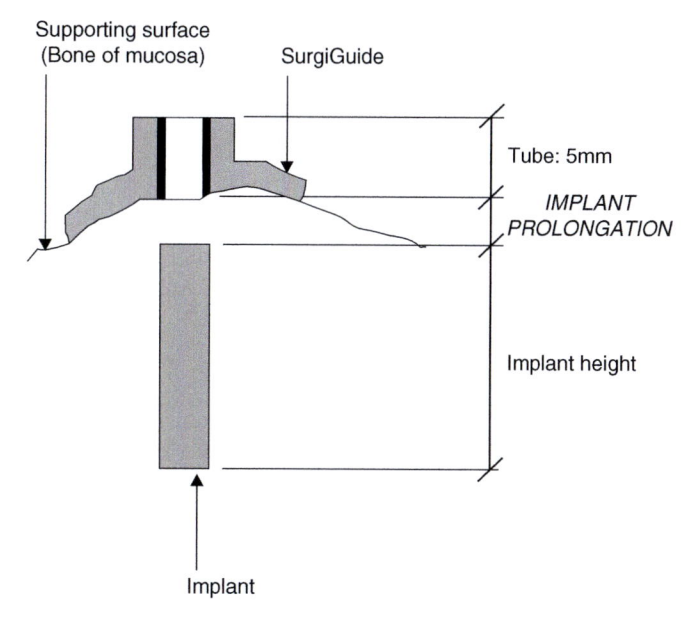

Figure 8.22A The drilling tube is positioned at the highest point of the bone crest above the planned implant position. The implant prolongation is the distance from the planned implant platform to the highest point of the bone crest. This distance is determined by the largest diameter CAD/CAM guide and is the same for each CAD/CAM guide of the case. Reprinted with permission from Mandelaris and Rosenfeld, 2009b.

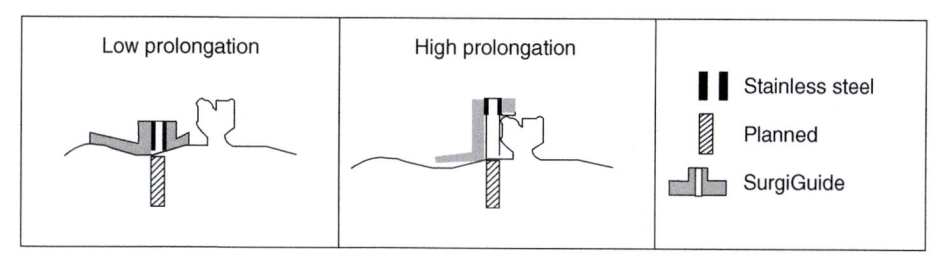

Figure 8.22B If an implant is positioned close to an adjacent tooth, it might be impossible to fixate the tube next to the tooth, and the tube as such has to be positioned above the tooth. This is known as a "high tube prolongation." Reprinted with permission from Mandelaris and Rosenfeld, 2009b.

prosthetic treatment requirements but also identifies the most likely surgical guide support necessary at the time of implant placement. The nature of the guide support underscores the importance of accurate diagnostics, a properly seated and verified scanning appliance, and proper scanning protocols. Support options can include bone, tooth, tooth/mucosa, or mucosa. Included in the guide support options is consideration of either dual or single scan protocols, which was discussed previously. In each instance a radiolucent interocclusal bite registration ensures full seating and stabilization of the scanning appliance at the time the CT/CBCT study is taken. Figures 8.15A, 8.17A, and 8.29 demonstrate a tooth-mucosa vacuform–based scanning appliance and a mucosal supported differential gradient (Tardieu) scanning appliance, each with radiolucent interocclusal bite registrations for CBCT imaging.

Selection of guide fixation strategies is most often considered for totally guided implant delivery systems which utilize bone, mucosa, or tooth/mucosa guide support. While fixation can be used for tooth-supported guides, its use is less frequent.

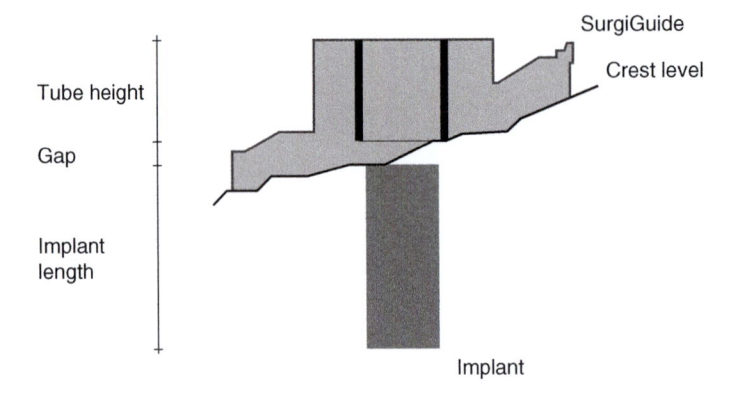

Picture: tube at heighest crest point above implant

Figure 8.22C Drilling depth for CAD/CAM guide assisted osteotomy site preparation. Drilling length = implant length + gap + tube height. Reprinted with permission from Mandelaris and Rosenfeld, 2009b.

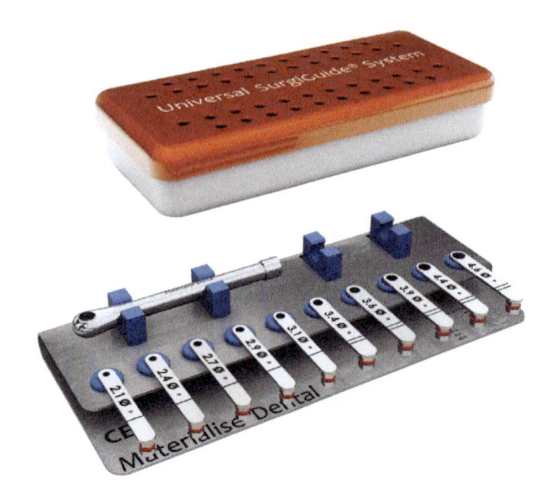

Figure 8.23 Partially guided CAD/CAM guidance system showing reduction key set that will be introduced into a single master tube, allowing for one guide to be used. Courtesy of Materialise Dental; Glen Burnie, MD, USA.

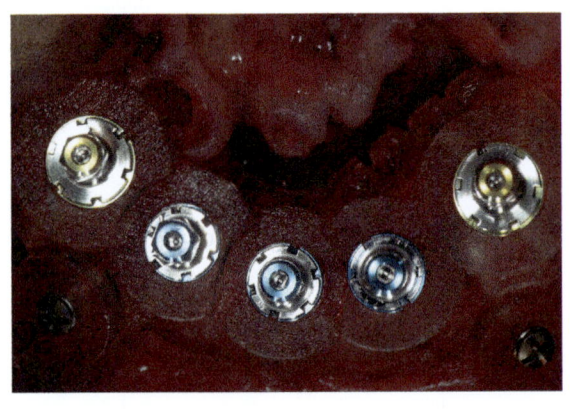

Figure 8.24 Totally guided, bone-supported CAD/CAM guidance system with rotational orientation control. Note alignment indices that allow for rotational control of the implant platform.

Totally guided delivery systems use a single RP surgical guide with either pin inserts or fixation screws to stabilize the guide (Figure 8.28). The use of an interocclusal verification bite registration of the surgical guide is helpful and can be fabricated from the preoperative mounted diagnostic models. This ensures the accurate placement and verification of the fixated guide. Figures 8.29, 8.30, and 8.31 demonstrate the use of a bite registration between the scanning appliance, stereolithographic RP virtual denture, and a patient's CAD/CAM surgical guide during minimally invasive immediate load surgery in the anterior mandible. This approach helps ensure the proper positioning of the CAD/CAM surgical guide and verifies positioning reproducibility/accuracy between the three appliances.

Mandelaris et al. (2010) described ten key elements influencing the ability to execute an accurate treatment outcome. These include but are not limited to the following:

1. Quality of the CT imaging, which includes panoramic, cross-sectional, and axial 2D views

Initial diagnostics for implant candidate
Clinical examination
Radiographic examination
Case type pattern determination
Preliminary patient consultation
Approval to proceed with diagnostic wax-up reflecting case type pattern

↓

Scanning appliance fabrication
Selection of case type pattern–directed scanning appliance
Fabrication of scanning appliance
Delivery to patient with bite registration as needed

↓

CT/CBCT imaging and planning software conversion
Determine single or dual scan protocol
Conversion of data set for use in planning software
Creation of appropriate anatomic segmentation/masks

↓

Definitive treatment planning process
Incorporate principles of restorative leadership and collaborative accountability
Preoperative consultation in an atmosphere of co-discovery and disclosure
Select and order surgical guide consistent with treatment plan

↓

Medical modeling
Surgical guide fabrication—selection either partial or full guidance
Select guide support surface
Fabrication of interim provisional prosthesis

↓

Surgery
Determine surgical access—flap or flapless
Implant placement—single or staged treatment
Placement of provisional restoration

↓

Definitive restoration and supportive peri-implant maintenance
Placement of definitive restoration
Recommendation of appropriate maintenance intervals

Figure 8.25   Implant treatment pathway.

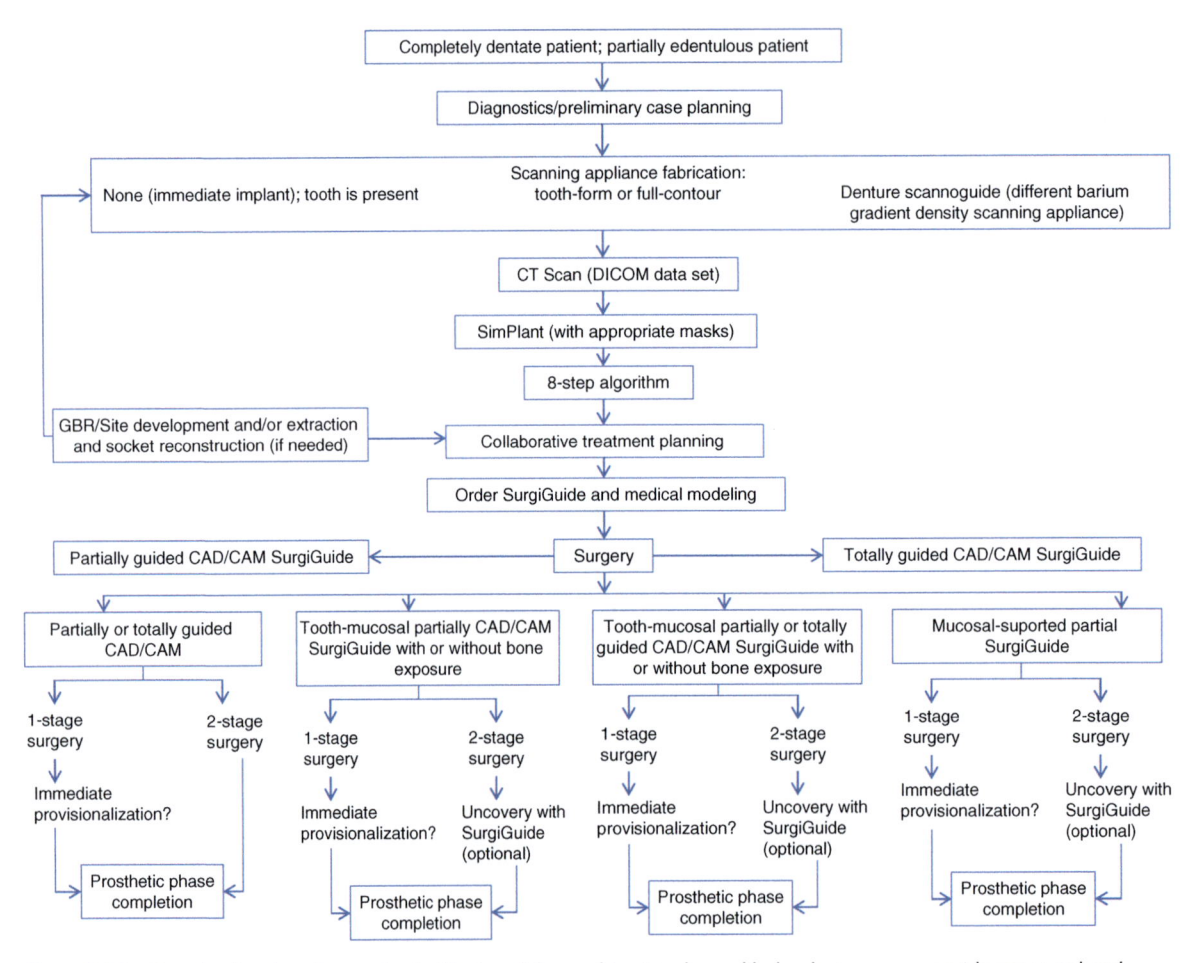

Figure 8.26 Completely edentulous patient with stereolithographic virtual mandibular denture scannoguide generated and stabilized with the bite registration used with the scannoguide.

2. Reliability of the 3D reconstruction that is created by the radiology technician using computer software
3. Quality of rapid prototype medical modeling
4. The challenge of determining the accurate position of thin crestal bone, which often competes with other radiodense structures (teeth, scanning appliances)
5. Regional anatomy characteristics
6. Dimensional stability of the stone model, which is optically imaged for tooth-supported cases
7. Accurate placement and stability of the scanning appliance at the time of imaging
8. Extent of imaging artifact
9. Movement and fit of the guide during surgical execution
10. Knowledge and experience in CT analysis and interpretation.

These key elements either alone or in combination can influence the accuracy of implant placement.

Implementation of CAD/CAM guidance into clinical practice

Implementation of new technology into clinical practice presents unique challenges. Change is often difficult. The most important guiding principle

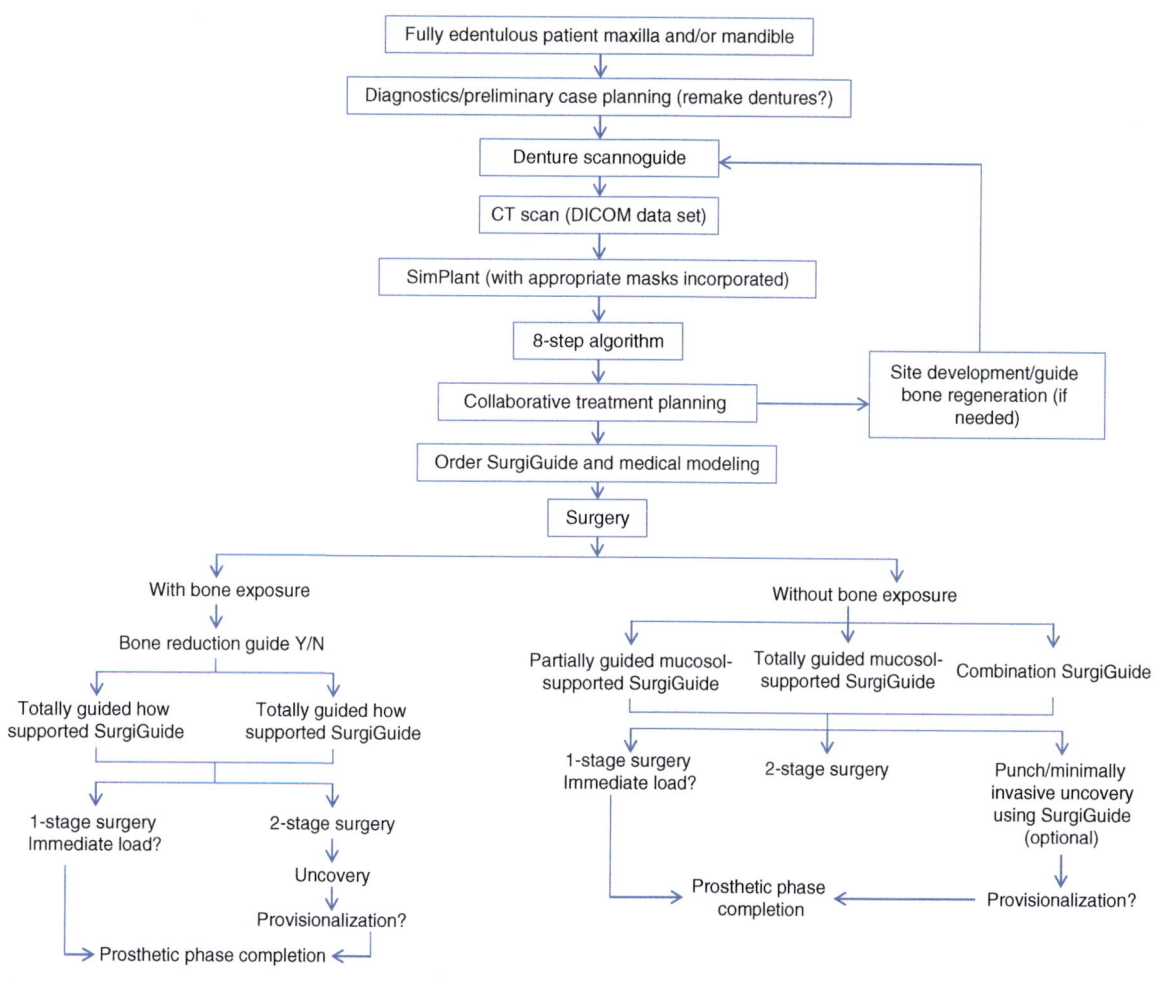

```
Fully edentulous patient maxilla and/or mandible
        ↓
Diagnostics/preliminary case planning (remake dentures?)
        ↓
Denture scannoguide ←──────────────────────┐
        ↓                                  │
CT scan (DICOM data set)                   │
        ↓                                  │
SimPlant (with appropriate masks incorporated)
        ↓                                  │
8-step algorithm                           │
        ↓                          Site development/guide
Collaborative treatment planning ──→ bone regeneration (if needed)
        ↓
Order SurgiGuide and medical modeling
        ↓
Surgery
   ↓                                        ↓
With bone exposure                    Without bone exposure
   ↓                                        ↓
Bone reduction guide Y/N          Partially guided / Totally guided / Combination
   ↓              ↓                mucosol-supported  mucosol-supported  SurgiGuide
Totally guided   Totally guided    SurgiGuide         SurgiGuide
how supported    how supported         ↓                 ↓                ↓
SurgiGuide       SurgiGuide        1-stage surgery   2-stage surgery  Punch/minimally
   ↓              ↓                Immediate load?                    invasive uncovery
1-stage surgery  2-stage surgery                                      using SurgiGuide
Immediate load?    ↓                                                  (optional)
   ↓            Uncovery                                                  ↓
   ↓            Provisionalization?    → Prosthetic phase ←       Provisionalization?
   └→ Prosthetic phase completion ←        completion
```

Figure 8.27 Completely edentulous patient with partial guidance, mucosal-supported CAD/CAM surgical guide in place. Positioning verified with the bite registration used with the scannoguide during imaging and with the virtual denture. Bite registration allows for cross-mounting accuracy and repeatability to be ensured.

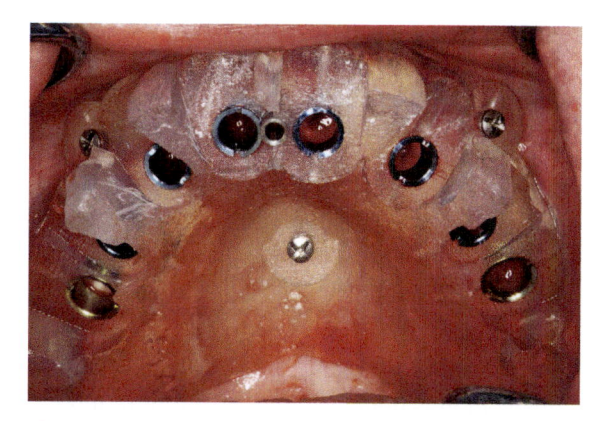

Figure 8.28 Totally guided, mucosal-supported CAD/CAM surgical guide with multiple fixation points to ensure stabilization.

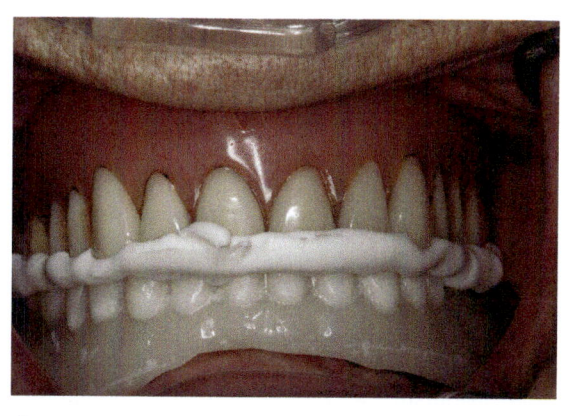

Figure 8.29 Completely edentulous patient with mandibular denture scannoguide in place stabilized with bite registration.

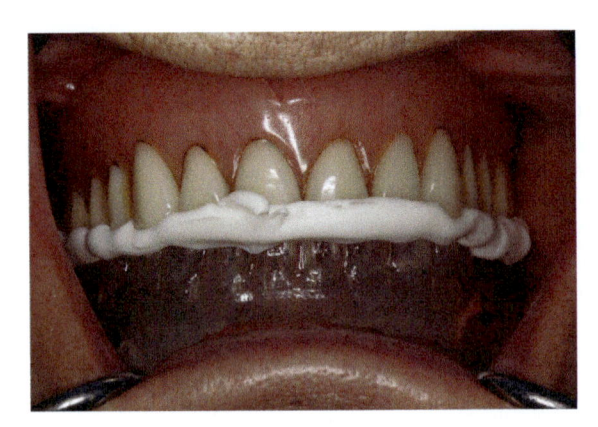

Figure 8.30 Completely edentulous patient with stereolithographic virtual mandibular denture scannoguide generated and stabilized with the bite registration used with the scannoguide.

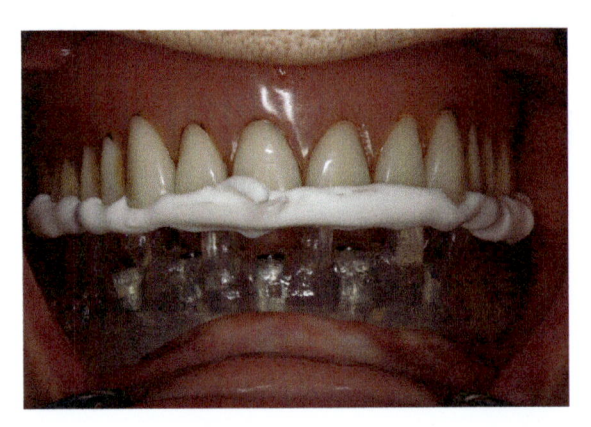

Figure 8.31 Completely edentulous patient with partial guidance, mucosal-supported, CAD/CAM surgical guide in place. Positioning verified with the bite registration used with the scannoguide during imaging and with the virtual denture. Bite registration allows for cross-mounting accuracy and repeatability to be ensured.

regarding new technology is that it is not a substitute for experience and sound clinical judgment. CBCT imaging and CAD/CAM technology is really a contemporary method of managing information. The implementation process comprises seven participants. These include (1) the prosthetic dentist, (2) the dental laboratory technologist, (3) the imaging center, (4) the CT/CBCT treatment plan, (5) the implant manufacturer, (6) the guide manufacturer, and (7) the surgeon. The guiding concepts of restorative leadership and collaborative accountability facilitate implementation of this technology.

Mandelaris and Rosenfeld (2008) have published a logical and progressive method for implementing this paradigm shift into practice. The first level of implementation strategy is to utilize CT/CBCT information to enhance treatment planning and surgical decision making. Learn how to recognize and interpret scan images. Scans offer comprehensive three-dimensional images when compared with traditional radiographs. When combined with interactive three-dimensional viewing and planning software, more predictable treatment planning occurs. Implant surgery can be performed using the traditional manual approach using a conventional surgical template. The scan provides significantly improved diagnostic and treatment planning data, thus better preparing the surgeon, prosthetic dentist, and patient for anticipated treatment. Figure 8.32A through K demonstrates the use of CT-based treatment planning for immediate implant placement + immediate nonocclusal function provisionalization in the esthetic zone while operating by manual (non-CAD/CAM surgical guidance) technique.

The second level of implementation strategy uses a bone-supported surgical guide (Figure 8.33A–C). This is an entry-level step into guided surgery that allows the surgeon to visualize, perform, and verify progress. The shift from nonguided surgery to this level of guidance is the smallest change from conventional surgery. The surgeon can visually confirm surgical progress, and if necessary, discontinue the use of the guide at a recoverable time during the surgery. It is recommended that a conventional template also be used during surgery as an adjunct to verify osteotomy-tooth position accuracy until a sufficient level of comfort and experience is achieved.

The third level of implementation strategy is the use of a tooth-supported drilling guide with or without bone exposure (Figure 8.21A, Figure 8.34 A–K). The clinician may or may not choose to visualize the surgical field to assess any deviation from the anticipated outcome. This could allow a minimally invasive approach to be considered. Figure 8.34 A–P demonstrates the use of a tooth-supported CAD/CAM surgical guide under the partially guided context. Minimally invasive implant placement + immediate nonocclusal provisionalization is demonstrated. Presurgical, model-based validation surgery is also performed as a

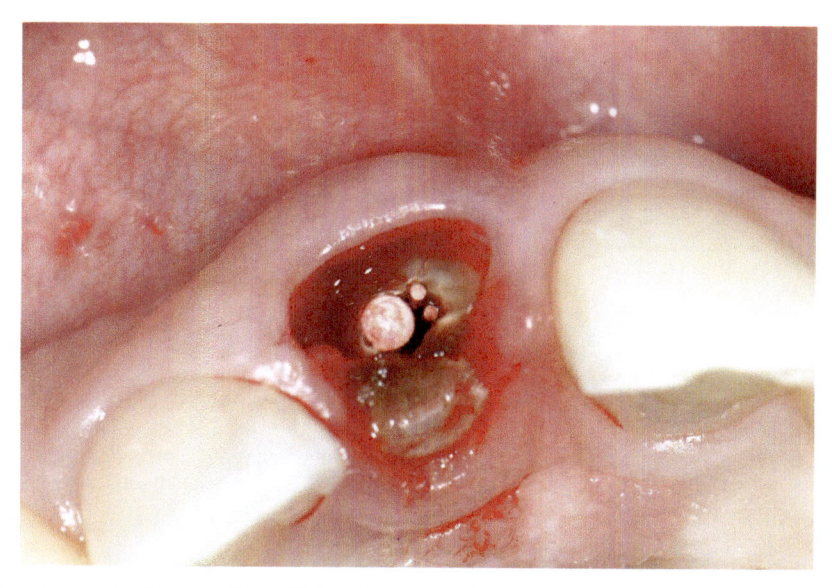

Figure 8.32A Clinical example of fractured #8 with hopeless prognosis.

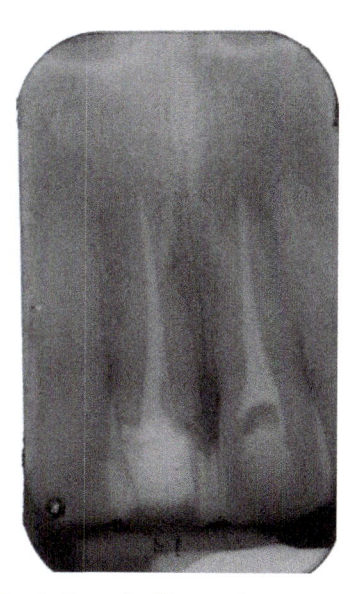

Figure 8.32B Radiograph of fractured #8.

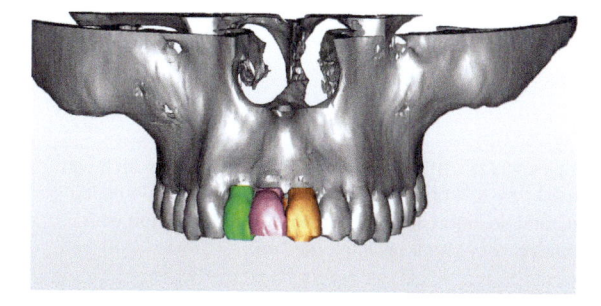

Figure 8.32C 3D reconstruction of the maxillary arch with masks created of #7, #8, and #9, and the maxilla/remaining natural dentition.

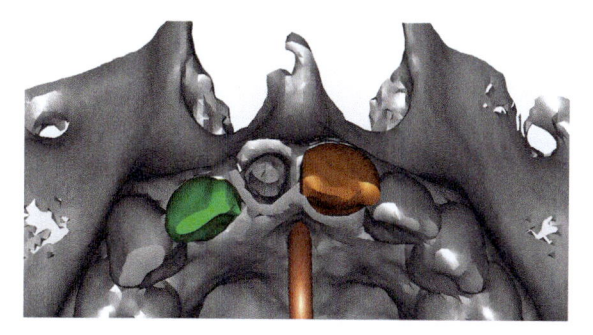

Figure 8.32D 3D reconstruction with mask of #8 toggle off to allow for simulated extraction and alveolus inspection.

dress rehearsal to the actual event. A provisional restoration (nonocclusal function) is also made prior to the surgery taking place (Figure 8.34C, D). If successive guide is used, the utilization of a conventional surgical template is recommended to verify osteotomy–tooth position accuracy. As

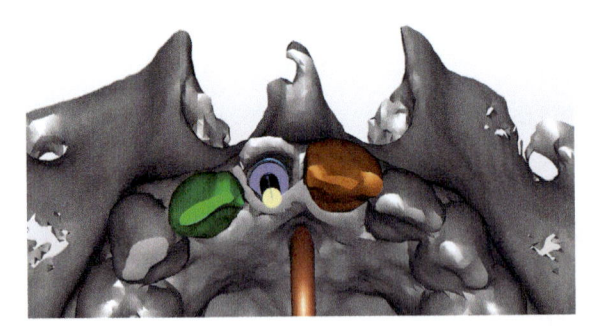

Figure 8.32E 3D reconstruction with mask of #8 toggle off and implant placed. Note implant:alveolus "gap," which may require management.

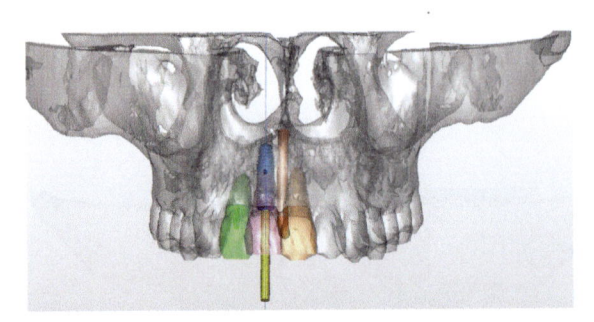

Figure 8.32F 3D reconstruction of the maxillary arch with masks created of #7, #8, and #9, and the maxilla/remaining natural dentition. Implant placed in the #8 position with transparency toggle switch turned on.

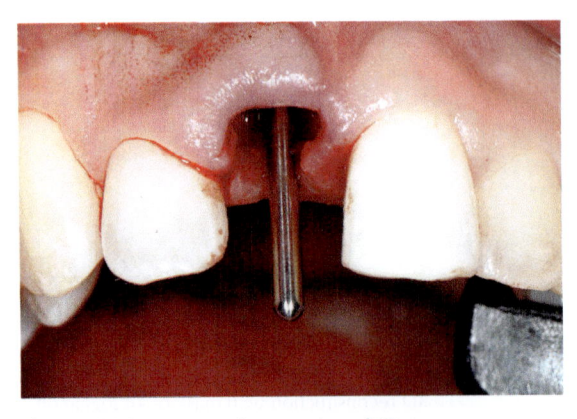

Figure 8.32G Atraumatic extraction of #8.

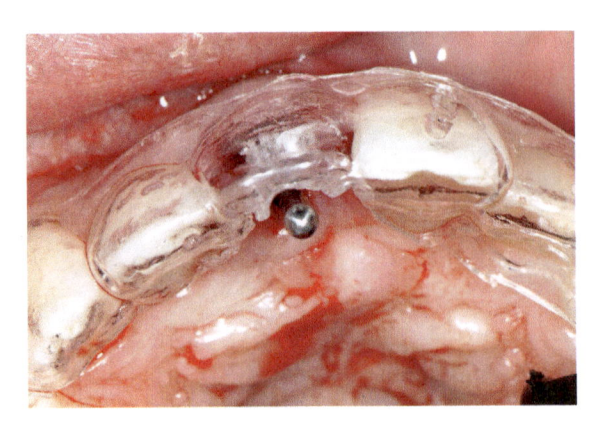

Figure 8.32H Manual osteotomy site preparation performed and positioning verification performed with conventional (non-CAD/CAM-generated) surgical template.

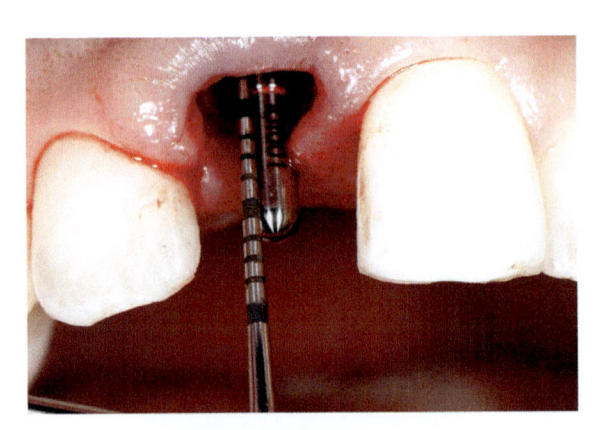

Figure 8.32I Manual implant placement and vertical positioning verified to ensure sufficient prosthetic emergence (vertical depth) established.

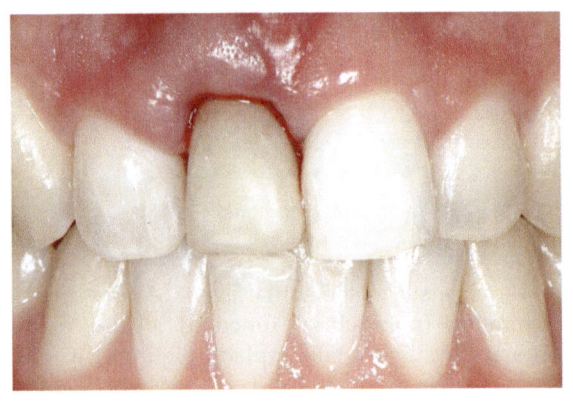

Figure 8.32J Immediate nonocclusal function provisionalization completed on #8.

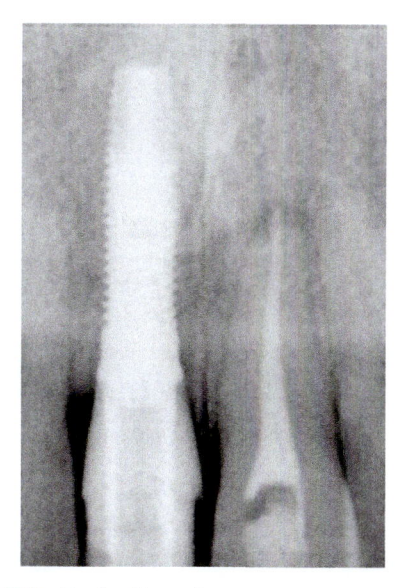

Figure 8.32K Final radiograph.

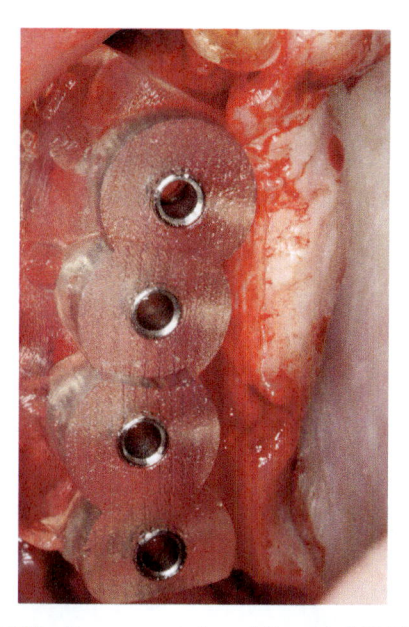

Figure 8.33B Bone-supported, partially guided CAD/CAM surgical guide seated on the edentulous ridge during open flap surgery.

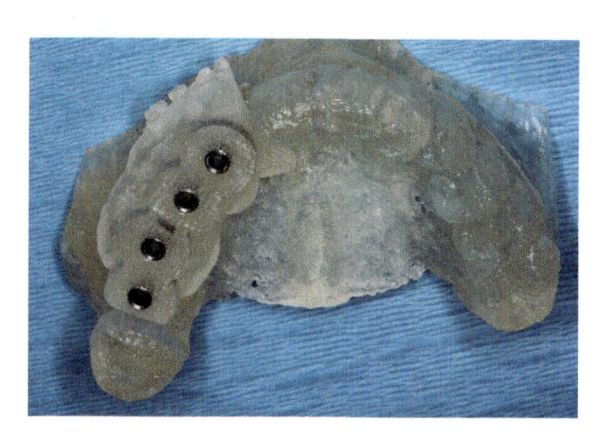

Figure 8.33A Bone-supported, partially guided CAD/CAM surgical guide seated on the stereolithographic rapid prototype medical model of the maxilla.

stated earlier, model surgery can also be performed prior to treatment to confirm accuracy with the planned outcome (Ganz, 2007).

In implementation strategies 2 and 3, partial guidance can be expanded to include a totally guided approach to osteotomy site preparation and implant delivery. Attempting surgery with complete guidance should be undertaken after acquiring experience in computer-guided implant

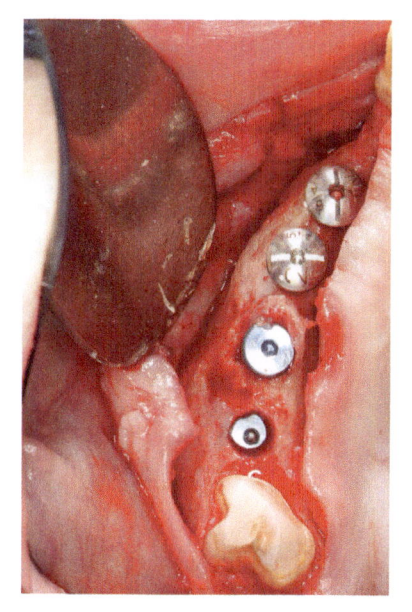

Figure 8.33C Osteotomy site preparation completed using bone-supported, partially guided CAD/CAM surgical guide. Implants placed manually at the #3, #4, #5, and #6 positions. Biologic shaping performed at #2.

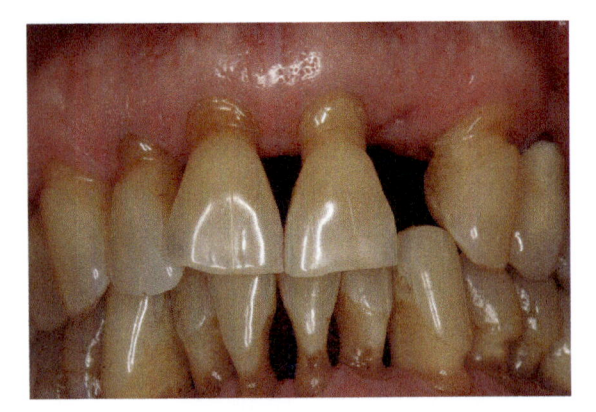

Figure 8.34A Clinical view of partial edentulism #10.

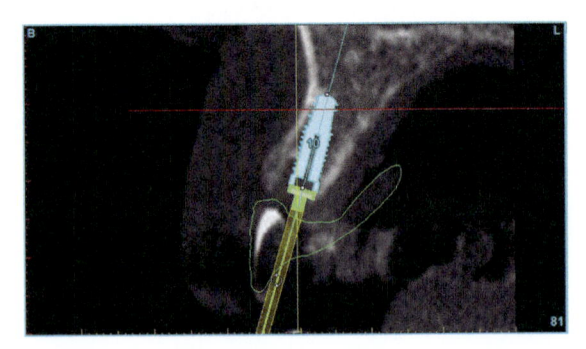

Figure 8.34B Cross-sectional view of #10 site. Virtual implant planning performed. Dual scan CBCT imaging protocol used. Green outline represents tooth position and denture flange.

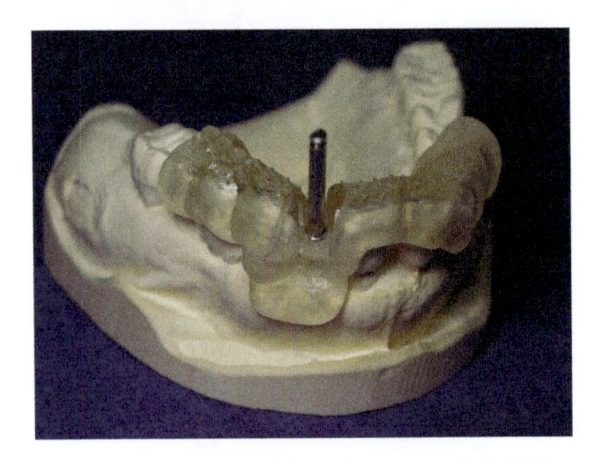

Figure 8.34C Partially guided, tooth-supported CAD/CAM surgical guide seated on stone model. Osteotomy site preparation performed in the stone model as a part of the presurgical workup and to develop an immediate nonocclusal function provisional prior to surgery. Note inspection windows allowing verification of complete seating of the guide.

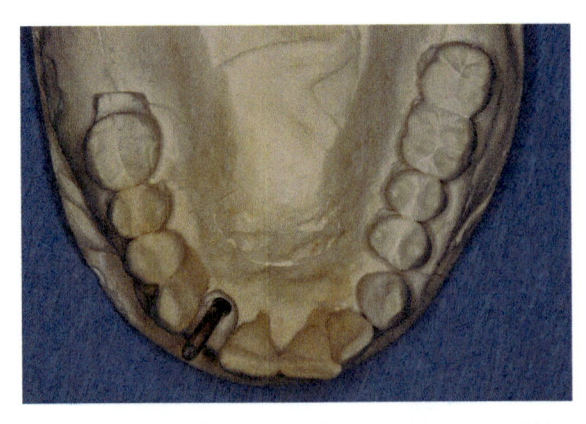

Figure 8.34D Guide pin inserted into osteotomy site within the stone model to verify angulation and overall positioning.

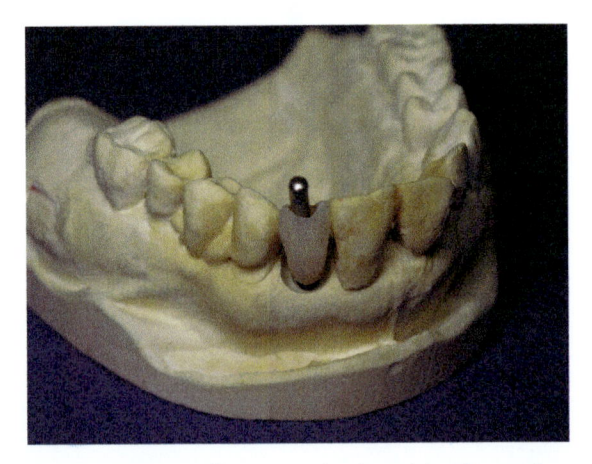

Figure 8.34E Immediate nonocclusal provisional created prior to surgery.

planning and surgery. The totally guided approach is less recoverable and therefore incurs the greatest risk potential, but it also offers the greatest rewards.

The fourth step is to use a guide that is placed directly on the edentulous mucosal tissue (Figure 8.35). A partially or completely guided approach can be taken. Successive guides, guides with successive reduction keys, and those incorporating totally guided implant delivery systems can be considered. Single surgical guides may be best served as fixated (Figure 8.24, Figure 8.28, Figure 8.36A). However, not all systems allow total guidance when using bone as support. With a system using total guidance, implants can be placed in a "flapless" manner (Figure 8.36A and B).

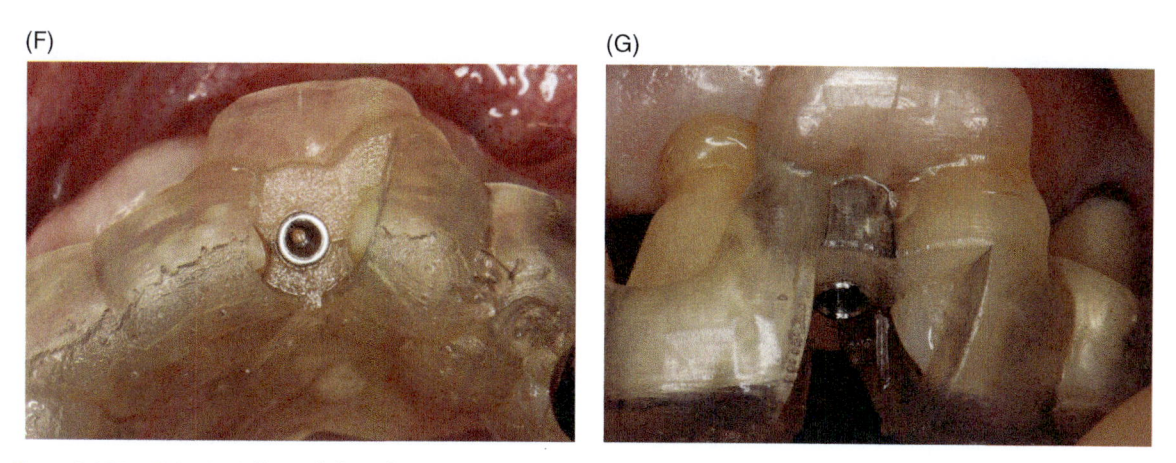

Figure 8.34F and G Partially guided, tooth-supported, CAD/CAM-generated surgical guide seated at the time of surgery. Note inspection windows allowing verification of complete seating of the guide.

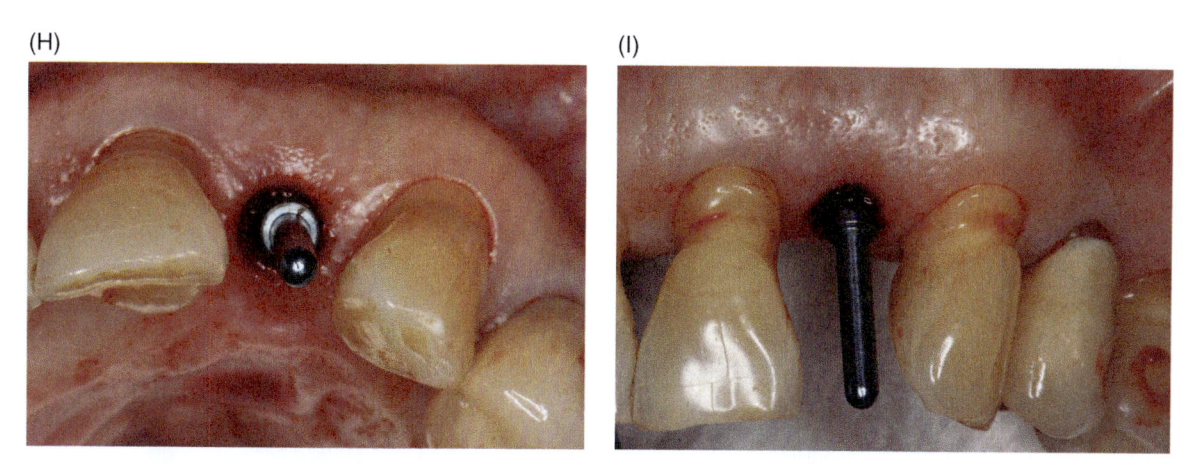

Figure 8.34H and I Guide pin in place demonstrating positional orientation of osteotomy site preparation performed without bone exposure of and via the partially guided, tooth-supported CAD/CAM surgical guide.

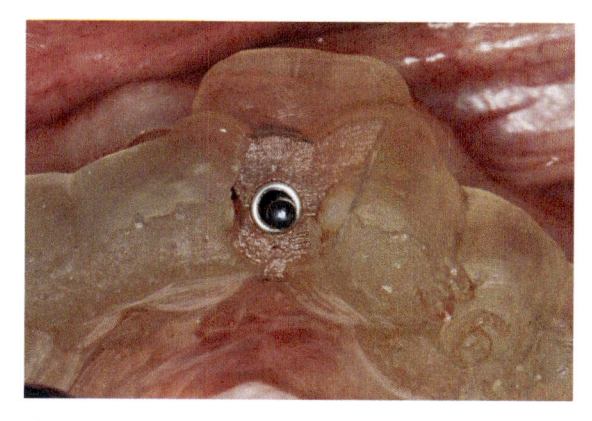

Figure 8.34J Guide pin in place through the seated partially guided, tooth-supported CAD/CAM surgical guide.

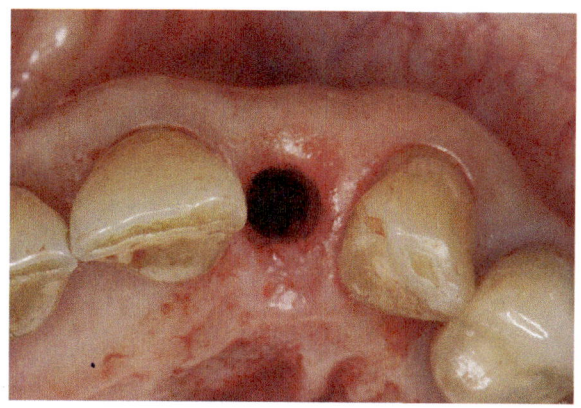

Figure 8.34K Osteotomy site preparation completed.

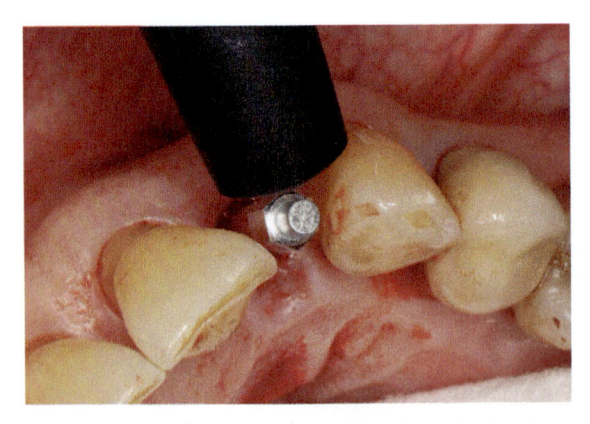

Figure 8.34L Manual implant placement performed and implant stability quotient measured (Implant stability meter by Osstell; Linthicum, MD, USA).

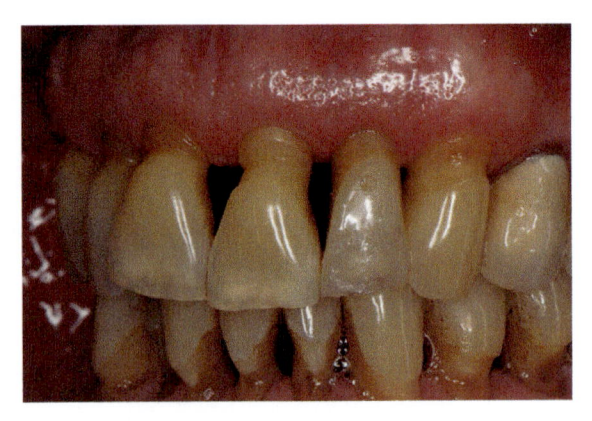

Figure 8.34O Immediate nonocclusal function provisionalization of #10 completed.

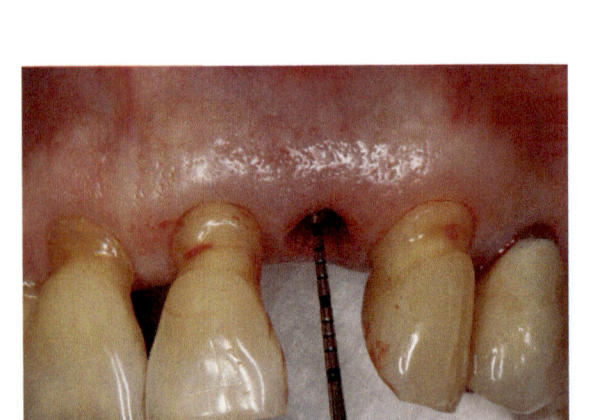

Figure 8.34M Vertical positioning of implant verified to ensure sufficient prosthetic emergence (vertical depth) established.

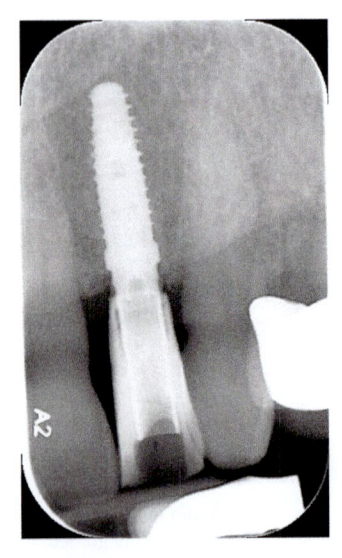

Figure 8.34P Postsurgical radiograph #10.

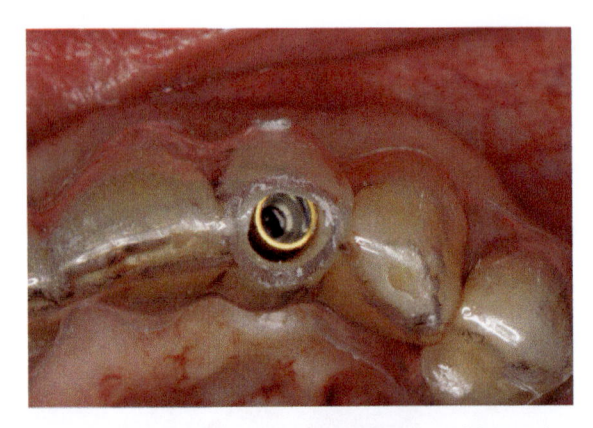

Figure 8.34N Implant emergence relative to prefabricated, immediate nonocclusal function provisional.

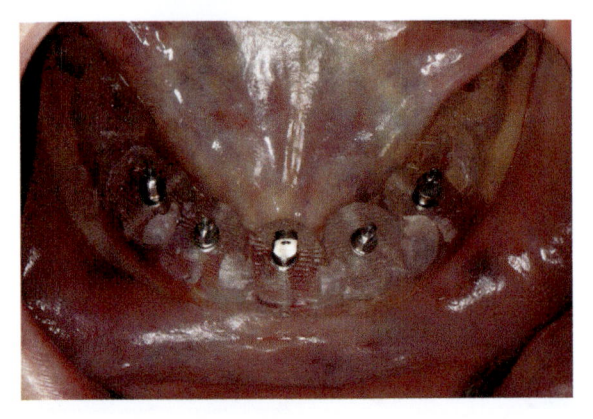

Figure 8.35 Partially guided, mucosal-supported CAD/CAM surgical guide.

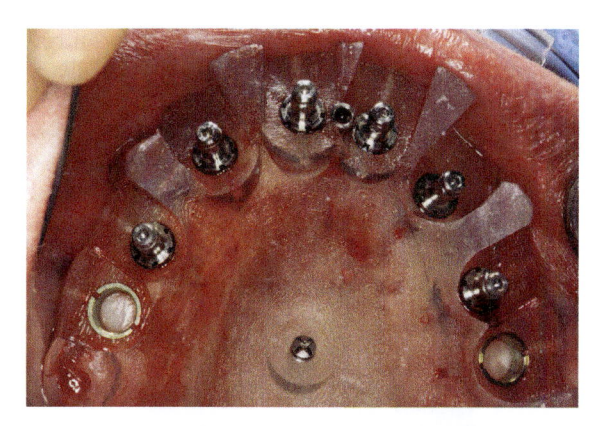

Figure 8.36A Totally guided, mucosal-supported CAD/CAM surgical guide with hex orientation allowed for and multiple fixation points used to ensure stabilization. Implants placed under total guidance and without bone exposure.

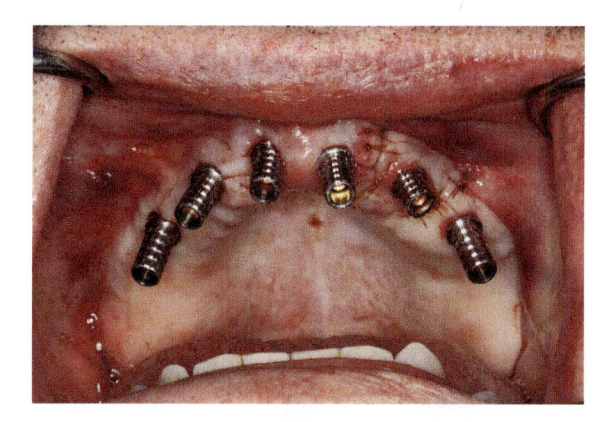

Figure 8.36B Flapless implant placement of six maxillary fixtures. Abutment placement and temporary cylinders in place to allow for immediate loading to proceed.

This is a true minimally invasive method of performing implant surgery and offers the clinical benefit of reduced patient morbidity. However, a blinded approach is associated with the highest risk and demands the most precise diagnostic prosthetic workup, scanning appliance fabrication, imaging quality, treatment planning, and surgical execution. Since it involves the greatest paradigm shift, it should be utilized by experienced clinicians. This paradigm shift requires the greatest leap of faith from conventional implant surgery. Last, it is recommended that all CAD/CAM surgical guides be preferentially disinfected with 80% alcohol or Octenidine using an incubation time of 15 minutes with ultrasonication before use in live surgery. This protocol has been shown to be the most effective approach at eliminating the growth of microorganisms such as *Pseudomonas aeruginosa, Acinetobacter vaumanni, Enterococcus faecalis, Enterococcus faecium, Staphylococcus aureus, Enterobacter cloacae, Escherichia coli,* and *Candida albicans* in vitro (Sennhenn-Kirchner et al., 2008).

Specialized guide design options

Bone reduction guides

Unfavorable intra- and interarch bone anatomy and patient-specific requirements for implant placement can complicate or negate the ability to use a minimally invasive CAD/CAM guidance approach (i.e., mucosal-supported surgical guide). The crestal bone width should accommodate the diameter of the planned implant. Ideally, the bone crest should allow for circumferential bone thickness of at least 1–2 mm circumferentially around the entire implant. Crestal bone width, at the level of the implant platform, is critical to the establishment of physiologic bone remodeling. It also is critical for the maintenance of soft tissue support. However, in many cases, thin crestal bone (associated with edentulous sites or in immediate implant cases) is present, precluding implant placement without vertical bone reduction. In conjunction with surgical planning software, the vertical bone height can be selectively reduced by using a bone reduction guide in order to establish bone width consistent with implant selection. In most cases the horizontal dimension of the residual ridge increases when measured inferiorly.

Osteoplasty is often needed to reduce unusable thin crestal bone until sufficient horizontal bone width is achieved. Traditionally, this has been an intuitive process, leading to manual osteotomy site preparation and implant placement. With the advent of bone-supported CAD/CAM bone reduction surgical guides, precision osteoplasty can be performed in order to ensure guide stability. The bone reduction will also allow the establishment of the shortest prolongation height consistent with osteotomy drill length and intraoral access. To accomplish accurate bone position and fit of the surgical guide, a manual approach is too inaccurate.

Bone reduction guides are stereolithographically generated CAD/CAM devices that allow for precisely guided osteoplasty to be performed. They are predominantly, but not exclusively, used in the anterior mandible during immediate load type cases or when the vertical position of implant placement requires a significant change from the patient's existing anatomy. They are used when the total depth of osteotomy site preparation cannot be accommodated with drilling systems due to excessive depth. The major advantage of a bone reduction guide is precision osteoplasty to optimize residual ridge anatomy to facilitate osteotomy site preparation. The main disadvantage of the bone reduction is its inherent weakness. This type of guide must have an open architectural design for surgical access. This design increases susceptibility to fracture or breakage. Additional disadvantages include visual seating verification, increased size of the surgical field, regional anatomic restrictions, and cost. Use of the bone reduction guide and its application in computer-guided surgery is illustrated through Figure 8.37A–Q.

Cutting pathway guide for lateral antroscopy of the maxillary sinus

Despite significant improvements made in CT imaging, difficulty in precisely creating the sinus window remains. The cutting path guide is a stereolithographically generated guide that facilitates precise osteotomy cuts, accurately defining the lateral boundaries of the maxillary sinus (Mandelaris et al., 2009). This technique uses three-dimensional CT imaging and computer software to presurgically outline the lateral boundaries of the maxillary sinus for antral bone grafting surgery. It can be used alone (Figure 8.38A–L) or in combination with partially or totally guided CAD/CAM surgical guides. (Figure 8.39A–C) The cutting paths can be verified in all planes of space to ensure that the planned osteotomy cuts will maximize the operator's ability to elevate the sinus membrane.

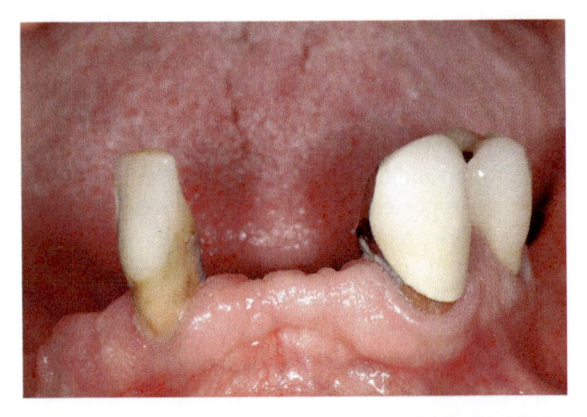

Figure 8.37A Clinical view of patient with partial edentulism in the mandible. Remaining natural teeth have poor prognoses.

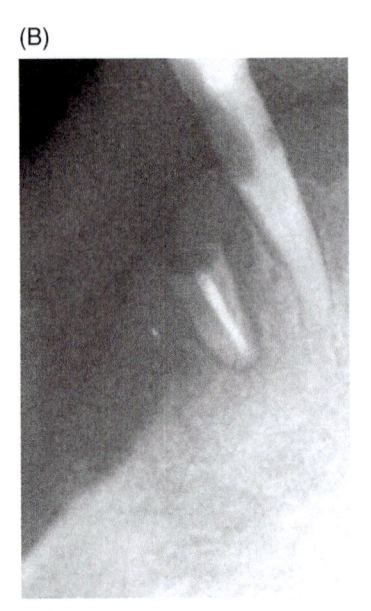

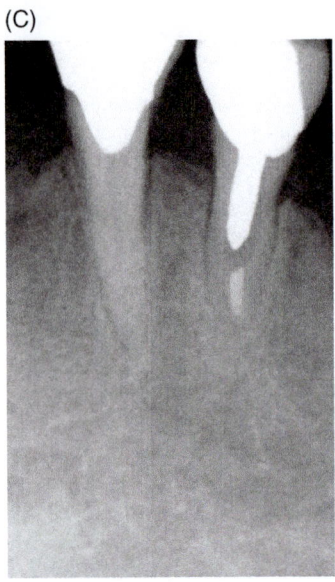

Figure 8.37B and C Radiographs of remaining mandibular dentition.

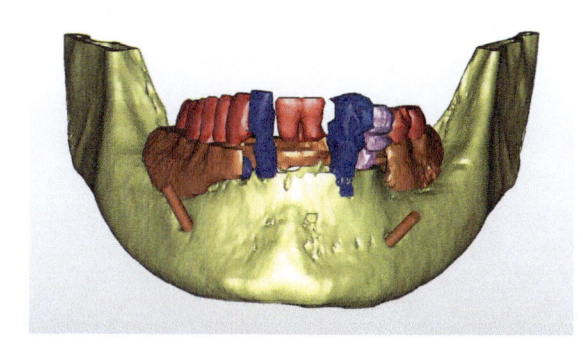

Figure 8.37D 3D reconstruction of mandible. Masks of mandible, remaining natural dentition, scan appliance dental anatomy (teeth), and surgical anatomy (denture base) created.

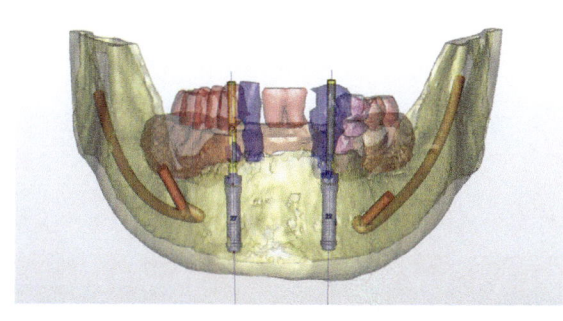

Figure 8.37E 3D reconstruction of mandible with transparency toggle switch engaged. Two interforamina implants have been placed to support a removable complete denture as the final prosthetic outcome goal.

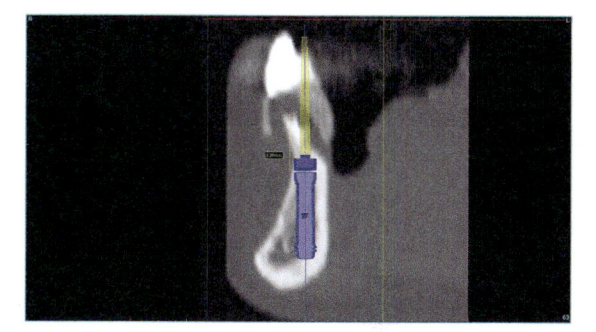

Figure 8.37F Cross-section view of implant positioning. Note the vertical positioning of the implant is 9 mm from the crest. Thin crestal bone requires significant osteoplasty in the vertical dimension to achieve a position where horizontal bone levels/position allow for implant placement. Also, note the differences in barium concentration between the denture flange (10%) and denture teeth (30%). Scan appliance is notably well seated as no air pocketing (radiolucencies) are noted.

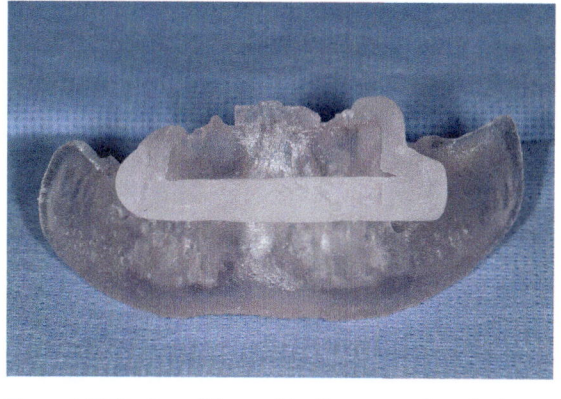

Figure 8.37G Stereolithographically generated medical model of postextraction, preosteoplasty anatomy with bone reduction guide.

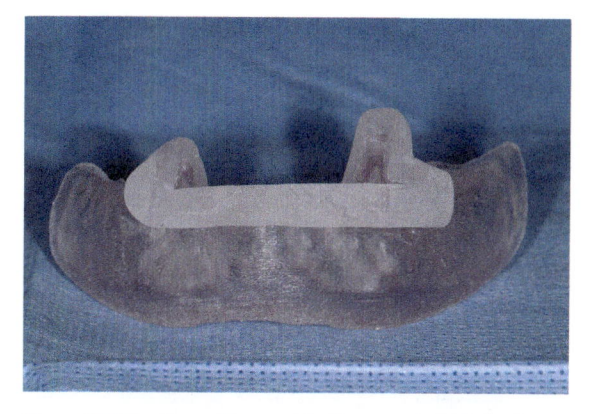

Figure 8.37H Stereolithographically generated medical model of postextraction, postosteoplasty anatomy with bone reduction guide. Bone reduction guide allows for precision osteoplasty to be performed.

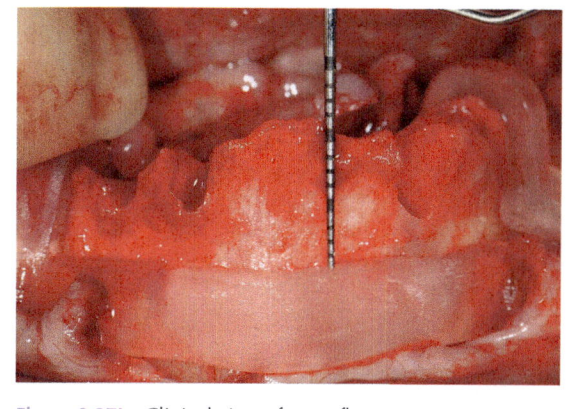

Figure 8.37I Clinical view of open flap surgery, postextraction anatomy. Bone reduction guide seated. 9 mm of unusable bone height.

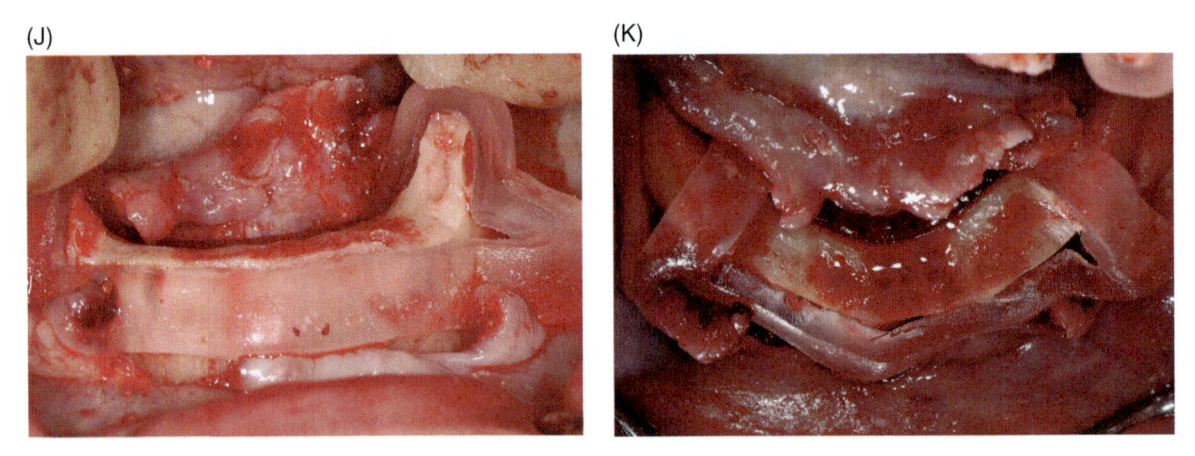

Figure 8.37J and K Precision osteoplasty performed and directed via bone reduction guide.

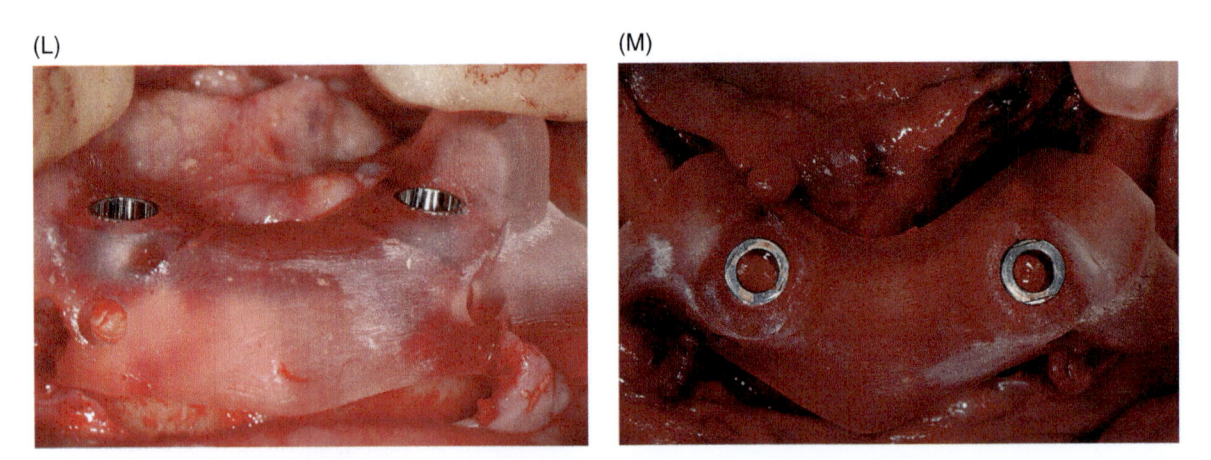

Figure 8.37L and M Totally guided, bone-supported CAD/CAM surgical guide in place on postosteoplasty anatomy in the mandibular anterior.

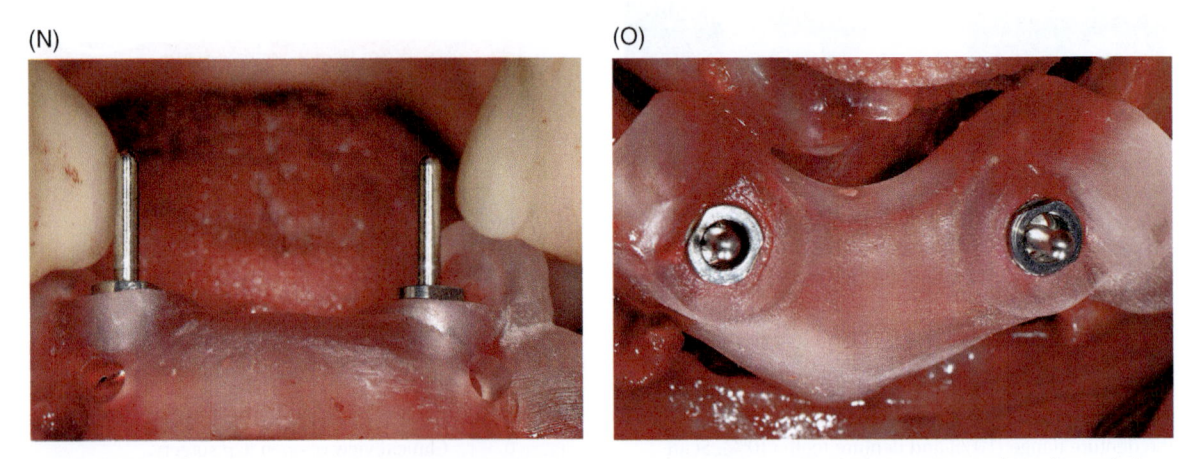

Figure 8.37N and O Direction guides in place to verify osteotomy site orientation within the bone-supported, totally guided CAD/CAM surgical guide.

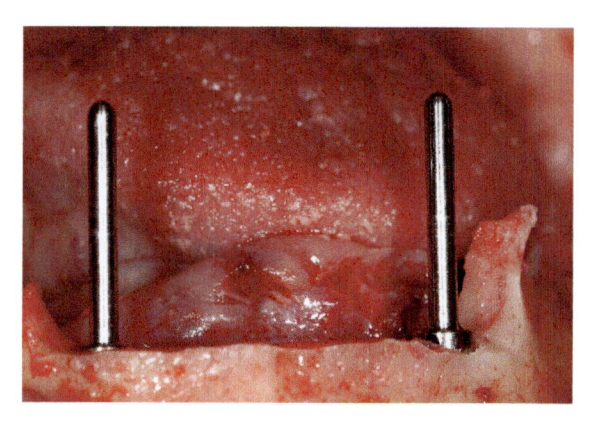

Figure 8.37P Totally guided CAD/CAM surgical guide removed and positioning verified.

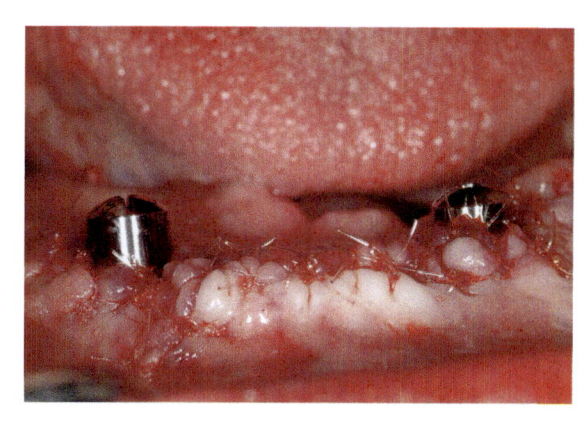

Figure 8.37Q Postsurgical view of implant placement #22 and #27, + healing abutments. Surgical field closed.

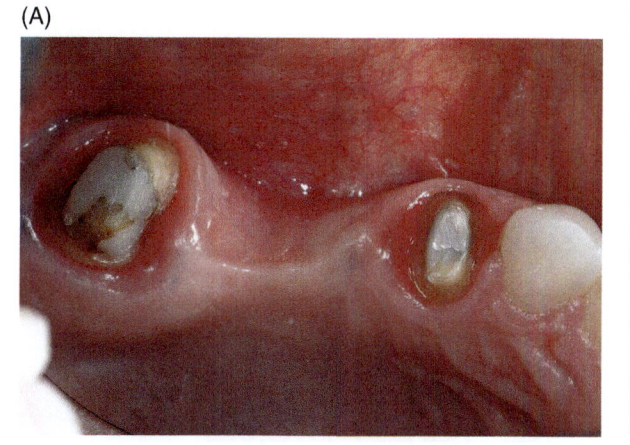

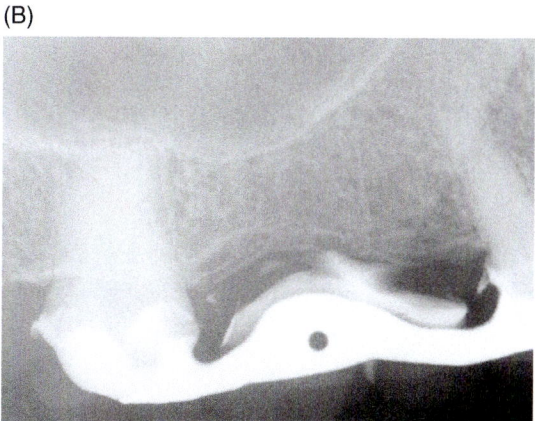

(A)

(B)

Figure 8.38A and B Preoperative view and initial radiographs. Partial edentulism #3 and #4. Reprinted with permission from Mandelaris and Rosenfeld, 2009a.

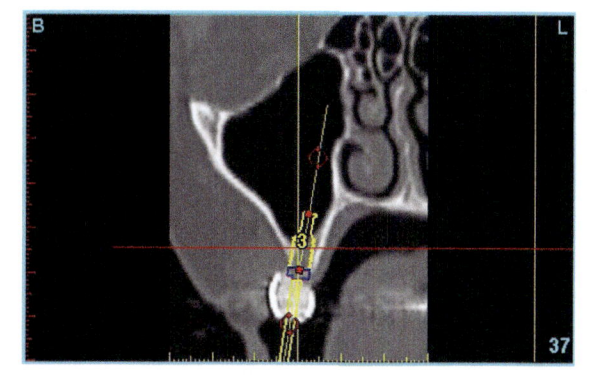

Figure 8.38C Cross-sectional CT images of implant position #3. A tooth-form scanning appliance demonstrates optimal, final tooth position in space. Disuse atrophy and residual ridge resorption are apparent as well as sinus pneumatization. Reprinted with permission from Mandelaris and Rosenfeld, 2009a.

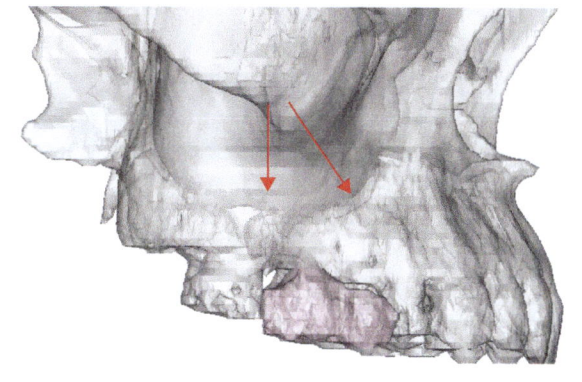

Figure 8.38D 3D image of the maxillary arch with tooth form scanning appliance in place (purple). Transparency tool is engaged and implants planned have been toggled off. The red arrows point to the anterior and inferior sinus boundaries. Reprinted with permission from Mandelaris and Rosenfeld, 2009a.

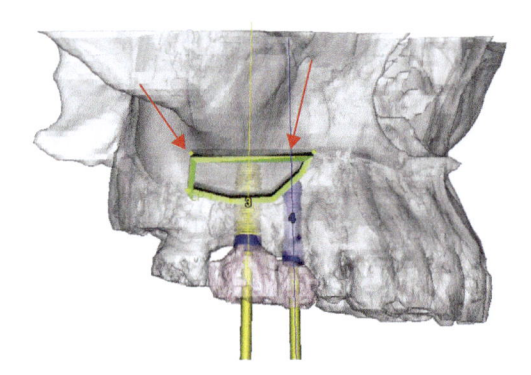

Figure 8.38E 3D reconstruction of the maxilla in Simplant OMS software and custom freeform cutting path outlining desired lateral window (red arrows). Reprinted with permission from Mandelaris and Rosenfeld, 2009a.

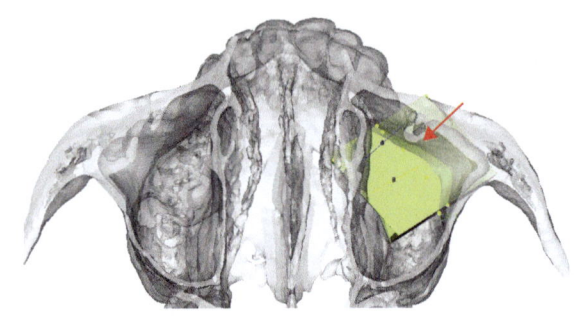

Figure 8.38F Superior view of 3D reconstruction of the maxilla in SimPlant OMS software and the same custom freeform cutting path visualized (red arrow). Reprinted with permission from Mandelaris and Rosenfeld, 2009a.

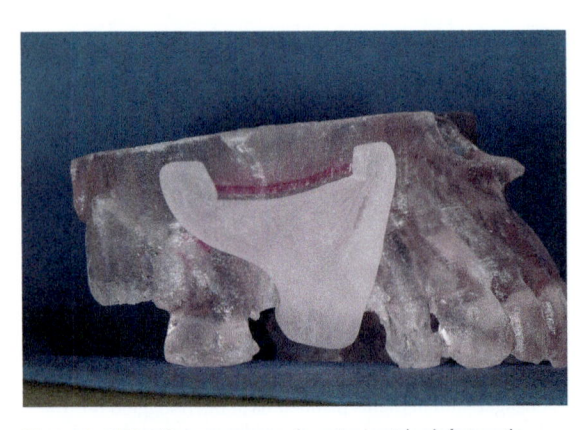

Figure 8.38G Bone-supported cutting guide defining the superior aspect of the planned lateral wall boundary. Reprinted with permission from Mandelaris and Rosenfeld, 2009a.

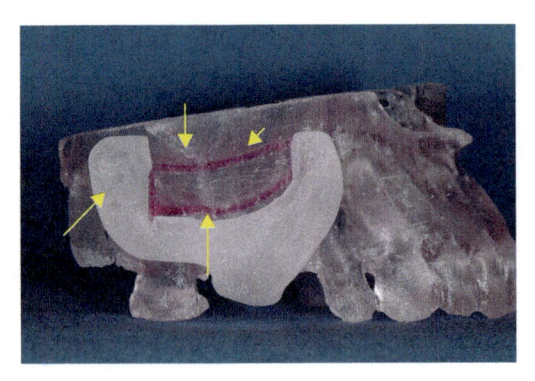

Figure 8.38H Medical model of the maxilla with custom freeform cutting path colorized in red (arrows). Bone-supported cutting guide defining the desired anterior, distal, inferior, and posterior lateral wall boundaries is seated. Note that the distal extent of the guide is rather obtrusive and will need to be modified to facilitate intraoperative surgical adaptation. Reprinted with permission from Mandelaris and Rosenfeld, 2009a.

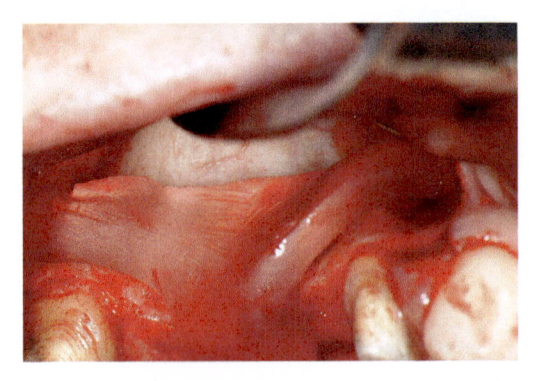

Figure 8.38I Bone-supported cutting guide in place defining the desired superior boundary. Reprinted with permission from Mandelaris and Rosenfeld, 2009a.

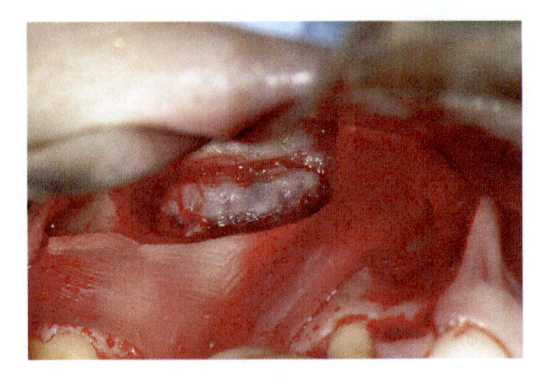

Figure 8.38J Bone-supported cutting guide in place following lateral window outlining and identification of membrane just prior to reflection. The anterior, distal, inferior, and posterior lateral wall boundaries are observed. Note that the distal aspect of the guide has been modified at the time of surgery to enable complete seating intraoperatively. Reprinted with permission from Mandelaris and Rosenfeld, 2009a.

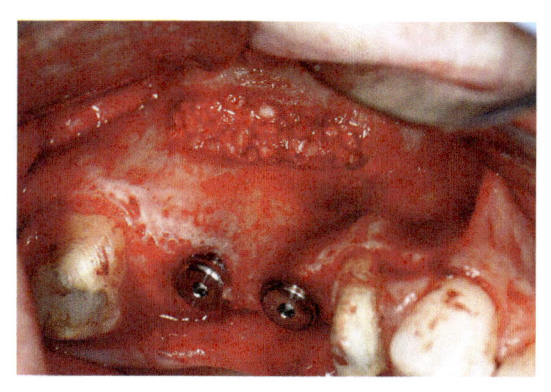

Figure 8.38K Bone-supported cutting guide removed and sinus bone grafting accomplished after verifying uneventful membrane reflection. Simultaneous implant placement has occurred manually. Reprinted with permission from Mandelaris and Rosenfeld, 2009a.

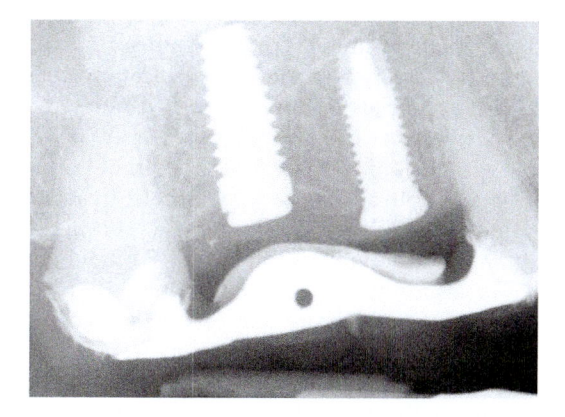

Figure 8.38L Direct postsurgical radiograph demonstrating complete fill of the bone graft at planned anterior portion of the antrum. Reprinted with permission from Mandelaris and Rosenfeld, 2009a.

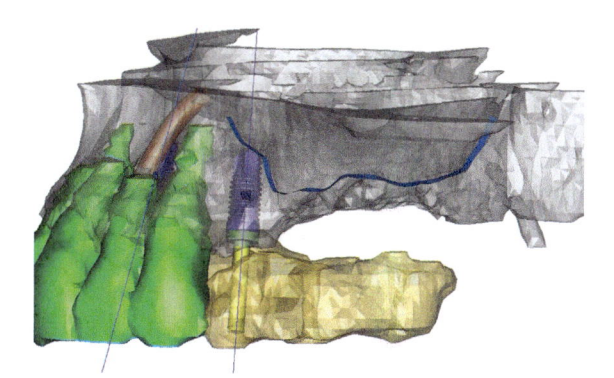

Figure 8.39A Transparency toggle tool activated. Inferior and anterior sinus boundaries outlined (blue line) in SimPlant OMS via custom freeform cutting path desired for maxillary left lateral window. Implant placement planned for #12. Reprinted with permission from Mandelaris and Rosenfeld, 2009a.

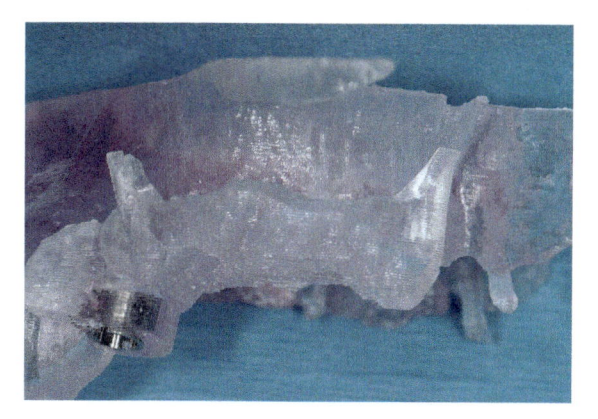

Figure 8.39B Stereolithographic tooth—bone-supported, totally guided CAD/CAM surgical guide combined with cutting guide to help outline the precise position of the inferior, distal, and anterior sinus boundaries desired to initiate Schneiderian membrane reflection. Reprinted with permission from Mandelaris and Rosenfeld, 2009a.

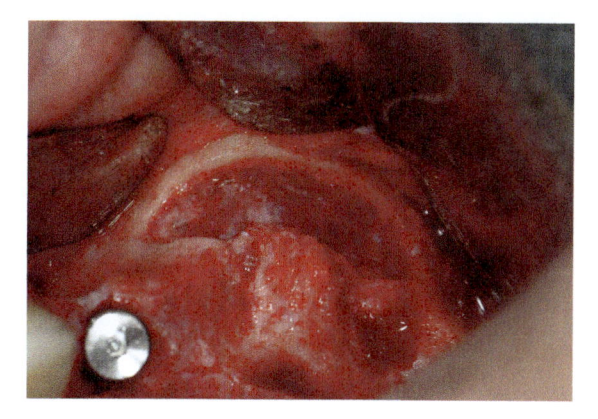

Figure 8.39C Intrasurgical confirmation of guided implant positioning and precise outlining of the lateral window prior to Schneiderian membrane reflection. Guided implant placement performed at #12. Reprinted with permission from Mandelaris and Rosenfeld, 2009a.

Surgical guide use for extraction of ankylosed teeth

Root resorption and ankylosis are pathologic entities that complicate extraction of teeth. Either partial or total controlled surgical guides can be used to remove internal tooth structure to allow atraumatic removal of teeth. The patient is imaged with either CT or CBCT scan protocols. The DICOM data are interfaced with viewing and planning

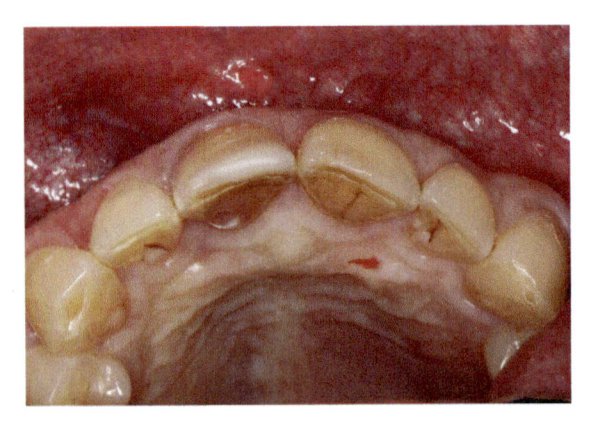

Figure 8.40A Presurgical view of ankylosed and nonrestorable #8.

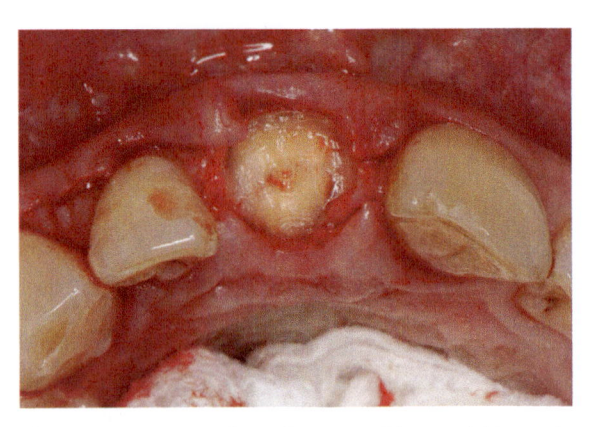

Figure 8.40C Minute flap reflection and fractured #8 noted.

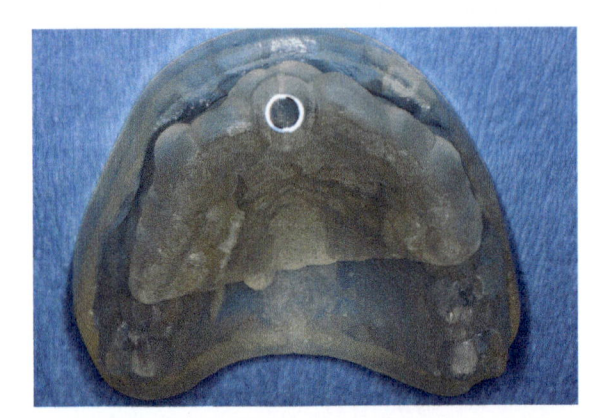

Figure 8.40B Tooth mucosal–supported, totally guided CAD/CAM surgical guide with medical model.

software. The guide design is developed, which allows osteotomies of increasing diameter to be introduced along the central long axis of the tooth. Once a sufficiently hollow root surface has been achieved, infracture of the residual tooth structure is easily accomplished. Figure 8.40A–J demonstrates the use of a CAD/CAM surgical guide for extraction of an ankylosed tooth.

Fully integrated surgical and restorative guides

A recent manufacturing breakthrough has enabled the implant team to take even fuller advantage of CAD/CAM technology. The possibility of developing an interim implant-supported prosthesis from only the patient's CT/CBCT study is now a reality. The fundamental principles of presurgical diagnostic case type pattern identification, selection of appropriate scanning appliance or virtual teeth from an implant library, and proper three-dimensional imaging set the stage for the delivery of both surgical and prosthetic treatment by merging several technologies. From the original dataset, fabrication of an RP model with receptacles for implant analogs along with representation of soft tissue serves as the working model for prosthesis fabrication. Once the prosthesis is fabricated it can be attached to the implants at the time of surgery. This process is efficient and simplifies the immediate delivery of teeth. While it is not the purpose of this chapter to discuss in detail this fully integrated surgical-prosthetic approach, clinical treatment examples are illustrated in Figure 8.41A–U and Figure 8.42A–Z.

Figure 8.43 demonstrates an example of the immediate smile model (Materialise Dental; Glen Burnie, MD, USA) for the mandibular arch in preparation for immediate loading implant surgery. Figure 8.44A–E demonstrate a case of the immediate smile model and bridge in preparation for immediate load implant surgery in the mandible. The immediate smile bridge is a polymethylmethacrylate appliance intended for provisionalization purposes and generated through CAD/CAM technology, CBCT DICOM volume, and computer software implant planning. (Materialise Dental, Glen Burnie, MD, USA).

(D)

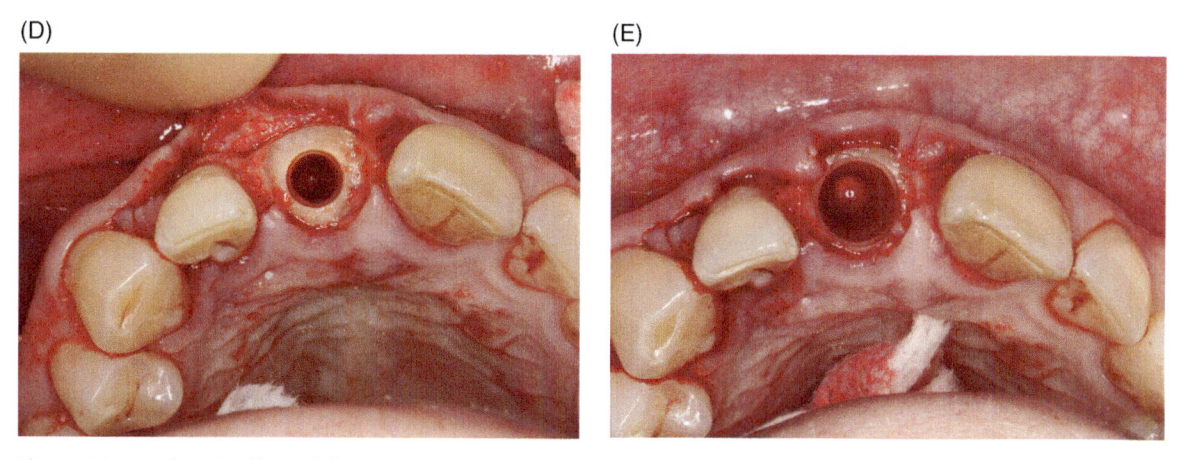

(E)

Figure 8.40D and E Totally guided osteotomy site preparation performed for #8 to implode ankylosed tooth.

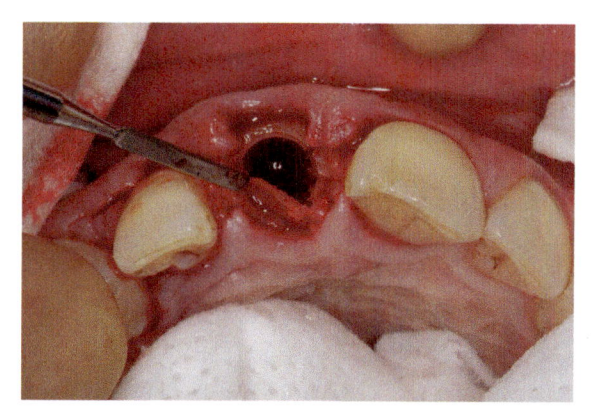

Figure 8.40F Removal of remaining tooth fragments after totally guided implosion of ankylosed tooth.

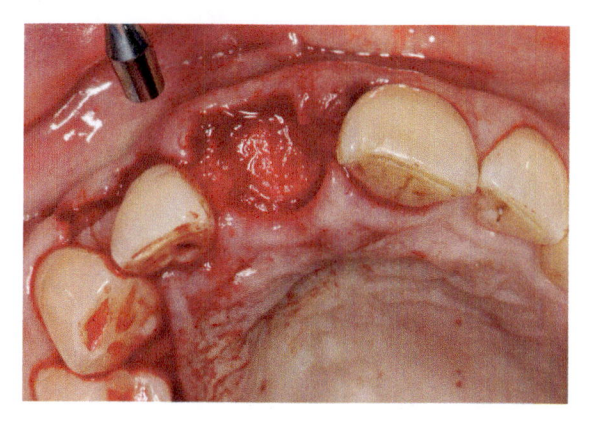

Figure 8.40H Socket preservation via rh-BMP2.

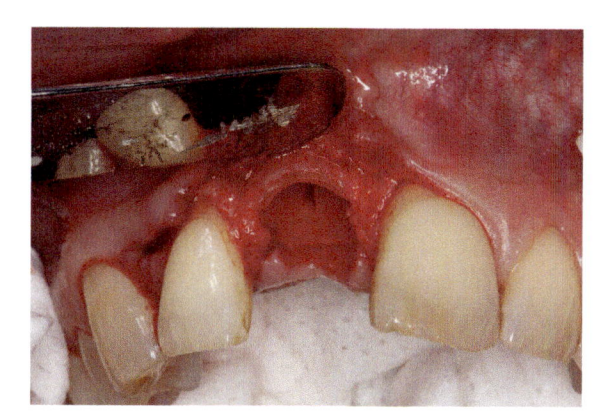

Figure 8.40G Extraction of #8 with an intact alveolus.

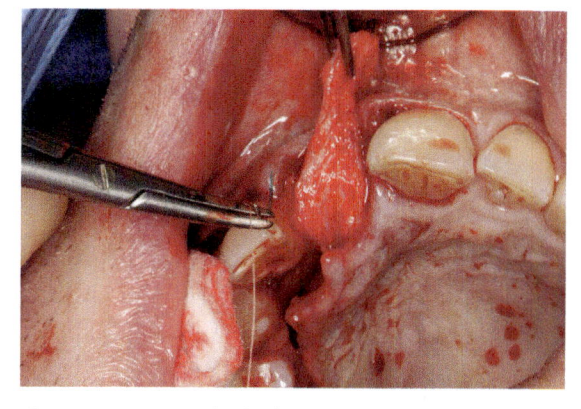

Figure 8.40I Rotated palatal pedicle connective tissue grafting performed to augment soft tissue and provide a primary wound closure of surgical site.

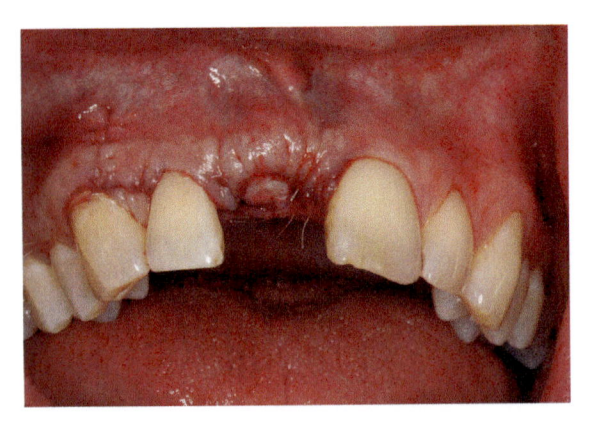

Figure 8.40J Sutures and surgical field closure.

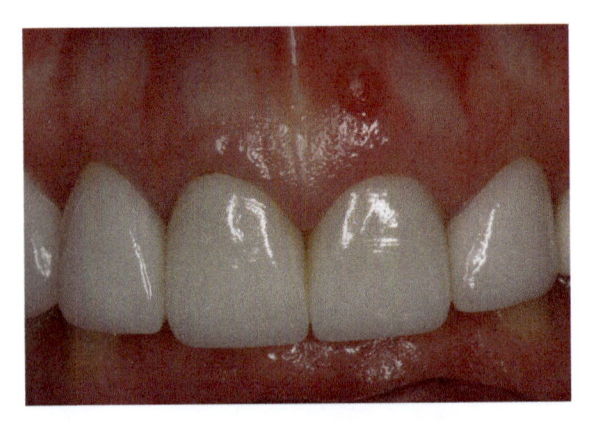

Figure 8.41A Clinical view of patient with parulis formation at #9.

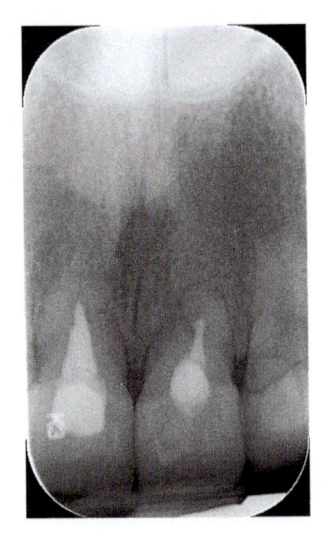

Figure 8.41B Radiographic view of #8–#9 demonstrating advanced external root resorption. Prognosis was determined to be poor for both teeth.

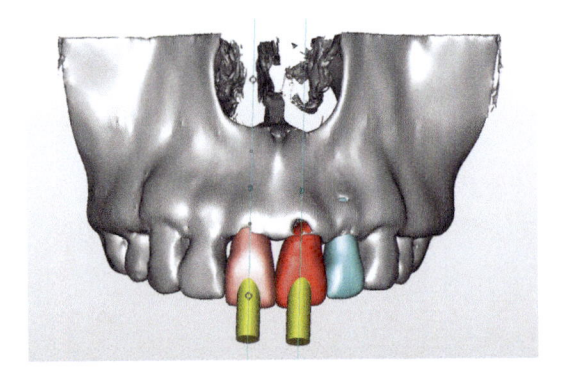

Figure 8.41C 3D reconstruction of CBCT with masks of the maxilla, natural teeth #8, #9, #10. Virtual implants placed at #8–#9.

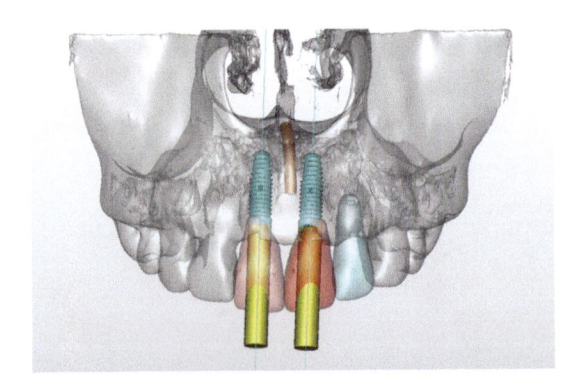

Figure 8.41D 3D reconstruction of CBCT with masks of the maxilla, natural teeth #8, #9, #10. Transparency toggle switch engaged. Virtual implants placed at #8–#9.

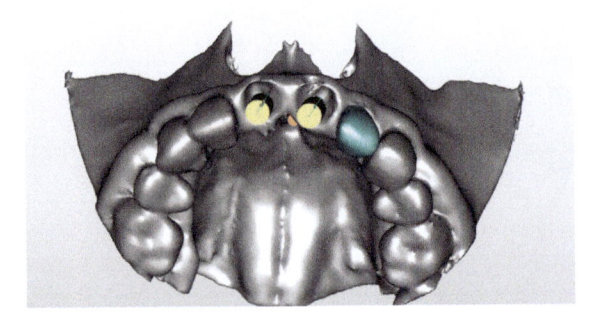

Figure 8.41E Occlusal view of 3D reconstruction with masks #8–#9 toggled off to simulate extraction. Implants placed and alveolus:implant discrepancy noted.

(F)

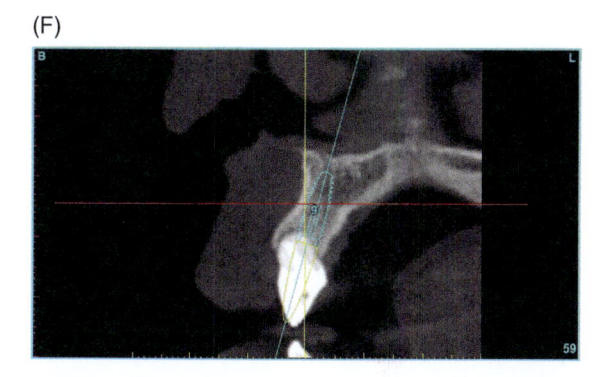

(G)

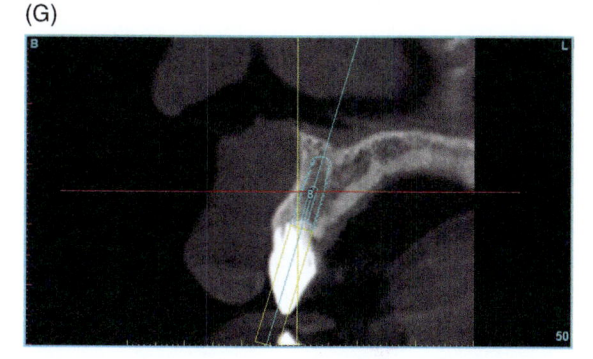

Figure 8.41F and G Cross-section view of sites #8–#9. Note the trajectory of the implants relative to the axial inclination of the teeth. Facial orientation is noted and will be compensated for in the prosthetic design. This interdisiciplinary discussion is made prior to surgery as a part of the workup and has an implication on vertical positioning of the fixtures.

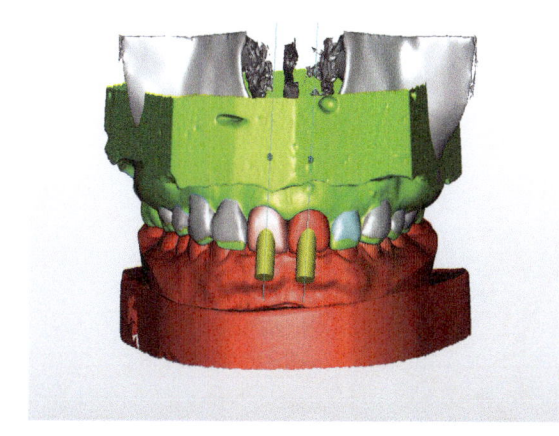

Figure 8.41H 3D reconstruction with optically imaged stone model interfaced in the maxilla. Optically imaged mandibular cast is also observed and articulated in the software program. Virtual implants placed at #8–#9 and facial trajectory confirmed.

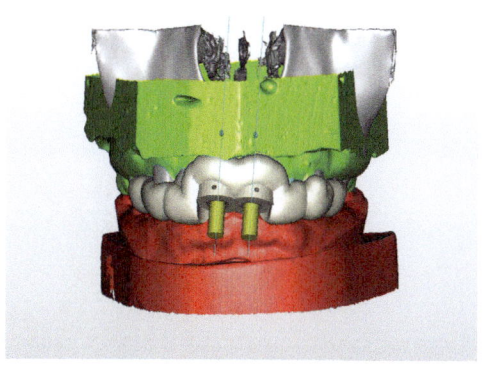

Figure 8.41I 3D reconstruction with optically imaged stone model interfaced in the maxilla. Optically imaged mandibular cast is also observed and articulated in the software program. Virtual implants placed at #8–#9 and facial trajectory confirmed. Simulated tooth-supported CAD/CAM surgical guide displayed.

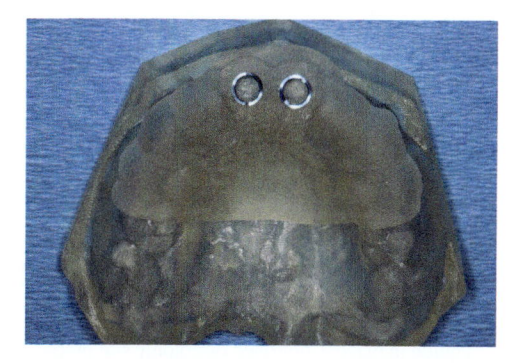

Figure 8.41J Tooth-supported, totally guided CAD/CAM surgical guide + medical model.

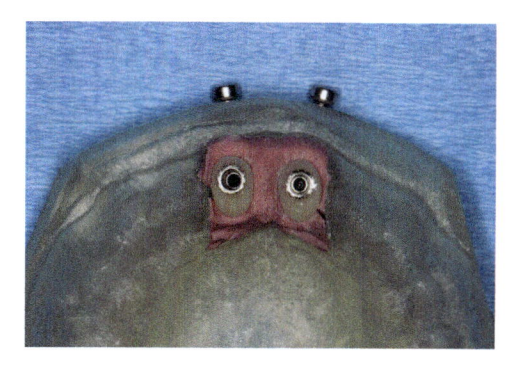

Figure 8.41K Immediate smile (Materialise Dental; Glen Burnie, MD, USA) model of the maxillary arch with planned osteotomy sites created, #8–#9. Silicone soft tissue representation in pink with lateral screws to secure analogs at #8–#9. Presurgically developed laboratory-made custom healing abutments in place.

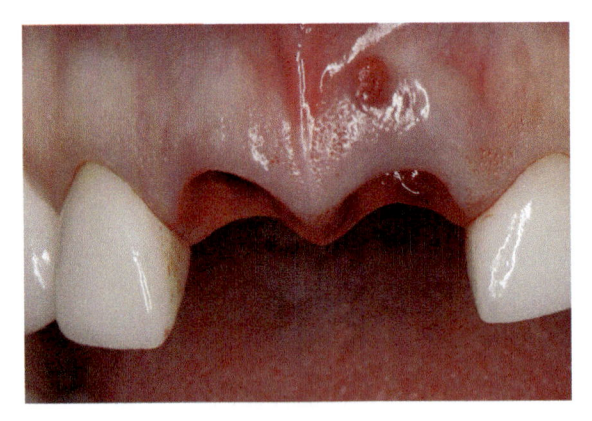

Figure 8.41L Extraction of #8–#9.

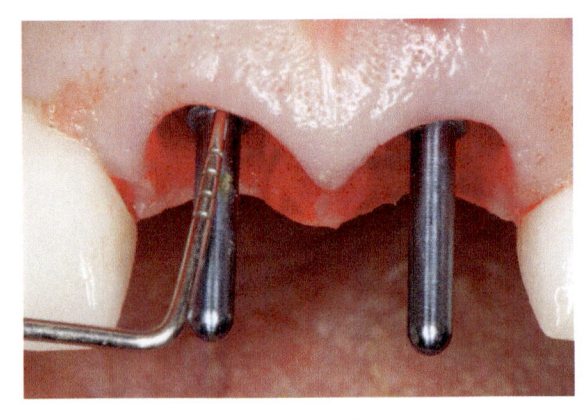

Figure 8.41O Guide pins positioned at sites #8–#9.

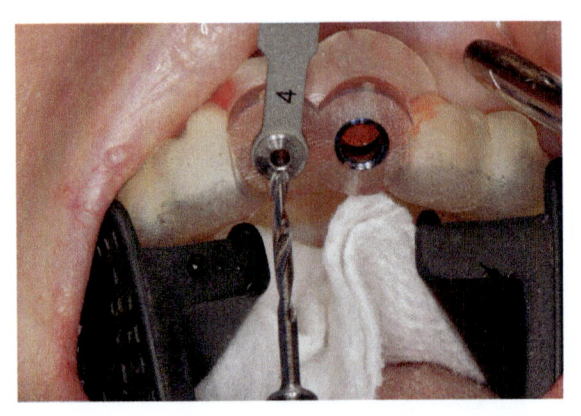

Figure 8.41M Tooth-supported, totally guided CAD/CAM surgical guide in place. Controlled osteotomy site preparation being performed.

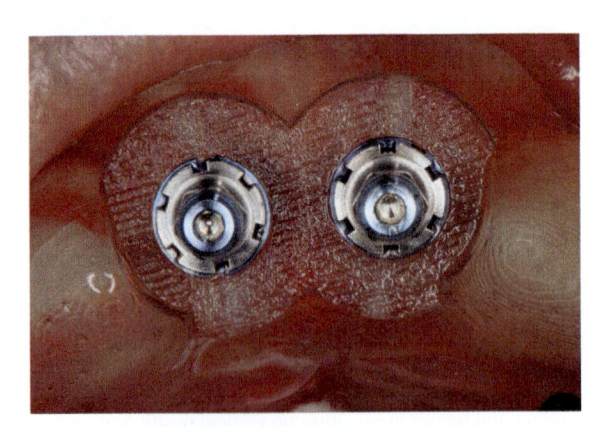

Figure 8.41P Totally guided implant placement with rotational control of implant platform.

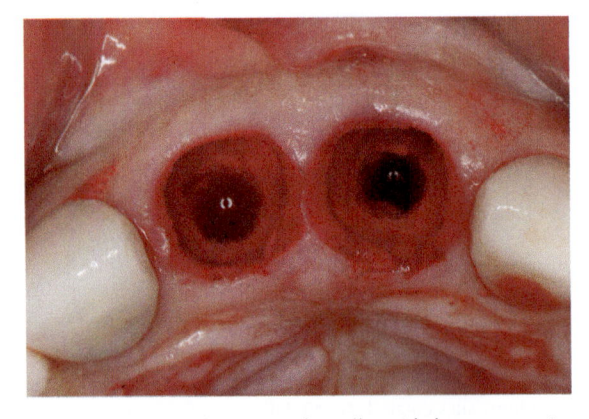

Figure 8.41N Tooth-supported, totally guided osteotomy site preparation completed, #8–#9.

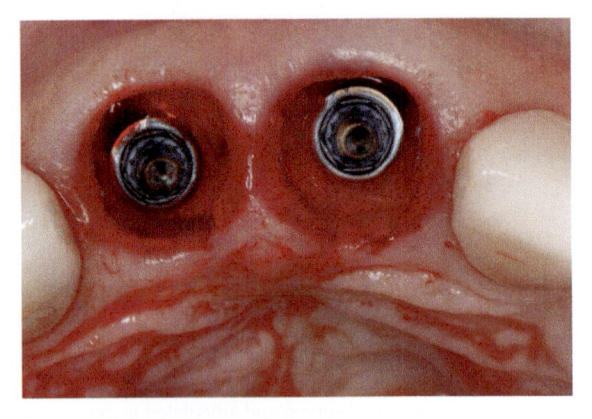

Figure 8.41Q Implant positioning.

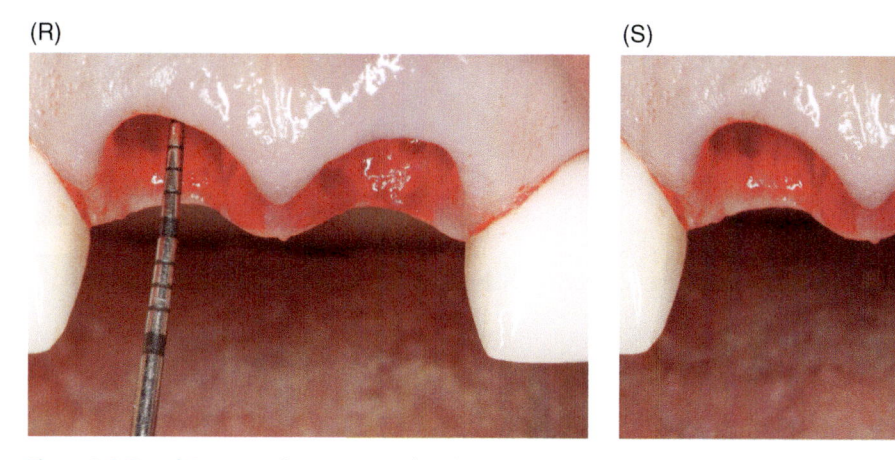

Figure 8.41R and S Vertical positioning of implants #8–#9 verified.

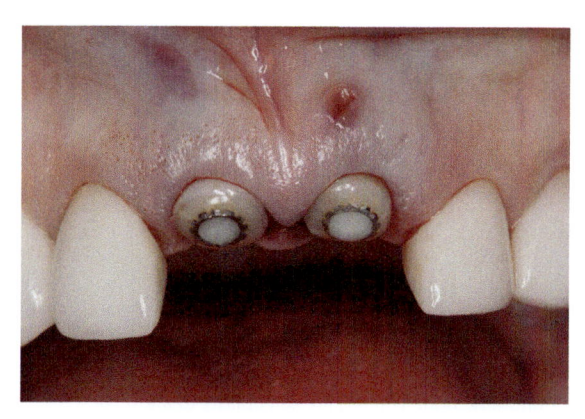

Figure 8.41T Presurgically developed, lab proceed custom healing abutments placed.

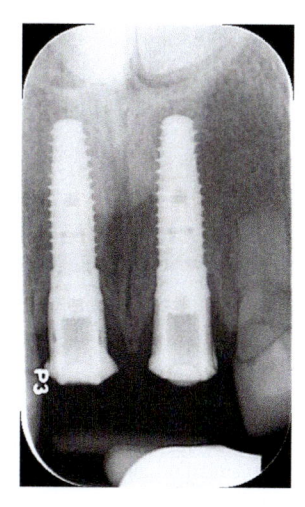

Figure 8.41U Postsurgical radiographs of immediate implants #8–#9.

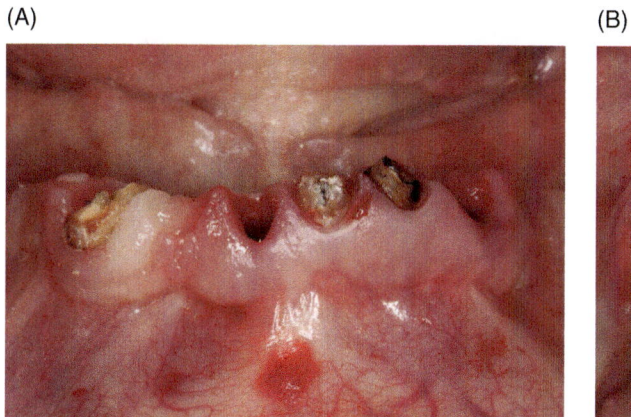

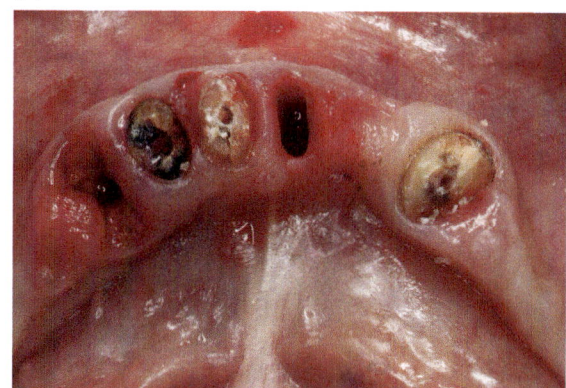

Figure 8.42A and B Initial examination of remaining hopeless mandibular natural dentition.

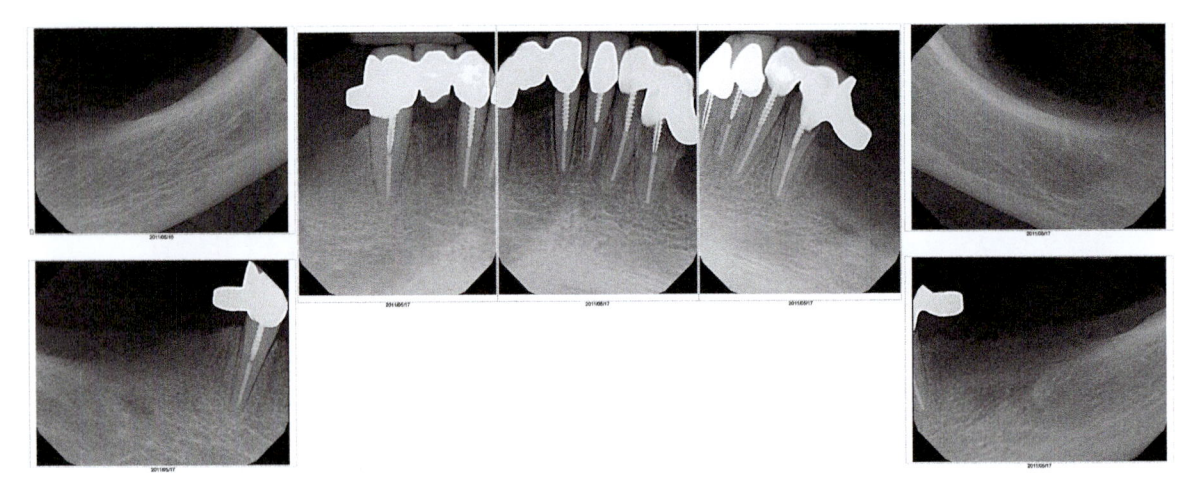

Figure 8.42C Radiographs of hopeless mandibular natural dentition.

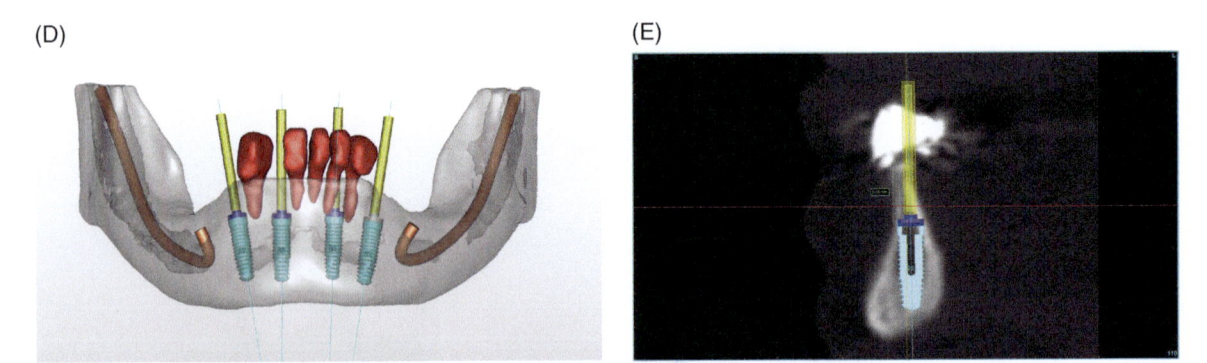

(D)

(E)

Figure 8.42D and E 3D and cross-sectional prosthetically directed implant planning for immediate load surgery in the mandible. Note the vertical position of the implant platform. 9 mm of unusable bone will require osteoplasty to allow for sufficient implant width.

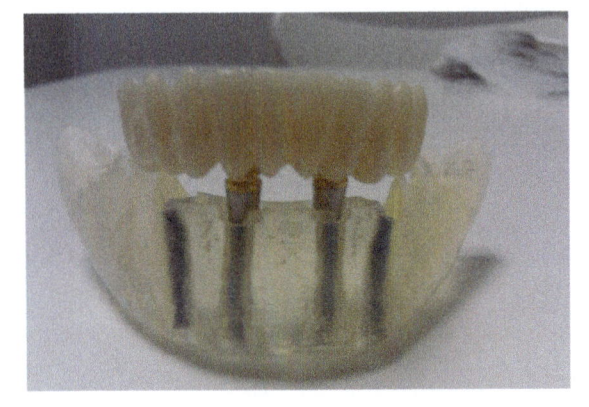

Figure 8.42F Mandibular immediate smile model with silicone soft tissue removed and analogs placed into planned positions. Abutments placed on anterior implants with temporary cylinders and immediate smile bridge seated.

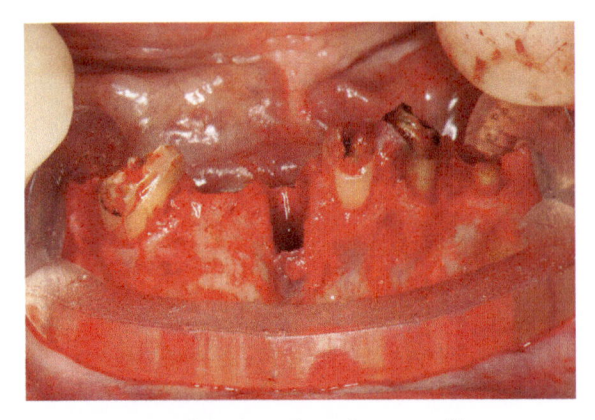

Figure 8.42G Full-thickness flap reflection and bone reduction guide in place for precision osteoplasty.

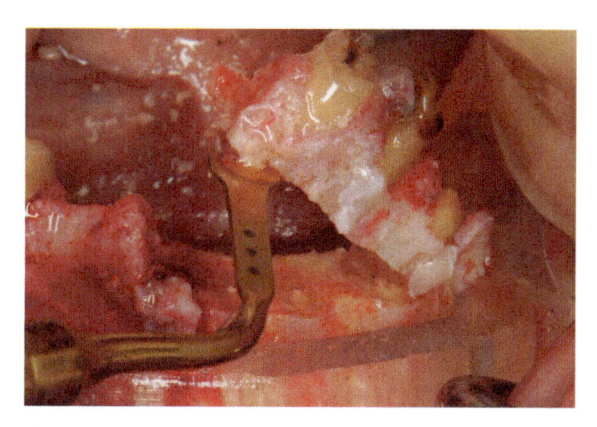

Figure 8.42H Presurgically planned bone segment removed en bloc via piezosurgery and guided by bone reduction guide.

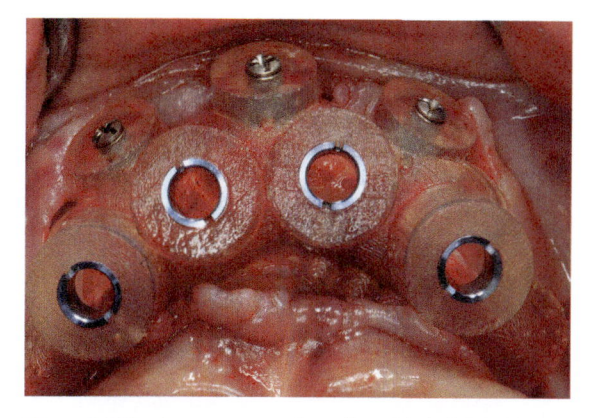

Figure 8.42K Bone-supported, totally guided CAD/CAM surgical guide in place and further stabilized through three fixation screws.

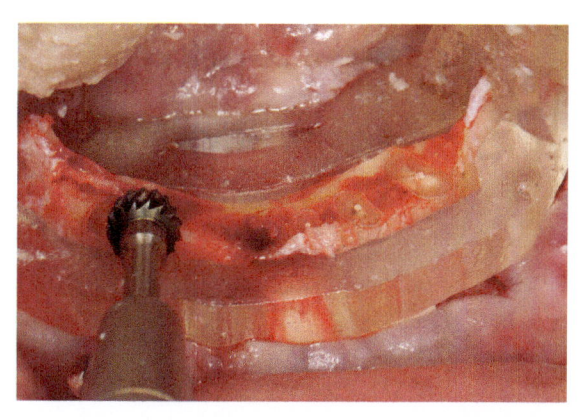

Figure 8.42I Final precision osteoplasty performed and as directed by the bone reduction guide.

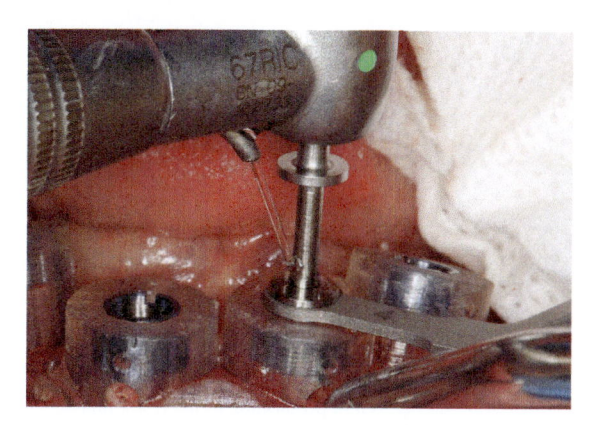

Figure 8.42L Totally guided implant surgery—osteotomy site preparation.

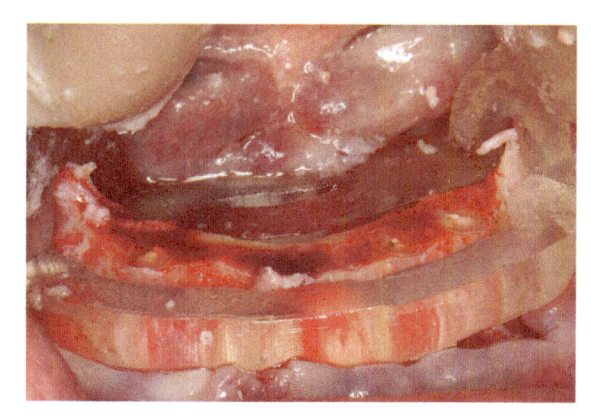

Figure 8.42J Osteoplasty is verified using the bone reduction guide. Its accuracy is critical to the next step.

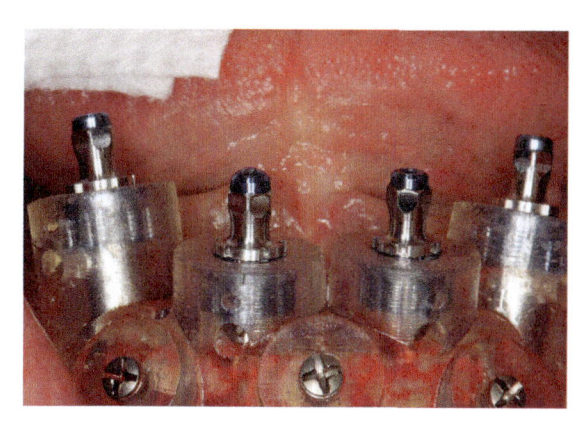

Figure 8.42M Totally guided implant placement—implants delivered.

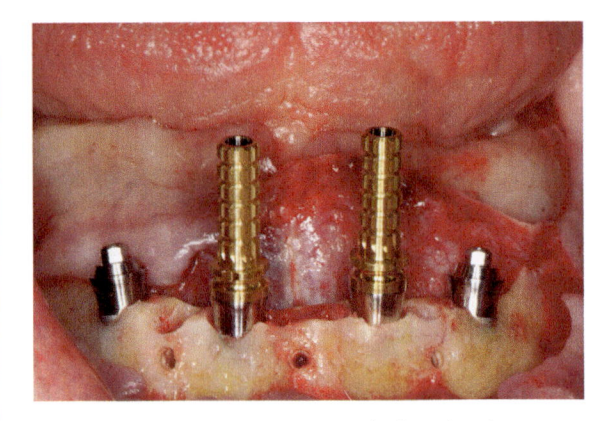

Figure 8.42Q Anterior temporary cylinders placed.

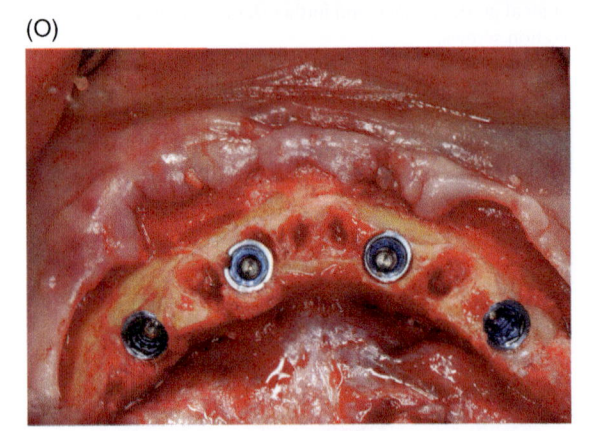

Figure 8.42N and O Final positioning of interforamina implants.

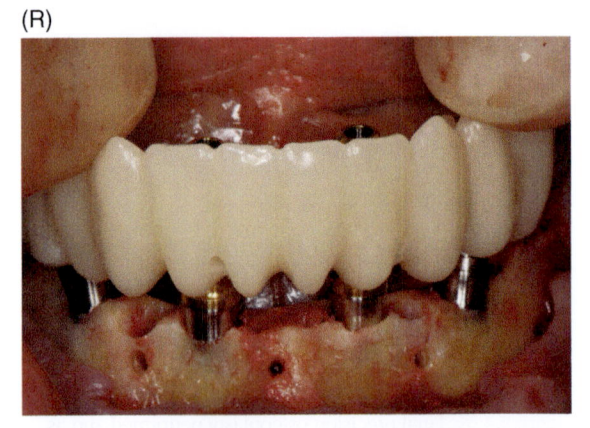

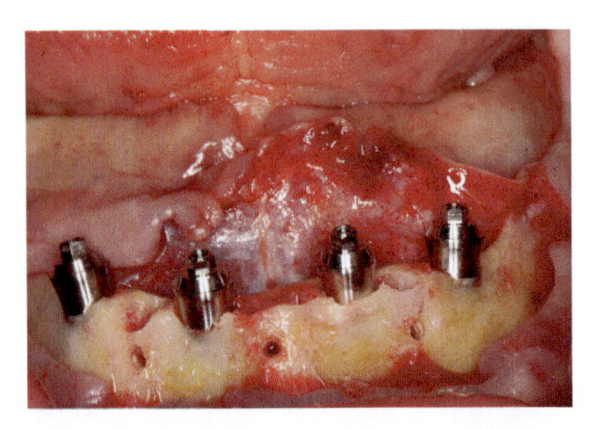

Figure 8.42P Abutments placed.

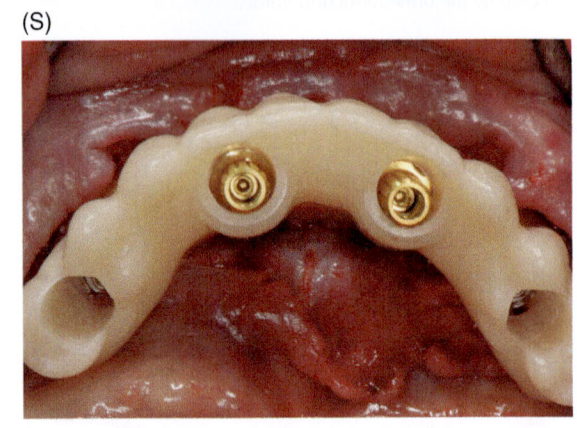

Figure 8.42R and S Immediate smile bridge tried on over the two temporary cylinders.

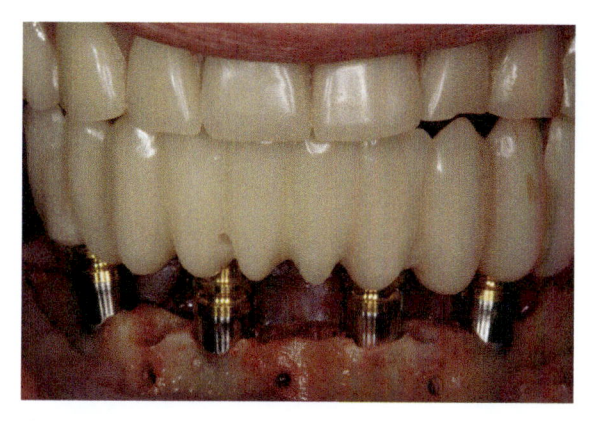

Figure 8.42T Posterior two temporary cylinders placed within prosthesis and then seated to abutments. Distal orientation of posterior fixtures does not allow for parallelism which is compensated through angulated abutment. Introducing the temporary cylinders through the prosthesis minimizes fracture potential within the provisional prosthesis.

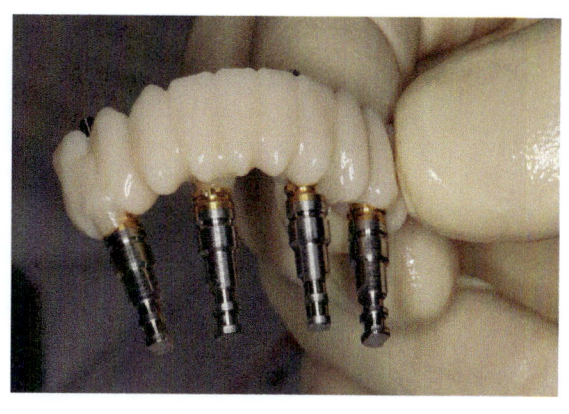

Figure 8.42W Following setting of the resin, prosthesis is picked up and finished and polished in the laboratory.

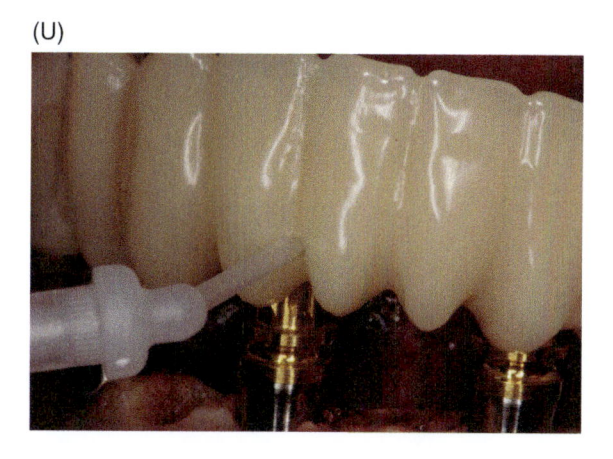

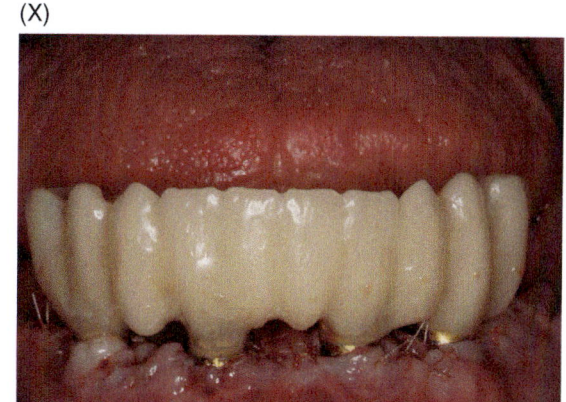

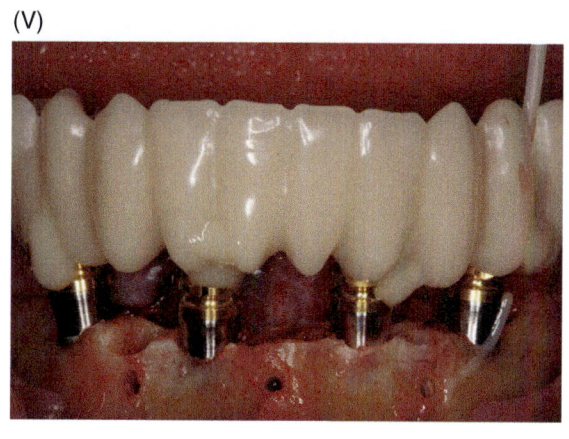

(U)

(X)

(V)

(Y)

Figure 8.42U and V Self-curing resin injected into lateral channels are within the polymethylmethacrylate CAD/CAM-generated bridge.

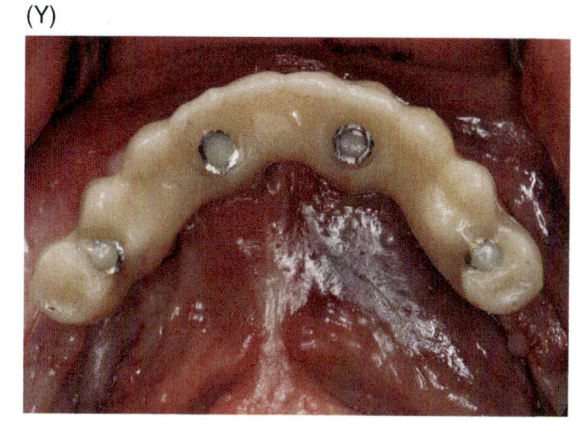

Figure 8.42X and Y Completed immediate load prosthesis and sutures.

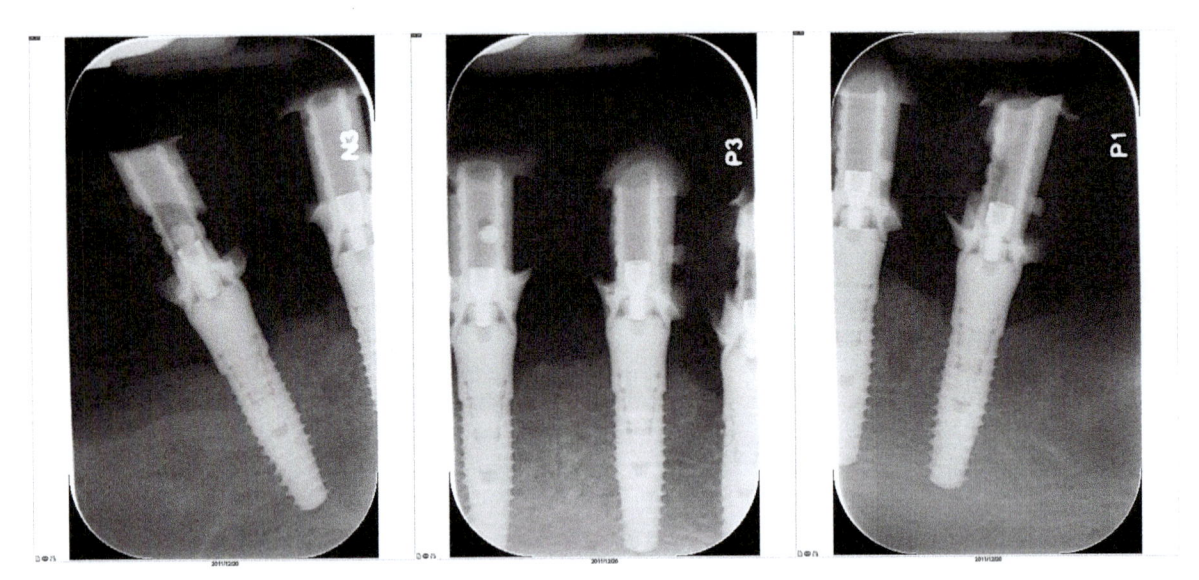

Figure 8.42Z Direct postsurgery radiographs.

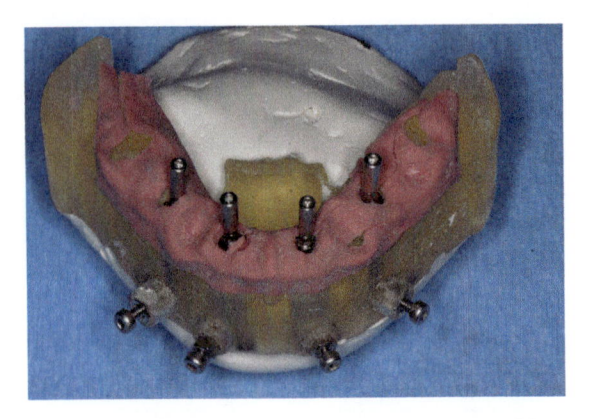

Figure 8.43 Mandibular immediate smile medical model with silicone soft tissue in place, analogs positioned with guide pins in place. Lateral screws noted on the buccal peripheral aspect of the medical model to secure analogs. Model will be mounted against maxillary arch to maintain vertical dimension of occlusion.

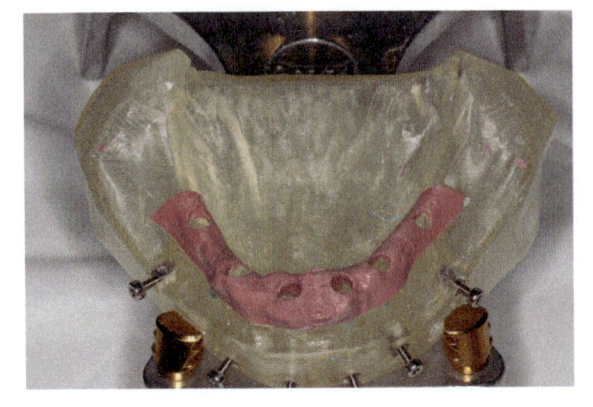

Figure 8.44A Mandibular immediate smile medical model with silicone soft tissue in place, and six osteotomy sites noted for the positioning of implant analog at presurgically planned positions. Lateral screws noted on the buccal peripheral aspect of the medical model to secure analogs.

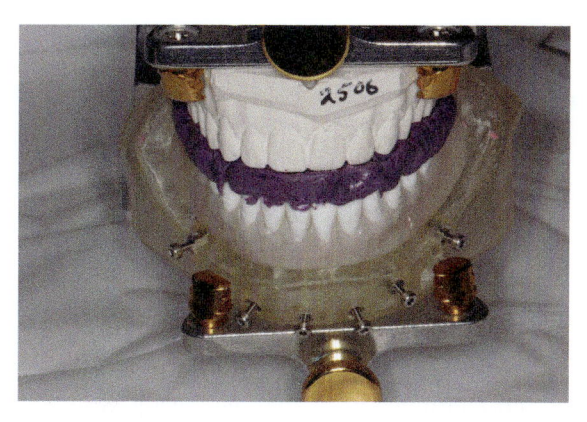

Figure 8.44B Mandibular immediate smile medical model with silicone soft tissue in place, scanning appliance seated and case mounted with radiolucent interocclusal bite registration.

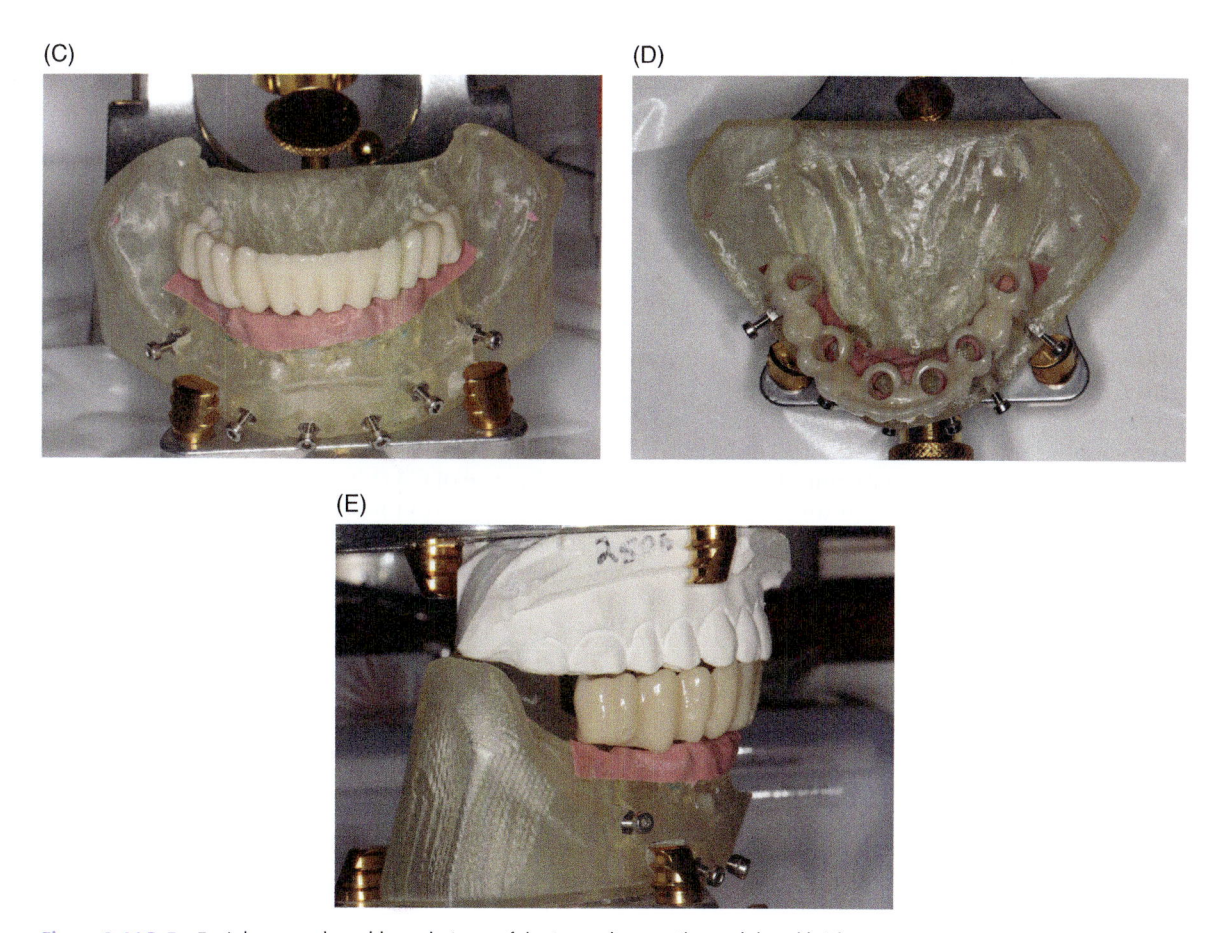

(C)

(D)

(E)

Figure 8.44C–E Facial, occusal, and lateral views of the immediate smile model and bridge.

Discussion

Perhaps the most underappreciated aspect of this technology is the ability for the implant team to manage complex information in an organized and objective manner. This helps define roles and responsibilities of patient care, allowing the implant team to consult with patients in an atmosphere of informed consent and disclosure. With the advent of in-office CBCT scanning machines, access to volumetric imaging data has become simpler and easier.

Implant placement has been and continues to be manually driven for most clinicians. Research over the past decade has unequivocally demonstrated that this approach to osteotomy site preparation is the least accurate method of implant treatment compared to approaches utilizing computer-generated RP surgical guides (Valente et al., 2009; Meloni et al., 2010). While less than optimal implant placement may appear to be rather trivial at the time of operation, the prosthetic reconciliation required to compensate can lead to a less than satisfactory prosthetic outcome and complicate patient care on many levels (Beckers, 2003).

Incorporating CAD/CAM guidance into implant practice offers many advantages for the treatment team as well as patients. The greatest value is that preoperative rather than intraoperative planning drives treatment. This can provide the treatment team sufficient time for planning by using accurate intuitive tools for case planning to achieve superior and consistent results. Compromises, modifications, alterations, and cost considerations can be evaluated, discussed, and negotiated before initiating treatment. This reduces aggravation, complications, and misunderstandings. Future applications will facilitate faster, more comfortable, and more predictable implant dentistry.

The most important aspect of patient care is an accurate diagnosis and treatment strategy that addresses the needs and concerns of both the patient and implant team. The ability to incorporate the prosthetic outcome into a CT dataset marks a collaborative breakthrough between the implant surgeon and restorative prosthetic dentist. Roles and responsibilities can now be clearly defined. This is the fundamental basis for a paradigm shift in implant dentistry. In our opinion the restorative leadership process allows implementation of the collaborative accountability concept, which is becoming the emerging standard of care in implant dentistry.

It should be stated that the use of CT scanning technology is not limited to so-called complex cases. Each and every implant surgery has its unique nuances affecting treatment outcomes. The ability to interpret CT radiographs is proportional to familiarity and its clinical application is related to experience. Rapid prototyping and stereolithographic medical modeling applications have opened an entirely new approach to the field of dental implantology. Last, it is important to recognize that CAD/CAM-based surgical guidance cannot be considered a substitute for adequate training, sound clinical judgment, experience, or expertise (van de Velde et al., 2008; Block and Chandler, 2009). It is not the technology that drives the care of our patients; rather, it is the management of information that is the true breakthrough.

Conclusions

1. Management of diagnostic and clinical information using 3D volumetric data is transforming oral health care.
2. The use of CAD/CAM technology in implant therapy provides great benefits in diagnostic, surgical, and restorative aspects of patient care.
3. Pretreatment analysis incorporating the principles of case type pattern identification is fundamental to developing an accurate diagnosis and treatment plan.
4. Restorative leadership and collaborative accountability provide the necessary framework for effective communication for all participants in the treatment process.
5. Selection, fabrication, and effective use of a scanning appliance is the fundamental method of incorporating surgical and prosthetic information into a volumetric dataset.
6. Volumetric scanning protocols can include single or dual scan strategies. Each strategy has its indications and benefits.

7. Surgical guides can be categorized as partial or total guidance systems. The surgeon has the responsibility to understand the advantages and disadvantages and where best to implement their use.
8. Surgical guides can be supported by bone, teeth, teeth/mucosa, or mucosa. The surgeon has the responsibility to understand the characteristics and indications of each type of guide support.
9. Surgical guides have the potential to deliver minimally invasive or flapless surgery, depending upon the case type pattern.
10. Specialized surgical guides can be used to manage complex surgical procedures.
11. Fully integrated surgical and restorative guides can simplify immediate delivery of teeth in partial and fully edentulous patients.
12. The technology discussed in this chapter is not a substitute for experience and clinical judgment. Rather, the technology facilitates more effective management of information to enhance collaborative patient care.

References

Armheiter, C., Scarfe W.C., and Farman, A.G. (2006). Trends in maxillofacial cone-beam computed tomography use. *Oral Radiology*, 22(2): 80–5.

Barker, T., Earwaker, W., and Lisle, D. (1994). Accuracy of stereolithographic models of human anatomy. *Australian Radiology*, 38(2): 106–11.

Basten, C., and Kois, J. (1996). The use of barium sulfate for implant templates. *Journal of Prosthetic Dentistry*, 76: 451–4.

Beckers, L. (2003). Positive effect of SurgiGuides on total cost. *Materialise Headlines*, 1: 3.

Block, M.S., and Chandler, C. (2009). Computed tomography-guided surgery: Complications associated with scanning, processing, surgery, and prosthetics. *Journal of Oral & Maxillofacial Surgery*, 67(Suppl 3): 13–22.

Campbell, S., Theile, R., Stuart, G., Cheng, E., et al. (2002). Separation of craniopagus joined at the occiput. Case report. *Journal of Neurosurgery*, 97: 983–7.

Cheng, A., and Wee, A. (1999). Reconstruction of cranial bone defects using alloplastic implants produced from stereolithographically-generated cranial model. *Annals of the Academy of Medicine*, 20: 692–6.

de Almeida, E.O., Pellizzer, E.P., Goiatto, M.C., et al. (2010). Computer-guided surgery in implantology: Review of basic concepts. *Journal of Craniofacial Surgery*, 21: 1917–21.

DiGiacomo, G.A., Cury, P.R., deAraujo, N.S., et al. (2005). Clinical applications of stereolithographic surgical guides for implant placement: Preliminary results. *Journal of Periodontology*, 76: 503–7.

Erickson, D., Chance D., Schmitt S., et al. (1999). An opinion survey of reported benefits from the use of stereolithographic models. *Journal of Oral Maxillofacial Surgery*, 57(9): 1040–3.

Ganz, S.D. (2003). Use of stereolithographic models as diagnostic and restorative aids for predictable immediate loading of implants. *Practical Procedures and Aesthetic Dentistry*, 15: 763–71.

Ganz, S.D. (2007). CT-derived model based surgery for immediate loading of maxillary anterior implants. *Practical Procedures and Aesthetic Dentistry*, 19: 311–18.

Gopakumar, S. (2004). RP in medicine: A case study in cranial reconstructive surgery. *Rapid Prototyping Journal*, 10: 207–11.

Israelson, H., Plemons, J., Watkins, P., et al. (1992). Barium-coated surgical stents and computer-assisted tomography in the preoperative assessment of dental implant patients. *International Journal of Periodontics & Restorative Dentistry*, 12: 52–61.

Jung, R.E., Schneider, D., Ganeles, J., et al. (2009). Computer technology applications in surgical implant dentistry. A systematic review. *International Journal of Oral Maxillofacial Implants*, 24(Suppl): 92–109.

Mandelaris, G.A., and Rosenfeld, A.L. (2008). The expanding influence of computed tomography and the application of computer guided implantology. *Practical Procedures and Aesthetic Dentistry*, 20(5): 297–306.

Mandelaris, G.A., and Rosenfeld, A.L. (2009a). Alternative applications to guided surgery. Precise outlining of the lateral window in antral sinus bone grafting. *Journal of Oral & Maxillofacial Surgery*, 67(Suppl 3): 23–30.

Mandelaris, G.A., and Rosenfeld, A.L. (2009b). Surgi-Guide options. In: P.B. Tardieu and A.L. Rosenfeld (eds.), *The Art of Computer Guided Implantology* (pp. 67–88). Chicago: Quintessence.

Mandelaris, G.A., Rosenfeld, A.L., King, S., et al. (2010). Computer guided implantology for precision implant positioning. Combining specialized stereolithographically generated drilling guides and surgical implant instrumentation. *International Journal of Periodontics & Restorative Dentistry*, 30(3): 274–81.

Mandelaris, G.A., Rosenfeld, A.L., and Tardieu, P.B. (2009). Clinical cases. In: P.B. Tardieu and A.L. Rosenfeld (eds.), *The Art of Computer Guided Implantology* (pp. 113–78). Chicago: Quintessence.

Mecall, R.A. (2009). Computer-guided implant treatment pathway. In: P.B. Tardieu and A.L. Rosenfeld (eds.), *The Art of Computer Guided Implantology* (pp. 89–111). Chicago: Quintessence.

Mecall, R.A., and Rosenfeld, A.L. (1992). The influence of residual ridge resorption patterns on implant fixture placement and tooth position. Part II: Presurgical determination of prosthesis type and design. *International Journal of Periodontics & Restorative Dentistry*, 12: 32–51.

Mecall, R.A., and Rosenfeld, A.L. (1996). Influence of residual ridge resorption patterns on fixture placement and tooth position. Part III: Presurgical assessment of ridge augmentation requirements. *International Journal of Periodontics & Restorative Dentistry*, 16: 322–37.

Meloni, S.M., De Riu, G., Pisano, M., et al. (2010). Implant treatment software planning and guided flapless sugery with immediate provisional prosthesis delivery in the fully edentulous maxilla. A retrospective analysis of 15 consecutively treated patients. *European Journal of Oral Implantology*, 3(3): 245–51.

Popat, A. (1998). Rapid prototyping and medical modeling. *Phidas Newsletter*, 1: 10–12.

Rosenfeld, A.L., Mandelaris, G.A., and Tardieu, P.B. (2006a). Prosthetically directed implant placement using computer software to ensure precise placement and predictable prosthetic outcomes. Part I: Diagnostics, imaging and collaborative accountability. *International Journal of Periodontics & Restorative Dentistry*, 26(3): 215–21.

Rosenfeld, A.L., Mandelaris, G.A., and Tardieu, P.B. (2006b). Prosthetically directed implant placement using computer software to ensure precise placement and predictable prosthetic outcomes. Part II: Rapid prototype medical modeling and stereolithographic drilling guides requiring bone exposure. *International Journal of Periodontics & Restorative Dentistry*, 26(4): 347–53.

Rosenfeld, A.L., Mandelaris, G.A., and Tardieu, P.B. (2006c). Prosthetically directed implant placement using computer software to ensure precise placement and predictable prosthetic outcomes. Part III: Stereolithographic drilling guides that do not require bone exposure and the immediate delivery of teeth. *International Journal of Periodontics & Restorative Dentistry*, 26(5): 493–9.

Sarment, D., Al-Shammari, K., and Kazor, C. (2003). Stereolithographic surgical templates for placement of dental implants in complex cases. *International Journal of Periodontics & Restorative Dentistry*. 23: 287–95.

Sarment, D., Sukovic, P., and Clinthorne, N. (2003). Accuracy of implant placement with a stereolithographic surgical guides. *International Journal of Oral Maxillofacial Implants*, 18: 571–7.

Schneider, D., Marquardt, P., Zwahlen, M., et al. (2009). A systemic review on the accuracy and the clinical outcome of computer-guided template-based implant dentistry. *Clinical Oral Implant Research*, 20(Suppl 4): 73–86.

Sennhenn-Kirchner, S., Weustermann, S., Mergeryan, H., et al. (2008). Preoperative sterilization and disinfection of drill guide templates. *Clinical Oral Investigations*, 12: 179–87.

Spielman, H. (1996). Influence of the implant position on the aesthetics of the restoration. *Practical Procedures and Aesthetic Dentistry*, 8: 897–904.

Swaelens, B. (1999). Drilling templates for dental implantology. *Phidas Newsletter*, 3: 10–12.

Tardieu, P.B. (2009). Scanning appliances and virtual teeth. In: P.B. Tardieu and A.L. Rosenfeld (eds.), *The Art of Computer Guided Implantology* (pp. 47–57). Chicago: Quintessence.

Valente, F., Schiroli, G., and Sbrenna, A. (2009). Accuracy of computer-aided oral implant surgery: A clinical and radiographic study. *International Journal of Oral Maxillofacial Implants*, 24: 234–42.

van Assche, N., van Steenberghe, D., Guerrero, M., et al. (2007). Accuracy of implant placement based on pre-surgical planning of three dimensional cone-beam images: A pilot study. *Journal of Clinical Periodontology*, 34(9): 816–21.

van de Velde, T., Glor, F., and De Bruyn, H. (2008). A model on flapless implant placement by clinicians with different experience level in implant surgery. *Clinical Oral Implants Research*, 19: 66–72.

van Steenberghe, D., Malevez, C., van Cleynenbreugel, J., et al. (2003). Accuracy of drilling guides for transfer from three-dimensional CT based planning to placement of zygoma implants in humans. *Clinical Oral Implants Research*, 14(1): 131–6.

Vrielinck, L., Politis, C., Schepers, S., et al. (2003). Image based planning and clinical validation of zygoma and pterygoid implant placement in patients with severe bone atrophy using customized drill guides. Preliminary results from a prospective follow-up study. *International Journal of Oral Maxillofacial Surgery*, 32: 7–14.

Webb, P. (2000). A review of rapid prototyping (RP) techniques in the medical and biomedical sector. *Journal of Medical Engineering & Technolology*, 24(4): 149–53.

Wouters, K. (2001). Colour rapid prototyping. An extra dimension for visualizing human anatomy. *Phidas Newsletter*, 6: 4–7.

9 Assessment of the Airway and Supporting Structures Using Cone Beam Computed Tomography

David C. Hatcher

Sleep disordered breathing (SDB), including obstructive sleep disordered breathing (OSDB) and upper airway resistance syndrome (UARS), is often associated with obstruction or increased airway resistance and cannot be diagnosed with cone beam CT scan (CBCT). Cone beam CT has a role in the anatomic assessment of the airway and the structures that support the airway (Hatcher, 2010a). Polysomnograms are currently the gold standard for diagnosis of SDB, but CBCT has an adjunctive role to assess the dimensions (size and shape) of the airway anatomy and to identify sites in and adjacent to the airway that may contribute to a change in airway dimensions (Kushida et al., 2005). OSDB and UARS affect the upper airway, including the nasal airway, nasopharynx, oropharynx, and hypopharynx. The nasal airway extends from the nares to the posterior nasal choanae. The nasopharynx extends from the posterior nasal choanae to a horizontal plane extending posterior from the palatal plane. The oropharynx includes the area posterior to the soft palate and tongue. The hypopharynx is the site between the tongue base (base of epiglottis) and larynx.

Background

Three-dimensional imaging studies of patients with obstructive sleep apnea (OSA) have indicated a reduction in cross-sectional area (CSA) of the airway when compared to non-OSA individuals (Ogawa et al., 2007). Li et al. (2003) have demonstrated a relationship between the likelihood of OSA and airway CSA. The probability of airway obstruction is low in adults when the airway CSA is greater than 110 mm^2, medium between 52 and 110 mm^2, and high when the CSA is less than 52 mm^2. Ogawa et al. (2007) using CBCT found similar results. The OSA patients with a high BMI in the Ogawa study had airway dimensional differences (volume, CSA, and linear distances) when compared to the normal BMI control group. The average smallest CSA was 46 mm^2 in the OSA group and 147 mm^2 in the control group.

There has been recent progress in determining normal values for airway dimensions. Two separate studies have a combined study population of 1,159 individuals, comprising 753 females and 406 males (Smith, 2009; Chang, 2011). These studies acquired CBCT scans of craniofacial regions,

---

Cone Beam Computed Tomography: Oral and Maxillofacial Diagnosis and Applications, First Edition. Edited by David Sarment.
© 2014 John Wiley & Sons, Inc. Published 2014 by John Wiley & Sons, Inc.

including the skull base and mandible, of individuals positioned in an upright position. In these studies the airway volume, linear distances, and cross-sectional areas are calculated at multiple 1–2 mm intervals in a rostrocaudal direction using semiautomated software calibrated to examine this area. The age groups were stratified into the following groups: (1) ages 7–10.9, (2) ages 11–14.9 (3) ages 15–18, (4) ages 19–29, (5) ages 30–39, (6) ages 40–49, (7) ages 50–59, (8) ages 60 and older. The human airway increases in length, cross-sectional area, and volume during a rapid period of craniofacial growth with males showing greater dimensional change than females (Smith, 2009; Chang, 2011). The female airway did not significantly lengthen after the age of 15 while the male airway lengthened up to the age of 18 (Chang, 2011). The site of smallest cross-sectional area during period of facial growth tended to be bimodal with one site near the palatal plane and the other tangent to C4 vertebra. The female mean minimum CSA is 82 mm^2 for ages 7–10.9, 99 mm^2 for ages 11–14.9, and 118 mm^2 for ages 15–18 (Chang, 2011). In males the minimum CSA is 84 mm^2 for ages 7–10.9, 95 mm^2 for ages 11–14.9, and 137 mm^2 for ages 15–18 (Chang, 2011). In adults the minimum cross-sectional area is significantly different between males and females and is not influenced by age (Smith, 2009). The mean minimum cross-sectional area in males is 172 mm^2 and in females is 150 mm^2. The site of the minimum cross-sectional airway area moves superiorly in normal adult males and females with increasing age (Smith, 2009).

Airway dimensional relationships to airway resistance

The inhalation process is an active movement of the diaphragm and ribs to reduce the pressure in the lungs to a level lower than the external atmosphere. This moves air from higher (external atmosphere) to lower pressure (lungs). Resistance to airflow increases the pressure gradient between the lungs and external atmosphere and increases the respiratory effort required to move air into the lungs. Poiseuille's and Ohm's laws describe the relationships between airflow, resistance, and airway dimensions.

Poiseuille's law

Poiseuille's law ($R = 8nl/\pi r^4$, where R=resistance, n=viscosity, l=length, π=pi, and r=radius) shows that radius has a greater influence of resistance than other factors such as airway length.

Ohm's law

Ohm's law ($V = P_{mouth/nose} - P_{alveoli}/R$, where V=flow, P=pressure, and R=resistance) shows that increased airway resistance increases the pressure gradient between the mouth/nose and the alveoli. The increased resistance can impede air flow, increase respiratory effort, and may predispose the airway to collapse on the downstream side of the high-resistance site.

The airway dimensions, particularly small airway dimensions, are of clinical interest because they may contribute to SDB. Identifying small airways, site of narrowest constriction, and the factors that may contribute to the airway narrowing are in the domain of the three-dimensional imaging.

Purpose

The pathogenesis of SDB is heterogeneous and the purpose of this article to identify and discuss several imaging features associated with conditions that may contribute to OSDB and UARS. A stratified diagnostic process provides the opportunity to employ a therapy that targets the etiology.

Imaging

The airway anatomy can be imaged with a variety of methods that include lateral cephalometry, magnetic resonance imaging (MRI), computed tomography (CT), fluoroscopy, and more recently cone beam CT (Hatcher, 2010a). The methods include 2D and 3D imaging and imaging in supine and upright positions. CBCT was introduced into the North American dental market in May 2001 and thus created the opportunity for dentists to visualize the airway and adjacent anatomy in three dimensions (Hatcher, 2010b). Maturation or evolution of the CBCT systems have trended toward upright imaging, flat panel detectors, graphical (faster) processing, shorter scan times, pulsed dose, flat panel sensors, and smaller voxel sizes. CBCT provides high-resolution anatomic data of the airway space, soft tissue surfaces, and bones but does not provide much detail within the soft tissues adjacent to the airway. CBCT imaging is considered a state-dependent imaging method and not a dynamic method. The state-dependent imaging captures the anatomy in a static or nondynamic state. Dynamic motion of the soft tissues and bony structures occurs during respiration, sleep, swallowing, and airway obstruction, creating a change in size and shape of the airway.

During a CBCT scan the scanner (x-ray source and a rigidly coupled sensor) rotates, usually 360 degrees, around the head, acquiring multiple images (ranging from approximately 150 to 599 separate and unique projection views; Hatcher, 2010b). Raw image data are collected from the scan and reconstructed into a viewable format. The scan time can range between 5 and 70 seconds depending on machine brand and protocol setting. The x-ray source emits a low milli-Amperage (mA) shaped or divergent beam. The beam size is constrained (circular or rectangular) to match the sensor size but in some cases can be further constrained (collimated) to match the anatomic region of interest. The field of view for an airway study includes the rostral caudal area between the cranial base and menton. Following the scan, the resultant image set or (raw) data are subjected to a reconstruction process that results in the production of a digital volume of anatomic data that can be visualized with specialized software. The smallest subunit of a digital volume is a volume element (voxel). CBCT voxels are generally isotropic (x, y, and z dimensions are equal) and range in size from approximately 0.07 to 0.4mm per side. The average voxel size for an airway study is 0.3mm^3. Each voxel is assigned a grey scale value that approximates the attenuation value of the represented tissue or space.

Data visualization

The reconstructed volumes are ready for viewing using specialized software. The voxel volume can be retrieved and viewed with various viewing options. Visualization options include multiplanar or orthogonal (coronal, axial, sagittal) viewing angles. The data can be sliced as single voxel row or column at a time. The multiple voxel layers can be combined to create a slab and then visualized. It is possible to produce and visualize oblique and curved slices or slabs. The entire volume can be rendered and visualized from any angle. There are several techniques for visualizing a volume, including shaded surface display and volume rendering. All CBCT units are installed with viewing software, but third party software is also available for general viewing or specialized applications, such as implant planning, assessment for orthodontics, and airway assessment. Software optimized for airway assessment generally processes the image volume using the following steps: (1) select the region of interest, (2) segmentation of the airway volume, and (3) measurement of the airway anatomy. The airway measurements include volume, linear distance (anteroposterior and mediolateral), and cross-sectional area.

Dose

The effective dose is expressed as micro-Sieverts (μSv). The effective doses for CBCT machines are not homogeneous with dose variations related to the machine settings (mA, kVp, time), field of view, signal requirements, sensor type, pulse, or continuous exposure. The effective dose for CBCT (87 μSv) is greater than a cephalometric projection (14.2–24.3 μSv) but less than a conventional CT scan (860 μSv; Ludlow and Ivanovic, 2008; Ludlow et al., 2008).

Anatomic accuracy

A semiautomated software (3dMD Vultus) designed to extract linear measurements, cross-sectional areas, and volumes from CBCT volumes was calibrated against an air phantom of known dimension, and no significant differences were noted ($p = .975$; Schendel and Hatcher, 2010).

Facial growth and airway

Limitation of normal nasal respiration occurring during facial growth can alter the development of the craniofacial skeleton in humans and experimental animals. Severely reduced nasal airflow may lead to compensations that include an inferior positioning of the mandible, separation of the lips, increased interocclusal space, change in tongue posture, inferior positioning of the hyoid bone, anterior extension of the head and neck, increased anterior face height, increased mandibular and occlusal plane angles, posterior cross-bite, narrow maxillary arch, high palatal vault, narrow alar base, class II occlusion, modal shift from nasal to oral breathing, and a clockwise facial growth pattern. The facial phenotype described above, sometimes called adenoidal facies, can occur from an increased airflow resistance located in the nose or nasopharynx as outlined in animal studies. The differential diagnosis for this facial phenotype may include other etiologies. Conventional thinking suggests that small airway dimensions increase airflow resistance and this leads to abnormal or altered facial growth. Alternatively, a primary problem of abnormal facial growth may lead to a small airway and an increase in airway resistance. Airway dimensions have been shown to have a proportional relationship to jaw growth and facial growth pattern. In other words, small mandibular and/or maxillary growth is associated with a reduction in airway dimensions. The largest airway dimensions are associated with a counterclockwise facial and normal facial growth pattern; therefore, a smaller airway may be associated with a clockwise facial growth pattern and deficient jaw growth. Several congenital and developmental conditions may be associated with a reduction in mandibular growth and clockwise facial growth pattern (Stratemann et al., 2010; Stratemann et al., 2011). These altered mandibular growth conditions include juvenile onset degenerative joint disease (condylysis), juvenile idiopathic arthritis, condylar hypoplasia, and 1st and 2nd branchial arch syndromes. Of the conditions that limit mandibular growth, the most common is juvenile onset degenerative joint disease, distantly followed by juvenile idiopathic arthritis (Hatcher, 2010a).

Arthrides

Adolescent onset of degenerative joint disease or juvenile idiopathic arthritis can result in a limitation of mandibular growth, clockwise direction of mandibular growth, and compensations in the maxilla and cranial base. The small mandible and clockwise rotation of the mandible allows the tongue and hyoid to be posteroinferiorly displaced and ultimately diminish the airway dimensions. The mandibular growth changes include a reduction in the vertical dimensions of the condylar process, ascending rami, and body of the mandible. The lateral development of the mandible is reduced. There is an increase in the vertical dimension and decrease in the labiolingual dimensions of the anterosuperior regions of the mandible. The gonial angles are obtuse and the mandibular and occlusal plane angles are steep (Hatcher, 2011a, 2011b, 2011c; Figure 9.1, Figure 9.2).

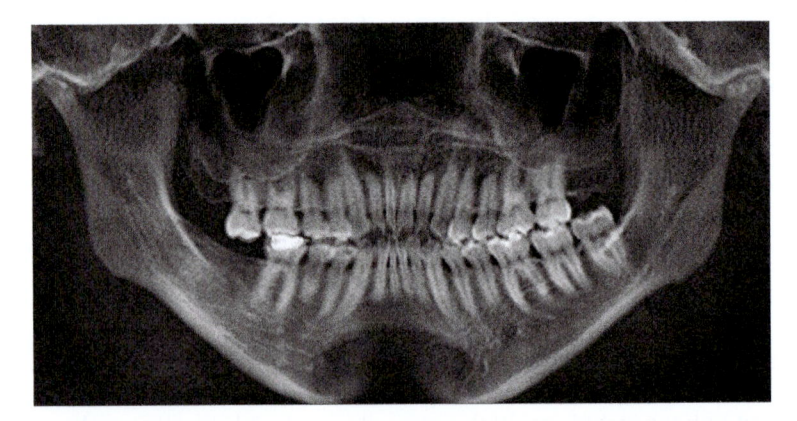

Figure 9.1A   Reconstructed panoramic projection for an adult female who has developmental onset degenerative joint disease, also known as condylysis (Hatcher, 2011a) or idiopathic condylar resorption. The condyles were small secondary to the degenerative process.

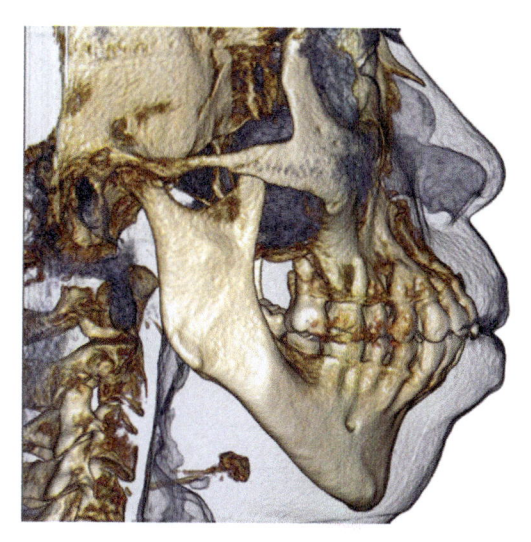

Figure 9.1B Lateral view of a volume-rendered CBCT scan of the same patient. This rendering shows the recessive mandible, steep mandibular plane, obtuse gonial angle, short condylar process, short ramus, and large vertical dimension of the anterior region of the mandible. This image shows a clockwise facial growth pattern.

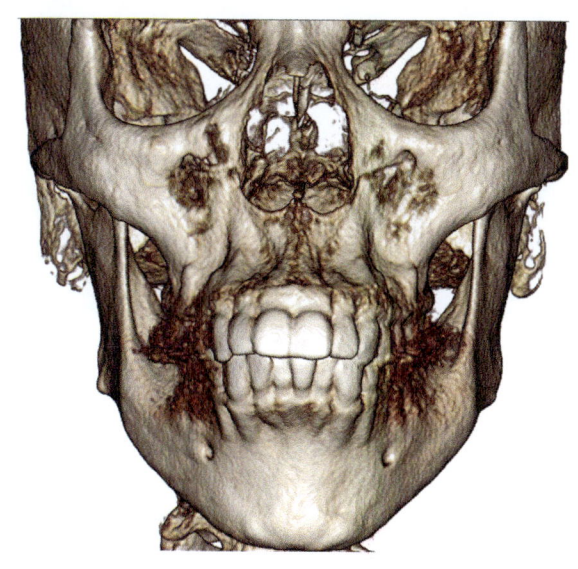

Figure 9.1C Frontal volume-rendered CBCT scan of the same patient that shows the narrowed transverse dimensions of the mandible and maxilla.

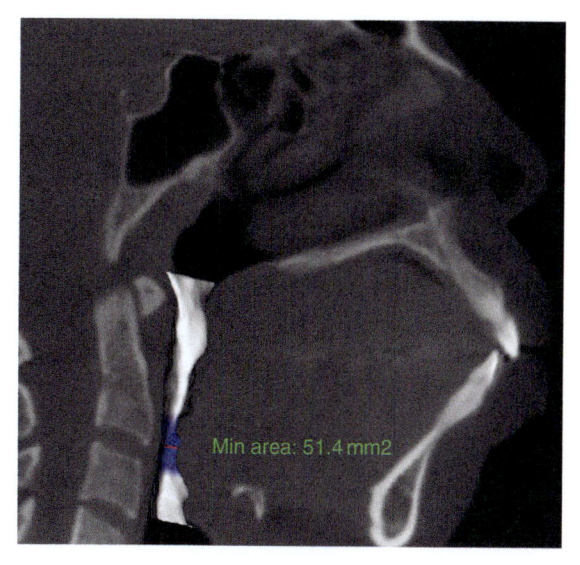

Figure 9.1D Midsagittal view of the same patient showing the airway. The clockwise facial growth pattern allows the menton region of the mandible and tongue to posteroinferiorly reposition and crowds the retroglossal airway dimensions. The minimum cross-sectional area of the airway is posterior to the tongue base and measured 51.4 mm².

Condylysis

Condylysis, also known as idiopathic condylar resorpton, osteoarthritis, degenerative joint disease, and progressive condylar resorption, is a localized noninflammatory degenerative disorder of TMJs that is characterized by lysis and repair of the articular fibrocartilage and underlying subchondral bone following the onset of purberty in females.

Natural history

Soft tissue changes precede osseous changes. The soft tissue changes include a nonreducing anteriorly displaced disc. The osseous changes begin with a loss of cortex along the anterosuperior surface of the condyle, followed by a cavitation defect and reduction in condylar volume. The active phase may be associated with a limited condylar motion and joint pain. The destructive phase is followed by a reparative phase that results in flattening and recortication of the defective surface (Hatcher Diagnostic Imaging Dental, 2011a; Figure 9.1).

Idiopathic juvenile arthritis

Juvenile arthritis is an autoimmune musculoskeletal inflammatory disease of childhood. The best diagnostic imaging clue is bilateral flat, deformed

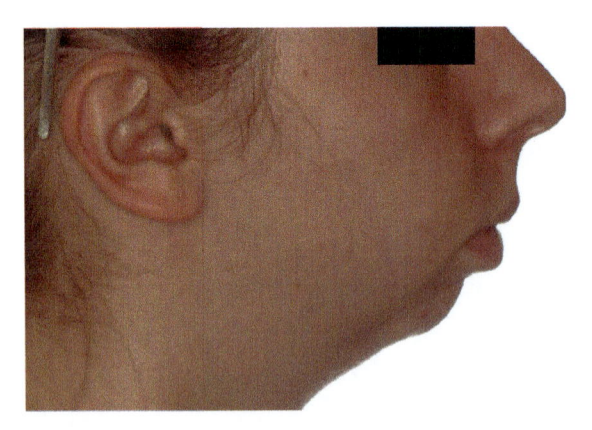

Figure 9.2A Lateral photograph of a 12-year-old female with juvenile idiopathic arthritis (Hatcher, 2011c). Note the recessive mandible and small maxilla creating a convex facial profile.

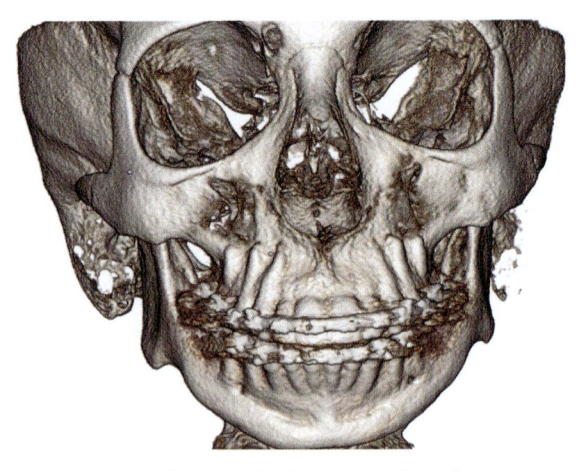

Figure 9.2C Volume-rendered CBCT in a frontal orientation. The mediolateral development of the mandible is small.

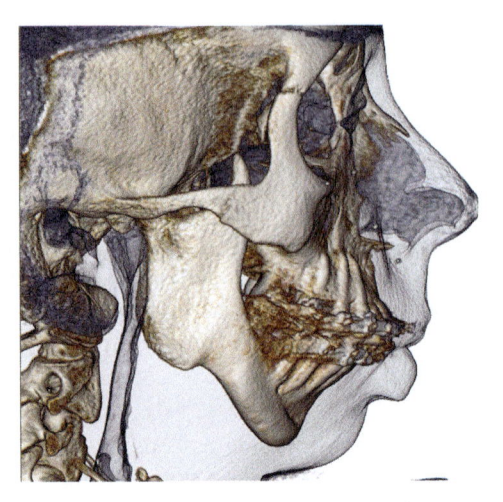

Figure 9.2B Volume-rendered CBCT in a lateral orientation showing the spatial relationships between the skeleton and overlying soft tissues. There is a convex facial profile. The mandibular and occlusal planes are steep. The gonial angles are obtuse. The menton is posteroinferiorly positioned. The condylar processes are very short.

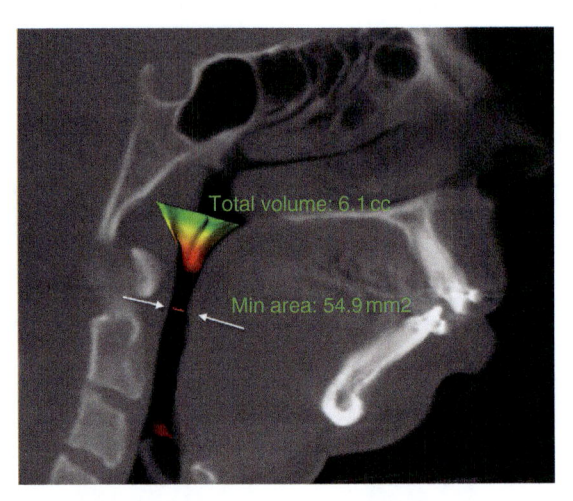

Figure 9.2D Midsagittal view of the airway that has a segmented airway and is colored to represent the cross-sectional areas. The smallest cross-sectional area is 54.9 mm² (white arrows). The hyoid bone is inferiorly repositioned.

mandibular condyles with wide glenoid fossae (Hatcher Diagnostic Imaging Dental, 2011c; Figure 9.2). The reduced mandibular development and associated clockwise facial growth pattern can result in repositioning of the tongue and hyoid bone, resulting in a reduction in airway dimensions.

Other contributions to a small airway may be from masses in the airway, selected cervical spine abnormalities, and selected abnormalities of the airway valves (nares, soft palate, tongue, and epiglottis (Hatcher, 2010a). The following image series will be used to illustrate the various scenarios that result in a reduction in airway dimensions. The images will be sorted by the following anatomic zones: nose, nasopharynx, and oral pharynx. The ability to achieve a specific diagnosis

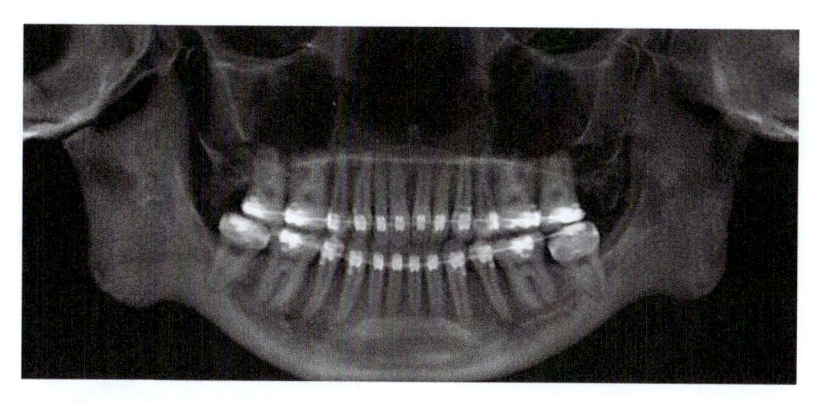

Figure 9.2E Reconstructed panoramic projection showing that the vertical dimensions of the condylar process, ascending rami, and body of the mandible are short. The coronoid processes are relatively long and superiorly repositioned. The antegonial notches are steep.

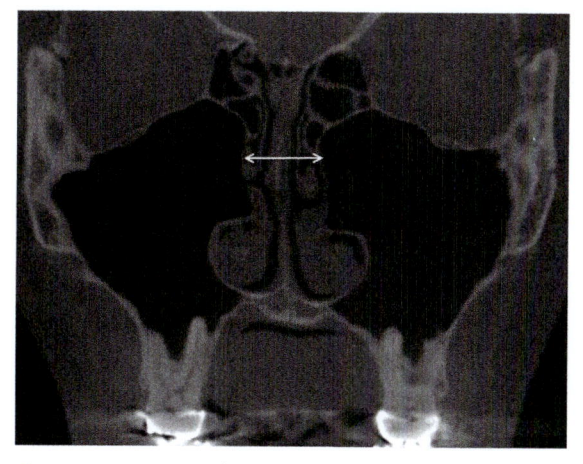

Figure 9.3A A coronal CBCT section showing mediolaterally narrow nasal fossae (white two-headed arrow). The narrow airway dimensions may increase airway resistance.

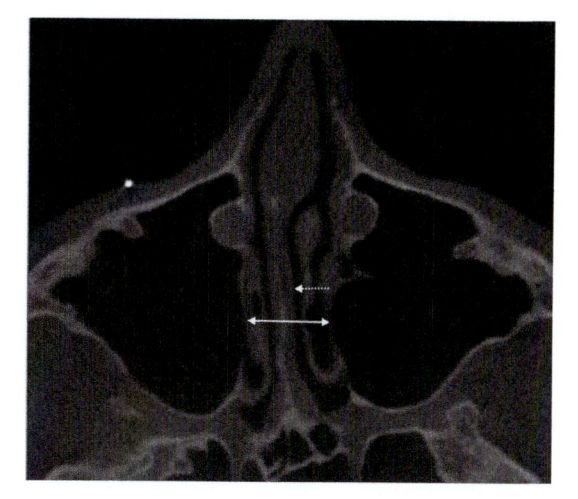

Figure 9.3B An axial CBCT section of the same patient showing the narrowed airway dimensions (white two-headed arrows) and a deviated septum (white dashed arrow).

may lead to a therapy that appropriately addresses the etiology of the small airway dimensions.

Nose

The evaluation of the nasal airway begins at the nares and extends posteriorly to the posterior nasal chonae. Nasal fossa (Figure 9.3), large turbinates (Figure 9.4), deviated nasal septum (Figure 9.5), small nares (Figure 9.6), nasal mucosal hypertrophy, and masses (Figure 9.5, Figure 9.6) may effectively increase air flow resistance.

Nasopharynx

Adenoids form in the posterosuperior region of the nasopharynx, and as they enlarge they extend toward the posterior nasal chonae and soft palate. In some patients the inferior turbinates may enlarge

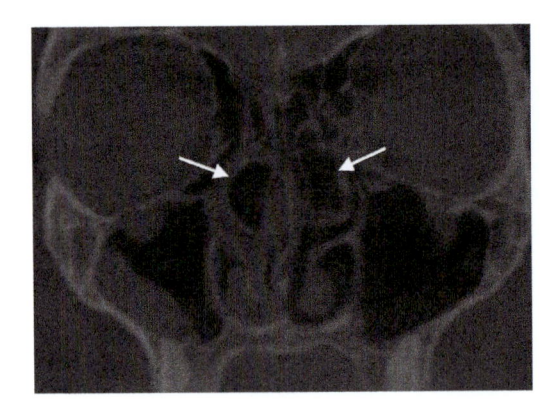

Figure 9.4A Coronal view through the midface and nasal fossae. The middle turbinates were pneumatized, called concha bullosa (white arrows), and this is an anatomic variation that may crowd the nasal fossa and increase resistance to airflow. Concha bullosa may also crowd the middle meatus and predispose to occlusion of the ostiomeatal unit.

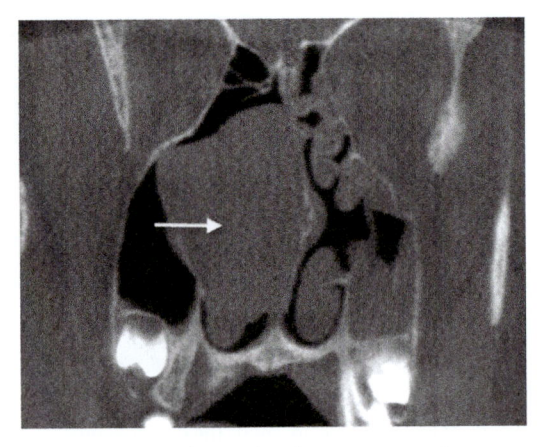

Figure 9.5B Coronal view showing mass occupying most of the right nasal fossa and expanding laterally to encroach on the maxillary sinus and medially to deviate the nasal septum toward the left, thus crowding the left nasal fossa.

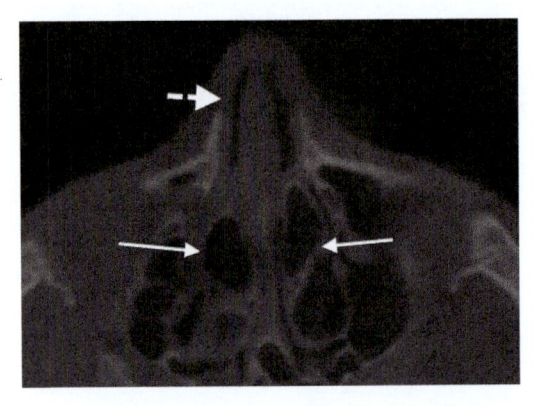

Figure 9.4B Axial view of the middle turbinates. The pneumatized middle turbinates were pneumatized (solid white arrows). The nares were constricted (dashed white arrow).

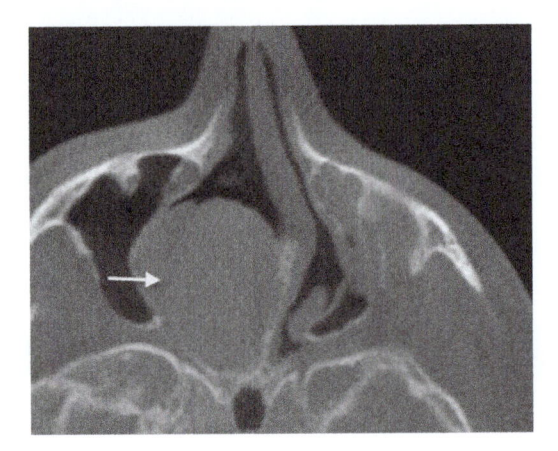

Figure 9.5C Axial section through the midface and nasal fossa. The schwannoma (white arrow) is expanding the right nasal fossa medially and laterally.

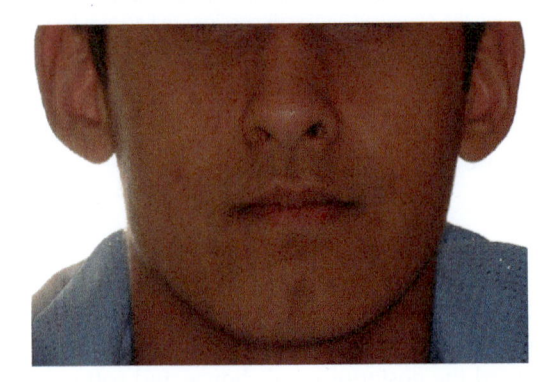

Figure 9.5A Facial photograph of 15-year-old male who had a mass within his right nasal fossa that was determined to be a schwannoma. A schwannnoma is a benign (99%) neural sheath tumor.

and extend posteriorly into the nasopharyx and occupy as much as 25% of the potential nasopharyngeal air space (Aboudara et al., 2003; Aboudara et al., 2009). The laterosuperior recesses of the nasopharynx, called the fossae of Rosenmuller, are sites that may give rise to neoplasms, such as a carcinoma. Adenoids will present as a midline mass (Figure 9.7), while a nasopharyngeal carcinoma will present as mass extending from a laterosuperior pharyngeal wall. Submucosal lesions, such as vascular lesions, may enlarge and produce a mass effect, reducing airway volume (Figure 9.6, Figure 9.7, Figure 9.8).

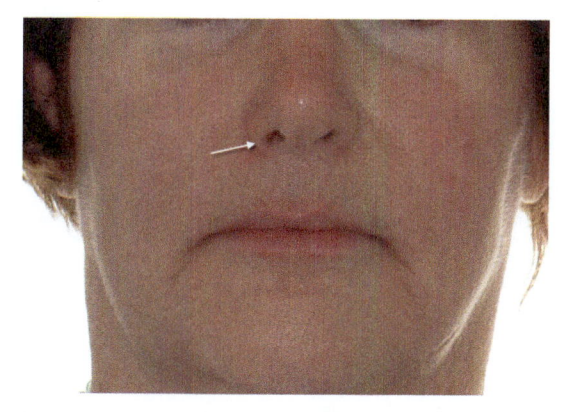

Figure 9.6A Facial photograph of 59-year-old female with narrow right nares and a right nasal fossa polyp.

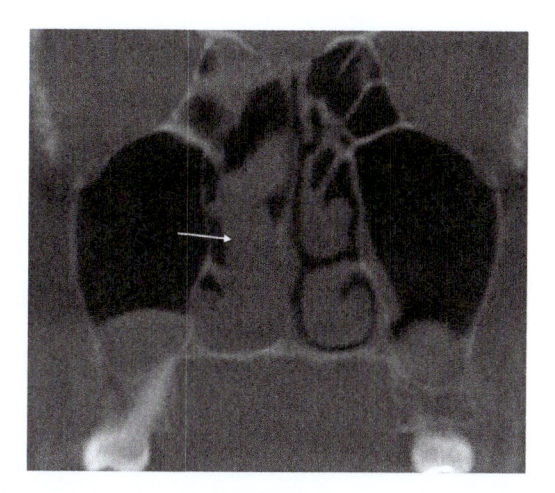

Figure 9.6B Coronal view showing a mass (polyp) nearly occluding the right nasal fossa without expanding the fossa (white arrow).

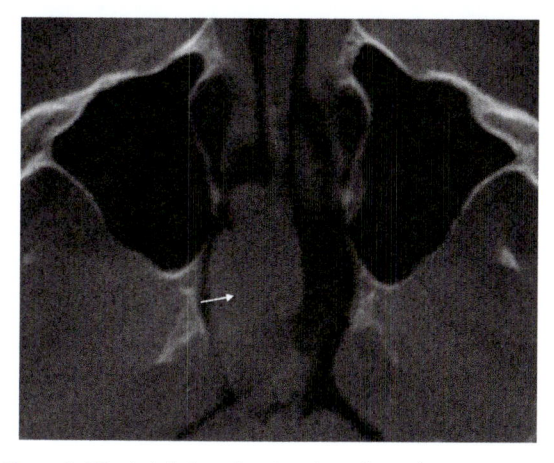

Figure 9.6C Axial view showing the polyp (white arrow) extending posteriorly into nasopharynx.

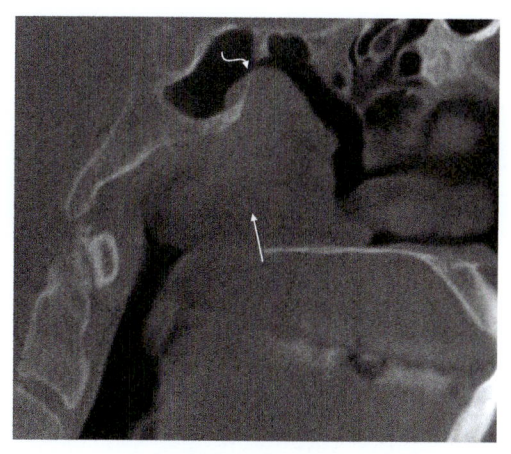

Figure 9.6D Sagittal view of polyp mass showing its location in the posterior half of nasal fossa and occupying most of the nasopharynx (white arrow). The mass extended through the ostium leading the sphenoid sinus (curved arrow).

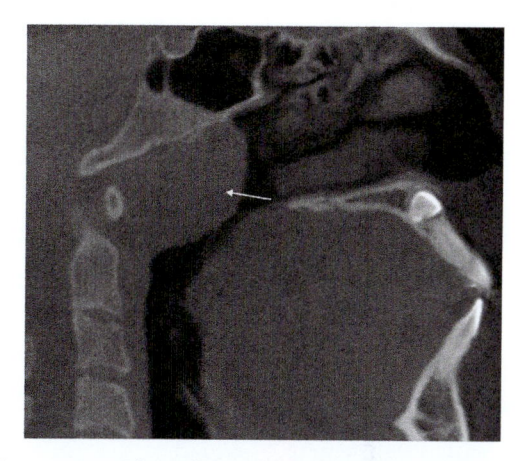

Figure 9.7A Midsagittal view showing adenoids extending from the posterosuperior regions of the nasopharynx (white arrow).

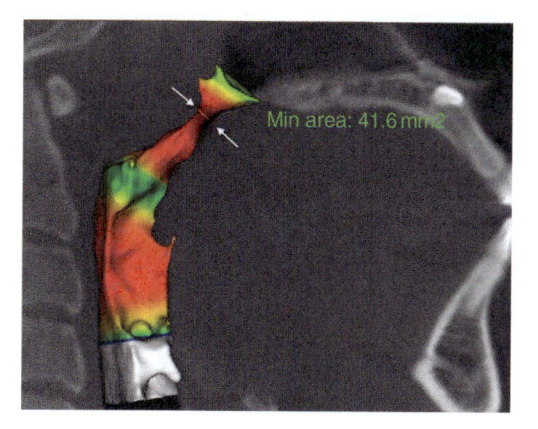

Figure 9.7B Sagittal section of airway that was segmented and measured (Anatomage, Inc). The white arrows show the site of the narrowest cross-sectional area (41.6 mm^2) located between the adenoids and soft palate.

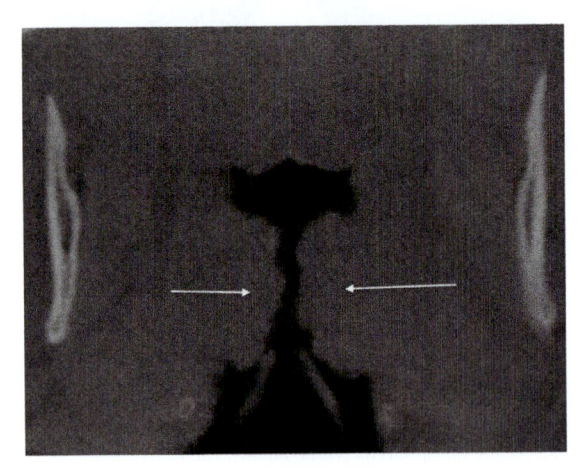

Figure 9.7C Coronal view of the oral and nasal pharynx. Tonsils are bilaterally extending from the lateral pharyngeal walls (white arrows). Note the large vertical and horizontal dimensions of these tonsils.

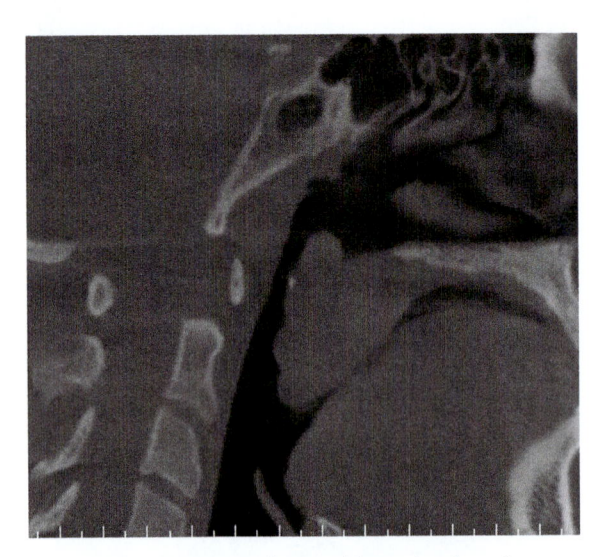

Figure 9.8A CBCT sagittal view of the oral and nasal pharyngeal airway space showing a hemangioma enlarging the soft palate and extending posteriorly to encroach on the airway space.

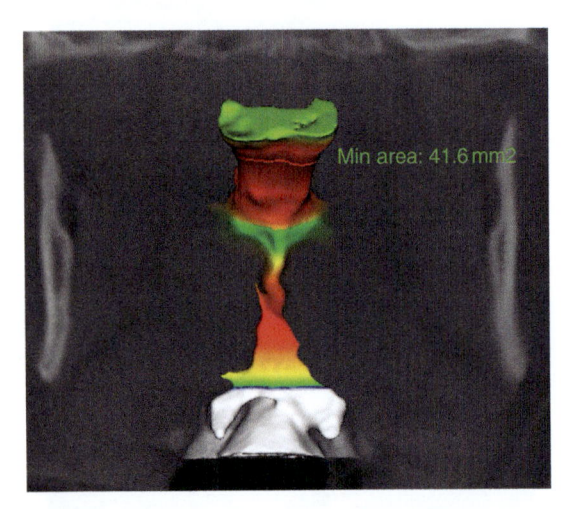

Figure 9.7D Coronal view of the oral and nasal pharynx showing a segmented and measured airway. The areas shaded in red and orange have a cross-sectional area below normal.

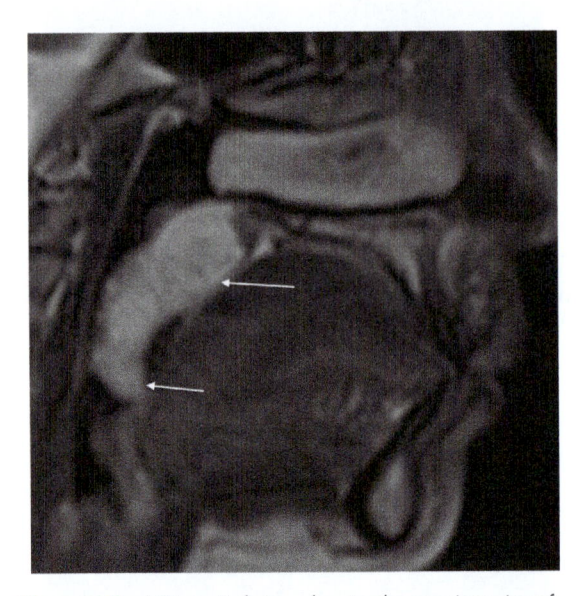

Figure 9.8B MRI sagittal view showing hemangioma in soft palate (white arrows) and narrowing the airway dimensions.

Oral pharynx

Enlargement of the tongue (Figure 9.9) or posterior displacement of the tongue may posteriorly displace the soft palate and reduce the airway dimensions. Masses extending from the tongue base (Figure 9.10) may reduce the size of the oropharyngeal air space. Changes in the cervical spine, including severe lordosis, horizontal misalignment of the vertebral bodies, and hyperostosis (diffuse idiopathic skeletal hyperotosis), may anteriorly deflect the posterior pharyngeal wall and reduce the airway dimensions (Hatcher, 2010a; Figure 9.11).

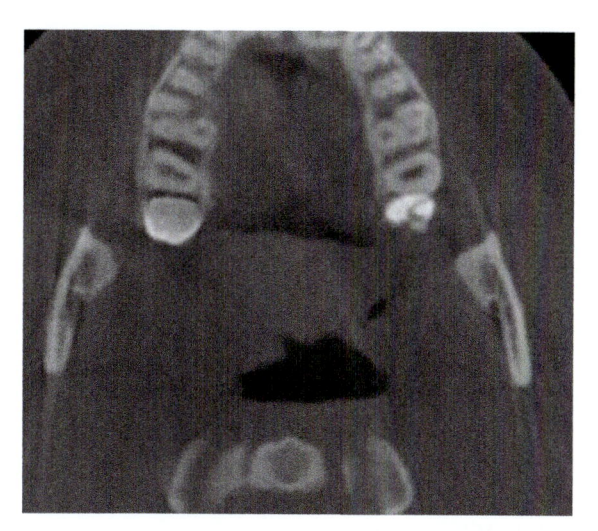

Figure 9.8C CBCT axial section showing the hemangioma enlarging the soft palate.

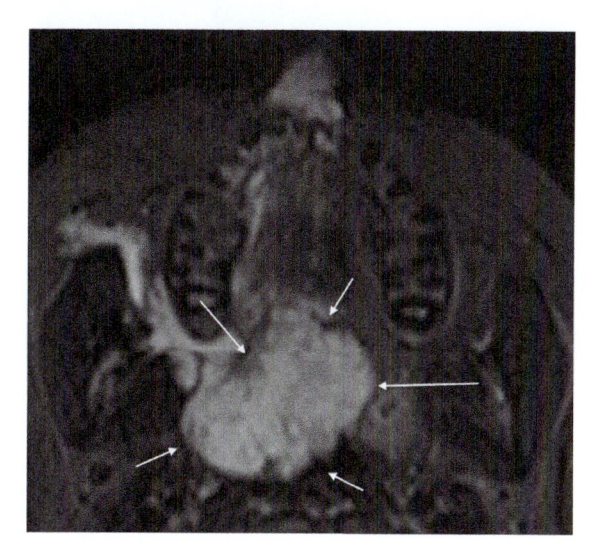

Figure 9.8D MRI axial view showing distribution of the hemangioma in the left palatal region (white arrows) and adjacent to the right alveolar process.

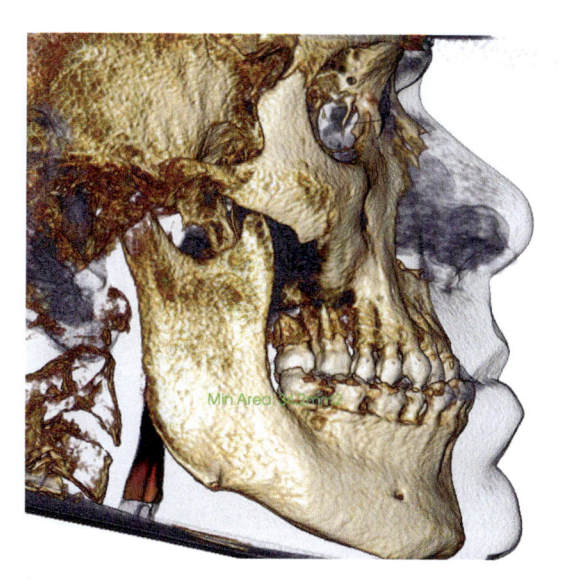

Figure 9.9A Volume-rendered CBCT scan shows a normal-sized maxilla and very large mandible. The mandibular teeth were in crossbite.

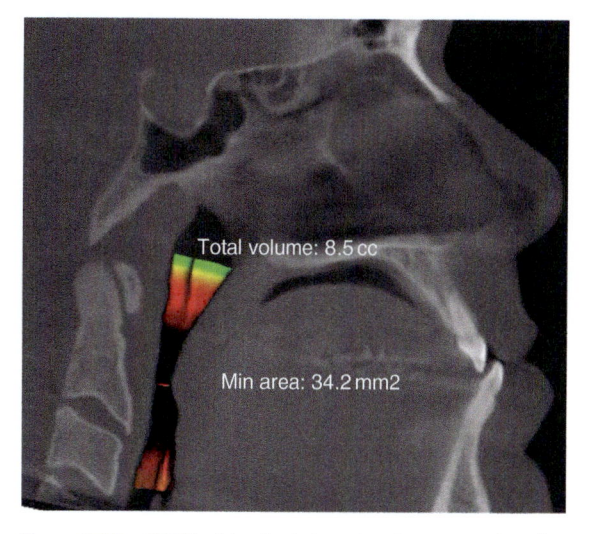

Figure 9.9B CBCT midsagittal view showing a retroglossal airway dimension with a minimal cross-sectional area of 34 mm². The reduction in airway dimensions was secondary to a very large tongue. Note the large sella turcica (AP dimension of 20 mm). This patient has acromegaly secondary to a pituitary adenoma.

Summary

Small airway dimensions may be a risk factor for obstructive sleep disordered breathing and upper airway resistance. The airway dimensions can be influenced by many factors, including age, gender, jaw growth, peripharyngeal fat deposits, tongue size, and airway masses. The use of CBCT, spatially accurate 3D imaging, creates the opportunity to

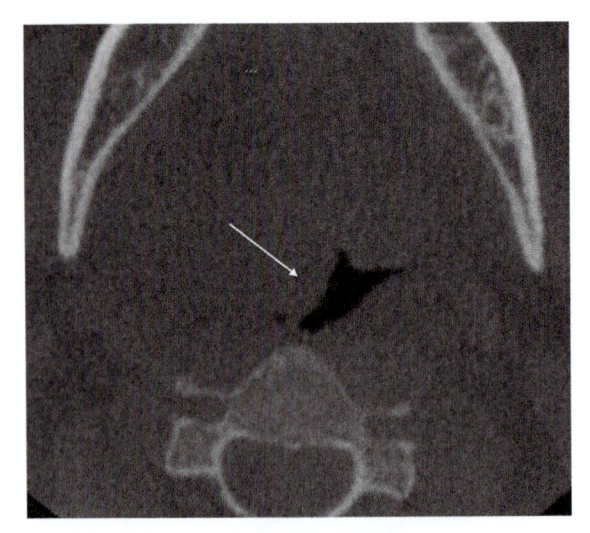

Figure 9.10A CBCT axial section showing a squamous cell carcinoma (SCCa; white arrow) extending from the right lateral side of the oral pharnynx.

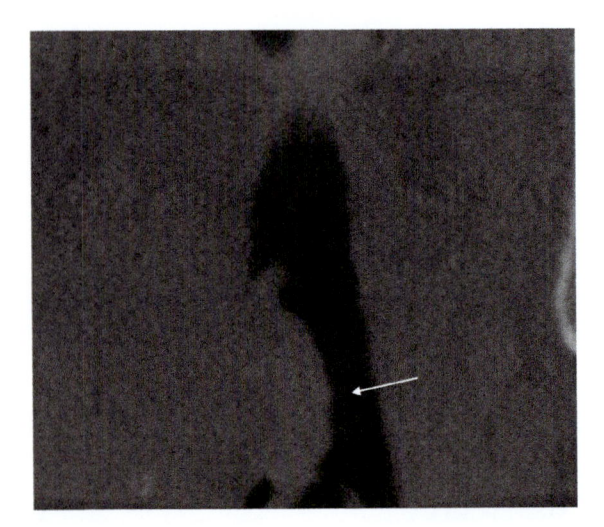

Figure 9.10B CBCT coronal view of same patient showing the airway encroachment by the SCCa (white arrow).

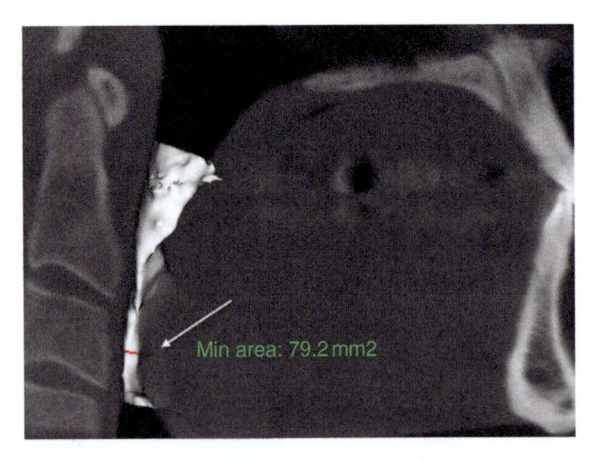

Figure 9.10C CBCT sagittal view showing that the smallest cross-sectional area of the airway (79.2mm²) is associated with the SCCa.

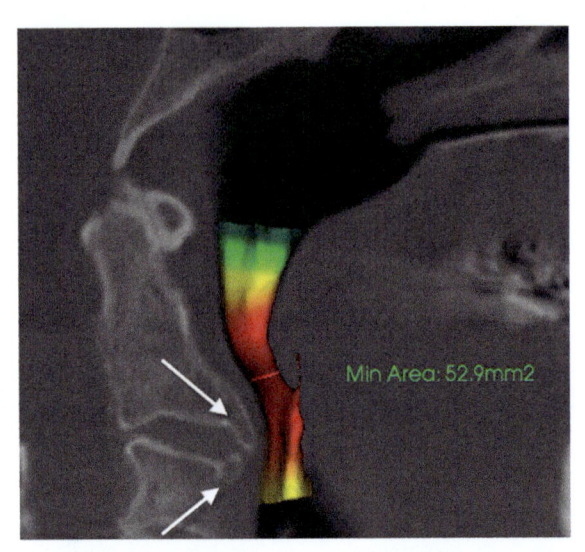

Figure 9.11 Midsagittal CBCT scan showing hyperostosis extending anteriorly from C2 and C3 vertebral bodies (white arrows). The hyperostosis has anteriorly displaced the posterior pharyngeal wall and reduced the size of the airway to 52.9mm².

assess the airway dimensions and to identify factors that have contributed to the diminution of airway size. A stratified diagnostic process and identification of the etiology of a small airway provide the opportunity to employ a therapy that targets the etiology.

References

Aboudara, C.A., Hatcher, D., Nielsen, I.L., and Miller, A.J. (2003). A three-dimensional evaluation of the upper airway in adolescents. *Orthodontics and Craniofacial Research*, 6(Suppl 1): 173–5.

Aboudara, C., Nielsen, I., Huang, J.C., Maki, K., Miller, A.J., and Hatcher, D.C. (2009). Comparison of evaluating the human airway using conventional two-dimensional cephalography and three-dimensional volumetric data. *American Journal of Orthodontics and Dentofacial Orthopedics*, 135: 468–79.

Chang, C.C. (2011). *Three-dimensional airway evaluation in 387 subjects from a university orthodontic clinic using cone beam computed tomography*. Thesis, University of Southern Nevada.

Hatcher, D.C. (2010a). Cone beam computed tomography: Craniofacial and airway analysis. *Sleep Medicine Clinics*, 5: 59–70.

Hatcher, D.C. (2010b). Operational principles for cone beam CT. *Journal of the American Dental Association*, 141(Suppl 3): 3S–6S.

Hatcher, D.C. (2011a). *Diagnostic imaging. Dental: Condylysis*. Salt Lake City, UT: Amirsys.

Hatcher, D.C. (2011b). *Diagnostic imaging. Dental: TMJ degenerative disease*. Salt Lake City, UT: Amirsys.

Hatcher, D.C. (2011c). *Diagnostic imaging. Dental: TMJ juvenile idiopathic arthritis*. Salt Lake City, UT: Amirsys.

Kushida, C.A., et al. (2005). Practice parameters for the indications for polysomnography and related procedures: An update for 2005. *SLEEP*, 28(4): 499–519.

Li, H.Y., Chen, N.H., Wan, C.R., et al. (2003). Use of 3-dimensional computed tomography scan to evaluate upper airway patency for patients undergoing sleep-disordered breathing surgery. *Oto-layrngol Head Neck Surg*, 1294–336.

Ludlow, J.B., Davies-Ludlow, L.E., and White, S.C. (2008). Patient risk related to common dental radiographic examinations: The impact of 2007 Internal Commission on Radiological Protection recommendations regarding dose calculation. *JADA*, 139: 1237–43.

Ludlow, J.B., and Ivanovic, M. (2008). Compariative dosimetery of dental CBCT devices and 64-slice CT for oral and maxillofacial radiology. *Oral Surg Oral Med Patholo Oral Radiol Endod*, 106(1): 106–14.

Ogawa, T., Enciso, R., Shintaku, W.H., Clark, G.T. (2007). Evaluation of cross-section airway configuration of obstructive sleep apnea. *Oral Surg Oral Med Oral Pathol Oral Radiol Endod*, 103: 102–8.

Schendel, S.A., and Hatcher, D.C. (2010). Automated 3-dimensional airway analysis from cone-beam computed tomography data. *Journal of Oral and Maxillofacial Surgery*, 68(3): 696–70.

Smith, J.M. (2009). *The normal adult airway in 3-dimensions: A cone-beam computed tomography evaluation establishing normative values*. MSc Thesis, University of Michigan.

Stratemann, S., Huang, J.C., Maki, K., Hatcher, D.C., and Miller, A.J. (2010). Methods for evaluating the human mandible using cone beam computed tomography (CBCT). *American Journal of Orthodontics and Dentofacial Orthopedics*, 137: S58–S70.

Stratemann, S., Huang, J.C., Maki, K., Hatcher, D.C., and Miller, A.J. (2011). Three dimensional analysis of the airway using cone beam computed tomography. *American Journal of Orthodontics and Dentofacial Orthopedics*, 140: 607–15.

10 Endodontics Using Cone Beam Computed Tomography

Martin D. Levin

Introduction

Endodontics is an image-guided treatment and, until recently, has been restricted to in-office periapical (PA) and panoramic radiographic assessments. However, these planar image projections suffer from inherent limitations: magnification, geometric distortion, compression of three-dimensional structures, and misrepresentation of structures. While a thorough history, clinical examination, and periapical radiograph are still essential elements of a presumptive diagnosis, the addition of tomographic imaging allows the visualization of the true extent of lesions and their spatial relationship to anatomic landmarks with high-dimensional accuracy (Figure 10.1; Patel et al., 2007; Cotton et al., 2007).

Radiographic imaging must rely on a risk and benefit analysis, whereby the degree of morbidity must be considered along with the consequences of patient exposure to ionizing radiation, misdiagnosis, or failure to diagnose. This requires knowledge of the potential diagnostic yield of additional radiographic imaging and the understanding that radiographic imaging will not provide a solution in all cases (Kau and Richmond, 2010). The most common radiolucencies of the jaws are inflammatory lesions of the pulp and periapical areas, namely, periapical periodontitis and radicular cysts (Scarfe et al., 2009; Weir, 1987; Tay, 1999). These lesions result from the intraradicular presence of microorganisms (Kakehashi et al., 1965) and begin as a periapical granuloma that sometimes forms a radicular cyst. While planar imaging generally provides better spatial resolution than three-dimensional radiography, surrounding bone density, X-ray angulation, image contrast, and the superimposition of structures often make interpretation of complex anatomy, morphologic variations, and surrounding structures difficult, with some periapical lesions not visible (Figure 10.2; Estrela, Bueno, Sousa-Neto, et al., 2008). Cone beam computed tomography (CBCT), on the other hand, allows for the three-dimensional assessment of the craniofacial complex for the visualization of pathologic alterations and anatomic structures without errors due to anatomic superimpositions, resulting in a significant reduction of false-negative results.

Endodontic disease

An understanding of endodontic disease begins with a review of the literature with special emphasis on systematic cross-sectional studies, which

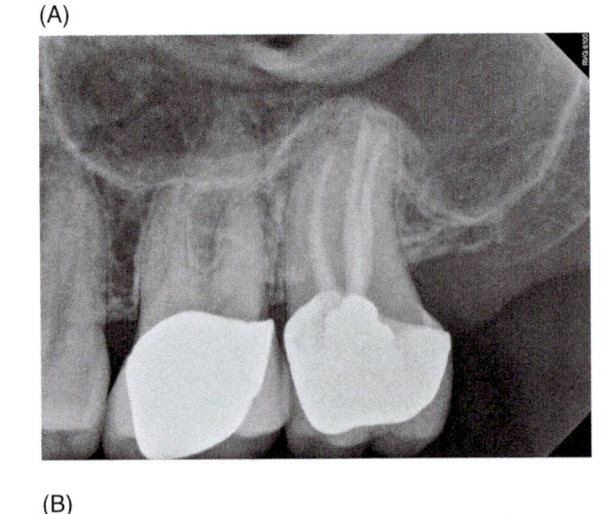

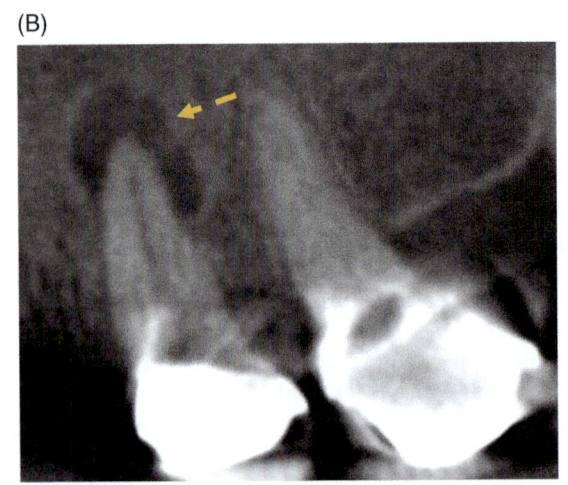

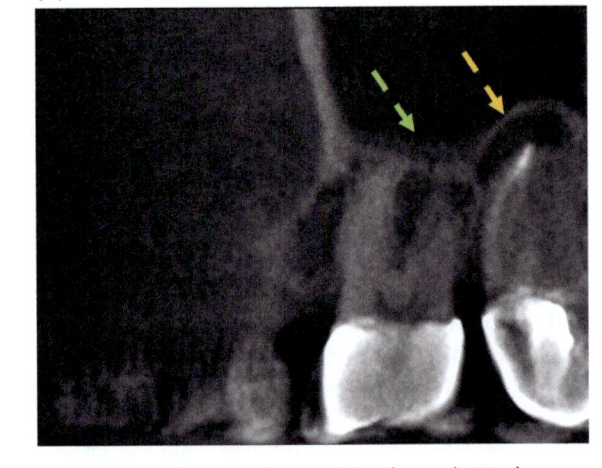

Figure 10.1 This series compares a periapical (PA) radiograph (A) of the maxillary right second molar with views of the same region using an LCBCT scan exposed to evaluate contradictory pulp test results. The limited field of view cone beam computed tomography (LCBCT) corrected sagittal view (B) of the palatal root shows a 6-mm well-defined oval-shaped radiolucency with a mildly corticated border, centered over the periapex of the palatal root, consistent with a radicular cyst or periapical abscess (yellow arrow).

Figure 10.2 This series shows a PA radiograph (A) of a previously endodontically treated maxillary left second molar with views of the same region using LCBCT exposed to assess contradictory findings. The corrected sagittal view (B) of the mesiobuccal root shows a 6-mm well-defined oval-shaped radiolucency with a mildly corticated border (yellow arrow), centered over the periapex of the mesiobuccal root, consistent with a radicular cyst or periapical abscess. The proximity of the lesion and the floor of the maxillary sinus and a limited mucositis (green arrow) are clearly depicted in this image. (Courtesy, Dr. Anastasia Mischenko, Chevy Chase, MD)

provide the highest level of evidence. A meta-analysis of 300,861 teeth from patient samples in modern populations, taken from 33 articles out of a total of 11,491 titles searched showed that 5% of all teeth had periapical radiolucencies and 10% were endodontically treated. Of the 28,881 endodontically treated teeth, 36% had periapical radiolucencies (Pak et al., 2012). However, the cross-sectional studies that were included cannot distinguish between healing and nonhealing radiolucencies. Although billions of teeth are retained through root canal treatment, the incidence of one radiolucency per patient and two root canal treatments per patient studied showed a surprisingly high level of disease. The majority of researchers criticized the quality of root canal treatment performed.

The loss of bone density around the apex of a tooth resulting from necrosis of the pulp is known as a periapical rarefying osteitis or apical periodontitis (AP). This radiolucency is a low-density or darkened area on a radiograph that indicates greater transparency to X-ray photons. The early phases of AP may be characterized by a widening of the periodontal ligament space followed by loss of the apical lamina dura. It shows endodontic lesions at the tissue level, where pathologic changes are macroscopic and do not correlate well with histologic findings (Barthel et al., 2004). Inflammatory lesions of the pulp and periapical areas are associated with an osteolytic process and remain radiolucent. Most endodontic lesions are unilocular, suggesting a local cause, while lesions that are multilocular or distributed throughout the jaws suggest a nonodontogenic or systemic cause (MacDonald, 2011). CBCT imaging also allows for the diagnosis of the occurrence and enlargement of periradicular lesions associated with individual roots of a multirooted tooth (Nakata et al., 2006). Some lesions, such as focal osseous dysplasia, may initially present as a radiolucency but subsequently may become partially opacified or completely radiopaque. Alterations of the supporting structures of teeth and associated lesions can be divided into the following outline:

- **Alterations in supporting structures of teeth**: Periapical radiolucencies, periapical radiopacities and mixed lesions, floating teeth, widened periodontal ligament space, lamina dura changes
- **Radiolucencies**: Well-defined unilocular radiolucencies, pericoronal radiolucencies without radiopacities, pericoronal radiolucencies with radiopacities, multilocular radiolucencies, generalized rarefaction
- **Radiopacities**: Well-defined radiopacities, ground-glass and granular radiopacities, generalized radiopacities
- **Periosteal reactions**

Aside from normal anatomic landmarks superimposed on teeth, AP or periapical rarefying osteitis can be confused with periapical cemental dysplasia, periapical scar, benign odontogenic tumors, osteomyelitis, and rarely, leukemia and metastasis.

The key to differentiating AP from the aforementioned lesions is vitality testing, where the tooth will be nonvital in cases associated with AP. While any odontogenic or nonodontogenic tumor can be superimposed on any tooth or teeth, the most common nonendodontic lesion is the keratocystic odontogenic tumor. These benign odontogenic tumors will have an intact lamina dura, may not be centered on the apex of the tooth, and can become secondarily infected if endodontic treatment was performed in error.

Not every case of pulpal necrosis is related to oral bacterial contamination via caries or by traumatic injury. An initial infection with varicella zoster virus or chickenpox can lead to subsequent expression in the form of herpes zoster, which can result in pulpal necrosis and AP (Worth et al., 1975). Another potential cause of pulpal necrosis is homozygous sickle cell anemia (SCA). In a study by Demirbaş et al. (2004), 36 patients with SCA, a genetically related systemic disease, and 36 patients without SCA as controls were evaluated for the presence of nonvital teeth. Fifty-one (6%) of the teeth with no history of trauma and no restorations were nonvital, with 67% of these teeth showing radiographic evidence of AP.

CBCT imaging is especially useful for the visualization of the lesional borders of radiolucencies without the superimposition of other structures. Differentiating common periapical lesions from other more aggressive types of pathologic entities is a routine task made easier and more precise by the use of CBCT. Well-defined lesional borders suggest an odontogenic cyst, benign neoplasm, or slow-growing lesion that is remodeling the surrounding bone; however, the lack of a well-defined lesional border is often consistent with a more infective or aggressive, invasive-type lesion. Some pathologic alterations with indistinct borders are not aggressive lesions, like reactive bone lesions such as condensing osteitis and idiopathic osteosclerosis. Mixed lesions associated with odontogenic tumors are surrounded with capsules, as often seen with an odontoma, cementoblastoma, supernumerary tooth, or embedded root tip. Analysis of intraosseous lesions should include an assessment of the definition of the lesional interface, uniformity and thickness of the reactive bone layer around the lesion, and the nature of the attachment of the lesional tissue to the surrounding bone.

Radicular cysts, for example, may exhibit a mostly corticated border with areas of ill-defined border consistent with an infected cyst, which is in contrast to more aggressive pathoses such as a malignancy (Bouquot, 2010).

The radiographic diagnosis of the true nature of an endodontic lesion has been shown to be somewhat elusive. Bashkar (1966) reported on the histology of periapical lesions, finding cystic degeneration in 42% of cases examined. Lalonde and Luebke (1968) determined the presence of cysts associated with endodontic lesions to be 44%. P. Nair et al. (1996) evaluated 256 extracted teeth and found that 35% were associated with periapical abscesses, 50% with granulomas, and only 15% were associated with cysts, which were composed of both 9% true apical cysts and 6% pocket cysts. Becconsall-Ryan et al. (2010) performed a retrospective analysis of the accuracy of clinical examination and the radiographic appearance of inflammatory radiolucent lesions of the jaws. Using histopathology as the criterion standard, they showed that in 17,038 specimens collected over a 20-year period in New Zealand, 29.2% were radiolucent jaw lesions, of which 72.8% were inflammatory. The largest group of radiolucent jaw lesions analyzed was AP (59.7%), followed by radicular cysts (29.2%). The mean age of the cohort study was 44 years old, with male and female equally represented. The study concluded that the provisional diagnosis before histopathologic evaluation was accurate for only 48.3% of periapical granulomas and 36% of radicular cysts. They concluded that while the incidence of cystic change in periapical lesions of endodontic origin is high at 30%, inflammatory radiolucent lesions cannot be accurately diagnosed from clinical presentation or radiographic appearance alone. In an additional study, Becconsall-Ryan and Love (2011) determined that the five most common radiolucent lesions of the jaws were periapical granuloma, radicular cyst, dentigerous cyst, hyperplastic dental follicle, and keratocystic odontogenic tumor. While it has been shown by Becconsall-Ryan and others that differentiating periapical granuloma from radicular cyst by clinical presentation or radiographic appearance alone was impossible, the studies by Becconsall-Ryan et al. were conducted with periapical and/or panoramic imaging alone, without the benefit of three-dimensional imaging techniques (personal communication, Robert Love, January 12, 2011).

Advantages of limited field of view CBCT in endodontics

The newest CBCT units are available in large, medium, limited, or adjustable field of view (FOV) configurations. The FOV is controlled by the detector size, beam projection geometry, and beam collimation. CBCT units that offer either limited field of view (LCBCT) or that can be collimated to sizes of approximately 6×6 cm or smaller generally offer three main advantages over medium and large FOV scanners, including (1) a lower radiation dose, (2) a higher spatial resolution, and (3) a smaller area of responsibility, as described below.

The aim of all radiographic imaging is to aid in the diagnosis of disease while exposing the patient to as little radiation as possible. Since most endodontic assessments are restricted to a quadrant or sextant of the jaw, LCBCT scans should be considered whenever possible to reduce radiation exposure in compliance with the ALARA principle (As Low As Reasonably Achievable). Choosing the smallest possible FOV, the lowest mA setting with the shortest exposure time is preferred. Dose optimization procedures should include custom exposure protocols based on patient body size; use of personal protective torso apron and, where applicable, a thyroid collar; adherence to quality control guidelines; and machine calibration performance recommendations.

CBCTs offering limited FOVs and dedicated limited FOV units generally produce images with higher spatial resolution than medium or large FOV units because acquisition occurs innately as high-resolution volumetric data. Newer scanners allow the clinician to select FOVs that best suit the imaging requirements for the task at hand, and range from 5×5 cm up to and including 17×13.5 cm. This projection data can then be sectioned nonorthogonally, allowing the best chance of lesion detection (Michetti et al., 2010). This allows visualization of lesion boundaries and radicular features that will aid in the assessment of pathologic alterations to the teeth and supporting structures.

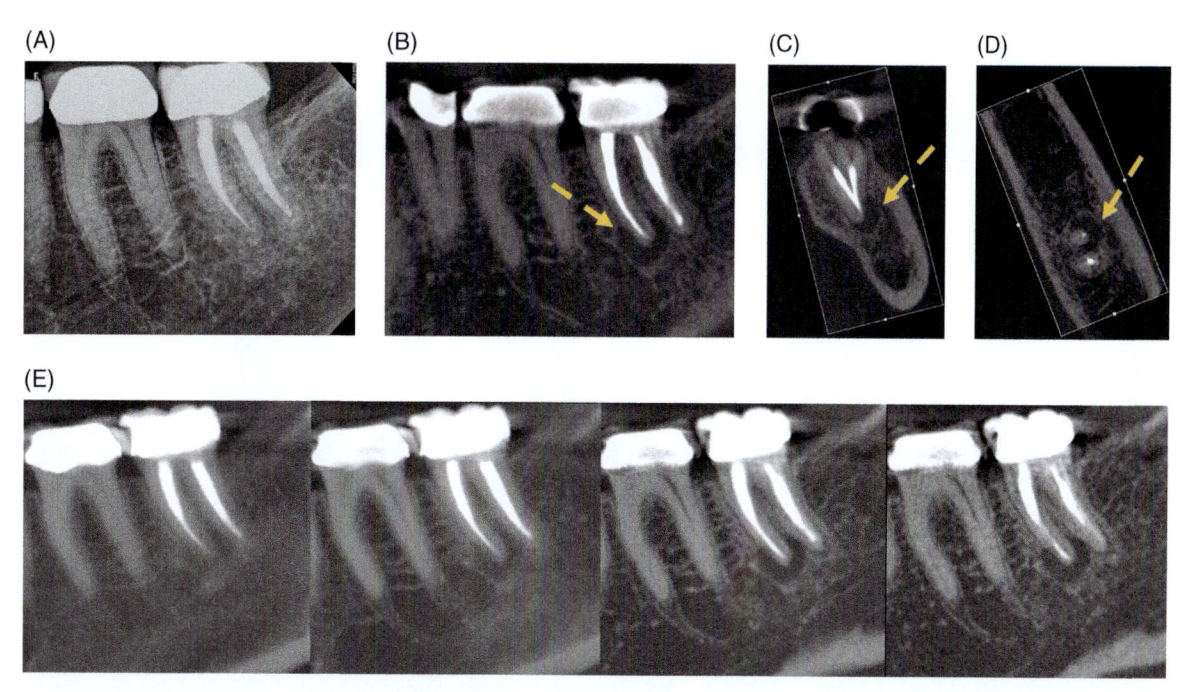

Figure 10.3 This 64-year-old female patient presented with a nonlocalized dull ache in the mandibular left posterior region. Endodontic testing revealed slight sensitivity to percussion and bite stick at the mandibular left second molar. The periodontal findings were normal and the patient's medical history was noncontributory. The PA radiograph (A) shows the previous endodontic treatment with no apparent lesion. An LCBCT was exposed to elucidate the contradictory findings, with the sagittal view (B) showing a lesion measuring 6 mm with a well-defined, mildly corticated border, centered over the periapex. The corrected coronal (C) and axial view (D) show the same lesion centered on the physiologic terminus of the root canal on the buccal aspect of the mesial root, 2 mm coronal to apex, consistent with radicular cyst or periapical abscess. The same case demonstrates how different slice thicknesses, with decreasing superimposition, affect lesion visualization (E).

The clinician ordering a CBCT study is responsible for interpreting the entire image volume (Carter et al., 2008). LCBCT units produce volumetric datasets that demonstrate small areas of the dentition and maxillofacial skeleton, limiting the area imaged. This greatly reduces interpreter responsibility because areas like the cranial base, spinal column, and airway are not imaged. The reduced image volume size also requires less time to interpret the image, which may result in lower costs to the patient.

Radiographic imaging is essential during each stage of endodontic treatment. CBCT imaging use should be limited to those cases that are justified by the patient's medical history and clinical examination and where lower dose conventional dental imaging cannot provide adequate information. Routine use of CBCT for endodontic assessments and for screening is not considered an acceptable practice (SEDENTEXCT, 2011). Periapical imaging may be required at all stages of endodontic treatment, including preoperative, intraoperative, and postoperative phases (Figure 10.3). Tomographic assessments can often provide valuable additional information in each of these phases of treatment.

Preoperative CBCT assessment of the teeth and alveolar hard tissue provides information on the effects and extent of periapical disease, the morphology of the dentition (Figure 10.4), the location of significant anatomical structures, and other diagnostic tasks, such as the location and extent of resorption lesions.

Intraoperative use of CBCT allows for the visualization and triangulation of calcified canals, the visualization of anatomic anomalies, and guidance during periapical surgery.

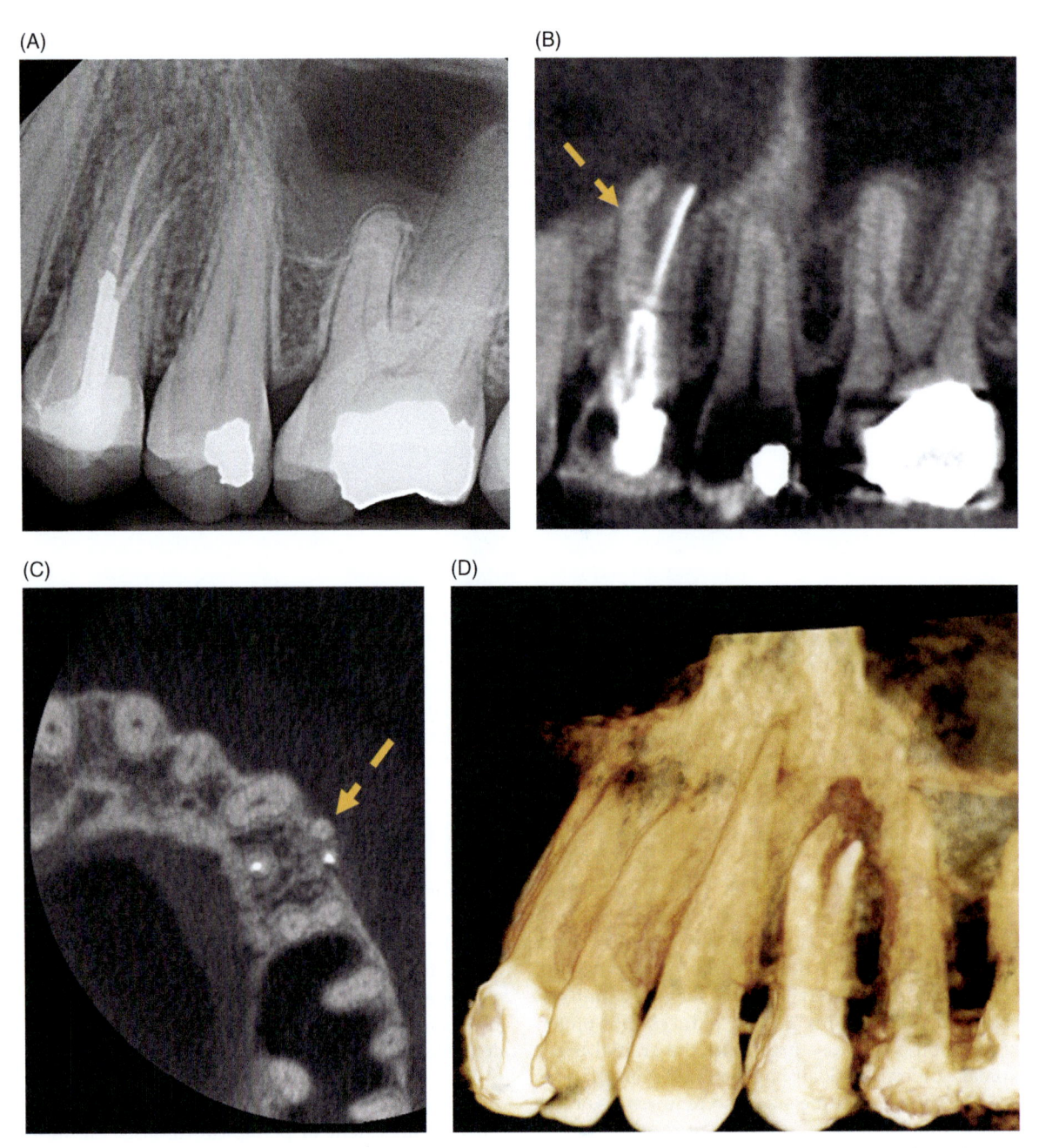

Figure 10.4 Many anatomic anomalies are difficult to assess with PA radiography alone. This patient was referred for evaluation and possible treatment of the maxillary left first bicuspid. A PA (A, partial image) was exposed and no obvious cause for the patient's continued postoperative discomfort was determined. An LCBCT was exposed, showing an untreated mesiobuccal canal in the sagittal (B), axial (C), and the reconstructed surface-rendered views (D). (Courtesy, Dr. Rajeev Gupta, Toms River, NJ)

The use of PA radiography for the temporal assessment of disease progression is often challenging because serial imaging requires standardization of beam geometry, detector placement, and radiation exposure parameters. CBCT allows for more accurate assessment of healing, which may be especially useful in assessing medically complex patients and may lead to earlier interventions.

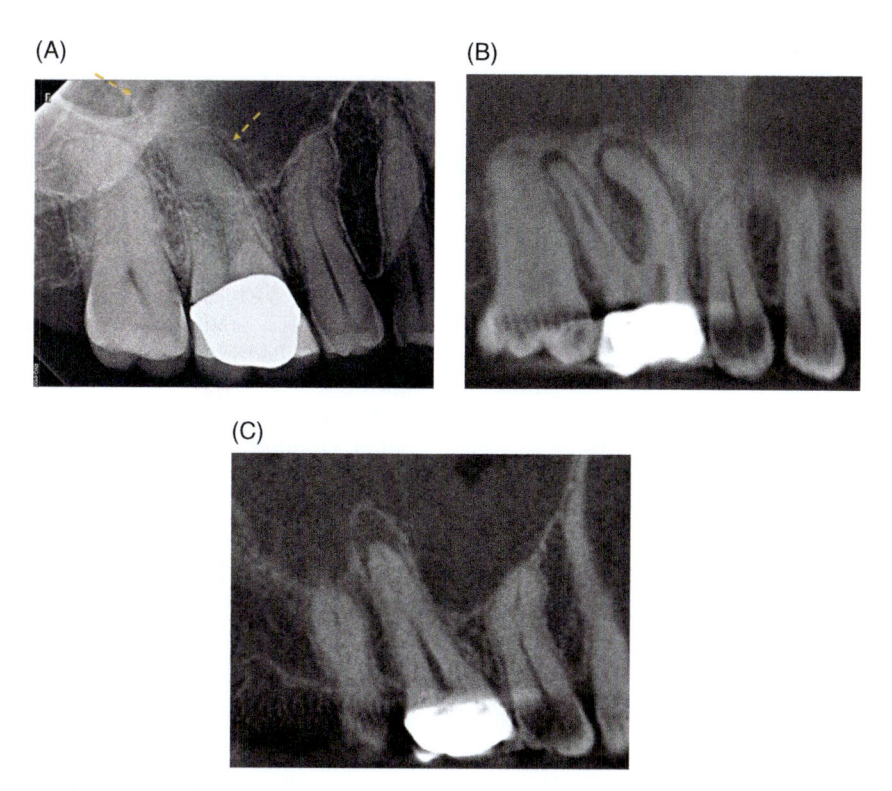

Figure 10.5 This PA radiograph (A) of a maxillary right first molar illustrates the difficulty in assessing the true nature of many periradicular lesions and their comorbid conditions. Although a periradicular periodontitis is visible on the mesiobuccal and palatal roots in the initial PA radiograph, the lesion on the distobuccal root (B), the osteoperiostitis on the palatal root (C), and the possibly associated moderate mucositis are not apparent.

Limitations of 2D imaging in endodontics

The ability to detect changes in periradicular structures is critical to endodontic diagnosis and the assessment of healing (Figure 10.5). Conventional radiography projects three-dimensional structures onto a two-dimensional image. This results in visualization of tissue features in the mesiodistal plane but not in the buccolingual plane. The often-cited classic study by Bender and Seltzer (2003a, 2003b) demonstrated the limitations of intraoral radiography for the detection of periapical lesions. Using human cadaver mandibles, their study revealed that in order for a lesion to be visible radiographically, the interface between the cancellous bone and cortical bone must be engaged.

Many subsequent studies have underscored the difficulty of detecting periapical lesions using planar imaging. Goldman et al. (1972) studied inter- and intraobserver differences when interpreting periapical radiographs. Later studies have shown only limited success in viewing some early changes in the cancellous bone alone, but they are dependent on bone density and the location of the lesion (S.J. Lee and Messer, 1986). Wide disagreement between observers was found, and when the same observers viewed the same films at a second session, there was only 19%–80% agreement between the two evaluations. These radiographic limitations are summarized in a review by Huumonen and Ørstavik (2002), in which they state that such limitations exist, in part, because radiographs are 2D in nature and clinical or biological features may not be reflected in radiographic changes. Essentially, conventional imaging suffers from the superimposition of "shadows" as projected on a detector, creating a 2D representation of a 3D object.

Periradicular bone loss can be detected with a higher accuracy with CBCT than with conventional radiography (de Paula-Silva et al., 2009). In a study of 888 patients involving 1,508 teeth, CBCT detected more AP than either panoramic or PA imaging, with the presence of advanced lesions correctly identified with conventional two-dimensional radiography (Estrela, Bueno, Leles, et al., 2008).

Although a low-dose tool to survey the jaws, panoramic imaging has several well-documented shortcomings. They are flat, two-dimensional, superoinferior or posteroanterior images that suffer from the superimposition of structures, distortion, and magnification errors. Direct measurements of objects on panoramic images are inaccurate. By contrast, CBCT images capture anatomic entities in three dimensions and can be viewed by digital selection of the region of interest with great accuracy. In a recent study published by Stratemann et al. (2008), linear measurements of skulls comparing calipers and CBCT imaging revealed only a 1% relative error.

When the lesion detection rate afforded by 2D imaging was compared to CBCT image data, additional clinically relevant findings were apparent, allowing the undistorted visualization of the maxillofacial complex, paranasal sinuses, and the relationship of anatomic structures in three dimensions (Pinsky et al., 2006). Velvart et al. (2001) showed that in a sample of 50 patients referred for possible endodontic surgery, volumetric imaging was able to identify all surgically diagnosed periapical lesions versus only 78% with periapical imaging. In a comparison of the accuracy of CBCT, CCD sensors, and film-based images for the detection of periapical bone defects artificially created in ten frozen pig jaws, Stavropoulos and Wenzel (2007) reported that there were few, if any, differences between the CCD sensors and film. However, CBCT showed better sensitivity (54%) and diagnostic accuracy (61%) than the CCD sensors. CCD sensors showed 23% sensitivity and 39% accuracy, while conventional radiographs had 28% sensitivity and 44% accuracy. The investigators point out that digital enhancement may result in limited improvement in the detection of periapical bone defects. When overall sensitivity for panoramic and periapical radiographs were tested to identify periradicular rarefactions, Estrela, Bueno, Leles, et al. (2008) found that these planar imaging techniques showed a relatively high probability of false negative results. Even when two periapical images with a 10-degree difference in horizontal beam angulation were compared with limited field of view LCBCT images for the detection of experimentally induced periapical lesions in jaw specimens, LCBCT was deemed superior in accuracy (Soğur et al., 2012).

Most CBCT imaging used for endodontic assessments will require voxel sizes smaller than 0.125 mm in order to provide adequate spatial resolution or detail. Because these images will require longer exposure times, the radiographic dosage will increase. This dosage increase can be offset by using a smaller FOV, which is often possible with CBCT units with either a limited FOV or with the option to collimate the FOV.

The determination of effective treatment is somewhat clouded by our inability to assess many lesions with PA imaging (Figure 10.6) and further degraded by a wide variation in our abilities to systematically assess even basic PA radiography. In a study performed by Sherwood (2011), 20 general practitioners were presented with two sets of questionnaires. The first asked which features they would interpret and the second consisted of 30 randomly selected PAs to assess. Fewer than 50% said they would interpret canal morphology, open apex, resorption, fracture, number of roots, and lamina dura. In the second questionnaire, 90% missed grade 1 or 2 periapical changes, resorption, and canal calcification, and more than 80% missed extra roots and root curvature buccally; most strikingly, no general practitioners were able to assess the periodontal ligament width changes.

Limiting geometric distortion is difficult with intraoral periapical imaging because positioning the paralleling guides and image receptors properly is rarely achieved. According to Vande Voorde et al. (1969), at least a 5% magnification of the feature being radiographed is to be anticipated because of the divergent nature of the X-ray beam and the distance between the object and the receptor.

Limitations of limited field of view CBCT in endodontics

When compared to conventional imaging for endodontic assessments, known limitations of CBCT include increased radiation dose, diminished spatial resolution, and imaging artifacts. Artifact generation is an area that continues to confound endodontic interpretation in some instances. This impediment should be considered when selecting cases for endodontic consideration.

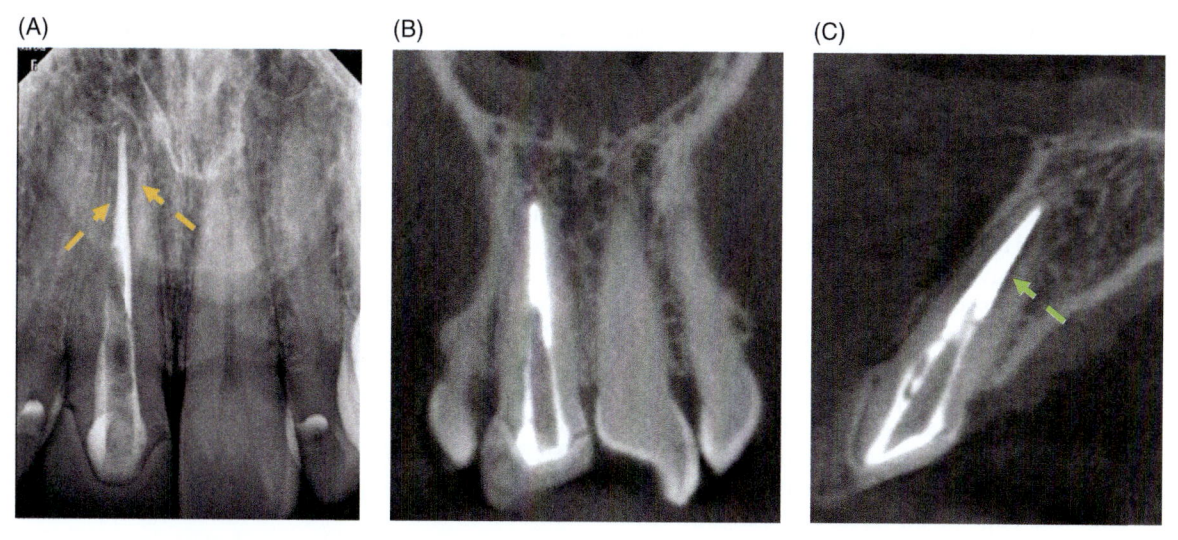

Figure 10.6 The dentition and supporting structures are subject to superimposition error, especially evident in everyday endodontic treatment. The PA radiograph (A) of this asymptomatic maxillary right central incisor appears to show a resorptive lesion at the apical third of the root (yellow arrow). An LCBCT was exposed to verify the presence of a resorptive lesion, with the corrected coronal (B) and sagittal views (C) showing normal root and supporting tissues, indicating that no treatment is required. There is a beam hardening artifact resulting in a dark area along the palatal aspect of gutta percha (green arrow).

Radiation dosage

Radiation exposure for dental imaging is usually measured by calculating the effective dose in micro-Sieverts (μSv), a parameter that attempts to quantitatively evaluate the biologic effects of ionizing radiation. Other exposure parameters such as kVp (kilovolt peak) and mAs (milliamp seconds), pulsed or continuous beam, rotation geometry, the size of the tissue being irradiated, beam filtration, number of basis images, and other factors all affect dose. Many CBCT units allow adjustment of exposure factors such as the kVp, mA, and FOV, while beam filtration and nature of the X-ray beam are not. The effective dose, based on the International Commission on Radiological Protection (ICRP, 1990) allows comparison of different CBCT units. In general, selecting the smallest FOV possible will result in the lowest dose. When imaging teeth in the maxilla, for example, collimating the beam to avoid the mandible will greatly reduce the effective dose since the thyroid and salivary glands contribute in large measure to the calculation algorithm (Ludlow and Ivanovic, 2008; Ludlow et al., 2008). Additional dose savings can be expected by reducing the degree of rotation from 360 to 180 and reducing voxel size settings.

Spatial resolution

Spatial resolution for CBCT imaging (approximately 1.25–6.5 line pairs/mm) is lower than either film-based (approximately 20 line pairs/mm) or digital intraoral radiography (approximately 8–20 line pairs/mm; Farman and Farman, 2005), but the lower resolution of CBCT images is offset by elimination of superimposition errors and the advantage of undistorted volumetric representations of the teeth and jaws that are viewable from any angle. Since CBCT relies on isotropic, non-planar geometry and true 3D reconstructions, the spatial resolution is excellent in all three dimensions (MacDonald, 2011) but is still diminished by partial volume averaging and other artifacts. Research by Bauman et al. (2011) demonstrated that multiobserver use of CBCT for the detection of mesiobuccal canals increased from 60% at 0.40 mm voxel resolution to more than 93% accuracy at 0.12 mm voxel resolution. In general, smaller voxel sizes will result in better spatial resolution and improved detection of features important in endodontic treatment.

Image artifacts

The diagnostic yield of CBCT imaging is sometimes affected by "beam hardening" artifact, caused when low energy photons are absorbed by material of high density, such as restorative materials, gutta percha, intracanal posts, implants, and retrograde amalgams. The resulting image can show two different but associated phenomena: (1) cupping, caused by the exaggerated attenuation of the beam as it passes through the center of a radiodense material in contrast to less attenuation as it passes through the edge of the same material, such as a post; and (2) dark streaks and bands, related to the direction of the beam as it passes through very radiodense objects, such as two adjacent obturated root-filled canals in close proximity. According to Katsumata et al. (2007, 2009), beam hardening artifact may be more problematic with LCBCT units.

Partial volume artifacts result from radiodense objects that are outside of the region of interest but within the area covered by the beam geometry. An implant in the mandibular first molar position, for example, may corrupt a mandibular anterior image volume, even though it is not in the field of view (R.D. Lee, 2008). Metal artifacts will cause streaking if they are in the field of view, especially dental restorations and amalgam retrogrades. This artifact can cause significant beam attenuation, resulting in bright and dark streaks.

Misregistration artifacts due to patient movement are common in CBCT imaging (Figure 10.7). Improper patient stabilization will result in suboptimal images since high-resolution images will register even small motions (Barrett and Keat, 2004). Positioning the patient in the sitting position is recommended whenever possible, to reduce this detrimental effect.

CBCT has not been judged more useful in determining obturation length or homogeneity. When six observers used LCBCT, PSP plates, and F-speed film to study 17 extracted permanent mandibular incisor teeth, they found that both PSP plates and F-speed film were superior to LCBCT (Soğur et al., 2007). While CBCT should not be exposed for the detection of caries, it can be helpful in select cases where root amputations or furcal involvements require 3D analyses.

As with any X-ray imaging modality, CBCT images should always be evaluated for any deviation from normal when performing a clinical evaluation (SEDENTEXT, 2009). Research has shown that CBCT was superior to F-speed film for the detection of proximal caries depth, but dose, cost, and availability will continue to make PA imaging the criterion standard for these assessments (Palomo et al., 2006).

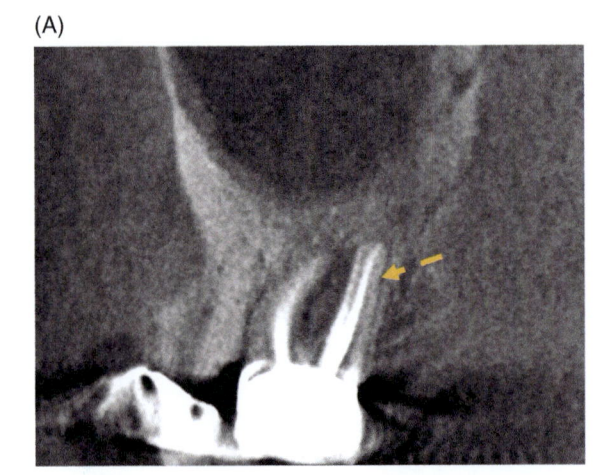

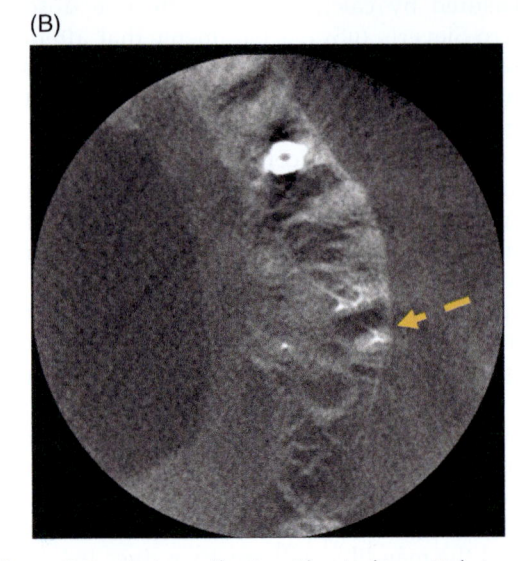

Figure 10.7 Motion artifact is evident in this sagittal view of an maxillary left first molar distobuccal root (A) and the starburst pattern associated with the gutta percha obturation material evident in the axial view of the same volume (B).

Endodontic applications of CBCT

Two-dimensional radiographic imaging is still one of the most commonly used diagnostic tools in endodontics, although many studies have shown that interpretation of changes in the root-supporting structures is not reliable (Molven et al., 2002; Saunders et al., 2000). The use of CBCT in endodontics is an important tool in the identification of critical anatomic structures and their relation with roots and periapical lesions (Estrela, Bueno, Sousa-Neto, et al., 2008). CBCT can provide additional information that cannot be obtained in any other way, but it should not be considered as a substitute for two-dimensional imaging. Advancements in CBCT imaging are on the horizon, promising to reduce radiation dose and improve resolution, readability, and functionality of CBCT imaging. These improvements include sophisticated algorithms that allow segmentation of different features of the dentition and maxillofacial skeleton which will enhance visualization (Figure 10.8).

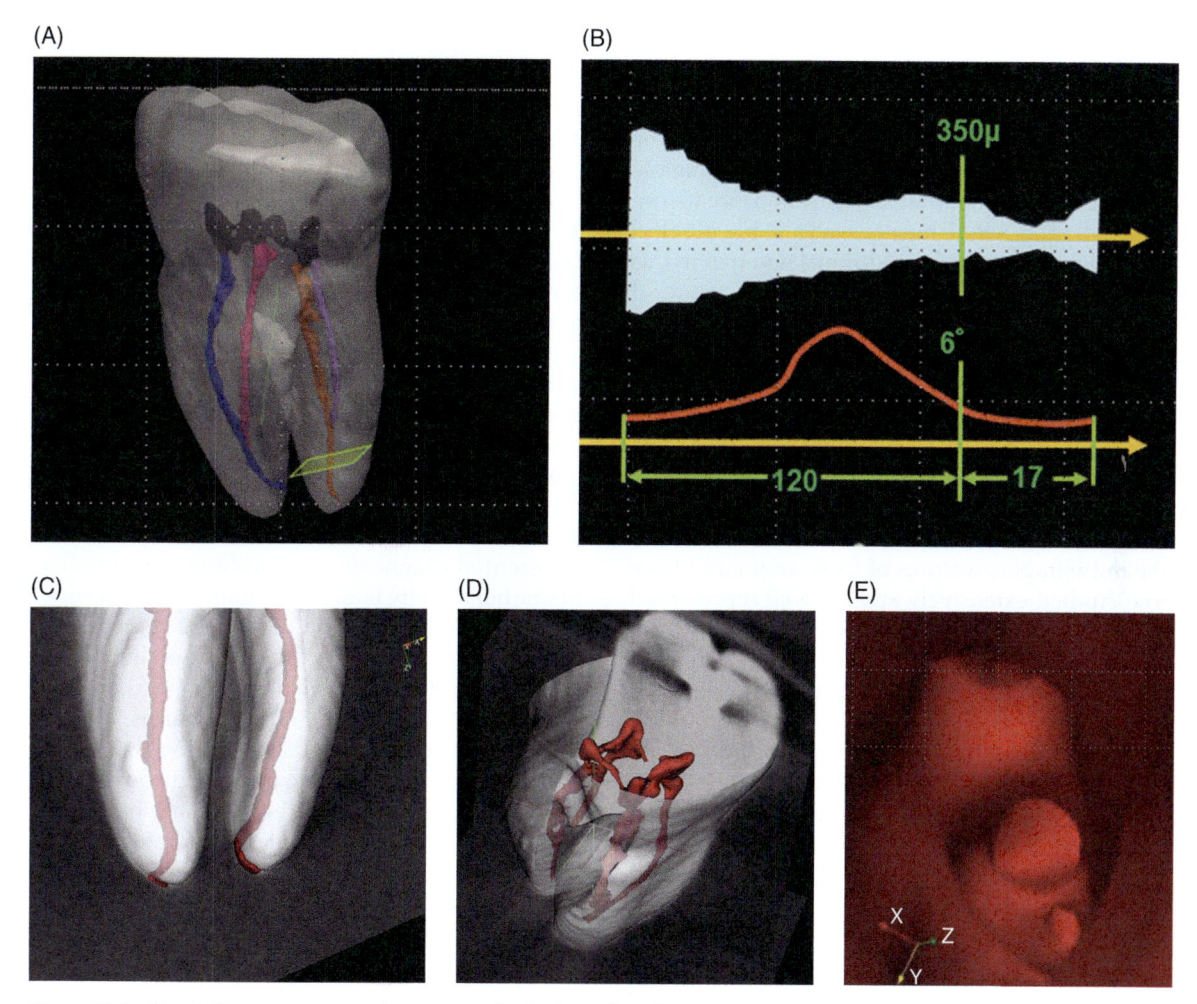

Figure 10.8 The ability to segment and measure individual canals is demonstrated in this in vitro series, exposed with an LCBCT and processed with special software (Courtesy, Carestream Dental, LLC, Atlanta GA). The individual canals are segmented (A), then sliced with an obliquely positioned plane, showing the resulting cross-sectional measurements of the canal size (B). The available spatial resolution is further demonstrated by this 0.076 mm image showing the root canal morphology (C). Additional segmentation algorithms applied to the same molar dataset show the root canals in red (D) and a portion of the canal interior captured from a virtual endoscopy (E).

The following applications of CBCT in endodontics are based on the 2010 Joint Position Statement of the American Association of Endodontics and the American Academy of Oral and Maxillofacial Radiology, "Use of Cone-Beam Computed Tomography in Endodontics." The last section describing the assessment of endodontic treatment outcomes was not included in this joint position statement.

1. Evaluation of anatomy and complex morphology

While no systematic studies with large sample sizes justify the routine use of CBCT imaging for the assessment of endodontic anatomy, and the use of the operating microscope may adequately reveal root canal anatomy without exposure to ionizing radiation, CBCT may prove valuable in select cases. There is a need for additional research in this area of endodontic practice.

A. Anomalies

Dental anomalies include dens invaginatus (DI), short roots, microdontia taurodontism, gemination, supernumerary teeth dentinogenesis iperfecta, agenesis, and malformations resulting from trauma. The radiographic features of these anomalies have been studied extensively and are well represented in the literature, showing that deviations from normal anatomy can cause difficulties in diagnosis and treatment. CBCT provides detailed information that can allow visualization of the root morphology, resulting in better treatment planning and postoperative assessments (Nair and Nair, 2007).

DI is a developmental anomaly that may not only require endodontic treatment, it may also complicate endodontic therapy. It has been postulated that DI results from the infolding of the dental papilla prior to tooth calcification (Silberman et al., 2006; Bishop and Alani, 2008). Usually affecting the permanent maxillary lateral incisors, followed by maxillary central incisors, premolars, canines, and least frequently molars, DI has a wide range of morphologic variations (Neves et al., 2010). According to Oehlers's (1957) classification, DI can be divided into three groups, with the most complex cases classified as type III, with extension of an enamel-lined invagination through the root to form an additional apical or lateral foramen. CBCT allows for the detailed three-dimensional visualization of the anomalous tooth and can facilitate the successful management of these anomalies.

Normal variants in the human dentition include many examples where the apical foramen is not coincidental with the root apex (Figure 10.9; Grande et al., 2008). Morphologic analysis has shown that the root apex is round only 35% of the time; the apical foramen is round 52.9% of the time; and is oval shaped 25.2% of the time (Martos et al., 2010). The location of the major foramen was in the center of the root in 58.4% of the teeth examined. Their largest diameter is in the buccolingual direction (Martos et al., 2009; M.K. Wu and Wesselink, 2001; M.K. Wu et al., 2000), making visualization with periapical radiography nearly impossible. It is well known that every tooth in the human dentition presents with occasional anomalous features. All of these factors complicate endodontic assessments by planar radiographic means alone (Baratto Filho et al., 2009).

Normal variants in the jaws include the mandibular salivary gland defect (Stafne bone cavity) and idiopathic osteosclerosis (dense bone island, enostosis, focal osteopetrosis; Figure 10.10). Both the Stafne bone cavity and idiopathic osteosclerosis can usually be assessed by using periapical or panoramic imaging but occasionally confuse the differential diagnosis of endodontic lesions. The Stafne bone cavity is an asymptomatic radiolucency usually found in routine panoramic radiographs. Similar defects associated with the sublingual and parotid gland have been described (Richard and Ziskind, 1957). Usually found in males with an incidence of between 0.10% and 0.48%, Stafne bone cavities often develop at middle age (Correll et al., 1980) as an extension of the submandibular salivary gland. They are unilateral, radiolucent, and usually corticated (Prapanpoch and Langlais, 1994) ovoid defects anterior to the angle of the mandible. While two-dimensional imaging is often sufficient for diagnosis, confirmatory CBCT imaging is recommended in atypical cases, whereby distinguishing this defect from a periapical lesion is imperative (Branstetter et al., 1999).

Idiopathic osteosclerosis, also a normal variant in the jaws, is a well-defined nonexpansile, homogeneous radiopacity with radiolucent periphery.

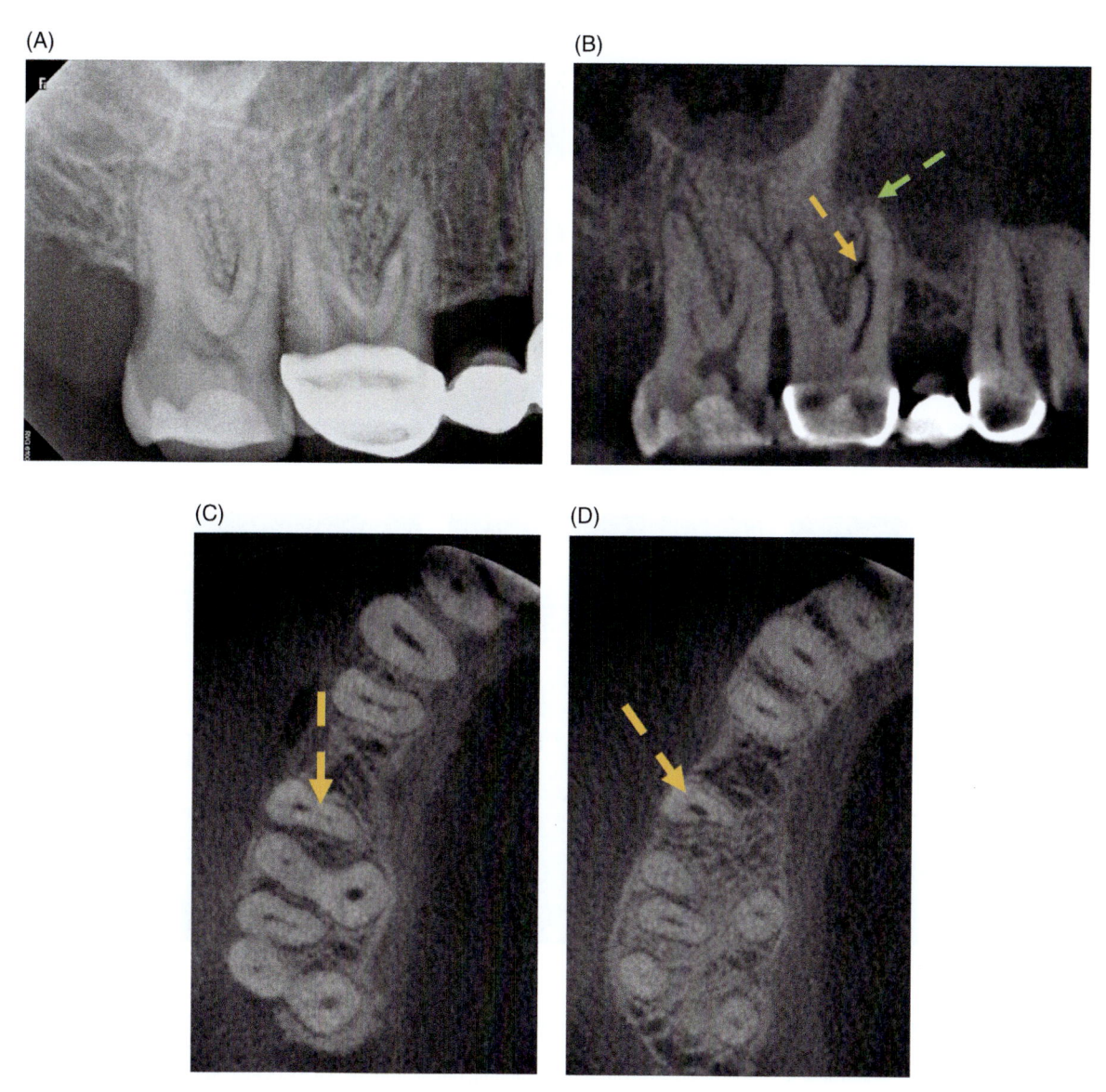

Figure 10.9 This comparison of a PA radiograph (A) with tomographically-generated views demonstrates the improved visualization provided. A sagittal section through the mesiobuccal root (B) shows the aberrant root morphology associated with the separate location of the physiologic apex (yellow arrow) and the radiographic apex (green arrow). The axial view (C) shows a mesiobuccal and mesioaccessory canal connected by a ribbon shaped isthmus (yellow arrow), and the oval shaped canal form (D) at the physiologic apex. The largest diameter is in the buccopalatal direction, making visualization with PA radiography nearly impossible.

It is usually closely associated with roots and can be easily confused with condensing osteitis, periapical cemental dysplasia, hypercementosis, and Gardner Syndrome (Basaran and Erkan, 2008). In a report by McDonnell (1993), idiopathic osteosclerosis affects females twice as often as males. In this cohort of 107 patients with 113 lesions analyzed, idiopathic osteosclerosis involved the mandible in 96.5% of cases, with the bicuspids and molar areas most commonly affected. Bony

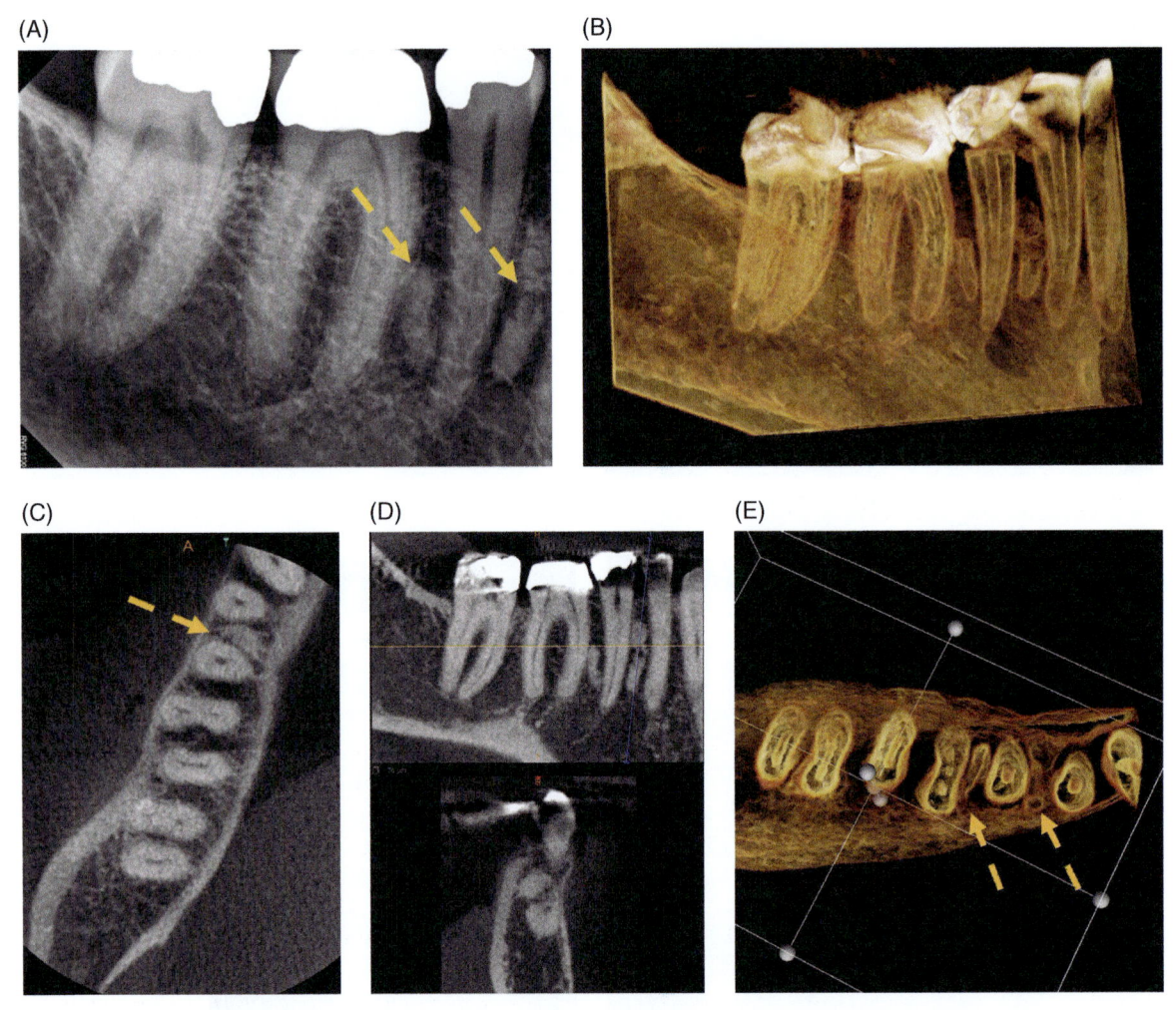

Figure 10.10 This 60-year-old male Caucasian patient presented for evaluation and possible endodontic treatment for nonlocalized pain in the mandibular posterior region. (A) The PA radiograph showed normal periapical tissues, a carious lesion and bifid canal structure on tooth #29, and two regions of idiopathic osteosclerosis. (B–E) These usually incidental findings are confirmed and well identified using an LCBCT; they are uniformly hyerdense foci of compact bone located in cancellous bone and demonstrate a spiculated structure (yellow arrow) with no surrounding rarefaction, typical of benign idiopathic osteosclerosis.

resorption was found in 9.7% of the cases and usually affected the succedaneous first molar.

B. Root curvatures

Thorough chemomechanical preparation and obturation of the root canal system are the principle steps necessary for successful root canal treatment. The purpose is to remove all of the pulpal tissue and canal debris from the root canal space while also removing infected inner layers of canal wall dentin. In endodontic cases where the canal configuration is relatively straight in its long axis and round in cross-section, our goal might be achieved using conventional hand and rotary-driven endodontic files. However, the cleaning, shaping, and disinfection of canals that are flat and oval-shaped in cross-section, as well as curved canals, represent a significant clinical challenge in endodontic treatment. According to a study by Siqueira and Rôças (2008), AP is caused by bacterial populations within the root canal that should be eliminated or at least reduced to levels that allow periapical healing. Metzger et al. (2009) determined that rotary file instrumentation left up to 60% of canal walls unaffected. Complex canal anatomy with compound curves, dilacerations, and other morphological variations are difficult to assess with two-dimensional radiographs, especially if the root curves in a direction perpendicular to the plane of the detector. Cunningham and Senia (1992) showed that 100% of 100 mandibular first and second molars examined had curvatures in both a buccolingual and mesiodistal direction with #8K files inserted. To better understand the extent of root curvatures, Estrela, Bueno, Sousa-Neto, et al. (2008) used CBCT imaging to plot the loci of three mathematical points within a root using specialized software. Understanding the severity of the canal curvatures allows for better treatment planning strategies, which may reduce the chances of instrument fracture and canal transportations (Lopes et al., 2008).

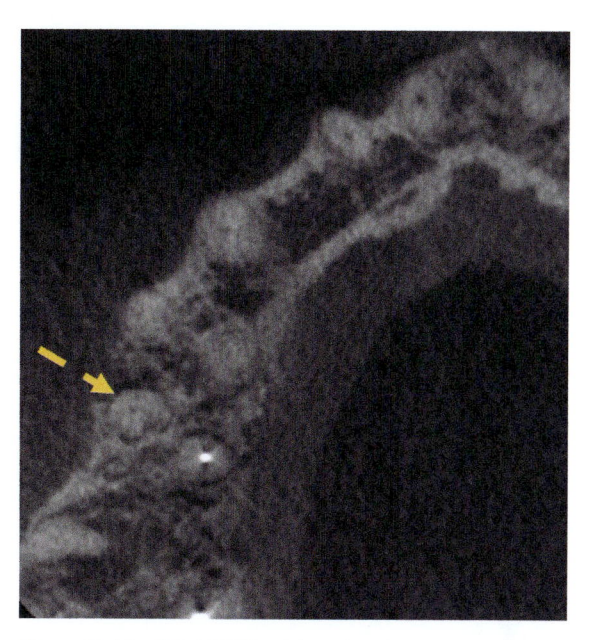

Figure 10.11 This LCBCT axial section demonstrates the identification of an untreated buccal canal of a maxillary right second bicuspid (yellow arrow) using a 76-micron voxel size.

C. Missed/accessory canals

High-resolution CBCT images improve the identification and localization of accessory root canals over conventional radiography, so the precise location and the morphology can be understood (Figure 10.11; Cohenca et al., 2007). Use of the operating microscope and CBCT imaging has been shown to be an important aid in the visualization of root canal orifices. In an investigation by Baratto Filho et al. (2009), three different methods were used to investigate the internal morphology of the root canals in maxillary first molars: ex vivo, clinical, and CBCT. In the ex vivo evaluation of 140 extracted teeth using an operating microscope, a second mesiobuccal canal was located in 92.9% of the teeth, with 17.4% of these canals judged nonnegotiable. During the clinical assessment of 291 teeth in this dental school cohort study, 95.63% of teeth exhibited a second mesiobuccal canal, with 27.5% being nonnegotiable. CBCT showed 90.9% of the teeth had an additional mesiobuccal canal. They concluded that the maxillary first molars exhibit significant variation and that the operating microscope and CBCT were good methods to assess their internal anatomy. In a limited study by Matherne et al. (2008), 72 teeth were exposed with 2D digital radiographic detectors, and these images were evaluated by three endodontists. Comparing the evaluation with CBCT images analyzed by an oral and maxillofacial radiologist, the endodontists failed to identify one or more root canal systems in approximately 40% of the teeth.

Human teeth generally conform to specific morphometric patterns, but there are known variants that have a predilection among different racial groups, with mandibular premolars being the most difficult to treat endodontically (Slowey, 1979). In these cases, CBCT evaluations can be invaluable.

D. Additional roots

Human teeth have been extensively analyzed. Wide variations have been found in the root and root morphology, with many of these variations being dependent upon ethnicity (Michetti et al., 2010; Sert and Bayirli, 2004) and gender (Serman and Hasselgren, 1992). Using CBCT examinations, Wang et al. (2010) examined the root and canal morphology of 558 mandibular first permanent molars in a western Chinese population. Using Vertucci's criteria, they found that 51.4% had four canals and 25.8% had a separate distolingual root. In a study of 744 Taiwanese patients, Tu et al. (2009) evaluated 123 permanent mandibular first molars. They found that 33.33% of these teeth had an extra distolingual root that could affect the success of endodontic procedures. Compared to an earlier 2D study by Tu et al. (2007), only 21.1% and 26.9%, respectively, had three-rooted mandibular first molars. The apparent differences between their 2D and 3D findings could possibly be attributed to the failure to detect the third root by conventional radiographic techniques.

2. Differential diagnosis

A. Contradictory or nonspecific clinical signs and symptoms

Diagnosis and treatment of acute and chronic orofacial pain can be challenging because of the complex interrelationships of different structures in the head and neck region as well as the absence of pathologic alterations to implicate the cause of the pain. One of these conditions has been termed "phantom tooth pain," "atypical odontalgia," or "atypical facial pain," and more recently, "chronic continuous dentoalveolar pain (CCDAP)" by the Orofacial Pain Special Interest Group of the International Association for the Study of Pain (Green and Murray, 2011). The diagnostic hallmarks of this condition are (1) chronic, continuous pain (8 hours/day, ≥15 days per month or ≥3 months' duration); (2) pain localized in the dentoalveolar region; and (3) pain not caused by another disorder. These patients suffer from neuropathic pain, defined as pain as a result of a lesion or disease that affects the actual nerves that convey touch, pressure, pain, and temperature information to the brain (Figure 10.12; Treede et al., 2008). The pain is often reported after dental treatment, is considered not to be of questionable odontogenic origin, and may affect these patients' psychological well-being and quality of life (List et al., 2007).

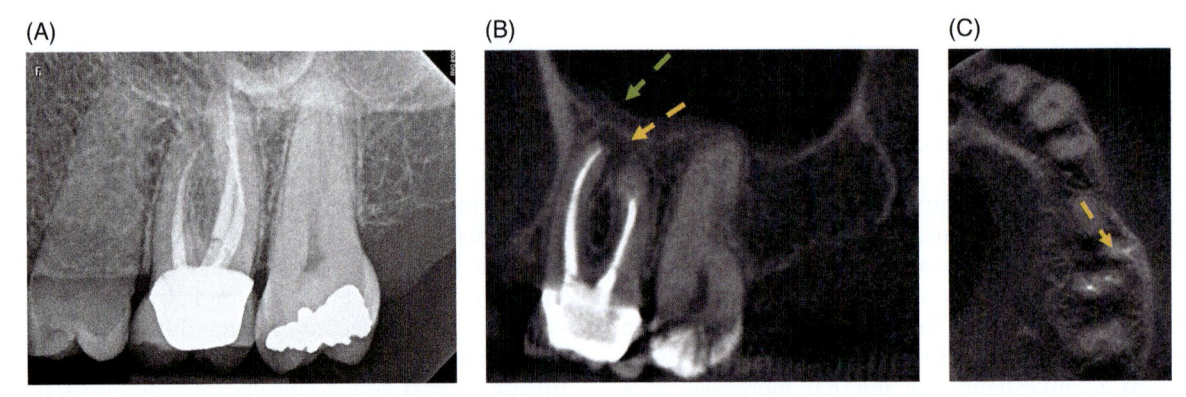

Figure 10.12 This 60-year-old female patient presented with a history of longstanding chronic discomfort in the area of the maxillary left first molar, exacerbated when her cheek touched her tooth, after a crown cementation procedure. Three subsequent crowns were placed by three different dentists to attempt to alleviate her symptoms. Finally, endodontic treatment was performed by others. No change in her symptoms was obtained. This author evaluated the patient and all objective tests were normal. A PA radiograph (A) was exposed and an anesthetic test with topical xylocaine applied in the vestibule greatly diminished her symptoms for 15 minutes, consistent with a diagnosis of peripherally mediated neuropathic pain. An LCBCT was then exposed to assess the teeth and supporting structures in the region. The scan volume was normal except for a periradicular radiolucency centered on the apex of the mesiobuccal root, shown in a corrected sagittal view (B) associated with a missed mb2 canal, shown on the corrected axial view (C), consistent with a periapical periodontitis or radicular cyst. The patient was referred to an oral pain specialist for consultation. A diagnosis of neuropathic pain, left maxilla, was confirmed. The treatment plan consisted of medical treatment of the neuropathic pain with subsequent treatment of the periapical lesion, which was not contributing to her symptoms. Instead of starting with a tricyclic, which is standard treatment, she opted for topical medications, ketamine, ketoprofen, and amitriptyline. Her symptoms have improved and she has since been changed to topically applied ketamine, gabapentin, and clonidine. Successful endodontic retreatment was then performed, but only the application of the topical medication continues to provide relief.

A high degree of specialization in dental medicine and taxonomic difficulties and uncertainties also can lead to errors. The best results may only be realized with an interdisciplinary approach to treatment (Rechenberg et al., 2011; Woda and Pionchon, 1999) including tomographic imaging. Difficulty in visualizing pathologic features using planar radiographic imaging has been supported by many studies. The use of CBCT is helpful in many of these cases, where periradicular radiolucency has not affected the cortical bone, or areas that do not show discontinuity of the periodontal membrane because of the superimposition of structures. The majority of patients with CCDAP had no pathologic findings.

It has been postulated that injuries to nerves after restorative or endodontic treatment can precipitate deafferentation of peripheral sensory neurons in the trigeminal nerve, leading to this pain condition. Sometimes a "neuroma" develops, allowing nerve impulses to fire off spontaneously in cases where all of the known noxious stimuli have been removed or have healed. The trigeminal ganglion and the trigeminal subnucleus caudalis can also become activated. Persistent pain is experienced by these patients without any identifiable causation, mimicking a toothache when in fact this is a manifestation of referred pain which involves neoplastic changes in the brain (Sessle et al., 2008; Greene, 2009). There is a great deal of overlap between the nociceptive pain symptoms of pulpitis, symptomatic AP, and CCDAP. These pain conditions are difficult to distinguish from one another and often rely on radiographic findings. CCDAP is a diagnosis by exclusion and requires the taking of a careful history, comprehensive examination, and planar and tomographic radiography. CBCT is an invaluable resource for definitively ruling out radiographic evidence of jaw lesions in these cases, where planar imaging may suffer from superimposition error. In a study reported by Pigg et al. (2011), 25 patients were evaluated with conventional radiography and CBCT. Of these cases, 20 patients presented with CCDAP of more than 6 months' duration after orthograde or surgical endodontic treatment, and 5 patients had symptomatic AP. The investigators concluded that CBCT improved the reliability of radiographic assessments, with 60% of patients with CCDAP showing no bony lesions detected with either conventional or CBCT examinations. In addition, CBCT showed 17% more periapical rarefactions than with conventional radiography.

Nonodontogenic pain can be caused by many other conditions; a partial list includes periodontalgia, myofascial pain, myalgia, TMJ, neurovascular pain, herpes zoster, maxillary sinusitis, pain of psychogenic origin, angina pectoris, myocardial infarction, temporal arteritis, neuralgias (e.g., peripheral and central), sialolithiasis, and neoplastic diseases. Planar and especially CBCT imaging modalities can be extremely useful in ruling out odontogenic causation.

B. Poorly localized symptoms associated with an untreated or previously endodontically treated tooth with no evidence of pathosis

Early diagnosis and management of patients with poorly localized or previously treated endodontic lesions in the absence of radiographic pathosis is necessary to alleviate nonspecific pain. Patient encounters should begin with a thorough review of the medical and dental history, chief complaint, and physical and radiographic examination. Diagnosis is frequently accomplished with adherence to basic principles of endodontic testing (Hyman and Cohen, 1984). A recent study by Newton et al. (2009) evaluated the value of all testing and imaging parameters used during endodontic diagnosis. Measuring the sensitivity, specificity, and predictive value of each method, they showed that while imaging was the most commonly used diagnostic procedure, interpretation of periradicular changes were considered unreliable. Since volumetric assessments of teeth and supporting structures have been shown to be useful even when conventional imaging is normal, the value of this technology cannot be underestimated.

C. Cases where anatomic superimposition of roots or areas of the maxillofacial skeleton hinders the performance of task-specific procedures

The identification of anatomic structures and the pathologic alterations associated with endodontic disease are an important benefit of using volumetric imaging (Estrela, Bueno, Sousa-Neto, et al., 2008). CBCT has been shown by Low et al. (2008) to be significantly more sensitive in detecting periapical lesions that extend into the maxillary sinus when compared to periapical and panoramic imaging. Using two examiners to evaluate 156 roots of maxillary posterior teeth that were referred for possible apical surgery, the CBCT images showed 34% more lesions compared to conventional periapical radiography. They concluded that periapical lesions were the most difficult to assess when associated with maxillary second molars and roots closest to the maxillary sinus. Especially useful when assessing multirooted teeth and teeth in the maxillary posterior, CBCT leads to a better understanding of the true nature of dentoalveolar pathoses, such as periapical disease, the location of fractures, and the characterization of resorptive lesions (Patel, 2009). Estrela, Bueno, Leles, et al. (2008) found that in a population of more than 1,500 teeth with endodontic disease, the prevalence of this pathosis visible on conventional radiographs was only 17%, with panoramic radiographs showing 35% and CBCT imaging showing 63%, suggesting that tomographic imaging is especially useful in the visualization of periradicular rarefactions and their relationship to individual roots.

Meaningful assessments of endodontic disease and associated comorbidities using planar imaging are difficult in the area of the maxillary sinus. The maxillary sinus is a pyramid-shaped area. It is the largest of the paranasal sinuses and the most likely to be affected by odontogenic pathoses. The floor of the maxillary sinus is formed by the alveolar process of the maxilla and is usually level with the floor of the nose. The proximity of the maxillary posterior teeth causes maxillary sinusitis in approximately 10% to 12% of all cases of sinusitis (Malokey and Doku, 1968). Misdiagnosis of maxillary sinusitis caused by odontogenic disease is well known, the basis of which is thought to be related to the innervation provided to the mucus membranes by the postganglionic parasympathetic nerve originating from the greater petrosal nerve (a branch of the facial nerve) and its proximity to the superior alveolar (anterior, middle, and posterior) nerves, branches of the maxillary nerve (Cymerman et al., 2011; Hassan et al., 2009; Yuan et al., 2009).

D. Nonodontogenic and odontogenic lesions

The use of CBCT for the assessment of nonodontogenic lesions is an extensive area of interest. There are many pathologic alterations that appear in the proximity of the teeth that require differentiation from endodontic pathoses in order to reach an accurate diagnosis and proper treatment plan. The differential diagnosis depends on a careful history and examination that must include pulp vitality testing as well as periodontal and radiographic evaluations. Careful analysis is necessary to distinguish endodontic conditions from nonodontogenic pathoses. It requires a thorough understanding of the pathogenesis of diseases that affect the oral cavity and a vigilant radiographic interpretation of the often confusing conditions listed below.

Nonodontogenic

- **Cysts, nonodontogenic**: aneurysmal bone cyst, nasopalatine duct cyst, nasolabial cyst, simple bone cyst (traumatic)
- **Fibro-osseous lesions**: periapical cemental dysplasia, florid cemento-osseous dysplasia, cemento-ossifying fibroma, fibrous dysplasia
- **Neoplasm, benign, nonodontogenic**: central hemangioma, osteoid osteoma, osteoblastoma, osteoma, nerve sheath tumor, neurofibromatosis type I, desmoplastic fibroma
- **Neoplasm, malignant, nonodontogenic**: metastasis, osteosarcoma chondrosarcoma, primary intraosseous carcinoma, central mucoepidermoid carcinoma, Burkitt lymphoma, non-Hodgkin lymphoma, multiple myeloma, Ewing sarcoma, leukemia
- **Tumorlike lesions**: central giant cell granuloma, Langerhans histiocytosis

Odontogenic

- **Cysts**: dentigerous cyst, lateral periodontal cyst, residual cyst, buccal bifurcation cyst
- **Neoplasm, benign**: odontoma, adenomatoid odontogenic tumor, ameloblastoma, ameloblastic fibroma, ameloblastic fibro-odontoma, calcifying epithelial odontogenic tumor, calcifying cystic odontogenic tumor, cementoblastoma,

odontogenic myxoma, central odontogenic fibroma, keratocystic odontogenic tumor, basal cell nevus syndrome
- **Neoplasm, malignant**: malignant ameloblastoma, ameloblastic carcinoma

The assessment and possible treatment of odontogenic and nonodontogenic radiolucent lesions of the teeth and supporting structures often require different management strategies. Endodontic treatment or retreatment depends on the accurate assessment of periapical radiographs. For example, the superimposition of the incisive foramen or a nasopalatine duct cyst can lead to unnecessary or delayed treatment, since they may simulate periapical pathosis. Confounding the difficulty in accurate assessment of the nasopalatine region is the substantial variation of the nasopalatine duct and its associated foramina. When 2D and 2D/3D observational strategies were compared by Mraiwa et al. (2004), interpretation of the canal morphology was significantly different, and there was important variation in morphology and dimensions. Endodontic assessment of the maxillary central incisors using only conventional radiography is compounded by the projection of the upper openings of the incisive canal onto the apices of the maxillary central incisors. Most incisive canals have two foramina superiorly and exit in one foramen inferiorly (Song et al., 2009). Cases of up to six foramina, variously called the foramina of Scarpa and Stensen (Langland et al., 2002), have been described, leading to superimposition error especially in cases resulting from a low nasal fossa and high angulation (Sicher, 1962).

The nasopalatine duct cyst (NPDC), when present, is in close association with the apices of the maxillary central incisors, leading to difficulty in establishing an accurate diagnosis with conventional imaging alone, especially when the central incisors have been endodontically treated or a preoperative endodontic diagnosis is unavailable. NPDC, the most common nonodontogenic cyst, is a unilocular, rounded corticated lucent lesion in the midline maxilla arising from the spontaneous proliferation of epithelial remnants of the nasopalatine duct. It is usually an asymptomatic incidental finding but can cause pain and swelling. NPDC must be differentiated from a large nasopalatine foramen, AP or radicular cyst arising from a tooth with a necrotic pulp, residual cyst, central giant cell granuloma, keratocystic odontogenic tumor, and dentigerous cyst to affect proper treatment (Faitaroni et al., 2011).

E. Endodontic assessment of nonhealed cases

AP results from inflammation of periapical alveolar bone and is opposed by the host's attempt to prevent enlargement. After endodontic treatment, success is measured by the absence of symptoms, normal objective tests, and periapical radiographic confirmation of healing. Most teeth with AP demonstrate healing after orthograde endodontic treatment, but AP may persist after treatment, appear after treatment, or reemerge after having healed (Vieira et al., 2011). Measuring endodontic healing using 2D radiographic assessments has been shown to be inconsistent (Figure 10.13; Goldman et al., 1974; Zakariasen et al., 1984), even when two PAs are exposed from different angles (Soğur et al., 2012). Wound healing after nonsurgical and surgical endodontic therapy is similar, but postsurgical healing is faster (Kvist and Reit, 1991). In nonsurgical endodontic therapy, macrophages remove bacteria, necrotic cells, and tissue debris through biologic processes, whereas surgical debridement removes these inflammatory irritants during the operative procedure (Lin et al., 1996). Ng et al. (2007) found that only 57% of outcome studies evaluated showed both clinical and radiographic healing. The remaining 43% of the reports were measured by radiographic examination alone. According to M.K. Wu et al. (2009), in many of these studies, published as recently as 2008, no limitations of periapical radiography were disclosed. CBCT and histologic (Brynolf, 1967) assessments of these findings have called this methodology into question. Teeth in different anatomical positions may have variations in cortical bone thickness. In addition, the location of the root apex of certain teeth may vary as to its distance to the junction of the cancellous and cortical bone, resulting in variations in lesion visibility as detected in conventional radiography (Figure 10.14). To some extent, this may invalidate some of the objective findings as seen in conventional periapical radiography as a consistent means of measuring AP. Paula-Silva

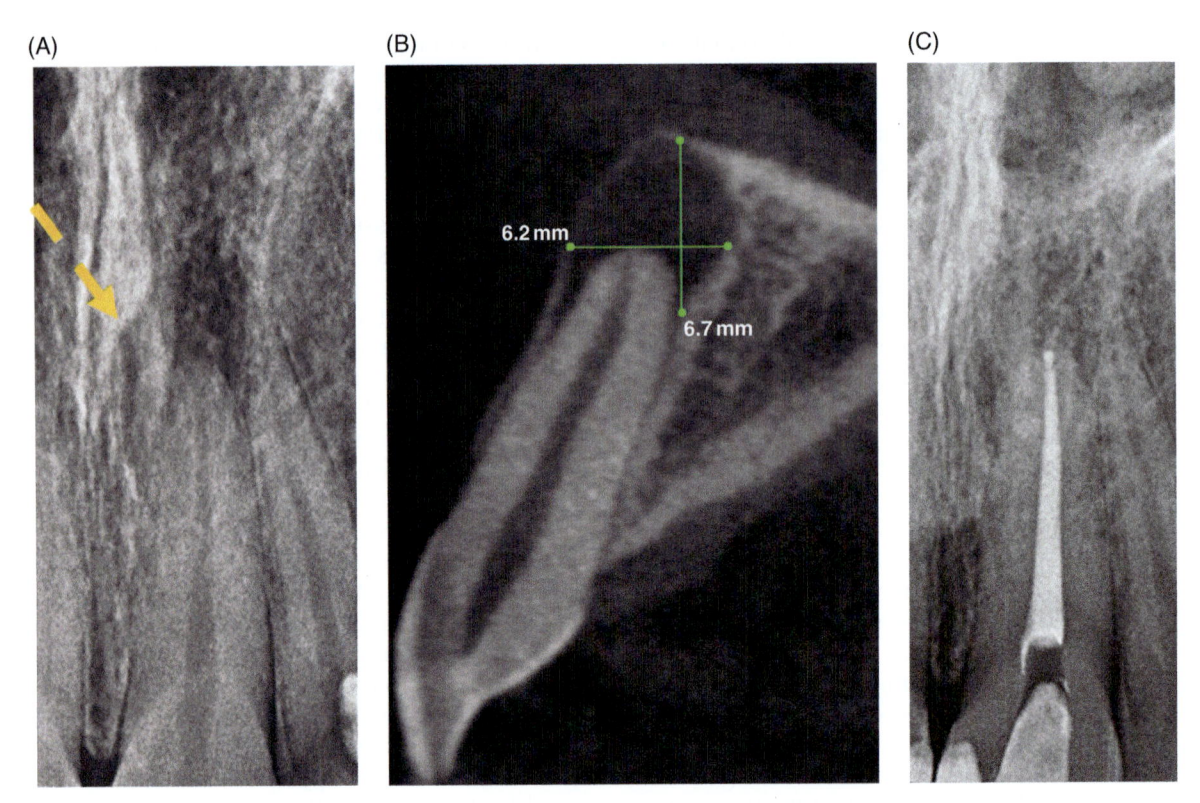

Figure 10.13 This 32-year-old female patient presented for evaluation and possible treatment 6 weeks after trauma to her maxillary left central incisor. The tooth was sensitive to percussion and palpation at the periapical area, was nonresponsive to thermal tests, and showed significant mobility. The periodontal findings were normal and the patient's medical history was noncontributory. The initial PA radiograph (A, portion of PA), showed a periapical periodontitis (yellow arrow) consistent with a periapical abscess. An LCBCT (B) was exposed to rule out a root and/or alveolar fracture possibly associated with the acute trauma suffered. It showed an approximately 6-mm diameter, well-defined periapical radiolucency with noncorticated border, with the lesion centered over the apex, consistent with a periapical abscess or radicular cyst. The maxillary left central incisor was endodontically treated and a postobturation PA radiograph was exposed. (C) On check-up examination after 3 months, the patient complained of sensitivity to chewing and touch associated with the same tooth. It was sensitive to percussion and bite stick, and was in hyper-occlusion.

et al. (2009) used histological evaluation as the criterion standard to evaluate the predictive value of CBCT scans for diagnosing AP. They found that whenever a histologic lesion was detected by either periapical or CBCT imaging, inflammation was present. Periapical radiography detected AP in 71% of roots, CBCT detected AP in 84% of roots, and histologic examination detected AP in 93% of roots.

Progression and regression of AP can be difficult to interpret. Healing is defined as the complete cessation of symptoms clinically and elimination of any radiographic radiolucency. The presence of an "apical scar" is rare in cases of orthograde endodontic treatment but is more common in cases after surgery, especially in the maxillary anterior region (Molven et al., 1987). It has also been seen that teeth showing a condensing osteitis or sclerotic bone before endodontic treatment will return to a normal bone appearance or not progress after endodontic treatment (Eliasson et al., 1984).

F. Vertical root fracture

Most root fracture cases fall into two main categories, vertical root fractures usually associated with chronic trauma caused by normal function, and horizontal root fractures usually associated with acute trauma

(D) (E) (F)

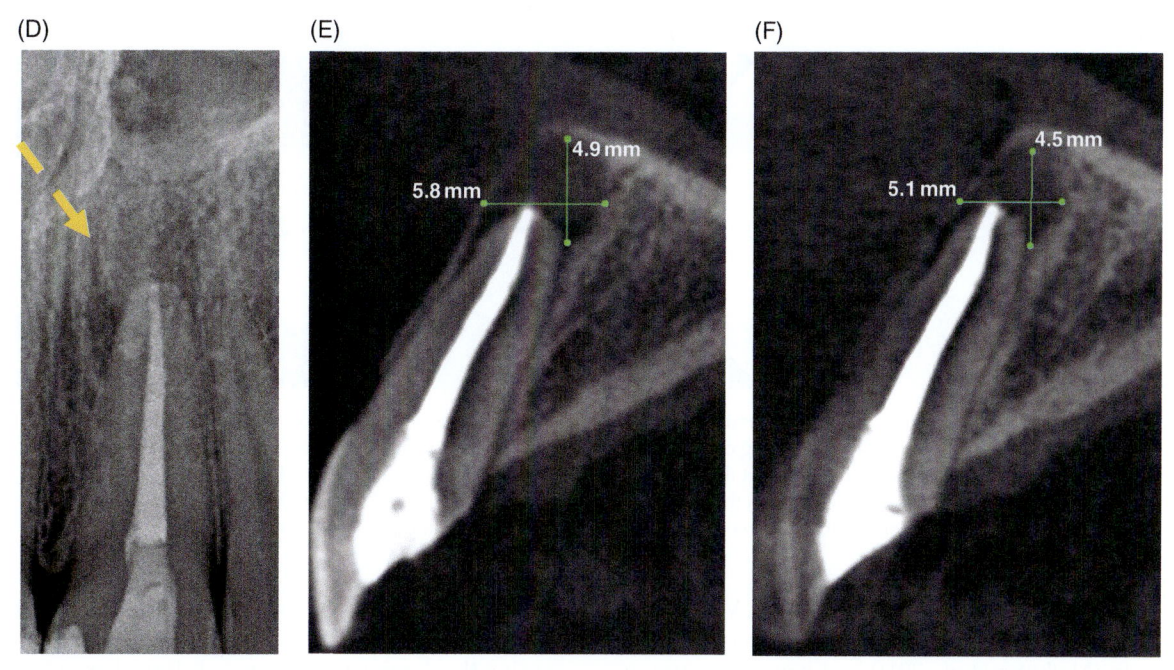

4.9 mm
5.8 mm

4.5 mm
5.1 mm

Figure 10.13 (*Continued*) A PA radiograph was exposed (D, portion of PA), showing a possible increase in lesion size (yellow arrow). An LCBCT (E, F) was then exposed, showing a reduction of the lesion size, consistent with healing. Another LCBCT was exposed at a 6-month check-up appointment (F), showing a lesion approximately 4.5–5 mm in diameter, consistent with healing.

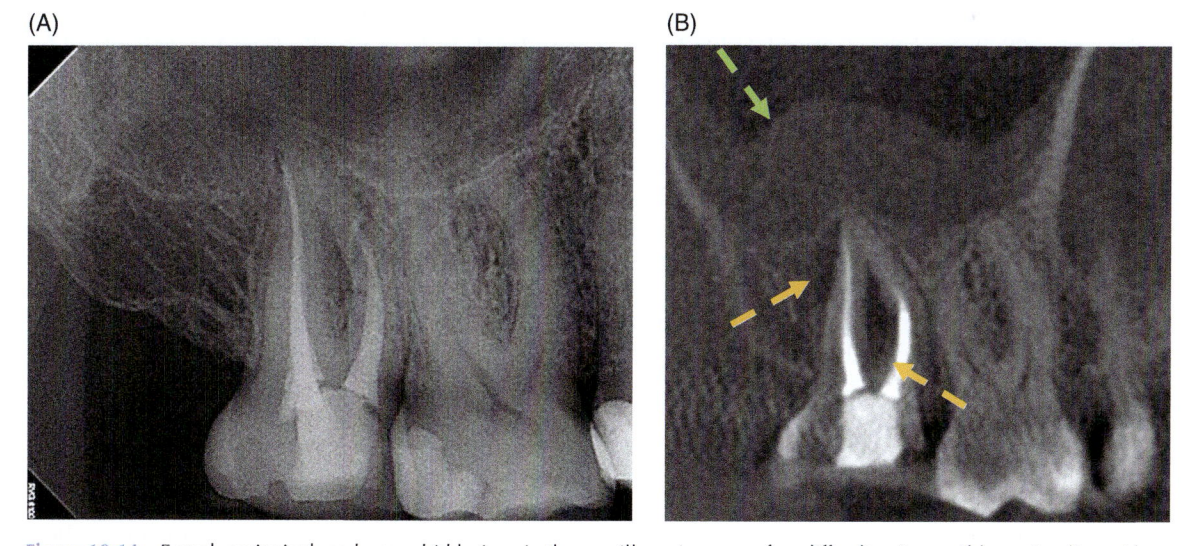

(A) (B)

Figure 10.14 Furcal, periapical, and comorbid lesions in the maxillary sinus are often difficult or impossible to visualize with PA radiography alone. In this endodontically treated maxillary right second molar, the PA image shows a short obturation in the mesial root along with a widened periodontal membrane at the terminus of the palatal root (A). This sagittal section (B) through the same region clearly shows the periradicular periodontitis affecting the furcal and periapical areas (yellow arrows), as well as a moderate mucositis possibly associated with this periradicular lesion (green arrow).

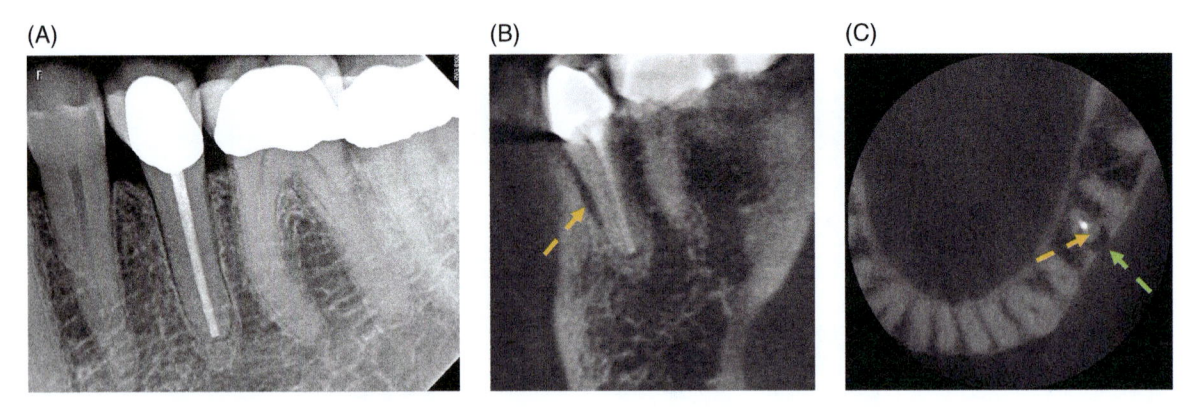

Figure 10.15 This symptomatic, vertically fractured mandibular left second bicuspid did not show a fracture on the PA radiograph (A), nor transillumination or staining of the exposed portion of the root, and probed normally upon periodontal examination. There was a condensing osteitis at the periapex that measured approximately 6 mm. LCBCT imaging, sagittal view, showed a vertical radiolucency extending from the crest of the alveolus to the junction of the middle and apical third of the root (B), and a periradicular periodontitis (C, green arrow) bisected by the vertical fracture (yellow arrow).

to anterior teeth, most often in children. Vertical root fractures (VRF) involve the dentin, cementum, and pulp (Malhotra et al., 2011) and have an enormous impact on treatment outcome (Figure 10.15). There have been a number of systematic reviews on the detection of vertical root fractures using CBCT, seven of which were laboratory studies using extracted teeth. These studies showed a significantly higher diagnostic accuracy with CBCT when compared with PA radiography. These results were tempered by lower sensitivity and specificity related to lower resolution scans and artifact generated by the presence of root fillings and posts.

Patients may present with pain and swelling, radiographic evidence of a periapical and lateral radiolucency, or the presence of a deep isolated periodontal defect in an area of otherwise normal findings. Unfortunately, diagnosis of root fracture is challenging because the signs and symptoms are not pathognomonic. The criterion standard is visualization of the fracture, either directly or with transillumination and/or staining with dye and lighted magnification (Edlund et al., 2011). But the diagnosis of VRF can present significant challenges because there is often a lack of specific signs, symptoms, or radiographic findings. VRFs have the highest prevalence in the 40–60-year-old age group, and the teeth most often affected are mandibular molars and maxillary premolars (Cohen et al., 2006).

The usefulness of LCBCT to assess root fractures has been detailed by multiple reports. A search of the current literature by Tsesis et al. (2010) showed that there is very little evidence-based data concerning the diagnostic accuracy of clinical or radiographic studies in endodontically treated teeth. They concluded that the determination of a VRF is more of a "prediction" than an absolute diagnosis. VRFs can be incomplete or complete and extend through the long axis of the tooth toward the apex. Vertical root fractures comprise between 2% and 5% of crown/root fractures, can affect the root at any level, and are usually found in patients older than 40 years (Cohen et al., 2003). Mesiodistal fractures are rarely visualized with 2D radiographs because the X-ray beam must be within 4 degrees of the fracture plane to allow detection (Rud and Omnell, 1970). Hassan et al. (2009) reported that the accuracy of detecting VRFs was higher for CBCT than PAs, and that the reconstructed axial view was the most accurate (Kajan and Taromsari, 2012). In this investigation, 80 teeth were endodontically prepared and divided into artificially fractured and unfractured groups; each group was further divided into root-filled teeth and non-root-filled teeth. Four observers found that the sensitivity and specificity for VRF was 79.4% and 92.5% for CBCT and 37.1% and 95% for conventional radiography, respectively. The specificity of CBCT was reduced by the presence of endodontic filling, but accuracy was not reduced. The sensitivity and accuracy of PAs were reduced by the presence of root canal filling. In a 5-year follow-up study by Chen et al. (2008), 32.1% of nonsurgically endodontically treated teeth that were extracted suffered from vertical root fracture. In a study that examined 46,000 insurance claims, Fennis et al. (2002) showed that endodontically treated teeth had a higher incidence of VRF than nontreated teeth. Tang et al. (2010) suggested that endodontically treated teeth may undergo an increased incidence of VFR because of loss of tooth structure, stresses induced by endodontic and restorative procedures, access preparation, instrumentation and obturation of the root canal, post space preparation, and abutment selection. In a recent study by Mireku et al. (2010), 45 single-rooted teeth were endodontically treated, prepared for posts, and subjected to cyclic loading until fracture. They concluded that VRFs were most likely to occur in teeth with thin dentin and in teeth of older patients. CBCT has also been found to improve the diagnostic accuracy of detecting transverse or horizontal fractures.

LFOV with higher resolution have been shown to provide higher sensitivity and specificity when endodontic lesions are assessed, which may translate to better assessments of VRFs (Edlund et al., 2011; Liang et al., 2010). Many of the studies performed to date using CBCT imaging have relied on resolutions greater than 0.20 mm (200 microns) voxel size, which is more than two times larger than the lowest voxel size available today, 0.076 mm (76 microns). Voxel size is not the sole determinant of the resolving power of a scan, because the signal-to-noise ratio, bit depth, and other complex issues are also important factors. In a study authored by Özer (2011), 30 teeth with VRF and 30 teeth without VRF were examined using several voxel sizes to compare the diagnostic accuracy of CBCT scans with different voxel resolutions. Of the 0.125, 0.20, 0.30, and 0.40 mm voxel sizes, the 0.20 mm voxel size was deemed the best. The article does not specify the smallest native voxel size of the CBCT unit, leading to the possibility that 0.125 mm voxel size or smaller could provide for the best detection of VRFs. According to Hassan et al. (2010), the detection of VRFs using CBCT was better with the smaller voxel sizes studied. In cases of suspected VRF, Wenzel et al. (2009) compared a photostimulable storage phosphor plate system with CBCT and found that CBCT was more accurate, leading to the recommendation that CBCT scans be used when VRFs cannot be visualized but are suspected.

3. Intra- or postoperative assessment of complications

Instrument separation can occur at any stage of endodontic treatment, and in any canal location. In a study of 2,654 teeth with 6,154 canals treated at the Nanjing Medical University in Jiangsu, China, J. Wu et al. (2011) reported that the overall incidence of instrument separation was 1.1%, with molars having the highest incidence. The ability to triangulate and remove the separated instrument can sometimes depend on visualization of the position of the instrument, the likelihood of removal, and whether the instrument poses an impediment to healing or not. When a separated instrument that is lodged in the apical third of a root canal, the chances of retrieval are the lowest (Gencoglu and Helvacioglu, 2009), and assessment of canals that anastomose at the apical terminus may be adequately sealed by a treatment of the joining canal. CBCT has been used by this author to assess the location of separated instruments in cases referred for revision treatment (Figure 10.16), and to provide more reliable assessment of treatment options.

A. Calcified canal identification

The number of elderly patients in the U.S. population is rising, with 10,000 Americans reaching the age of 65 every day until 2030. This aging cohort of Americans makes up 26% of the total U.S. population (Pew Research Center, 2010) and will continue to want to preserve their dentition (Qualtrough and Mannocci, 2011). Geriatric patients will present challenges for dental clinicians as biologic and anatomic conditions are considered, including narrower canals (Goodis et al., 2001). Assessment and treatment of calcified canals can be assisted by the use of CBCT. Perioperatively, the location of calcified canals can be more precisely located with CBCT (Scarfe et al., 2009) and may help correct an off-course access to prevent root perforation. All multiplanar views may be helpful in the process of triangulation, with the application of a radiodense

(A) (B) (C) (D)

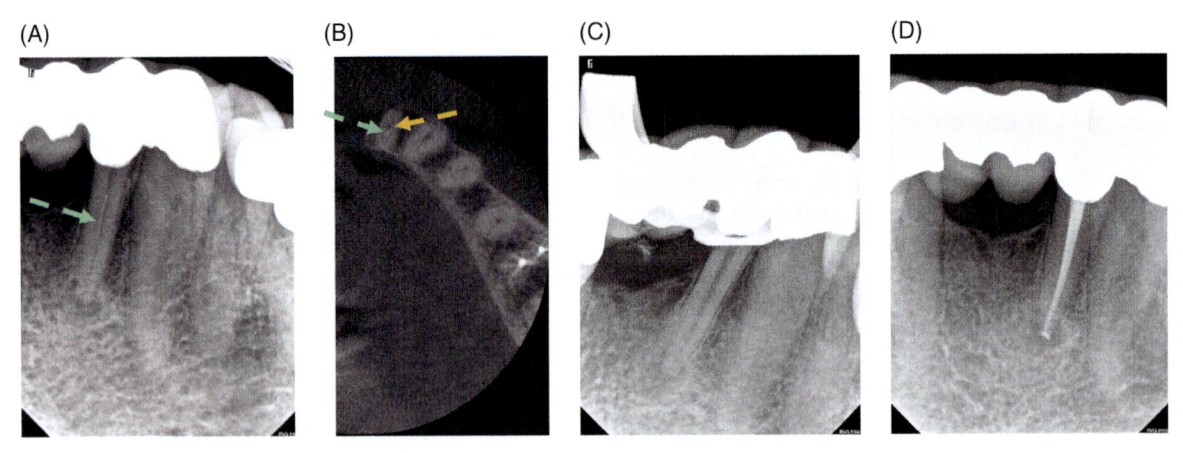

Figure 10.16 This 62-year-old female patient was referred for endodontic revision of the mandibular left lateral incisor after a periradicular lesion and separated instrument were revealed on a routine PA radiograph (A). An LCBCT was exposed, and the separated instrument (green arrow) was localized at the lingual aspect of the ribbon-shaped canal on the axial view (B). A bypass strategy (yellow arrow) to engage and elevate the separated instrument was successfully adopted, followed by routine biomechanical preparation and obturation. A PA was then exposed to verify the instrument removal (C) and assess endodontic treatment (D).

instrument or gutta percha cone used as an indicator to help triangulate.

B. Localization of perforations

Iatrogenic root perforations may be caused by a post or fractured instrument, and are often difficult to localize with conventional imaging. While PAs do not provide information concerning the buccolingual dimension, LCBCT allows the three-dimensional examination of the perforation (Young, 2007; Tsurumachi and Honda, 2007). Streaking, flare, and cupping artifacts resulting from root canal obturation and restorative materials, such as gutta percha, posts, and perforative repair materials, present challenges to the interpretation of root integrity. An approach advocated by Bueno et al. (2011) suggested that map-reading strategy of viewing sequential axial slices reduces the beam hardening effect. Newer root canal obturation materials may present lower streaking, flare, and cupping artifacts by virtue of a lower radiopacity profile.

4. Dentoalveolar trauma

Facial trauma results in dental injuries in approximately 48% of all traumatic injuries, with the male-to-female ratio associated with work-related injuries being 10:1 and violence being 8:1, respectively. Epidemiologic data suggests that facial trauma is common, with the dentition affected in 57.8% in household and play accidents, 50.5% in sports accidents, 38.6% in work-related accidents, 35.8% in acts of violence, 34.2% in traffic accidents, and 31% unspecified (Gassner et al., 1999).

Injuries to the orofacial complex can cause dental trauma resulting in the following injuries to the primary and permanent dentition: (1) infraction; (2) crown fracture, uncomplicated and complicated; (3) crown/root fracture; (4) root fracture; (5) concussion; (6) subluxation; (7) lateral luxation; (8) intrusion; (9) extrusion; and (10) avulsion. The extent of injury requires a systematic approach that evaluates the teeth, periodontium, and associated structures (Figure 10.17; Andreasen and Andreasen, 2000). A study by Wang et al. (2011) showed that the sensitivity and specificity of root fractures for PA radiography was 26.3% and 100%, respectively, whereas CBCT was 89.5% and 97.5%, respectively. CBCT images of root-filled teeth showed lower sensitivity and unchanged specificity, whereas 2D images showed the same sensitivity and specificity.

Triangulating the exact position of teeth displaced by dental trauma and the extent of root and alveolar fractures, if any, is difficult to accomplish using 2D imaging modalities alone (Figure 10.18). Additional complications include damage to other

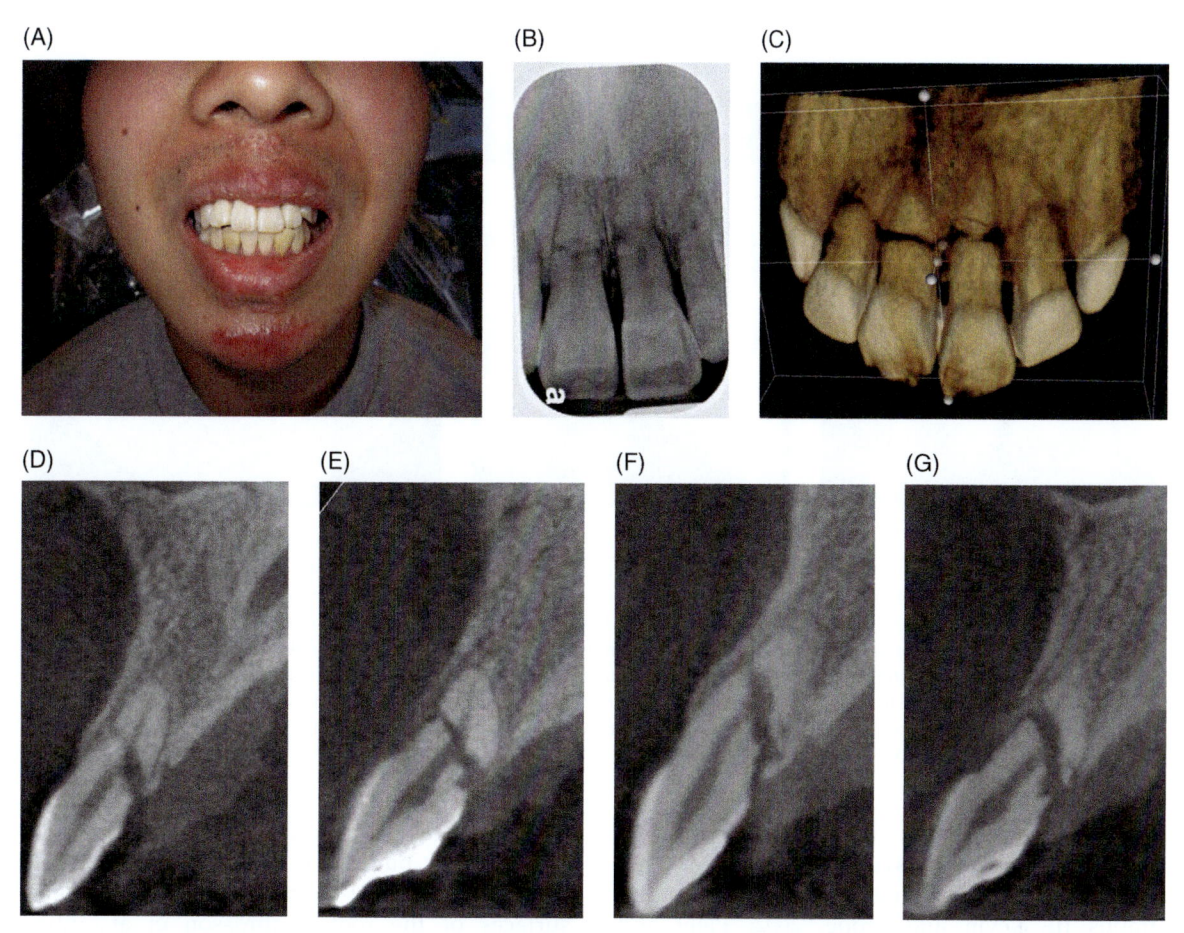

Figure 10.17 This 22 year old patient (A) was referred for evaluation and possible treatment nine months after the patient suffered horizontal root fractures to the maxillary lateral and central incisors as a result of a bicycle accident, shown in this accompanying film-based PA radiograph (B). A polyethylene splint was placed immediately after the accident, and the teeth remained asymptomatic, responded normally to pulp vitality testing, and the crowns remained normal in color. There is minimal mobility and normal periodontal probing. Each of the root-fractured teeth can be accurately monitored for future changes as a result of LCBCT assessment (C, cropped reconstructed view; D, the maxillary right lateral incisor; E, the maxillary right central incisor; F, the maxillary left central incisor; and G, the maxillary left lateral incisor).

perioral structures, such as the maxillary sinuses and nasal floor.

5. Resorption

Root resorption (RR) results in the loss of hard tissues from the action of multinucleated giant cells on teeth. In the primary dentition, RR is a normal physiologic process, except where resorption is premature, allowing the secondary dentition to erupt and enter function. Permanent teeth undergo RR in response to inflammation, but the exact mechanism remains unclear. RR is caused by orthodontic treatment, trauma, AP, neoplasia, or other factors that are considered a pathologic occurrence (Estrela et al., 2009; Cohenca et al., 2007). Types of root resorption are repair-related (surface), ankylosis-related (osseous replacement), infection-related (inflammatory), and extracanal invasive cervical resorption. Each of these forms of RR has a poor prognosis if the causative lesion is not treated (Patel et al., 2009).

Internal root resorption (IRR) is a relatively rare occurrence, characterized by structural changes of

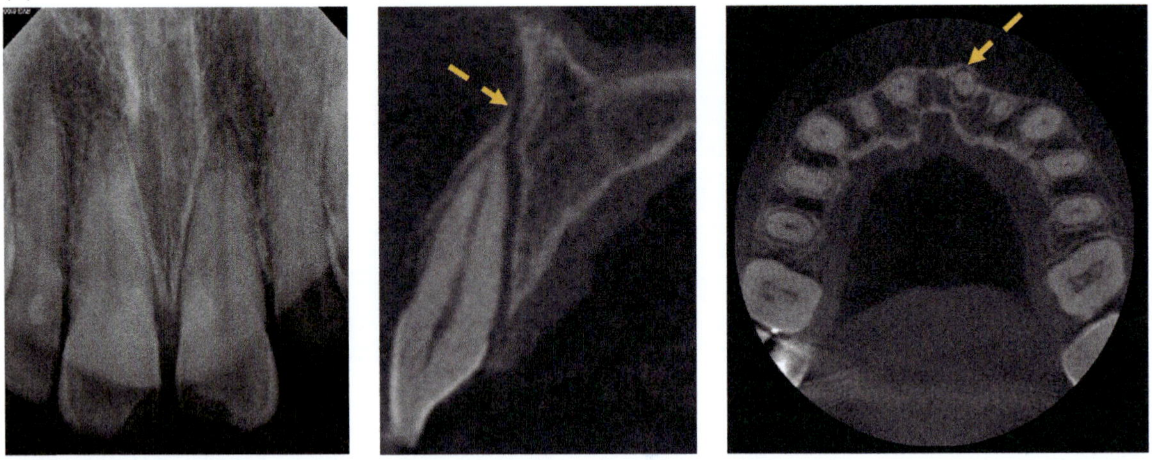

Figure 10.18 This patient was referred for evaluation and possible treatment of a lateral luxation injury to the maxillary left and right central incisors and maxillary left lateral incisor. A PA radiograph (A) was exposed, showing a periapical rarefaction and a Class II crown fracture at the maxillary left central incisor. There were Class II crown fractures on the maxillary right and left lateral incisors with normal responses to pulp testing. The maxillary left central incisor showed significant mobility consistent with a root and/or alveolar fracture. An LCBCT was exposed, showing labial displacement and widened periodontal membrane space of the maxillary left central incisor in the corrected sagittal (B) and axial views (C), consistent with a traumatic fracture of the alveolus in this region. There was a vertical alveolar fracture at the periapex (yellow arrow) through the facial cortical plate and nutrient channel leading to the root canal. The axial view confirms the displacement to the facial. (Courtesy, Dr. Anastasia Mischenko, Chevy Chase, MD)

the tooth that appear as a widening of the root canal. IRR is usually asymptomatic and is often detected on routine periapical and panoramic radiographs (L. Levin and Trope, 2002; Patel and Dawood, 2007). The pulp is nonvital in the area where the resorption is inactive and is vital or partially vital in the areas where the resorption is continuing, apical to the resorptive lesion. A uniform radiolucent enlargement of the pulp canal will include some part of the canal space, cause extensive destruction of the dentin, and will be filled with granulation tissue alone or in combination with mineralized tissues (Lyroudia et al., 2002).

External root resorption (ERR) results from the inflammatory response to mechanical damage to the attachment of a tooth, and is always associated with bony resorption (Figure 10.19). Differentiation between IRR and ERR is challenging, even with multiple changes in X-ray angulation. ERR can be classified as surface resorption, external inflammatory resorption, external replacement resorption, external cervical resorption, and transient apical breakdown (Patel and Ford, 2007). Difficult to view with conventional radiography, the early stages of ERR will sometimes be visible on the mesial and distal surfaces of roots, but ERR is unlikely to be visualized when it affects only the buccal, palatal, or lingual surfaces of the root (Sigurdsson et al., 2011). According to a study by Estrela et al. (2009), 48 periapical radiographs and CBCT scans were exposed on 40 patients. IRR was detected in 68.8% of periapical radiographs while CBCT scans showed 100% of the lesions. Conventional radiographs were only able to detect lesions between 1 mm and 4 mm in 52.1% of the images, whereas 95.8% of the lesions were detectable with CBCT. They concluded that using CBCT technology allowed more accurate and earlier detection of IRR. This finding was in agreement with other studies (Cohenca et al., 2007; Liedke et al., 2009) and demonstrates the value of tomographic analysis. In a study by Kim et al. (2003), the extent and location of the IRR was accurately reproduced with the fabrication of a rapid prototyping tooth model.

Voxel size is also an important factor that affects detection of RR. In a study by Liedke et al. (2009) different voxel resolutions were evaluated to detect simulated RR. The results showed that the smaller

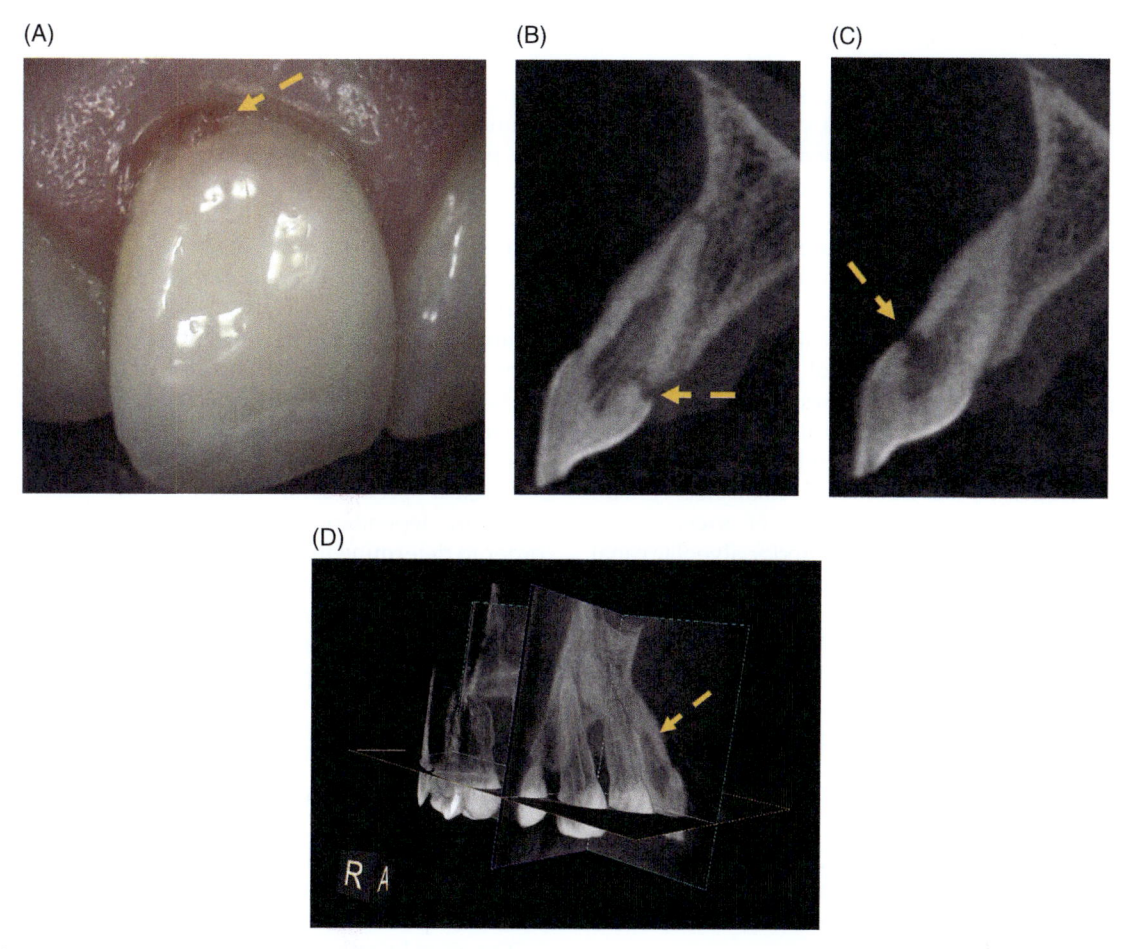

Figure 10.19 Extracanal cervical resorption resulted in a perforative defect at the facial aspect of this maxillary right central incisor (A). Corrected sagittal views of the palatal and facial lesions showing the sparing of the peritubular dentin are apparent in these images (B, C). A semitransparent reconstructed view shows the true extent of the lesion (D).

voxel resolutions were better than the larger voxel resolutions. While voxel size is an important consideration, the signal-to-noise ratio of different detectors and the processing algorithms also affect detection probability. While many in vitro studies on the ability of CBCT to detect RR have been performed, additional evaluations that use in vivo methodology will add to our knowledge.

6. Presurgical case planning

The introduction of CBCT imaging has greatly improved our understanding of the relationships of teeth, their associated pathoses, and important anatomic features such as the antra, mandibular canal, mental foramen, and lingual artery have a significant impact on surgical treatment planning. In surgical case assessments, the interpretation of planar images are limited by complex background patterns so often present in the maxillofacial skeleton.

When the detection of periradicular lesions with PA radiography was compared with CBCT imaging, Lofthag-Hansen et al. (2007) found 38% more lesions, even after PAs were exposed at two different angles. Low et al. (2008) and Bornstein et al. (2011) further highlighted the limitations of PA imaging by finding that 34% and 25.9%, respectively, of periradicular lesions were only detected with CBCT imaging. When PAs of periradicular lesions were compared to sagittal and coronal CBCT images, the PAs were statistically smaller than their CBCT counterparts, causing an underestimation of the true size of the defects.

Surgery requires precise treatment planning and safe operative procedures, especially when significant anatomical structures are at risk. Injury to the inferior alveolar nerve resulting from surgical complications such as mechanical injury including compression, stretching, laceration, and partial or total resection is not rare (Figure 10.20). Wesson and Gale (2003) showed that between 20% and 21% of patients suffered temporary neuropathies of the lower lip after endodontic surgery in the vicinity of the inferior alveolar nerve, with permanent issues occurring in 1% of cases.

The inability to detect the inferior alveolar canal with PA and panoramic radiography alone has been reported in numerous studies. Velvart et al. (2001) and Bornstein et al. (2011) showed that the inferior alveolar nerve canal could only be identified in 62.0% of 50 cases and 35.3% of 68 cases assessed with PA radiography, respectively. Angelopoulos et al. (2008) looked at 40 cases, in each comparing CBCT reformatted panoramic, direct digital panoramic, and storage phosphor panoramic radiographs. CBCT reformatted panoramic images were superior to the other two modalities and were free from magnification and superimposition error.

Understanding the relationship between the apex of the mandibular posterior teeth and the roof of the inferior alveolar nerve is complicated by the fact that the nerve canal, lined by cribiform bone, is only visible in 64.7% of PA radiographs. Access to the apices of mandibular molars is challenging because the mean cortical bone thickness is 1.7 mm and the mean access distance from the surface of the buccal plate to the apices of the teeth is 5.3 mm (Borstein et al., 2011).

The relationship of teeth, their associated pathoses, and important anatomic features such as the maxillary sinus, mandibular canal, and mental foramen have significant impact on surgical treatment planning. CBCT images provide unmatched visualization of these complex structures, so that each procedure can be planned appropriately. CBCT is also a great asset for determining the extent of postoperative healing. Because CBCT voxels are isotropic, image data can be sectioned nonorthogonally, allowing multiplanar reformations that allow the clinician to visualize tissue boundaries and accurately assess discontinuities in the periodontal membrane without superimposition. Christiansen et al. (2009) evaluated 58 teeth one week and one year after apical surgery for assessing healing in root-filled teeth. They found that more periapical bone defects were detected after one year on CBCT images than on periapical radiographs. While they did not attempt to measure how this information would impact success or failure, it was clear that CBCT imaging was superior to conventional imaging for the presence of AP.

Surgical procedures, especially on posterior teeth, are dependent on a thorough preparation in order to determine the thickness of the cortical and cancellous bone, the location of the roots within the bone, and the root morphology and inclination (Patel et al., 2007). Identifying and excluding cases with an unfavorable prognosis can reduce the risk for iatrogenic injury. Anterior teeth are not exempt from consideration of their proximity to important anatomic structures. Taschieri et al. (2011) evaluated 57 maxillary central and lateral incisors with CBCT imaging and found that the average central incisor measured 4.71 ± 1.26 mm from the anterior wall of the nasopalatine duct at a level of 4 mm from the apex.

The exact location of the palatal roots of the maxillary first and second molars are also difficult to visualize in the buccopalatal direction with periapical radiographs alone. An examination of the palatal roots of 100 extracted maxillary first and second permanent molars showed that 85% curved more than 10 degrees (Bone and Moule, 1986). The proximity of the root apices to the nasal floor and the inferior border of the maxillary sinus depth and the location of the palatal vault also play a role in determining surgical access.

The surgical management of overextensions of obturation materials and repair of perforating defects is another area where LCBCT can play an important adjunctive role (Shemesh et al., 2011; Bhuva et al., 2011). The overextension of root canal obturation materials that results in damage to the inferior alveolar nerve or mental nerve is an infrequent complication of endodontic treatment. Injury may occur from mechanical impingement or

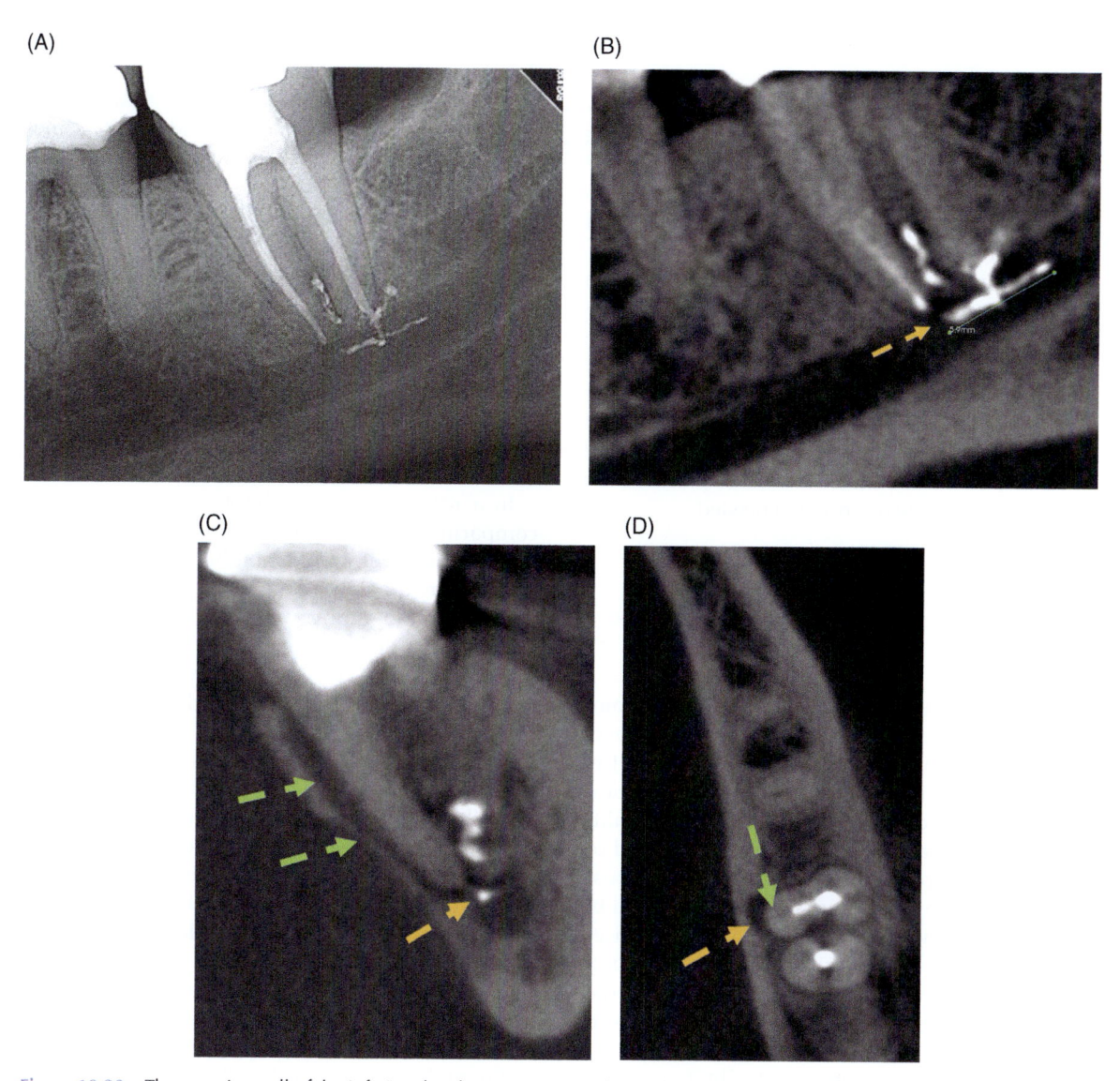

Figure 10.20 The superior wall of the inferior alveolar nerve (IAN) is located only 1.11 mm from the radiographic apex of the distal root of the mandibular second molar. This proximity and the somewhat porous nature of the cribiform bone lining the canal can lead to impingement of the IAN due to inadvertent overextension of obturation material, as shown in this PA image (A) of a 58-year-old male patient who was referred for evaluation and possible treatment. The dental history included a transient parasthesia IAN, shown in these corrected sagittal (B), coronal (C) and axial (D) views. The errant material was localized with LCBCT imaging (yellow arrows). Subsequent extraction was accomplished due to a periradicular periodontitis that extended from the apex of the root on the lingual (green arrows). Localization of the errant material and subsequent treatment plan choices were elucidated by LCBCT.

chemical effects (Escoda-Francoli et al., 2007) and can be localized and in some cases removed by surgical intervention. In an early case report using CBCT, Tsuramachi and Honda (2007) described the triangulation of a tooth with a fractured instrument that extended into the maxillary sinus. Since obturation materials extending into the maxillary sinus can promote sinusitis (Rud and Rud, 1998), their judicious removal can prevent associated comorbidities.

7. Dental implant case planning

Although a majority of endodontists limit their practice to endodontic treatment, a growing number are placing dental implants (<10%; Creasy et al., 2009). In a recent survey of practicing endodontists, 57.0% think that the scope of endodontic treatment should include implant placement (Potter et al., 2009). LCBCT is useful for implant site assessment, when clinical examination, casts, and conventional radiographs are inadequate to determine ridge dimensions, bone quality, and location of anatomic structures such as the mental foramen, inferior alveolar nerve, incisive canal, maxillary sinus, and floor of the nasal cavity. The appropriate FOV and voxel size should be selected to limit patient dose and still provide the information needed.

8. Assessment of endodontic treatment outcomes

Root canals systems are inherently complex. A systematic review (Ng et al., 2008) of 63 outcome studies has shown that four main factors influence healing: (1) the presence or absence of preoperative periradicular periodontitis, (2) density of obturation, (3) apical extent of root canal filling, and (4) quality of coronal restoration. These studies were based on planar radiography, and suffer from superimposition error, where radiolucent lesions are covered by thick cortical bone or are confined within the cancellous bone. New studies using CBCT imaging to assess healing are now providing improved sensitivity when detecting periradicular lesions, especially when high resolution is available.

It is generally accepted that CBCT provides improved sensitivity when detecting periradicular lesions. In a study by Velvart et al. (2001), 50 patients with persistent apical lesions were evaluated. There were 6 mandibular premolars and 44 mandibular molars, with a total of 80 roots. All 78 lesions diagnosed during surgery were also visible with the CBCT scans exposed, while PA images only showed 61 lesions. The mandibular canal could only be identified in 31 cases using PA radiography, whereas all mandibular canals were detected with CBCT. They concluded that CBCT provides additional beneficial information not available from PA radiography.

What is success and how can CBCT help with decisions about treatment outcomes? While the terms *success* and *failure* or *healed* and *nonhealed* are commonly used to describe the end result of root canal treatment, these terms may be problematic. M.K. Wu et al. (2011) describe a new terminology that includes *effective* and *ineffective*, where *effective* is defined as the absence of symptoms and complete or partial resolution of a periapical radiolucency at 1 year after treatment, or if no lucency was present, that the tooth remains asymptomatic at 1 year. If a periradicular lesion develops or enlarges and/or the signs or symptoms are present at 1 year postoperatively, revision should be recommended. Haalpasalo et al. (2011) suggests that a 1-year follow-up is too short to decide on the healing of some lesions.

In a recent study by Christiansen et al. (2009) comparing PA radiography with CBCT after apicectomy at 1 week and 12 months, the CBCT images were approximately 10% larger in coronal view than PA radiography, and CBCT showed more periradicular defects than PAs. While they did not draw conclusions on how this relates to success after root-end resection, improved visualization of the presence and size of lesions should help our guide our postoperative decisions.

In a study by M.K. Wu et al. (2009) of previously published systematic reviews of endodontic healing, a high percentage of cases believed to be healed by PA radiography showed apical periodontitis when viewed with CBCT. The periapical index was focused on radiographic and histologic assessments of maxillary anterior teeth, which subjects the data to misinterpretation because of the variation in the position of the root apex to the cortex and the thickness of this bone. This study further implicates PA radiography as a useful but flawed tool to assess treatment outcomes and certainly speaks to the need to reevaluate long-term longitudinal studies.

There are few case reports in the literature that have used limited field CBCT technology to assess the postoperative healing of endodontically treated teeth where 2D imaging has resulted in inconclusive findings. Liang et al. (2011) studied 74 patients with a total of 115 teeth (143 roots) that were endodontically treated and then followed up for 2 years. A multivariate regression analysis showed that CBCT detected periapical lesions more frequently (25.9% of roots) than with PA imaging (12.6% of roots). Additionally, CBCT analysis of obturation density, length of root canal filling, and treatment outcomes were different than the values determined with PA imaging. In a case study published by M. Levin and Mischenko (2010), three patients were evaluated with PA imaging followed by CBCT. In each case, the CBCT image clearly showed a reduction in the lesion size, and in the one case with an associated sinusitis, normal healing occurred. There is no question that CBCT is more sensitive that PA radiography in the detection of AP (Estrela, Bueno, Leles, et al., 2008).

There are several reports of the potential correlation between AP and cardiovascular disease. While this research has been inconclusive, a recent prospective study by Cotti et al. (2011) suggests that increased ADMA (asymmetrical dimethylarginine) levels and their relationship with poor endothelial flow reserve and increased IL-2 might suggest the presence of an early endothelial dysfunction in young adults with AP. There are other lesions that may affect systemic health, and patients with cardiac valvular prostheses and other conditions, total joint replacement, diabetes, and who are immunosuppressed because of cancer or rheumatoid arthritis may all be at greater risk of chronic periradicular lesions.

Acknowledgment

I wish to thank Ms. Angela Wang for her organizational assistance, and Drs. Barry Pass and Louis Berman for their help editing the manuscript. All of the PA images in this chapter were exposed with CS 6100 sensors and all of the CBCT images were exposed with CS 9000 3D units, manufactured by Carestream Dental, LLC, Atlanta, GA. (Disclosure: The author reports that he is a consultant to Carestream Dental, LLC).

References

Andreasen, J.O., and Andreasen, F.M. (2000). *Essentials of traumatic injuries to the teeth*, 2nd ed. Copenhagen, Denmark: Munksgaard and Mosby.

Angelopoulos, C., Hechler, T.S., Parissis, N., et al. (2008). Comparison between digital panoramic radiography and cone-beam computed tomography for the identification of the mandibular canal as part of pre-surgical dental implant assessment. *Journal of Oral and Maxillofacial Surgery*, 66: 2130–5.

Baratto Filho, F., Zaitter, S., Haragushiku, G.A., et al. (2009). Analysis of the internal anatomy of maxillary first molars by using different methods. *Journal of Endodontics*, 35: 337–42.

Barrett, J.F., and Keat, N. (2004). Artifacts in CT: Recognition and avoidance. *Radiographics*, 24(6): 1679–91.

Barthel, C.R., Zimmer, S., and Trope, M. (2004). Relationship of radiologic and histologic signs of inflammation in human root–filled teeth. *Journal of Endodontics*, 30: 75.

Basaran, G., and Erkan, M. (2008). One of the rarest syndromes in dentistry: Gardner Syndrome. *European Journal of Dentistry*, 2: 208–12.

Bauman, R., Scarfe, W., Clark, S., et al. (2011). Ex vivo detection of mesa-buccal canals in maxillary molars using CBCT at four different isotropic voxel dimensions. *International Endodontics Journal*, 44(8): 752–8.

Becconsall-Ryan, K., and Love, R.M. (2011). Range and demographics of radiolucent jaw lesions in a New Zealand population. *Medical Imaging Radiation Oncology*, 55(1): 43–51.

Becconsall-Ryan, K., Tong, D., and Love, R.M. (2010). Radiolucent inflammatory jaw lesions: a twenty year analysis. *International Endodontic Journal*, 43(10): 859–65.

Bender, I.B., and Seltzer, S. (2003a). Roentgengraphic and direct observation of experimental lesions in bone: I. *Journal of Endodontics*, 29: 702–6.

Bender, I.B., and Seltzer, S. (2003b). Roentgengraphic and direct observation of experimental lesions in bone: II. *Journal of Endodontics*, 29: 707–12.

Bhaskar, S. (1966). Periapical lesions: Types, incidence and clinical features. Oral Surgery-Oral Pathology Conference No 17. Walter Reed Army Medical Centre. *Oral Surgery, Oral Medicine and Oral Pathology*, 21: 657–71.

Bhuva, B., Barnes, J.J., and Patel, S. (2011). The use of limited cone beam computed tomography in the diagnosis and management of a case of perforating internal root resorption. *International Endodontic Journal*, 44(8): 777–86. Epub 2011 Mar 4.

Bishop, K., and Alani, A. (2008). Dens invaginatus. Part 1: classification, prevalence and aetiology. *International Endodontics Journal*, 41: 1123–36.

Bone, J., and Moule, A.J. (1986). The nature of curvature of palatal canals in maxillary molar teeth. *International Endodontic Journal*, 19(4): 178–86.

Bornstein, M., Lauber, R., Pedram, S., et al. (2011). Comparison of periapical radiography and limited cone-beam computed tomography in mandibular molars for analysis of anatomical landmarks before apical surgery. *Journal of Endodontics*, 37: 151–7.

Bouquot, J.E. (2010). Diagnostic oral pathology with computed tomography. In C.H. Kow and S. Richmond, eds., *Three-Dimensional Imaging for Orthodontics and Maxillofacial Surgery*. Chichester, UK: Wiley-Blackwell.

Branstetter, B.F., Weissman, J.L., and Kaplan, S.B. (1999). Imaging of a Stafne bone cavity: What MRI adds and why a new name is needed. *American Journal of Neuroradiology*, 20: 587–9.

Brynolf, I. (1967). A histological and roentgenological study of periapical region of human upper incisors. *Odontology Review*, 18(suppl 11): 1–97.

Bueno, M.R., Estrela, C., and Figueiredo, J.A. (2011). Map-reading strategy to diagnose root perforations near metallic intra-canal posts by using cone beam computed tomography. *Journal of Endodontics*, 37: 85–90.

Carter, L., et al. (2008). AAOMR executive opinion statement on performing and interpreting diagnostic cone beam computed tomography. *Oral Surgery, Oral Medicine, Oral Pathology, Oral Radiology and Endodontics*, 106(4): 561–2.

Chen, S.C., Chueh, L.H., Hsiao, C.K., et al. (2008). First untoward events and reasons for tooth extraction after nonsurgical endodontic treatment in Taiwan. *Journal of Endodontics*, 34: 671–4.

Christiansen, R., Kirkevang, L.L., Gotfredsen, E., et al. (2009). Periapical radiography and cone beam computed tomography for assessment of the periapical bone defect 1 week and 12 months after root-end resection. *Dentomaxillofacial Radiology*, 38(8): 531–6.

Cohen, S., Blanco, L., and Berman, L. (2003). Vertical root fractures. *Journal of the American Dental Association*, 134: 434–41.

Cohen, S., Berman, L.H., Blanco, L., et al. (2006). A demographic analysis of vertical root fractures. *Journal of Endodontics*, 32: 1160–3.

Cohenca, N., Simon, J., Mathur, A., et al (2007). Clinical indications for digital imaging in dento-alveolar trauma. Part 2: Root resorption. *Dental Traumatology*, 23(2): 105–13.

Correll, R.W., Jensen, J.L., and Rhyne, R.R. (1980). Lingual cortical mandibular defects: A radiographic incidence study. *Oral Surgery, Oral Medicine and Oral Pathology*, 50: 287–91.

Cotti, E., Dessi, C., Piras, A., et al. (2011). Association of endodontic infection with detection of an initial lesion to the cardiovascular system. *Journal of Endodontics*, 37(12): 1624–9.

Cotton, T.P., Geisler, T.M., Holden, D.T., et al. (2007). Endodontic applications of cone beam volumetric tomography. *Journal of Endodontics*, 33: 1121–32.

Creasy, J.E., Mines, P., and Sweet, M. (2009). Surgical trends among endodontists: The results of a web-based survey. *Journal of Endodontics*, 35: 30–4.

Cunningham, C.J., and Senia, E.S. (1992). A three dimensional study of canal curvatures in the mesial roots of mandibular molars. *Journal of Endodontics*, 18: 294–300.

Cymerman, J.J., Cymerman, D.H., and O'Dwyer, R.S. (2011). Evaluation of odontogenic maxillary sinusitis using cone beam computed tomography: Three case reports. *Journal of Endodontics*, 37: 1465–9.

Day, P., Duggal, M. A. (2003). Multicentre investigation into the role of structured histories for patients with tooth avulsion at their initial visit to a dental hospital. *Dental Traumatology*, 19(5): 243–7.

de Paula-Silva, F.W., Wu, M.K., Leonardo, M.R., et al. (2009). Accuracy of periapical radiography and cone-beam computed tomography scans in diagnosing apical periodontitis using histopathological findings as a gold standard. *Journal of Endodontics*, 35: 1009–12.

Demirbaş, K.A., Aktener, B.O., and Ünsal, C. (2004). Pulpal necrosis with sickle cell anemia. *International Endodontic Journal*, 37: 602–6.

Edlund, M., Nair, M.K., and Nair, U.P. (2011). Detection of vertical root fractures by using cone beam computed tomography: A clinical study. *Journal of Endodontics*, 37: 768–72.

Eliasson, S., Halvarson, C., and Ljunheimer, C. (1984). Periapical condensing osteitis and endodontic treatment. *Oral Surgery, Oral Medicine, Oral Pathology*, 57: 195.

Escoda-Francoli, J., Canalda-Sahli, C., Soler, A., et al. (2007). Inferior alveolar nerve damage because of overextended endodontic material: A problem of sealer cements biocompatibility? *Journal of Endodontics*, 33: 1484–9.

Estrela, C., Bueno, M.R., De Alencar, A.H., et al. (2009). Method to evaluate inflammatory root resorption by using cone beam computed tomography. *Journal of Endodontics*, 35(11): 1491–7.

Estrela, C., Bueno, M.R., Leles, C.R., et al. (2008). Accuracy of cone beam computed tomography and panoramic and periapical radiography for detection of apical periodontitis. *Journal of Endodontics*, 34: 273–9.

Estrela, C., Bueno, M.R., Sousa-Neto, M.D., et al. (2008). Method for determination of root curvature radius using cone-beam computed tomography images. *Brazilian Dental Journal*, 19(2): 114–8.

Faitaroni, L.A., Bueno, M.R., Carvalbosa, A.A., et al. (2011). Differential diagnosis of apical periodontitis and nasopalatine duct cyst. *Journal of Endodontics*, 37: 403–10.

Farman, A.G., and Farman, T.T. (2005). A comparison of 18 different X-ray detectors currently used in dentistry. *Oral Surgery, Oral Medicine, Oral Pathology, Oral Radiology and Endodontics*, 99(4): 485–9.

Fennis, W.M., Kuijs, R.H., Kreulen, C.M., et al. (2002). A survey of cusp fractures in a population of general dental practices. *International Journal of Prosthodontics*, 15: 559–63.

Gassner, R., Bosch, R., Tuli, T., et al. (1999). Prevalence of dental trauma in 6000 patients with facial injuries: Implications for prevention. *Oral Surgery, Oral Medicine, Oral Pathology, Oral Radiology and Endodontics*, 87: 27–33.

Gencoglu, N., Helvacioglu, D. (2009). Comparison of the different techniques to remove fractured endodontic instruments from root canal systems. *European Journal of Dentistry*, 3: 90–5.

Goldman, M., Pearson, A.H., and Darzenta, N. (1972). Endodontic success: Who's reading the radiograph? *Oral Surgery, Oral Medicine and Oral Pathology*, 33(3): 432–7.

Goldman, M., Pearson, A.H., and Darzenta, N. (1974). Reliability of radiographic interpretations. *Oral Surgery, Oral Medicine, Oral Pathology, Oral Radiology and Endodontics*, 38: 287–93.

Goodis, H.E., Rossall, J.C., and Kahn, A.J. (2001). Endodontic status in older U.S. adults. Report of a survey. *Journal of the American Dental Association*, 132: 1525–6.

Grande, N.M., Plotino, G., Pecci, R., et al. (2008). Micro-computerized tomographic analysis of radicular and canal morphology of premolars with long oval canals. *Oral Surgery Oral Medicine Oral Pathology Oral Radiology Endodontics*, 106: 70–6.

Greene, C.S. (2009). Neuroplasticity and sensitization. *Journal of the American Dental Association*, 140(6): 676–8.

Greene, C.S., and Murray, G.M. (2011). Atypical odontalgia. *Journal of the American Dental Association*, 142(9): 1031–2.

Haapasalo, M., Shen, Y., and Ricucci, D. (2011). Reasons for persistent and emerging post-treatment endodontic disease. *Endodontic Topics*, 18: 31–50.

Hasan, B., Metska, M.E., Ozok, A.R., et al. (2009). Detection of vertical root fractures in endodontically treated teeth by a cone beam computed tomography scan. *Journal of Endodontics*, 35: 719–22.

Hassan, B., Metska, M.E., Ozok, A.R, et al. (2010). Comparison of five cone beam computed tomography systems for the detection of vertical root fractures. *Journal of Endodontics*, 36: 126–9.

Huumonen S., and Ørstavik, D. (2002). Radiological aspects of apical periodontitis. *Endodontic Topics*, 1: 3–25.

Hyman, J.J., and Cohen, M.E. (1984). The predictive value of endodontic diagnostic tests. *Oral Surgery, Oral Medicine and Oral Pathology*, vol. 58.

International Commission on Radiological Protection. (1990). Recommendations of the International Commission on Radiological Protection: Adopted by the commission in November 1990. New York: Pergamon.

Joint Position Statement of the American Association of Endodontists and the American Academy of Oral and Maxillofacial Radiology. (2010). Use of cone-beam computed tomography in endodontics. Accessed 29 Dec 2011. http://www.aaomr.org/?page=AAOMRAAE.

Kajan, Z.D., and Taromsari, M. (2012). Value of cone beam CT in detection of dental root fractures. *Dentomaxillofacial Radiology*, 41: 3–10.

Kakehashi, S., Stanley, H.R., Fitzgerald, R.J., et al. (1965). The effects of surgical exposures of dental pulps in germ-free and conventional laboratory rats. *Oral Surgery, Oral Medicine and Oral Pathology*. 20: 340.

Katsumata, A., Hirukawa, A., Okumura, S., et al. (2007). Effects of image artifacts on gray-value density in limited-volume cone-beam computerized tomography. *Oral Surgery, Oral Medicine, Oral Pathology, Oral Radiology and Endodontics* 104: 829–36.

Katsumata, A., Hirukawa, A., Okumura, S., et al. (2009). Relationship between density variability and imaging volume size in cone-beam computerized tomographic scanning of the maxillofacial region: An in vitro study. *Oral Surgery, Oral Medicine, Oral Pathology, Oral Radiology and Endodontics* 107: 420–5.

Kau, C.H., and Richmond, S. (2010). *Three-dimensional imaging for orthodontics and maxillofacial surgery*. Oxford, UK: Wiley-Blackwell.

Kim, E., Kim, K.D., Roh, B.D., et al. (2003). Computed tomography as a diagnostic aid for extra canal invasive resorption. *Journal of Endodontics*, 29: 463–5.

Kvist, T., and Reit, C. (1991). Results of endodontic retreatment: a randomized clinical study comparing surgical and nonsurgical procedures. *Journal of Endodontics*, 25: 814.

Lalonde, E., and Luebke, R. (1968). The frequency and distribution of periapical cysts and granulomas. *Oral Surgery, Oral Medicine and Oral Pathology*, 25: 861–8.

Langland, O.E., Langlais, R.P., and Preece, J.W. (2002). *Principles of dental imaging*. Baltimore: Lippincott Williams & Wilkins.

Lee, R.D. (2008). Common image artifacts in cone beam CT. Summer 2008 AADMRT Newsletter. Accessed 29 Dec 2011. http://aadmrt.com/static.aspx?content=currents/lee_summer_08.

Lee, S.J., and Messer, H.H. (1986). Radiographic appearance of artificially prepared periapical lesions confined to cancellous bone. *International Endodontics Journal*, 19: 64–72.

Levin, L., and Trope, M. (2002). Root resorption. In: K.M. Hargreaves and H.E. Goodis, eds., *Seltzer and Bender's dental pulp* (pp. 425–48). Chicago: Quintessence.

Levin, M., and Mischenko, A. (2010). Limited field cone beam computed tomography: Evaluation of endodontic healing in three cases. *Alpha Omegan*, 103: 141–5.

Liang, X., Lambrichts, I., Sun, Y., et al. (2010). A comparative evaluation of cone beam computed tomography

(CBCT) and multi-slice CT (MSCT). Part II: On 3D model accuracy. *European Journal of Radiology*, 75: 270–4.

Liang, Y.H., Li, G., Wesselink, P.R., et al. (2011). Endodontic outcome predictors identified with periapical radiographs and cone-beam computed tomography scans. *Journal of Endodontics*, 37(3): 326–31.

Liedke, G.S., Silveira, H.E.D., Silveira, H.L.D., et al. (2009). Influence of voxel size in the diagnostic ability of cone beam tomography to evaluate simulated external root resorption. *Journal of Endodontics*, 35: 233–5.

Lin, L.M., Gaenglerm, P., Langeland, K. (1996). Periapical curettage. *International Endodontic Journal*, 29: 220.

List, T., Leijon, G., Helkimo, M., et al. (2007). Clinical findings and psychosocial factors in patients with atypical odontalgia: a case-control study. *Journal of Orofacial Pain*, 21: 89–98.

Lofthag-Hansen, S., Huumonen, S., Gröndahl, K., and Gröndahl, H.G. (2007). Limited cone-beam CT and intraoral radiography for the diagnosis of periapical pathology. *Oral Surg Oral Med Oral Pathol Oral Radiol Endod*, 103(1): 114–9.

Lopes, H.P., Moreira, E.J.L., Elias, C.N., et al. (2008). Cyclic fatigue of Protaper instruments. *Journal of Endodontics*, 33: 55.

Low, K.M.T., Dula, K., Burgin, W., et al. (2008). Comparison of periapical radiography and limited cone-beam tomography in posterior maxillary teeth referred for apical surgery. *Journal of Endodontics*, 34: 557–62.

Ludlow, J.B., Davies-Ludlow, L.E., White, S.C. (2008). Patient risk related to common dental radiographic examinations: The impact of 2007 International Commission on Radiological Protection recommendations regarding dose calculation. *JADA*, 139(9): 1237–43.

Ludlow, J.B., Ivanovic, M. (2008). Comparative dosimetry of dental CBCT devices and 64-slice CT for oral and maxillofacial radiology. *Oral Surgery, Oral Medicine, Oral Pathology, Oral Radiology and Endodontics*, 106(1): 106–14.

Lyroudia, K.M., Dourou, V.I., Pantelidou, O.C., et al. (2002). Internal root resorption studied by radiography, stereomicroscope, scanning electron microscope and computerized 3D reconstructive method. *Dental Traumatology*, 18: 148–52.

MacDonald, J. (1997). In: R. Novelline, *Squire's Fundamentals of Radiology*, 5th ed. (chap. 9 and wiki). Harvard University Press.

MacDonald, D. (2011). *Oral & Maxillofacial Radiology*. Oxford, UK: Wiley-Blackwell, Oxford UK.

Malhotra, N., Kundabala, M., and Acharaya, S. (2011). A review of fractures: Diagnosis, treatment and prognosis. *Dental Update*, 38: 615–24.

Maloney, P.L., and Doku, H.C. (1968). Maxillary sinusitis of odontogenic origin. *Journal of the Canadian Dental Association*, 34: 591–603.

Martos, J., Ferrer-Luque, C.M., Gonzalez-Rodrıguez, M.P., et al. (2009). Topographical evaluation of the major apical foramen in permanent human teeth. *International Endodontics Journal*, 42: 329–34.

Martos, J., Lubian, C., Silveira, L.F., et al. (2010). Morphologic analysis of the root apex in human teeth. *Journal of Endodontics*, 36: 664–7.

Matherne, R.P., Angelopoulos, C., Kulild, J.C., et al. (2008). Use of cone-beam computed tomography to identify root canal systems in vitro. *Journal of Endodontics*, 34: 87–9.

McDonnell, D., (1993). Dense bone island: A review of 107 patients. *Oral Surgery, Oral Medicine and Oral Pathology*, 76(1): 124–8.

Metzger, Z., Huber, R., and Slavescu, D. (2009). Healing kinetics of periapical lesions enhanced by the apexum procedure: A clinical trial. *Journal of Endodontics*, 35(2): 153–9.

Michetti, J., Maret, D., Mallet, J.P., et al. (2010). Validation of cone beam computed tomography as a tool to explore root canal anatomy. *Journal of Endodontics*, 36: 1187–90.

Mireku, A.S., Romberg, E., Fouad, A.F., et al. (2010). Vertical fracture of root filled teeth restored with posts: The effects of patient age and dentine thickness. *International Endodontic Journal*, 43: 218–25.

Molven, O., Halse, A., Fristad, I. (2002). Long-term reliability and observer comparisons in the radiographic diagnosis of periapical disease. *International Endodontics Journal*, 35: 142–7.

Molven, O., Halse, A., Grung, B. (1987). Observer strategy and the radiographic classification of healing after endodontic surgery. *International Journal of Oral Maxillofacial Surgery*, 16: 432–9.

Mraiwa, N., Jacobs, R., Van Cleynenbreugel, J., et al. (2004). The nasopalatine canal revisited using 2D and 3D CT imaging. *Dentomaxillofacial Radiology*, 33(6): 396–402.

Nair, M.K., and Nair, U.P. (2007). Digital and advanced imaging in endodontics: A review. *Journal of Endodontics*, 33(1): 1–6.

Nair, P., Pajarola, G., and Schroeder, H. (1996). Types and incidence of human periapical lesions obtained with extracted teeth. *Oral Surgery, Oral Medicine, Oral Pathology, Oral Radiology and Endodontics*, 81: 93–102.

Nakata, K., Naitoh, M., Izumi, M., InamotoK, et al. (2006). Effectiveness of dental computed tomography in diagnostic imaging of periradicular lesion of each root of a multi-rooted tooth: A case report. *Journal of Endodontics*, 32(6): 583–7.

Neves, F.S., Luana, C.B., Solange, M.D., et al. (2010). Dens invaginatus: A cone beam computed tomography case report. *Journal of Health Science Institute*, 28(3): 249–50.

Newton, C.W., Hoen, M.M., Goodis, H.E., et al. (2009). Identify and determine the metrics, hierarchy, and predictive value of all the parameters and/or methods used during endodontic diagnosis. *Journal of Endodontics*, 35(12): 1635–44.

Ng, Y.-L., Mann, V., Rahbaran, S., et al. (2007). Outcome of primary root canal treatment: Systematic review of the literature—Part 1. Effects of study characteristics on probability of success. *International Endodontics Journal*, 40: 921–39.

Ng, Y.-L., Mann, V., Rahbaran, S., et al. (2008). Outcome of primary root canal treatment: Systematic review of the literature—Part 2. Influence of clinical factors. *International Endodontics Journal*, 41: 6–31.

Oehlers, F.A. (1957). Dens invaginatus, Part I: Variations of the invagination process and association with anterior crown forms. *Oral Surgery, Oral Medicine and Oral Pathology*, 10: 1204–18.

Ozer, S.Y. (2011). Detection of vertical root fractures by using cone beam computed tomography with variable voxel sizes in an *in vitro* model. *Journal of Endodontics*, 37: 75–79.

Pak, J.G., et al. (2012). Prevalence of periapical radiolucency and root canal treatment: A systematic review of cross-sectional studies. *Journal of Endodontics*, 38: 1170–6.

Palomo, J.M., Kan, C.H., Palomo, L.B., et al. (2006). Three-dimensional cone beam computerized tomography in dentistry. *Dentistry Today*, 25(11): 130–5.

Patel, S. (2009). New dimensions in endodontic imaging: Part 2. Cone beam computed tomography. *Journal of Endodontics*, 42(6): 463–75. Epub 2009 Mar 2.

Patel, S., and Dawood, A. (2007). The use of cone beam computed tomography in the management of external cervical resorption lesions. *International Endodontic Journal*, 40(9): 730–7.

Patel, S., Dawood, A., Ford, T., et al. (2007). The potential applications of cone beam computed tomography in the management of endodontic problems. *International Endodontic Journal*, 40: 818–30.

Patel, S., Dawood, A., Wilson, R., et al. (2009). The detection and management of root resorption lesions using intraoral radiography and cone beam computed tomography: An in vivo investigation. *International Endodontic Journal*, 42: 831–8.

Patel, S., and Ford, T.P. (2007). Is the resorption external or internal? *Dental Update*, 34: 218–29.

Paula-Silva, F.W., Wu, M.K., Leonardo, M.R., et al. (2009). Accuracy of periapical radiography and cone-beam computed tomography scans in diagnosing apical periodontitis using histopathological findings as a gold standard. *Journal of Endodontics*, 35: 1009–12.

Pew Research Center. (2010). Accessed 3 Feb 2012. And http://pewresearch.org/databank/dailynumber/?NumberID=1150

Pigg, M., List, T., Petersson, K., et al. (2011). Diagnostic yield of conventional radiographic and cone beam computed tomographic images in patients with atypical odontalgia. *International Endodontics Journal*, 44(12): 1092–101.

Pinsky, H.M., Dyda, S., Pinsky, R.W., et al. (2006). Accuracy of three dimensional measurements using cone beam CT. *Dentomaxillofacial Radiology*, 35: 410–6.

Potter, K.S., McQuistan, M.R., Williamson, A.E., et al. (2009). Should endodontists place implants? A survey of U.S. endodontists. *Journal of Endodontics*, 35: 966–70.

Prapanpoch, S., and Langlais, R.P. (1994). Lingual cortical defect of the mandible: An unusual presentation and tomographic diagnosis. *Dentomaxillofacial Radiology*, 23: 234–7.

Qualtrough, A.J., and Mannocci, F. (2011). Endodontics and the older patient. *Dental Update*, 38: 550–62.

Rechenberg, D.K., Kruse, A., Grätz, K.W., et al. (2011). Chronic orofacial pain (OFP) of different origin: A case report [Article in French, German]. Schweiz Monatsschr Zahnmed, 121(9): 839–48.

Richard, E.L., and Ziskind, J. (1957). Aberrant salivary gland tissue in the mandible. *Oral Surgery, Oral Medicine and Oral Pathology*, 10: 1086–90.

Rud, J., and Omnell, K. (1970). Root fractures due to corrosion. Diagnostic aspects. *Scandinavian Journal of Dental Research*, 78: 397–403.

Rud, J., and Rud, V. (1998). Surgical endodontics of upper molars: Relation to the maxillary sinus and operation in acute state of infection. *Journal of Endodontics*, 24: 260–1.

Saunders, M.B., Gulabivala, K., Holt, R., et al. (2000). Reliability of radiographic observations recorded on a proforma measured using inter- and intra-observer variation: A preliminary study. *International Endodontics Journal*, 33: 272–8.

Scarfe, W.C., Levin, M.D., Gane, D., et al. (2009). Use of cone beam computed tomography in endodontics. *International Journal of Dentistry*, doi: 10.1155/2009/634567.

SEDENTEXCT. (2009). Radiation protection: CBCT for dental and maxillofacial radiology. Provisional guidelines. A report prepared by the SEDENTEXCT project. Accessed Aug 2009. www.sedentexct.eu.

SEDENTEXCT. (2011). Radiation Protection No. 172, Cone beam CT for dental and maxillofacial radiology (evidence-based guidelines), SEDENTEXCT Project Consortium, 2011, The Seventh Framework Programme of the European Atomic Energy Community (Euratom), Accessed 15 Oct 2012. http://www.sedentexct.eu/content/guidelines-cbct-dental-and-maxillofacial-radiology.

Serman, N.J., and Hasselgren, G. (1992). The radiographic incidence of multiple roots and canals in human mandibular premolars. *International Endodontics Journal*, 25: 234–7.

Sert, S., and Bayirli, G.S. (2004). Evaluation of the root canal configurations of the mandibular and maxillary permanent teeth by gender in the Turkish population. *Journal of Endodontics*, 30: 391–8.

Sessle, B.J., Lavigne, G.J., Lund, J.P., et al. (2008). Mechanisms of neuropathic pain. In: B.J. Sessle, G.J. Lavigne, J.P. Lund, and R. Dubner, eds., *Orofacial pain: From basic science to clinical management*, 2nd ed (pp. 53–9). Hanover Park, IL: Quintessence.

Shemesh, H., Cristescu, R.C., Wesselink, P.R., et al. (2011). The use of cone-beam computed tomography and digital periapical radiographs to diagnose root perforations. *Journal of Endodontics*, 37: 513–6.

Sherwood, I.A., (2011). Pre-operative diagnostic radiograph interpretation by general dental practitioners for root canal treatment. *Dentomaxillofacial Radiology*, 41(1): 43–54.

Sicher, H. (1962). Anatomy and oral pathology. *Oral Surgery, Oral Medicine and Oral Pathology*, 15: 1264–9.

Sigurdsson, A., Trope, M., and Chivian, N. (2011). The role of endodontics after dental traumatic injuries. In: K.M. Hargreaves and S. Cohen, eds., *Pathways of the pulp*, 10th ed (pp. 620–54). St Louis: Mosby.

Silberman, A., Cohenca, N., and Simon, J.H. (2006). Anatomical redesign for the treatment of dens invaginatus type III with open apexes: A literature review and case presentation. *Journal of American Dentistry Association*, 137(2): 180–5.

Siqueira, J.F., and Rôças, I.N. (2008). Clinical implications and microbiology of bacterial persistence after treatment procedures. *Journal of Endodontics*, 34(11): 1291–1301.

Slowey, R.R. (1979). Root canal anatomy: Road map to successful endodontics. *Dental Clinics of North America*, 23: 555–73.

Soğur, E., Grondahl, H.G., and Baksi, B.G. (2012). Does a combination of two radiographs increase accuracy in detecting acid-induced periapical lesions and does it approach the accuracy of cone beam computed tomography scanning? *Journal of Endodontics*, 38: 131–6.

Soğur, E., Baksi, B.G., Gröndahl, H.G. (2007). Imaging of root canal fillings: A comparison of subjective image quality between limited cone-beam CT, storage phosphor and film radiography. *International Endodontic Journal*, 40: 179–85.

Song, W.C., Jo, D.I., Lee, J.Y., et al. (2009). Microanatomy of the incisive canal using three-dimensional reconstruction of microCT images: An ex vivo study. *Oral Surgery, Oral Medicine, Oral Pathology, Oral Radiology and Endodontics*, 108(4): 583–90.

Stavropoulos, A., and Wenzel, A. (2007). Accuracy of cone-beam dental CT, intraoral digital and conventional film radiography for the detection of periapical lesions. An ex vivo study in pig jaws. *Clinical Oral Investigations*, 11(1): 101–6.

Stratemann, S.A., Huang, J.C., Maki, K., et al. (2008). Comparison of cone beam computed tomography imaging with physical measures. *Dentomaxillofacial Radiology*, 37: 80–93.

Tang, W., Wu, Y., and Smales, R.J. (2010). Identifying and reducing risks for potential fractures in endodontically treated teeth. *Journal of Endodontics*, 36: 609–17.

Taschieri, S., Weinstein, T., Rosano, G., et al. (2011). Morphological features of the maxillary incisors roots and relationship with neighboring anatomical structures: Possible implications in endodontic surgery. *International Journal of Oral and Maxillofacial Radiology* [Epub ahead of print].

Tay, A.B. (1999). A 5 year survey of oral biopsies in an oral surgical unit in Singapore: 1993–1997. *Annals of the Academy of Medicine* [Singapore], 28: 665–71.

Treede, R.D., Jensen, T.S., Campbell, J.N., et al. (2008). Neuropathic pain: Redefinition and a grading system for clinical and research purposes. *Neurology*, 70(18): 1630–5.

Tsesis, I., Rosen, E., Tamse, A., et al. (2010). Diagnosis of vertical root fractures in endodontically treated teeth based on clinical and radiographic indices: A systematic review. *Journal of Endodontics*, 36: 1455–8.

Tsurumachi, T., and Honda, K. (2007). A new cone beam computerized tomography system for use in endodontic surgery. *International Endodontic Journal*, 40: 224–32.

Tu, M.G., Tsai, C.C., Jou, M.J., Chen, W.L., Chang, Y.F., Chen, S.Y., et al. (2007). Prevalence of three-rooted mandibular first molars among Taiwanese individuals. *J Endod*, 33(10): 1163–6.

Tu, M.G., Huang, H.L., Hsue, S.S., et al. (2009). Detection of permanent three-rooted mandibular first molars by cone-beam computed tomography imaging in Taiwanese individuals. *Journal of Endodontics*, 35(4): 503–7.

Vande Voorde, H.E., and Bjorndahl, A.M. (1969). Estimated endodontic "working length" with paralleling radiographs. *Oral Surgery, Oral Medicine, Oral Pathology, Oral Radiology and Endodontics*. 27: 106–10.

Velvart, P., Hecker, H., and Tillinger, G. (2001). Detection of the apical lesion and the mandibular canal in conventional radiography and computed tomography. *Oral Surgery, Oral Medicine, Oral Pathology, Oral Radiology and Endodontics*, 92: 682–8.

Vieira, A.R., Siqueira, J.F., Ricucci, D., et al. (2011). Dentinal tubule infection as the cause of recurrent disease and late endodontic treatment failure: A case report. *Journal of Endodontics*, 38: 250–4.

Wang, P., Yan, X.B., Zhang, W.L., et al. (2011). Detection of dental root fractures by using cone-beam computed tomography. *Dentomaxillofacial Radiology*, 40: 290–8.

Wang, Y., et al. (2010). Evaluation of the root and canal morphology of mandibular first permanent molars in a western Chinese population by cone beam computed tomography. *Journal of Endodontics*. 36(11): 1786–9.

Weir, J.C., Davenport, W.D., and Skinner, R.L. (1987). A diagnostic and epidemiologic survey of 15,783 oral lesions. *Journal of the American Dental Association*, 115: 439–42.

Wenzel, A., Neto, F.H., Frydenberg, M., et al. (2009). Variable-resolution cone-beam computerized tomography with enhancement filtration compared with intraoral photo-stimulable phosphor radiography in detection of transverse root fractures in an in vitro model. *Oral Surgery, Oral Medicine, Oral Pathology, Oral Radiology and Endodontics*, 108: 939–45.

Wesson, C.M., and Gale, T.M. (2003). Molar apicoectomy with amalgam root-end filling: Results of a prospective study in two district general hospitals. *British Dental Journal*, 195: 707–14.

Woda, A., and Pionchon, P. (1999). A unified concept of idiopathic orofacial pain: Clinical features. *Journal of Orofacial Pain*, 13(3): 172–84; discussion 185–95.

Worth, B., Brooks, L.E., and Penick, C. (1975). Herpes zoster associated with pulpless teeth. *Journal of Endodontics*, 1(1): 32–5.

Wu, J., Lei, G., Yan, M., et al. (2011). Instrument separation analysis of multi-used ProTaper Universal rotary system during root canal therapy. *Journal of Endodontics*, 37: 758–63.

Wu, M.K., Shemesh, H., and Wesselink, P.R. (2009). Limitations of previously published systematic reviews evaluating the outcome of endodontic treatment. *International Endodontics Journal*, 42(8): 656–66.

Wu, M.K., Shemesh, H., and Wesselink, P.R. (2011). Letter to the Editor, *International Endodontic Journal*, 44(11): 1079–80.

Wu, M.K., and Wesselink, P.R. (2001). A primary observation on the preparation and obturation of oval canals. *International Endodontics Journal*, 34: 137–41.

Wu, M.K., Wesselink, P.R., and Walton, R.E. (2000). Apical terminus location of root canal treatment procedures. *Oral Surgery, Oral Medicine, Oral Pathology, Oral Radiology and Endodontics*, 89: 99–103.

Young, G.R. (2007). Contemporary management of lateral root perforation diagnosed with the aid of dental computed tomography. *Australian Endodontic Journal*, 33: 112–8.

Yuan, G., Ove, P.A., Hongkun, W., et al. (2009). An application framework of three-dimensional reconstruction and measurement for endodontic research. *Journal of Endodontics*, 35(2): 269–74.

Zakariasen, K.L., Scott, D.A., and Jensen, J.R. (1984). Endodontic recall radiographs: How reliable is our interpretation of endodontic success or failure and what factors affect our reliability? *Oral Surgery, Oral Medicine, Oral Pathology, Oral Radiology and Endodontics*, 57: 343–7.

11 Periodontal Disease Diagnosis Using Cone Beam Computed Tomography

Bart Vandenberghe and David Sarment

Periodontal diseases

Prevalence and progression

Periodontal diseases are inflammatory processes causing loss of tooth support. Loss of clinical attachment and alveolar bone lead to tooth exfoliation, generally over a long period of time. Chronic periodontitis affects up to 75% of the population in one form or another (Brown et al., 1989; Levy et al., 2003), while moderate periodontitis affects approximately one-half of the population. The prevalence, extent, and severity of this disease increase with age (Loe, 1967), but close to 10% of the population is susceptible to severe bone loss at a relatively young age. Because of population growth and aging, disease prevalence has not been decreasing over the last 20 years (Oliver and Heuer, 1995; Copeland et al., 2004). In addition, there is evidence that periodontal disease is a contributing factor to systemic illnesses such as heart and cerebrovascular diseases (Khader et al., 2004). Unfortunately, patterns of attachment loss are not predicable and can vary in location, frequency, and severity (Jeffcoat and Reddy, 1991). Various models of disease activity such as cyclic or burstlike progression patterns have surfaced over time, challenging the original linear hypothesis (Socransky et al., 1984), but none have proven accurate, suggesting that predictions are inadequate because of the complexity of disease progression. In addition, disease activity causes unpredictable bone loss, resulting in a complex surface topology (Figure 11.1).

This architecture is important to depict for diagnostic and treatment purposes. For example, loss of bone in interradicular areas has a greater likelihood to continue to progress. Similarly, treatment approaches may vary with bone morphology: periodontal surgical techniques such as osteoplasty with or without ostectomy as well as bone regeneration are highly dependent upon the convoluted topology resulting from disease progression. Yet, only surgical access allows for a true evaluation. This is due to limitations of two-dimensional radiographic imaging, only allowing for an incomplete evaluation of the periodontal anatomy. As a result, three-dimensional radiographic analysis has potential to enlighten the clinician and allow for enhanced diagnosis and treatment.

In this chapter, the limitations of traditional diagnostic methods are reviewed to demonstrate

---

Cone Beam Computed Tomography: Oral and Maxillofacial Diagnosis and Applications, First Edition. Edited by David Sarment.
© 2014 John Wiley & Sons, Inc. Published 2014 by John Wiley & Sons, Inc.

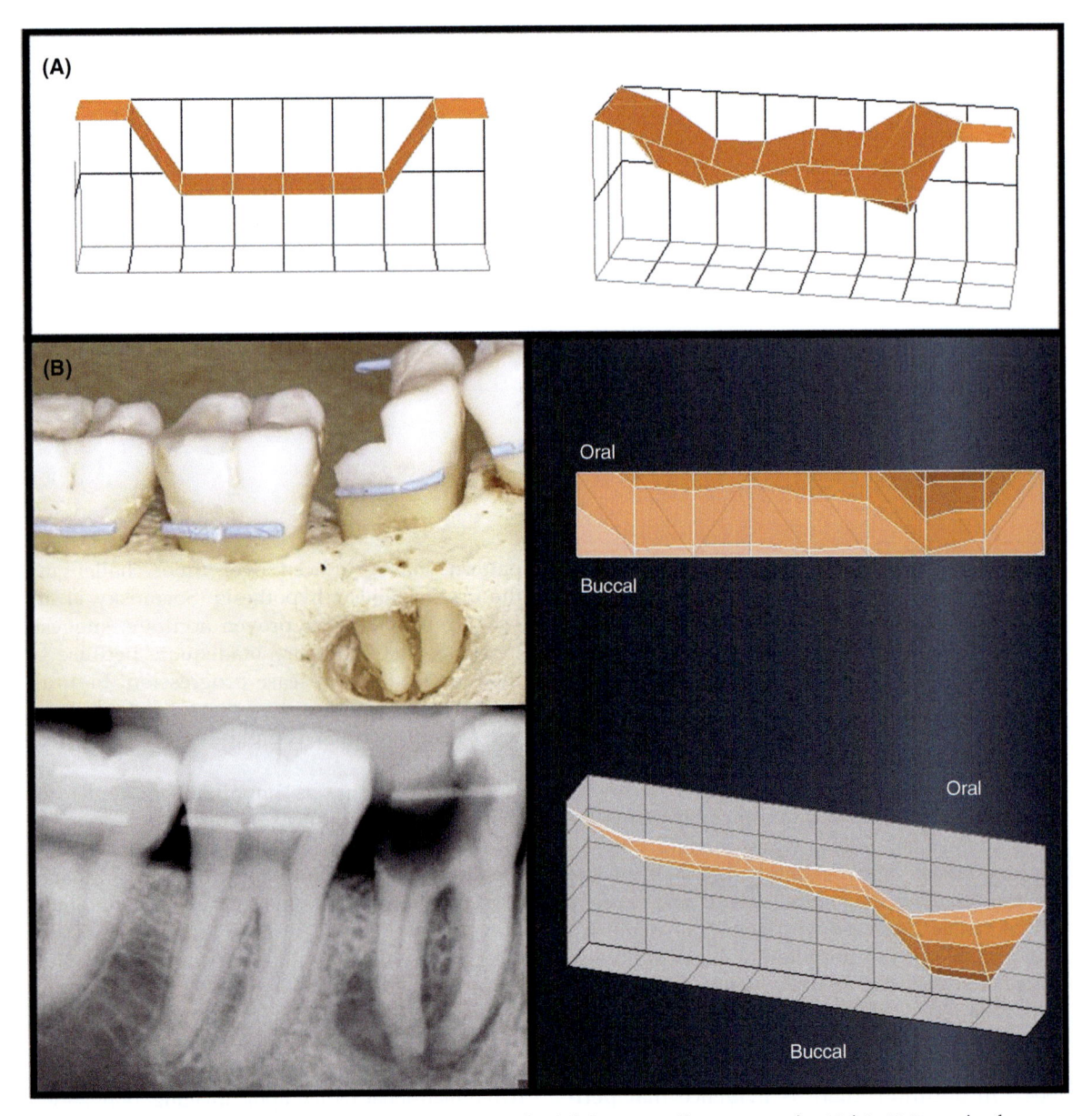

Figure 11.1 (A) Periodontal bone loss can be linear topography (left) but is usually more complex (right). (B) Example of an angular defect on a standardized dry skull (molar region). The periapical radiograph is of limited value. The topography calculated using CBCT is seen buccally (right, top) and the three dimensions (right, bottom).

the need for three-dimensional imaging. The impact of precise assessment on predicting future disease and treatment potential is briefly outlined. Next, three-dimensional imaging of periodontal tissues using computed tomography is introduced, followed by its potential to also impact treatment.

Traditional diagnostic methods

Clinical measurements

Clinical measurements include pocket probing depth, clinical attachment levels, bleeding, and suppuration on probing. These methods are well established, simple, and cost effective. They are utilized to establish the extent of disease as well as to predict disease progression. Although much diagnostic information can be obtained from the clinical examination and some important markers like tooth mobility and bleeding on probing are exclusively related to this examination, there are limitations to the use of clinical measurements alone.

Probing depth and clinical attachment measurements are subject to operator errors. Probing force, angle, and positioning around the tooth vary within the same examiner and in between examiners (Goodson, 1992). For probing depth and attachment level measurements, 2–3 mm of errors is common, resulting in limited ability to detect disease progression. In fact, examiners involved in clinical research, requiring more accurate measurements to study disease or treatment modalities, must undergo training and calibration sessions in the hope measurements can be standardized. Yet, even in such controlled environments, 1–2 mm errors are expected (Polson, 1997). In practice, methodology varies among providers within the same office: probe angulation and localization in the interdental area are common sources of discrepancy. For example, some clinicians prefer to record probing depth at the line angle, whereas others will look for the presence of craters interproximally. Similarly, attachment level depends on these parameters as well as the ability to define the cemento-enamel junction. More advanced measurement tools such as semiautomated probes have provided only limited additional benefits with similar precision, and are therefore rarely utilized (Armitage, 2004).

Because accuracy of pocket probing depths and clinical attachment levels is subject to large deviation errors in clinical practice, early detection of disease progression remains challenging (Cohen and Ralls, 1988). Supplemental clinical tests are at hand to address this issue. Although periodontal diseases are of bacterial origin, identification of specific pathogens is made difficult by the complexity of the flora. As a result, with the exception of rare forms of the disease, bacterial testing is a limited indicator of present or future disease. New strategies that test host response or tissue breakdown factors using discriminant analysis may improve the ability to predict future periodontal disease. Yet, the extent of disease as well as osseous morphology cannot be appreciated using these various tests (Giannobile et al., 2003). The use of a radiographic method to assess damage caused to hard tissues continues to play a central role in diagnosis.

Radiographic assessment

The most important purpose of the radiographic examination for periodontal diagnosis is to measure the alveolar bone level relative to the roots and determine the pattern and extent of bone loss. This not only impacts treatment decisions but also allows visualization of bony changes over time. In addition, the periodontal ligament space, lamina dura, periapical regions, and other related factors such as subgingival calculus can be depicted on radiographs (Tugnait et al., 2000; Mol, 2004).

There are three types of radiographic methods routinely used in dentistry: panoramic, bitewings, and periapical. Panoramic radiographs provide an overall picture of the periodontium but are susceptible to image distortion where patient positioning is critical. Their diagnostic value is therefore more limited than periapical radiographs (Pepelassi and Diamanti-Kipioti, 1997). The latter are—just like bitewings—projection radiographs that present a more detailed picture of the alveolar crest and other periodontal landmarks or pathologic conditions.

However, intraoral radiographs remain a two-dimensional projection of a three-dimensional disease. Ramadan and Mitchell (1962) confirmed that most funnel-shaped defects or lingually located defects cannot be detected. In addition, destruction of the buccal plate could not be distinguished from destruction of the lingual plate. Periodontal buccal or lingual defects are difficult to diagnose using radiographs only (Rees et al., 1971), and angular infrabony defects from vertical bone loss are underestimated by about 1.5 mm on average, with great variations (±2.6 mm; Eickholz and Haussman, 2000). One of the parameters often utilized for evaluation of periodontal stability is the appearance of a lamina dura. However, Manson (1963) using specimens and Greenstein et al. (1981) using patients and clinical longitudinal parameters found no evidence for such claim. In fact, Pauls and Trott (1966) suggested that a bone loss of 3 mm or more is necessary before it can be detected radiographically.

Sensitivity of radiography significantly improves when high-quality images are utilized. Many studies have explored the validity of digital radiography, as compared to conventional films (Wolf et al., 2001; Borg et al., 1997; Jorgenson et al., 2007), and found an equal or better detection of bone loss. The associated lower radiation dose and the ability to enhance images lead to better viewing, but intraoral radiography remains a 2D modality. Since no traditional technique describes complex periodontal defects, advanced methods have been introduced for research purposes. Digital subtraction radiography is one of them: it involves the acquisition of periapical radiographs at various time points, using reproducible angulation and exposure methods (Grondahl et al., 1983). Software is available to subtract the radiographs and underscore changes (Samarabandu et al., 1994). Although this technique is able to better detect changes for specific sites under clinical investigation (Reddy, 1997), it does not improve preoperative description of the patient's overall condition, and it is complex for routine clinical usage.

In summary, the diagnostic value of existing radiography is limited by its two-dimensional nature, and technical improvements cannot resolve this drawback.

Accuracy of intraoral radiography has been validated as an appropriate diagnostic tool for interproximal bone height measurements. Under standardized conditions and using proper positioning, interobserver variability is within 1 mm (Pecoraro et al., 2005). Clinical studies from Borg et al. (1997) reported deviations up to 1.5 mm, when compared to per-surgical measurements. Mean deviation might be approximately 1.5 mm; Pepelassi and Diamanti-Kipioti (1997) reported 80% of their measurements within 1 mm, 91% within 2 mm, and 96% within 3 mm. Overestimations were more significant in severe osseous defects and greater deviations were found in molar regions (Eickholz and Haussman, 2000).

Serial radiographs allow the practitioner to evaluate periodontal disease over time, but standardization of the exposure is required for correct interpretation. When positioning instruments and exposure parameters are properly used, 1 mm of crestal change might be detectable (Hausmann and Allen, 1997). Digital subtraction radiography has potential to identify mineral changes as small as 5%. However, this method is highly dependent upon angulation and exposure. In daily clinical practice, these parameters cannot be controlled, and radiography can only be utilized for evident diagnosis.

Advanced imaging for periodontal applications

Tuned aperture computed tomography

Due to the limitations of two-dimensional radiography, various three-dimensional techniques have been developed over time, with hopes to identify subtle osseous defects located buccally or lingually. Conventional tomography produces a 2-dimensional cross-section but is of poor diagnostic quality: identification of major structures such as the mandibular canal is as low as 20% of cases (Kassebaum et al., 1990). This is primarily due to the unavoidable blur inherent to the method. Furthermore, multiple slices are necessary to ensure that the region of diagnostic interest is sampled adequately. Because each slice is acquired successively, the process is time consuming, technique sensitive, and heavy in radiation (Tyndall and Brooks, 2000). To address these issues, tuned aperture computed tomography (TACT) was developed (Ruttimann et al., 1989), applying principles similar to that of linear tomography but utilizing traditional radiography. This method has shown good potential for detection of periodontal and peri-implant defects (Webber et al., 1997; Ramesh et al., 2001; Ramesh et al., 2002). However, it requires complex manipulation, so far unpractical to daily clinical use.

Traditional computed tomography

Computed tomography (CT) is a more sophisticated method for obtaining cross-sectional images without geometrical distortion. It is a modern and reliable technique for assessment of bone height and width, localization of the inferior alveolar canal, mental foramen, nasopalatine canal, or maxillary sinuses (Yang et al., 1999; Klinge et al., 1989). Although CT scanning has been used extensively for maxillofacial pathology, reconstruction, and implants (Preda et al., 1997), some intent has been made to utilize it for estimating alveolar bone loss. Langen et al. (1995) compared radiographs and axial CT scanning on dry skulls. The traditional radiograph could identify only 70% of defects, with a mean underestimation of 2.2 mm. In contrast, 100% of defects were seen with CT scanning, with an underestimation of 0.5 mm (Fuhrmann, Bücker, et al., 1995). Schliephake et al. (2003), investigating bone levels surrounding dental implants, also found that CT scanning was superior to radiography despite the presence of these dense metal objects. As expected, traditional CT scanning is not easily justified or practical in routine dentistry since radiation, cost, and machine complexity are significant.

Cone beam computed tomography

The introduction of cone beam computed tomography (CBCT) has revived interest in the use of three-dimensional radiography for periodontal applications. In spite of the obvious implementation of CBCT to implant and craniofacial surgical planning, its use is less evident for other dental applications such as periodontal diagnosis. In Figure 11.2, the left molar region of a maxillary cadaver jaw was imaged using intraoral radiography and CBCT.

On the standardized projection radiograph (Figure 11.2B), infrabony defects and furcation involvements of both molars are suspected, but no information can be derived on the exact interproximal, buccal, or palatal bone topography. However, reconstructions of sagittal, coronal, or oblique slices allow viewing of subtle defects (Figure 11.2C). An oblique reslicing of the data following the jaw's arch makes an overview of the periodontal bone possible at submillimeter slice thickness. By increasing the slice thickness (stacking several slices on top of each other), a panoramic reconstruction is simulated, at high resolution, without the drawbacks of a tomographic technique where image quality is degraded by overlaid anatomy. When scrolling through the sagittal, coronal, and axial slices, the exact extent of bone destruction can be assessed around each tooth. For a true three-dimensional evaluation, software allows rendering of CBCT data into a volume (Figure 11.3).

Requirements for periodontal applications

The use of CBCT for periodontal evaluation is controversial because of limited research and justification of its usefulness. Interestingly, this is also true for traditional radiography in periodontology (Tugnait et al., 2000). Much information can be derived from the clinical examination alone, but for more complex patterns of bone destruction and the multitude of modern regenerative treatment techniques, the three-dimensional exam is advantageous.

Radiation dose is within the range of an intraoral full-mouth series (Sukovic, 2003; Ludlow et al., 2003), while spatial resolution of CBCT can be as small as 75 microns. Even when using fast films or digital radiography, the exposure varies from 30 to 100 µSv (Ludlow et al., 2003; Ludlow et al., 2008). Radiation using CBCT examination is similar, although a greater range exists among units and settings such as the size of the field of view, kV, and mAs (Palomo et al., 2008; Pauwels et al., 2012).

The ability of CBCT to diagnose craters and furcations has been compared to 2-dimensional intraoral radiographs and found to be a superior imaging technique (Fuhrmann, Wehrbein, et al., 1995; Mengel et al., 2005; Misch et al., 2006; Vandenberghe et al., 2007a, 2008; Mol and Balasundaram, 2008). These encouraging results indicate that CBCT may be a desirable method where complex periodontal defects are inadequately assessed clinically and radiographically (Figure 11.4).

Furthermore, CBCT might be utilized for treatment outcome assessment. For example, Grimard et al. found that CBCT is superior to intraoral radiographic in postoperative evaluation of periodontal regeneration (Grimard et al., 2009). Three-dimensional analysis of defects, especially using volumetric measurements, may thus provide a more accurate tool to monitor osseous lesions. Note that similar studies have also focused on peri-implant bone loss (Schliephake et al., 2003). Table 11.1 compares clinical and radiographic parameters for periodontal diagnosis.

Alveolar bone loss: measurement accuracy

When scanning the patient using CBCT along the occlusal plane, axial slices are obtained parallel to the occlusal plane. The orthogonal cross-sections

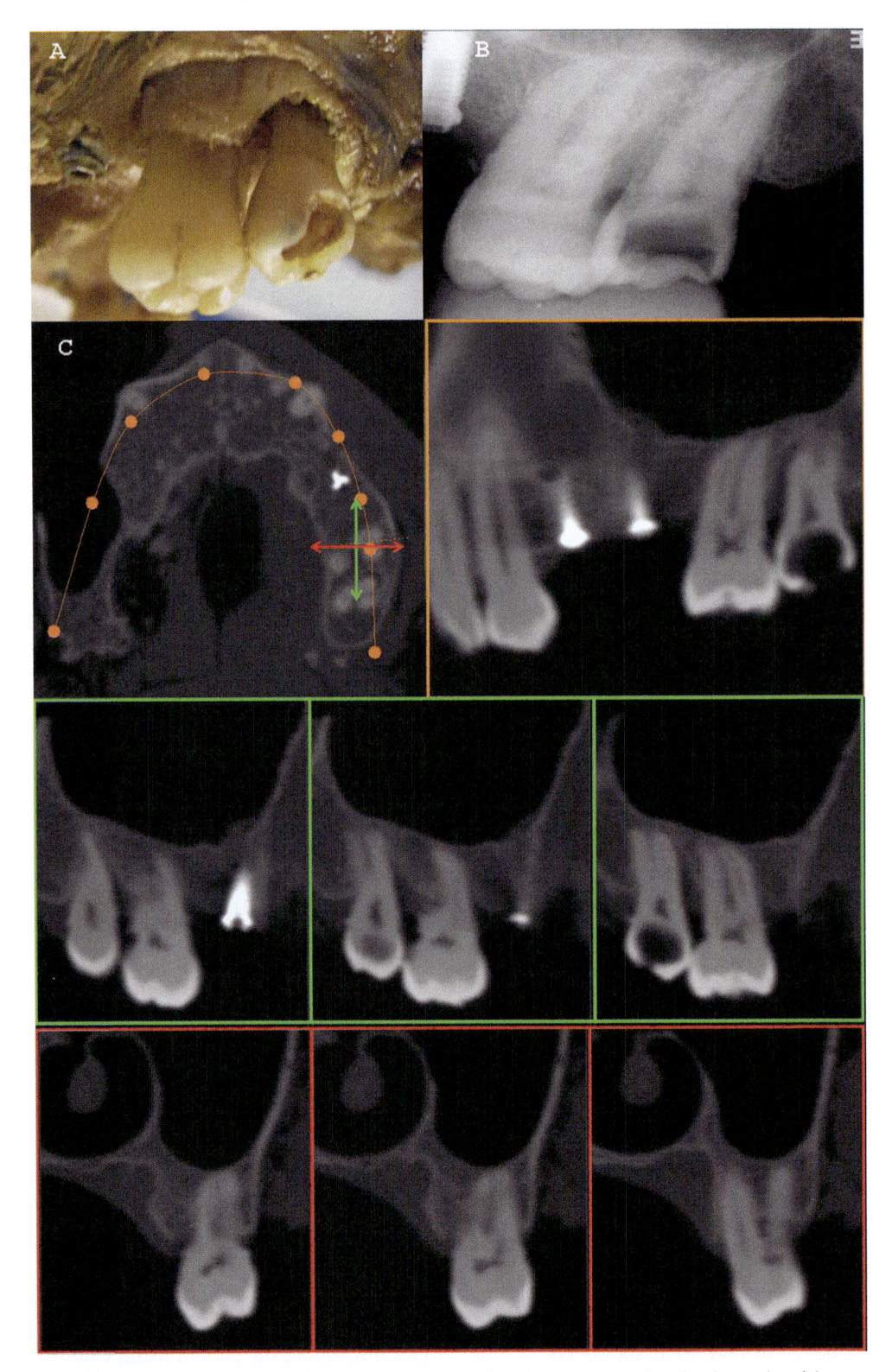

Figure 11.2 (A) The bony defect would only become apparent after flap elevation. (B) Intraoral radiography of the same region only shows a projection of infrabony defects and furcation involvement. (C) A CBCT slice with oblique reslicing curve (orange), sagittal slices (green), and coronal slices (red) allows for interactive scrolling through the three-dimensional defects for topography determination.

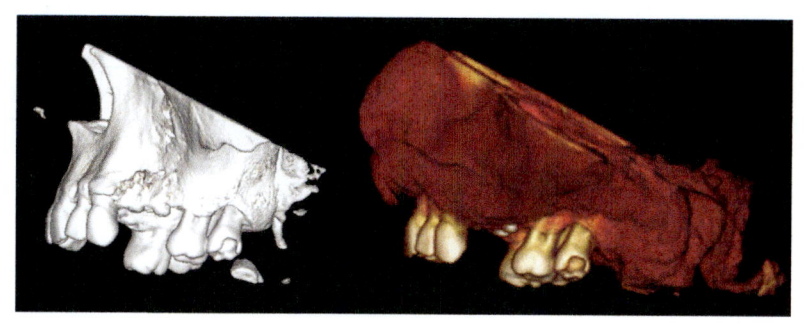

Figure 11.3 Software allows the user to render 3D volumes of the acquired 3D dataset. The stack of slices is displayed as a volume, but careful interpretation is required because the rendering depends on chosen settings.

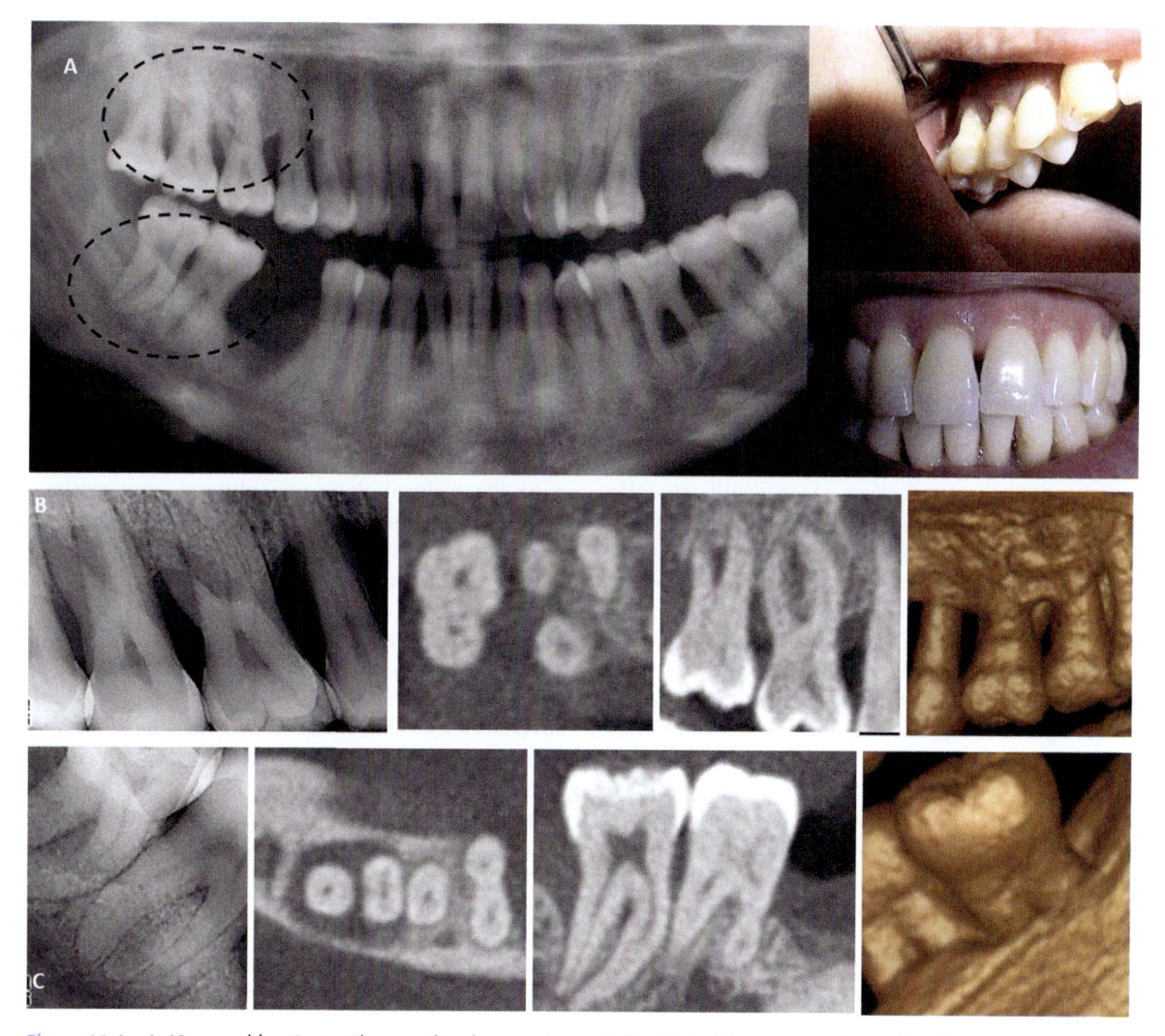

Figure 11.4 A 40-year old patient with generalized aggressive periodontitis. (A) Panoramic radiograph and clinical probing reveal severe periodontal bone loss. (Courtesy of Pierre Koumi) (B) Maxillary right molars on intraoral radiographs (left) and CBCT images, the latter revealing the exact furcation involvements. (C) Mandibular right molars on intraoral radiograph and CBCT images, the latter revealing the exact defect morphology around the molars.

Table 11.1 Visualization of important periodontal features using existing methods and CBCT.

	Clinical	Intraoral XR	CBCT
Plaque	++	—	—
Gingival inflammation	++	—	—
Pocket depths/attachment level	++	—	—
Bone level	—	+	++
Infrabony craters	+	+	++
Furcation involvements	+	+	++
Follow-up of regenerative therapy	+	+	++
Mobility	++	—	—
Local factors (calculus, overhang, caries)	++	++	+[a]
Lateral abcess	++	—	—
Periapical abcess	—	+	++
Periodontal ligament space	—	++	+[b]
Lamina dura	—	++	+[b]
Trabecularization	—	++	+[b]

+ = adequate method; ++ = best method; a dash denotes that the specific evaluation cannot be done.
a. Metallic restorations cause artifacts and may obscure the image. Detection of caries on CBCT is limited, especially at initial stages.
b. These factors depend on the CBCT unit and scanning protocol; for modern units with higher spatial resolution, a better depiction is likely.

that are recalculated from the dataset are perpendicular to these axial slices. As a result, alveolar bone loss measurements will be approximately perpendicular to the occlusal plane. However, if the patient is not scanned along the occlusal plane, alveolar bone level measurement deviations will most likely increase since orthogonal slices would no longer be perpendicular to the occlusal plane. Figure 11.5 illustrates that slight deviations in patient positioning, away from the occlusal plane, will generate orthogonal cross-sections perpendicular to the reconstruction axis but not the occlusal plane. Figure 11.5A shows CBCT scanning with the plane of occlusion parallel to the grid and the corresponding views on sagittal, axial, and cross-sections. Figure 11.5B shows the same views with a five-degree inclination of the occlusal plane. Consequently, all other images are affected. More importantly, bone loss measurements are significantly different. In fact, because of individual angulations, the long axis of each tooth must be found prior to performing a bone level measurement.

When reformatting the volume and aligning it with the occlusal plane, new oblique cross-sections will be generated, counteracting for this alignment deviation.

This angulation is important during the initial evaluation, and positioning of the patient is essential. The panoramic reconstruction is generated, consisting of an oblique reslicing along the curvature of the jaw on an axial slice at the level of the alveolar crest. This image manipulation is the standard view for implant site analyses to which the same principle applies when measuring the alveolar ridges. Yet for periodontal measurements, multiple individual sites need to be measured per tooth, and the long axes of teeth are often not aligned to this occlusal plane because of pathological tilting or strong lingual orientation of mandibular molars. Therefore, a more individualized image manipulation is needed for an accurate measurement of bone loss (Figure 11.6).

While first-generation software did not allow for real-time oblique reslicing and thus requiring

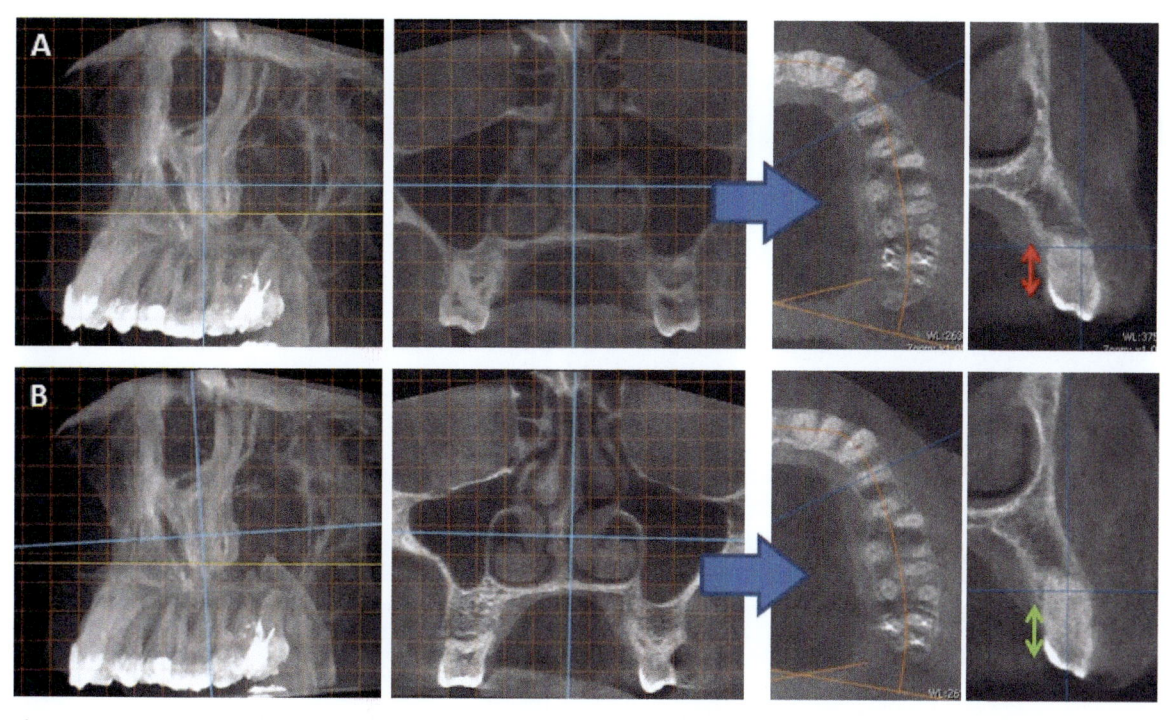

Figure 11.5 Clinical CBCT scan of the maxilla with the patient's occlusal plane (A) parallel to the grid, and (B) with a 5-degree angulation. Note how this small change impacts other views and measurements of bone loss (red and green arrows).

a new volume reconstruction as illustrated in Figure 11.5, latest upgrades accommodate real-time reconstruction along the long axis of teeth. Panoramic reconstruction and rapid measurement of the bone levels are now easily achieved. Care should be given in hospital environments where CBCT cross-sections are sent to a specific PACS system that does not allow for this kind of manipulation without having the entire specific dataset: prior to sending the images, adequate reconstruction is necessary.

In the studies below, although correct positioning is often used, small deviation differences may thus be caused not only by the error of an observer's anatomical landmark identification but also by the degree of standardization of measurements. Just like the paralleling technique of intraoral radiographs, CBCT data need correct standardization.

Mengel et al. (2005) compared periodontal measurements (fenestrations, dehiscences, and furcations) on periapical radiographs, panoramic films, CT, and CBCT in animal and human mandibles to their corresponding histologic specimens. They reported mean height discrepancies of 0.29 mm for intraoral radiographs and 0.16 mm for CBCT. These small deviation errors are due to an elaborate standardization where the teeth's occlusal surfaces were reduced for better alignment. Although the level of accuracy might not be reproducible clinically, this study highlights the geometric accuracy of CBCT. Using a geometric model, Marmulla et al. (2005) reported a similar accuracy (0.13 mm ± 0.09 S.D.) with a maximum deviation of 0.3 mm. Lascala et al. (2004) using large measurements of skulls in vitro found errors varying from 0.07 mm to 0.2 mm.

Misch et al. (2006) compared linear measurements of artificially created periodontal defects on CBCT images and periapical radiographs. They reported a mean error of 0.41 mm for measurements on CBCT. Again, a small measurement error was found, although the natural dentition was used to identify occlusal planes of dry skulls. The study also reported that CBCT measurements are as accurate as direct measurements using a periodontal probe, and as reliable as radiographs for interproximal areas. Yet, because buccal and lingual defects could not be diagnosed with

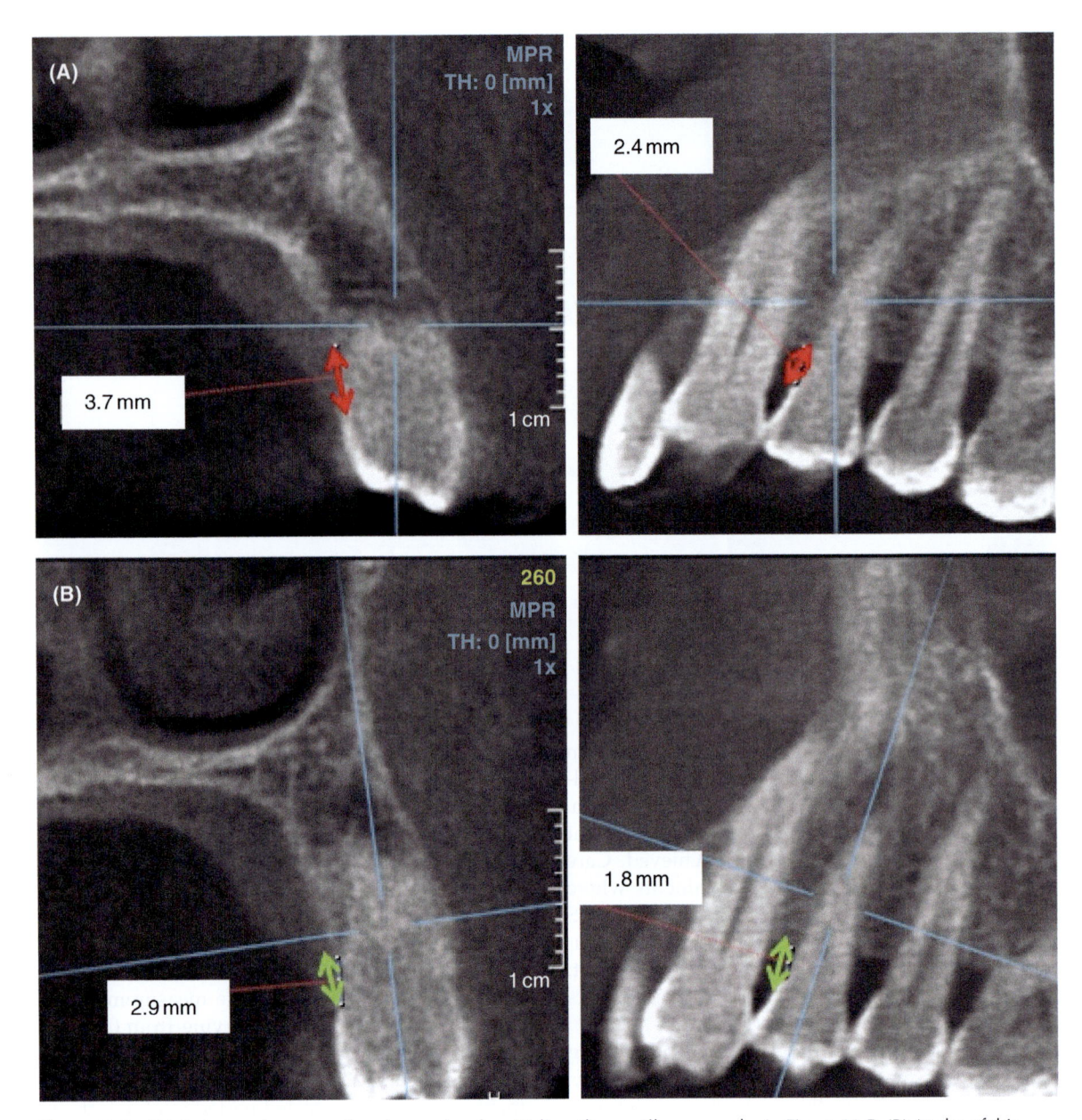

Figure 11.6 (A) Orthogonal cross-sections (coronal and sagittal) on the maxillary premolar in Figure 11.5. (B) Angles of this cross-section were modified to find the long axis of the tooth. Note how different the measurements are.

radiography, CBCT was a superior technique. Although no difference was found between intraoral radiographs and CBCT, the visualization of gutta percha fiducials along the infrabony defects on the radiographic images facilitated identification of cemento-enamel junctions, which would be more difficult in a clinical setting, resulting in greater errors, especially for intraoral radiography.

Mol and Balasundaram (2008) assessed the accuracy of alveolar bone height measurements on dry skulls without the use of radiographic markers along the defects, and categorized the results by

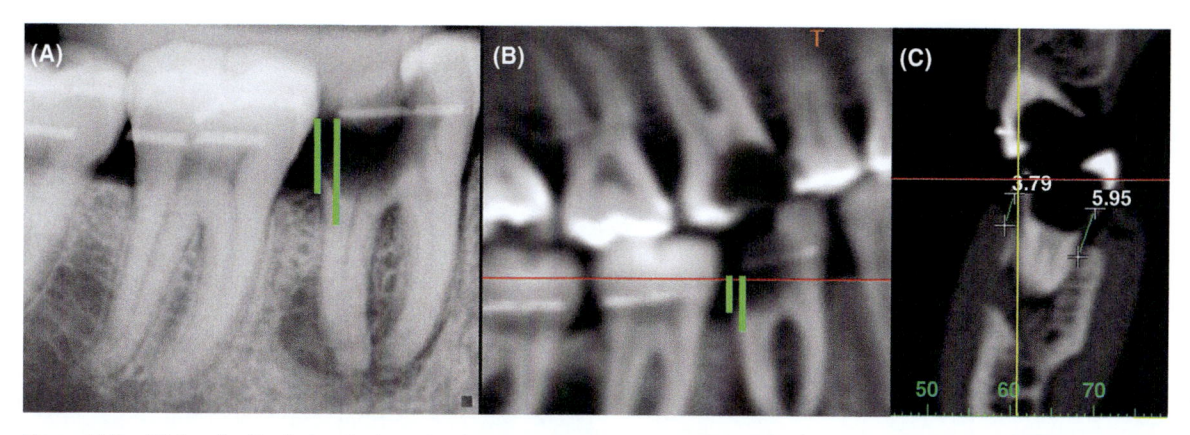

Figure 11.7 (A) Standardized alveolar bone level measurements on intraoral digital radiographs. (B) a 5.2-mm thickness CBCT slice, reformatted along the alveolar crest to simulate a panoramic reconstruction and (C) on a 0.4-mm cross-sectional slice.

tooth groups. They reported measurements varying between 1.16 and 2.24 mm using radiography, versus variations of 0.91 to 1.95 mm with CBCT. For the mandibular anterior region, it was concluded that both modalities have limited accuracy because of the specific anatomy of the region: bony plates are thin and the alveolar bone tapers towards the crest. The authors stated that the use of an older machine might have contributed to their observation because submillimeter detection and enhanced contrast are critical when cortical bone is thin and the bucco-lingual crestal thickness is reduced. However, it must be noted that in this study measurements were carried out on 1-mm cross-sections, while the actual spatial resolution of most CBCT systems is below 0.4 mm.

The influence of a cross-section's thickness was investigated by Vandenberghe et al. (2007a). When assessing naturally occurring periodontal bone defects of human cadaver jaws on a 5.2 mm orthogonal cross-section (simulating a high-resolution panoramic reconstruction) measurements, deviations between 0.13 and 1.67 mm were found. These were not significantly different from intraoral measurements, which ranged from 0.19 to 1.66 mm. In a second study (Vandenberghe et al., 2008), these 5.2-mm reconstructed cross-sections were thus compared with measurements on 0.4-mm cross-sections (see Figure 11.7). For intraoral radiography, errors varied from 0.01 to 1.65 mm. When using 5-mm-thick panoramic reconstructions, errors varied from 0.03 to 1.69 mm but decreased to a range of 0.04 to 0.9 mm when using 0.4-mm-thick reconstructions.

These in-vitro studies all support the use of CBCT to measure alveolar bone levels. Furthermore, latest generations of CBCT technology with submillimeter slices would likely yield better results. To date, there is sparse clinical research comparing radiography to CBCT. Naito et al. (1998) assessed 186 sites on 9 patients for periodontal bone loss and found no significant difference in measurements, compared to bone sounding. de Faria Vasconcelos et al. (2012) compared bone loss measurements on intraoral radiographs and CBCT images of patients referred for periodontal evaluation and found the latter to be more precise. Nevertheless, the impact of CBCT periodontal diagnosis, choice of treatment protocols, or evaluation of postsurgical outcome remains anecdotal. Despite the high(er) precision of CBCT for alveolar bone loss measurements, other diagnostic markers that are more likely to influence treatment outcome, such as bone defect topography, have to be explored and considered in the application of CBCT for periodontal diagnosis.

Infrabony defects and furcation involvement

Two-dimensional radiography is particularly limited in detecting furcation involvement and infrabony defects, although these anatomic features are essential to periodontal diagnosis and prognosis (Muller et al., 1995; Walter et al., 2011; Figure 11.8). In contrast, CBCT has good potential

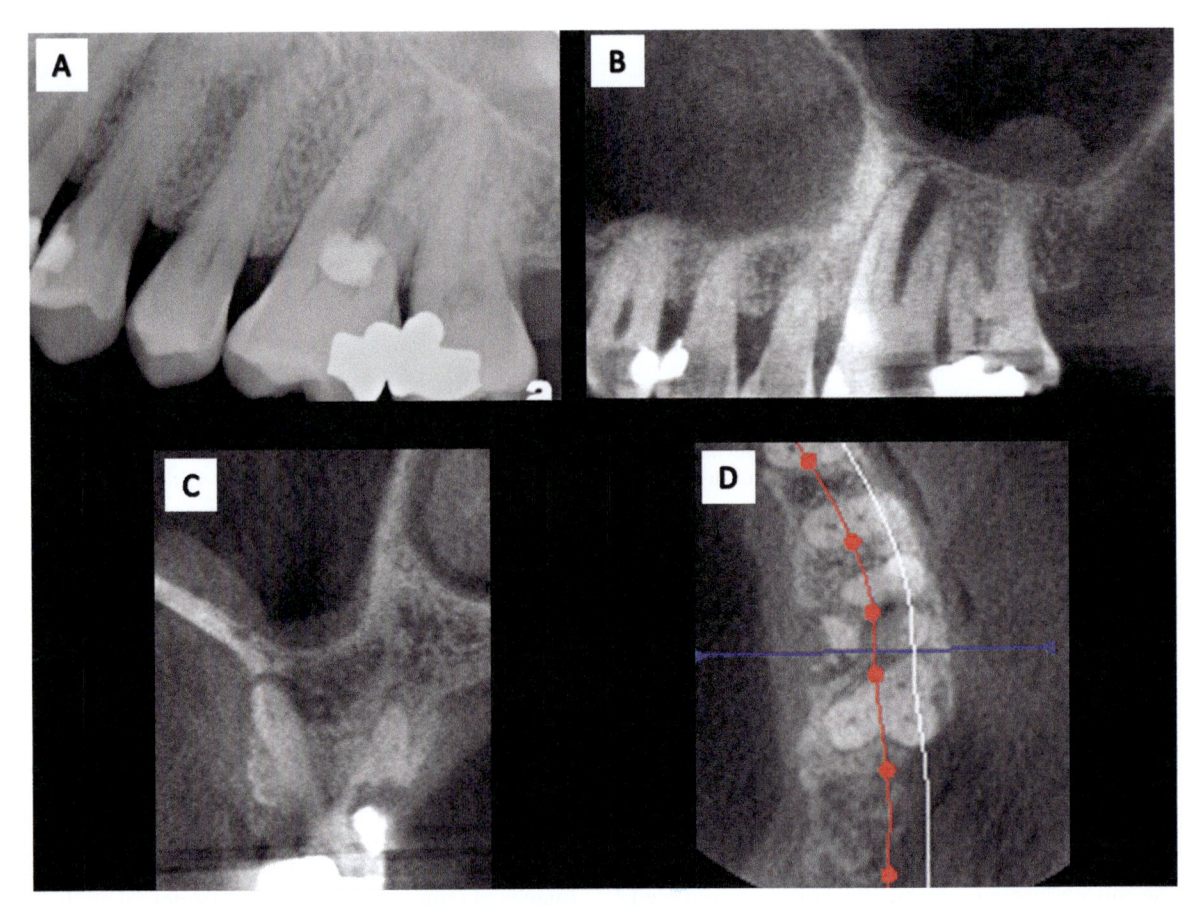

Figure 11.8 (A) Intraoral radiograph of a maxillary first molar shows bone loss centered on the disto-buccal root. (B–D) A CBCT uncovers a more significant lesion, as well as root resorption on the palatal root.

and investigators have attempted to demonstrate its superiority.

Fuhrmann, Wehrbein, et al. (1995), using human cadaver jaws and artificially produced infrabony defects, compared intraoral radiographs with high-resolution CT and found that only 60% of infra-alveolar bony defects were identified on radiographs, whereas 100% could be distinguished using CBCT. This is similar to the findings of Misch et al. (2006), where 67% of infrabony defects were detected on the intraoral radiographs, compared to 100% with CBCT. Fuhrmann et al. (1997) also investigated the detection of furcation involvements using high-resolution CT and found that 21% were detected using intraoral radiographs, while 100% were detected using CT.

Vandenberghe et al. (2007b) studied the actual topography of crater and furcation involvements on intraoral and CBCT images. Observers were asked to classify the craters according to the number of bony walls (0 = no defect, 1 to 4 = 1 to 4 wall defects) and furcation involvements. Only 69% of crater defects and 58% of furcation involvements were identified using intraoral images, in contrast to 100% for both lesion types on CBCT images. For intraoral digital imaging, craters were classified correctly only 25% of the time, with a tendency to overestimate (62%). For CBCT, 80% of the craters and 100% of the furcation involvements were correctly classified. A recent in-vitro study from Noujeim et al. (2009) confirms that CBCT provides a more accurate detection of periodontal lesions than intraoral radiography.

Similar in vivo findings had already been suggested in 2001 by Ito et al. (2001), reporting on a single patient who underwent CBCT scanning before periodontal regenerative surgery, and again one year after the procedure. As expected, the regenerative outcome and defect morphology were clearly visible on CBCT. A few years later, the clinical studies by Walter et al. have demonstrated the accuracy of CBCT in the detection of furcation-involved teeth (Walter et al., 2010) and the usefulness of CBCT in decision making for furcation surgery (Walter et al., 2009; Walter et al., 2012). Walter et al. (2009) reported on 12 patients with generalized chronic periodontal disease. After completion of the initial therapy consisting of scaling and root planing, maxillary molars scheduled for periodontal surgery were further examined using CBCT. Interestingly, treatment planning was refined 60% to 80% of the time once three-dimensional imaging was obtained, in particular when furcations were affected. Furthermore, in their next study, Walter et al. (2012) investigated the financial benefit, consisting of treatment costs and time, of CBCT-based imaging for treatment of furcation-involved maxillary molars and found a significant reduction, especially for second molars with elaborate treatment plan. They do suggest, however, that CBCT as an additional diagnostic tool is only justified when more invasive treatment choices are planned. Similarly, for interproximal infrabony defects, a recent study from Takane et al. (2010) investigated the usefulness of CBCT in vivo, during presurgical planning. When using two-dimensional intraoral radiographs, preparation of surgical membranes could not be achieved while trimming time was more significant. Using CBCT, adequate defect evaluation and membrane trimming could be achieved prior to surgery.

Other periodontal landmarks and subjective image analysis

Radiographic examination also provides information on the presence of a lamina dura, the periodontal ligament space, the trabecular pattern of periodontal bone, the periapical region, and other factors such as overhang restorations or the presence of subgingival calculus. Although Hashimoto et al. (2003; 2006) found that CBCT was superior to conventional helical CT for subjective evaluation of lamina dura, periodontal ligament space, and pulp cavity, they recognized that CBCT was limited in contrast resolution. Using cadaver jaws, Vandenberghe et al. (2008) asked observers to rate the ability to identify the lamina dura and trabecular patterns as well as the perception of contrast. For all variables, intraoral radiography scored significantly better than CBCT. Ozmeric et al. (2008) estimated CBCT in the detection of the periodontal ligament space. Although both intraoral radiography and CBCT were able to detect a thickness greater than 200 μm nearly 100% of the time, gaps smaller than 200 μm were less visible using CBCT. In addition, Liang et al. (2010) compared subjective image quality evaluations of five different CBCT units to multislice computed tomography (MSCT) and found that image quality was comparable or even superior to MSCT. Lamina dura delineation, periodontal space, and trabeculation were most difficult to assess and showed significant variation among different machines. For instance, in a recent study from Kamburoğlu et al. (2011), dental landmarks like the lamina dura scored much better on CBCT images acquired with modern units at small voxel sizes (<0.2 mm). Besides the continuous improvement in image quality of modern CBCT units, it is quite obvious that the acquisition protocol is an important contributing factor to the visibility of such small structures. Figure 11.9 shows axial slices of a cadaver maxillary canine region scanned at high resolutions with four different CBCT units. Even though similar voxel sizes are used for optimal periodontal ligament space or lamina dura rating comparisons, differences in trabecular depiction are evident.

Bone density and periodontal disease

One particularly intriguing aspect of periodontal disease is its likely link to systemic changes in bone density. Although a relationship has been documented for many years, the advent of in-office head and neck computed tomography is opening new venues for research and clinical applications.

Osteoporosis may be detectable in part using dental radiography. Attempts to utilize panoramic or periapical images have been reported (White et al., 2005; Lindh et al., 2008; Devlin et al., 2007). On the other hand, osteoporotic women may have less mandibular bone mass and density, more tooth

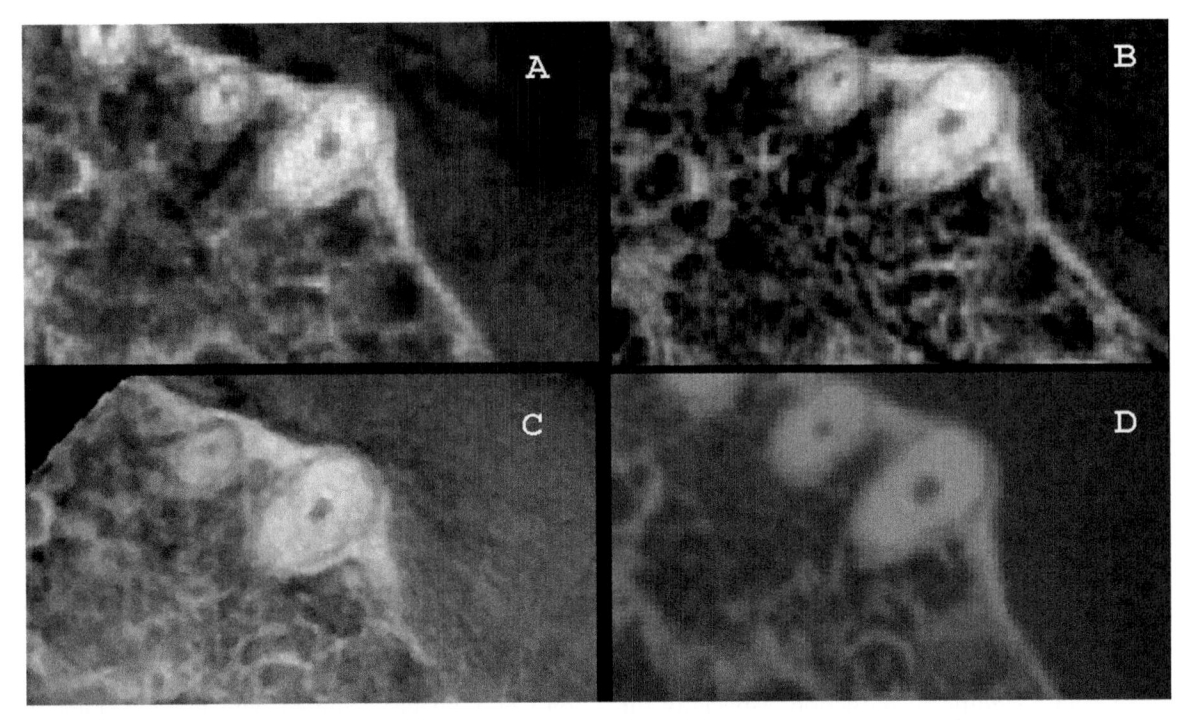

Figure 11.9 Axial slices of a maxillary cadaver canine region scanned with (A) Scanora 3D (0.2 mm, 85kV, 8mA), (B) PaX-Uni3D (0.2 mm, 85kV, 6mA), (C) Accuitomo 3D (0.125 mm, 80kV, 4mA), and (D) I-CAT next generation (0.25 mm, 120kV, 5mA).

loss, and more edentulism when compared with aged-matched individuals (Geurs, 2003; Mattson et al., 2002; Nicopoulou-Karayianni et al., 2009). Overall, studies suggest that treatment with estrogen replacement therapy may slow down bone loss at the mandible (Narai and Nagahata, 2003). In addition, there is mounting evidence that periodontal disease is increased in the presence of osteoporosis, as suggested by various reports (Swoboda et al., 2008; Pepelassi et al., 2011). Inagaki et al. (2005) studied the efficacy of utilizing periodontal disease and tooth loss status to screen for low bone mineral density in a population of Japanese women. They found a positive association between decreasing bone mineral density and prevalence of periodontal disease in this population of women. They also concluded that tooth loss was significantly elevated in postmenopausal Japanese women with low bone mineral density and that their odds of periodontal disease increased as bone mineral density decreased. This study and others support an association between bone mineral density and periodontal status, suggesting the possible role of the dental clinician in the detection of osteoporosis. One common limitation of these studies is that radiographic modalities utilized to assess bone density were imperfect: two-dimensional projections can only provide limited density information since cortical plates and various regions of the trabecular bone are overlaid. Despite these limitations, it has been suggested that even traditional radiography such as panoramic films may be an imaging modality by which dentists can evaluate the dentition as well as screen for osteoporosis (White et al., 2005; Lindh et al., 2008; Devlin et al., 2007). Therefore, it is conceivable that a CBCT, in addition to dental evaluation, be utilized for screening low bone density to both detect a contributing factor to periodontal disease and detect undiagnosed osteopenia. Due to the nature of CBCT technology, Hounsfield units (HU) vary from machine to machine and between images on the same machine, depending on the patient size and position. Therefore, density measurements are an approximation and more research needs to be conducted for the use of bone density measurements on CBCT images. Interestingly, one clinical study from Song et al. (2009) measured CT

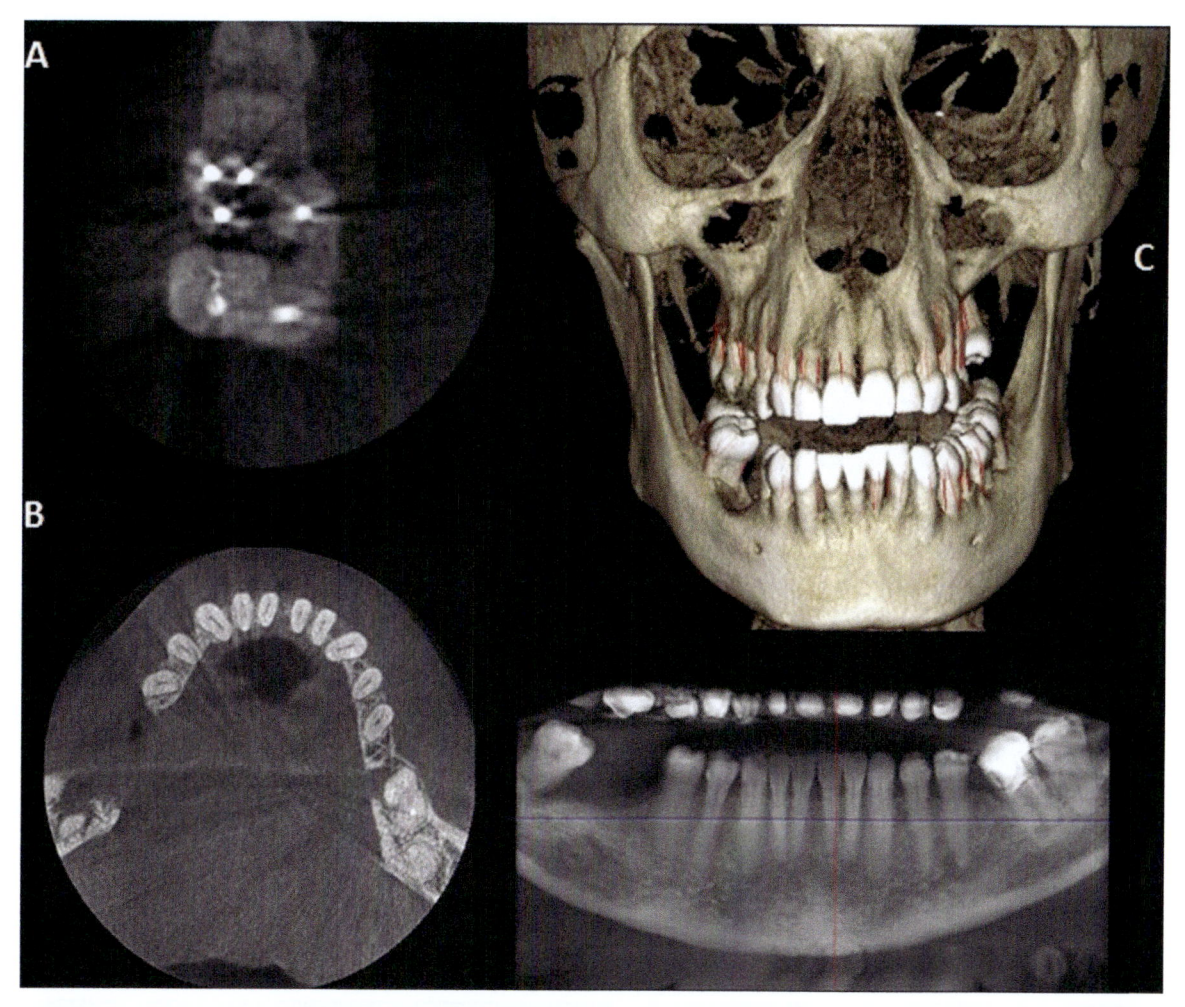

Figure 11.10 Various fields of view for periodontal applications. (A) Small field CBCT (4 × 4 cm, CS9000, Carestream Dental, France) for a combined endodontic-periodontal problem. (B) Medium field CBCT (8 × 6 cm, Cranex 3D, Soredex, Finland) of a mandibular jaw for implant site and periodontal diagnosis. (C) Large field CBCT (16 × 13 cm, KaVo 3D Exam, KaVo Dental GmbH, Germany) for generalized, aggressive periodontal disease in combination with sinus pathology.

numbers and thickness of compact bone around dental implants for correlation to primary stability and found CBCT values to be predictive of their stability. Koh and Kim (2011) also investigated the use of CT indices on CBCT images to assess bone mineral density and found it to be quite accurate in the assessment of osteoporotic women. However, Hua et al. (2009), using mandibular bone samples, seem to point out that methods like fractal analysis (trabecular pattern analysis) and bone area measurements may have potential in assessment of bone quality on CBCT images but that density measurements do not seem to be valid.

Future applications

Detectors and algorithms are being refined in order to improve soft tissue contrast and image quality in the vicinity of metals or dense objects such as endodontic treatments. Furthermore, it is important to determine optimal protocols for specific diagnostic tasks by keeping the ALARA principle in mind: achieving optimal image quality at the lowest radiation dose.

The field of view is an important variable for periodontal diagnosis since it is directly related to the radiation exposure. Depending on the clinical case, it may only be necessary to supplement the periodontal examination with a local 3D examination. In more complex cases with generalized and severe periodontal breakdown, where implant treatment is foreseen, a larger field of view should be desirable (see Figure 11.10).

Researchers are currently testing parameters to determine which specific settings are adequate for specific diagnostic tasks. Lowering the voltage and amperes as well as reducing exposure times and frame counts are among methods to reduce radiation while ensuring diagnostic quality. Figure 11.11 is an example of a standardized dry skull with soft tissue simulation at different exposure settings. Preliminary results reveal that image quality using low exposure parameters may be sufficient for adequate bone level measurements and/or subjective image quality ratings.

Despite the excellent spatial resolution of CBCT, contrast resolution is still limited. It is therefore impossible to discern between soft tissue types such as the cheeks or lips and the gingival tissues (see Figure 11.12A). In order to overcome this inconvenience, for instance for soft tissue profile assessment in aesthetic implant rehabilitation, a modified CBCT protocol can be applied consisting of patient scanning while wearing a lip retractor (Vandenberghe et al., 2010; Januario et al., 2008; Barriviera et al., 209). This separates the surrounding tissues from the gingiva and traps air around it, which makes them more visible on the CBCT image (see Figure 11.12B).

Januario et al. (2008) utilized this scanning method to successfully measure soft and hard tissue parameters: cemento-enamel junction to the gingival margin, bony crest to the gingival margin, and gingival thickness. These encouraging initial results provide evidence for further research on periodontal soft tissue assessments using a modified

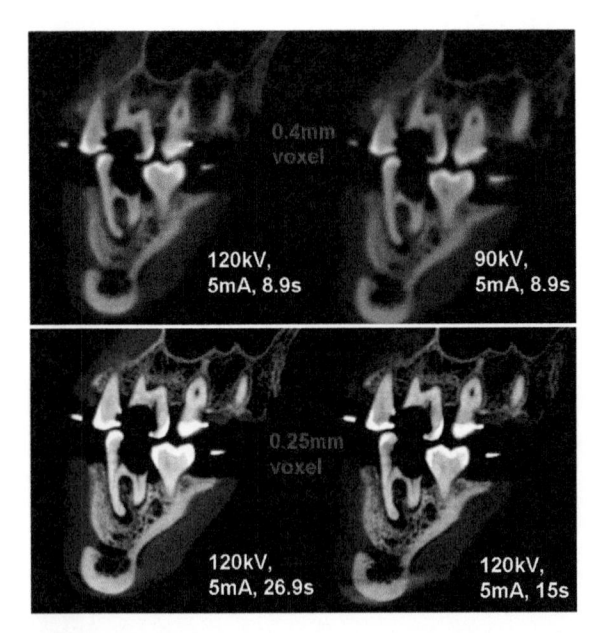

Figure 11.11 Dry skull with soft tissue simulation, scanned with different exposure parameters (i-CAT next generation).

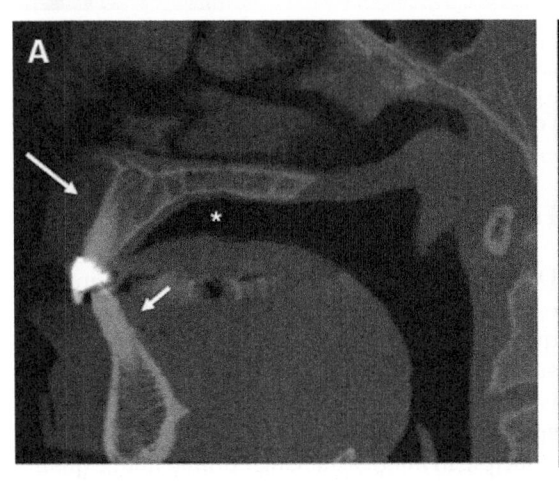

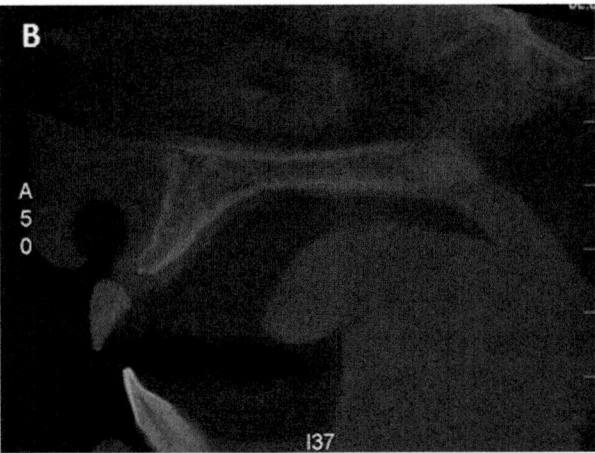

Figure 11.12 (A) Sagittal view with limited soft tissue contrast. White arrows show that, both buccally and lingually, no distinction between gingival and surrounding tissues can be made. The asterisk indicates the airway, which makes the palatal mucosa visible. (B) Sagittal slice of a patient scanned while wearing a lip retractor. Gingival tissues are more apparent.

CBCT scanning technique. Barriviera et al. (2009) also used this new scanning technique for assessments of the palatal mucosa thickness. This mucosa is the main donor site for soft tissue grafts in periodontal surgery. Determination of its thickness is clinical probing, which requires local anesthesia prior to surgery, thus limiting presurgical planning. In this clinical study, 31 patients were recruited and palatal mucosa thickness was measured at 40 different sites on each patient. The authors found different thicknesses depending on tooth type and age, which were similar to other studies using different assessment methods. They concluded that this modality is accurate for planning of periodontal surgery.

Few studies have addressed changes of alveolar bone levels after periodontal regenerative surgeries or implant therapy. Grimard et al. (2009) compared clinical, periapical radiographic, and CBCT measurements of bone level changes after periodontal regenerative surgery. Thirty-five intrabony defects on 29 patients were imaged before grafting, and again 6 months later. CBCT measurements correlated strongly with those performed during surgery, while intraoral radiographic measurements (calibrated with a millimetric grid) were less accurate.

Loss of bone volume can also be evaluated. Feichtinger et al. (2007) assessed bone resorption after site preservation using CT. They outlined bone on each slice by drawing its borders using dedicated software, and stacked them to obtain a small three-dimensional model of the local defect. This volume could then be compared to postsurgical scanning. Figure 11.13 shows scanning of a patient using CBCT at the time of site preservation

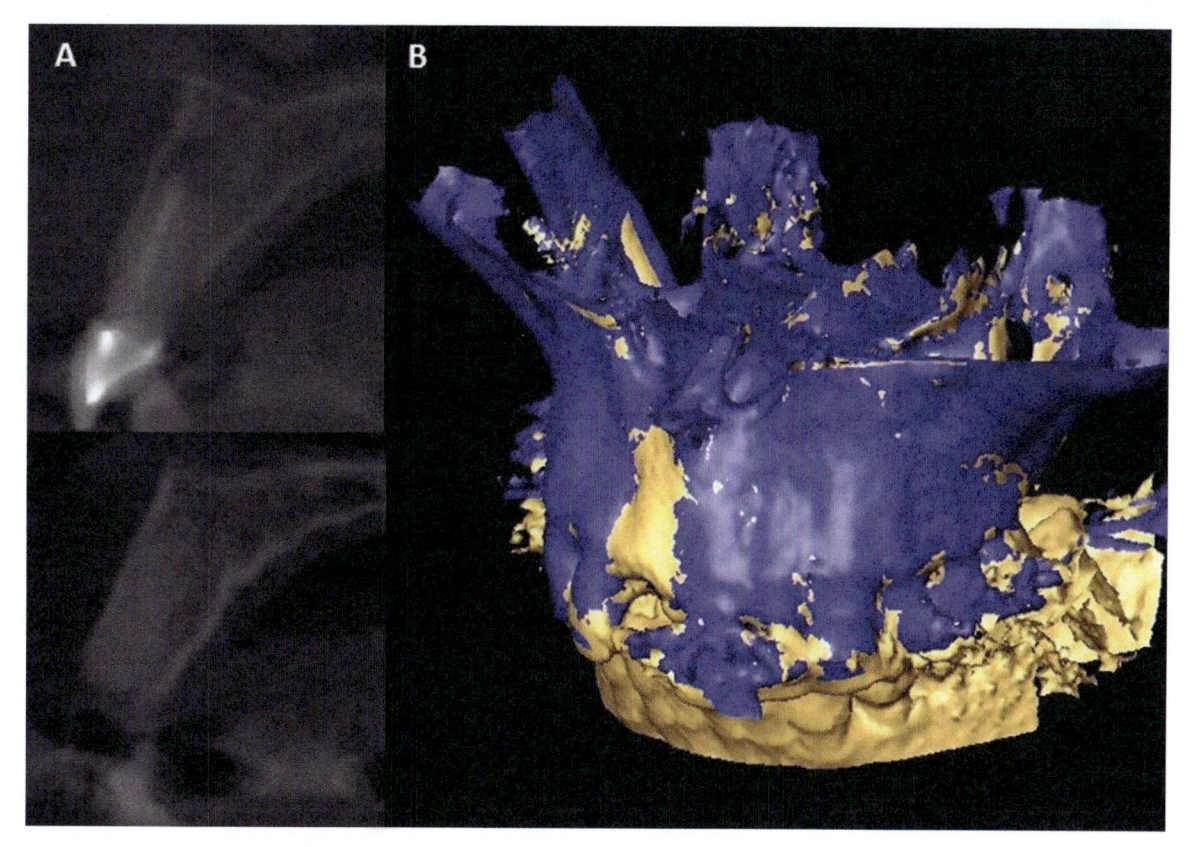

Figure 11.13 (A) Pre- and postextraction CBCT views of a patient's maxillary central incisor. A site-preservation technique was performed after extraction of the tooth. (Courtesy of Anthony Sclar) (B) Registered CBCT data of the maxillary central incisor. The prescan (taken at the time of site preservation, in yellow) and the postscan (6 months later, in blue) show a small local bone loss at the buccal plate.

of a central maxillary incisor, and 6 months later. CBCT datasets were overlaid to highlight local bone loss at the ridge.

Conclusion

Although CBCT has been available only for a few years, its periodontal applications are becoming evident. Despite the fact that periodontal disease affects a growing population due to aging and better maintenance of the natural dentition, diagnostic methods have only evolved at a slow pace. Biologic markers are site specific but reveal little of the osseous topography. As a result, surgical approaches continue to be empirical and decision making is often relegated to the surgical event. Three-dimensional imaging will likely improve patient understanding of their disease, enhance diagnosis, and assist clinicians in refining their treatment methods.

References

Armitage, G.C. (2004). Periodontal diagnoses and classification of periodontal diseases. *Periodontol 2000*, 34: 9–21.

Barriviera, M., et al. (2009). A new method to assess and measure palatal masticatory mucosa by cone-beam computerized tomography. *J Clin Periodontol*, 36(7): 564–8.

Borg, E., Gröndahl, K., and Gröndahl, H. (1997). Marginal bone level buccal to mandibular molars in digital radiographs from charge-coupled device and storage phosphor systems: An in vitro study. *Journal of Clinical Periodontol*, 24: 306–12.

Brown, L.J., Oliver, R.C., and Loe, H. (1989). Periodontal diseases in the U.S. in 1981: Prevalence, severity, extent and rate of tooth mortality. *J Dent Res*, 60: 363–70.

Cohen, M.E., and Ralls, S.A. (1988). Distributions of periodontal attachment levels, mathematical models and implications. *J Periodontol*, 15: 254–8.

Copeland, L.B., et al. (2004). Predictors of tooth loss in two US adult populations. *Journal of Public Health Dentistry*, 64(1): 31–7.

de Faria Vasconcelos, K., et al. (2012). Detection of periodontal bone loss using cone beam CT and intraoral radiography. *Dentomaxillofac Radiol*, 41(1): 64–9.

Devlin, H., et al. (2007). Diagnosing osteoporosis by using dental panoramic radiographs: the OSTEODENT project. *Oral Surg Oral Med Oral Pathol Oral Radiol Endod*, 104(6): 821–8.

Eickholz, P., and Haussman, E. (2000). Accuracy of radiographic assessment of interproximal bone loss in intrabony defects using linear measurements. *Eur J Oral Sci*, 108: 70–3.

Feichtinger, M., Mossbock, R., and Karcher, H. (2007). Assessment of bone resorption after secondary alveolar bone grafting using three-dimensional computed tomography: A three-year study. *Cleft Palate Craniofac J*, 44(2): 142–8.

Fuhrmann, R.A., Bücker, A., and Diedrich, P.R. (1995). Assessment of alveolar bone loss with high resolution computed tomography. *Journal of Periodontal Research*, 30(4): 258–63.

Fuhrmann, R.A., Bücker, A., and Diedrich, P.R. (1997). Furcation involvement: Comparison of dental radiographs and HR-CT-slices in human specimens. *J Periodontal Res*, 32(5): 409–18.

Fuhrmann, R.A., Wehrbein, H., et al. (1995). Assessment of the dentate alveolar process with high resolution computed tomography. *Dento-Maxillo-Facial Radiology*, 24(1): 50–4.

Geurs, N.C. (2003). Osteoporosis and periodontal disease progression. *Periodontol 2000*, 32: 105–10.

Giannobile, W.V., Al-Shammari, K.F., and Sarment, D.P. (2003). Matrix molecules and growth factors as indicators of periodontal disease activity. *Periodontol 2000*, 31: 125–34.

Goodson, J.M. (1992). Conduct of multicenter trials to test agents for treatment of periodontitis. *J Periodontol*, 63(12 Suppl): 1058–63.

Greenstein, G., et al. (1981). Associations between crestal lamina dura and periodontal status. *Journal of Periodontology*, 52: 362–6.

Grimard, B.A., et al. (2009). Comparison of clinical, periapical radiograph, and cone-beam volume tomography measurement techniques for assessing bone level changes following regenerative periodontal therapy. *J Periodontol*, 80(1): 48–55.

Grondahl, H.G., Grondahl, K., and Webber, R.L. (1983). A digital substraction technique for dental radiography. *Oral Surgery, Oral Medicine, Oral Pathology, Oral Radiology, & Endodontics*, 55: 96–102.

Hashimoto, K., Arai, Y., et al. (2003). A comparison of a new limited cone beam computed tomography machine for dental use with a multidetector row helical CT machine. *Oral Surgery Oral Medicine Oral Pathology Oral Radiology & Endodontics*, 95(3): 371–7.

Hashimoto, K., Kawashima, S., et al. (2006). Comparison of image performance between cone-beam computed tomography for dental use and four-row multidetector helical CT. *Journal of Oral Science*, 48(1): 27–34.

Hausmann, E., and Allen, K. (1997). Reproducibility of bone height measurements made on serial radiographs. *J Periodontol*, 68(9): 839–41.

Hua Y., et al. (2009). Bone quality assessment based on cone beam computed tomography imaging. *Clin Oral Implants Res*, 20(8): 767–71.

Inagaki, K., et al. (2005). Efficacy of periodontal disease and tooth loss to screen for low bone mineral density in Japanese women. *Calcif Tissue Int*, 77(1): 9–14.

Ito, K., et al. (2001). Clinical application of a new compact computed tomography system for evaluating the outcome of regenerative therapy: A case report. *J Periodontol*, 72(5): 696–702.

Januario, A.L., Barriviera, M., and Duarte, W.R. (2008). Soft tissue cone-beam computed tomography: A novel method for the measurement of gingival tissue and the dimensions of the dentogingival unit. *J Esthet Restor Dent*, 20(6): 366–73, discussion p. 374.

Jeffcoat, M.K., and Reddy, M.S. (1991). Progression of probing attachment loss in adult periodontitis. *J Periodontol*, 62: 185–9.

Jorgenson, T., et al. (2007). Comparison of two imaging modalities: F-speed film and digital images for detection of osseous defects in patients with interdental vertical bone defects. *Dentomaxillofac Radiol*, 36(8): 500–5.

Kamburoğlu, K., et al. (2011). Comparative assessment of subjective image quality of cross-sectional cone-beam computed tomography scans. *J Oral Sci*, 53(4): 501–8.

Kassebaum, D.K., et al. (1990). Cross-sectional radiography for implant site assessment. *Oral Surgery, Oral Medicine, Oral Pathology, Oral Radiology, & Endodontics*, 70: 674–82.

Khader, Y., Albashaireh, Z., and Alomari, M. (2004). Periodontal diseases and the risk of coronary heary and cerebrovascular diseases: A meta-analysis. *J Periodontol*, 75: 1046–53.

Klinge, B., Petersson, A., and Maly, P. (1989). Location of the mandibular canal: Comparison of macroscopic findings, conventional radiography, and computed tomography. *International Journal of Oral & Maxillofacial Implants*, 4: 327–32.

Koh, K.J., and Kim, K.A., et al. (2011). Utility of the computed tomography indices on cone beam computed tomography images in the diagnosis of osteoporosis in women. *Imaging Sci Dental*, 41(3): 101–6.

Langen, H.J., et al. (1995). Diagnosis of infra-alveolar bony lesions in the dentate alveolar process with high-resolution computed tomography: Experimental results. *Investigative Radiology*, 30(7): 421–6.

Lascala, C.A., Panella, J., and Marques, M.M. (2004). Analysis of the accuracy of linear measurements obtained by cone beam computed tomography (CBCT-NewTom). *Dentomaxillofac Radiol*, 33(5): 291–4.

Levy, S.M., et al. (2003). The prevalence of periodontal disease measures in elderly adults, aged 79 and older. *Special Care in Dentistry*, 23(2): 50–7.

Liang, X., et al. (2010). A comparative evaluation of cone beam computed tomography (CBCT) and multi-slice CT (MSCT): Part I. On subjective image quality. *Eur J Radiol*, 75(2): 265–9.

Lindh, C., et al. (2008). The use of visual assessment of dental radiographs for identifying women at risk of having osteoporosis: the OSTEODENT project. *Oral Surg Oral Med Oral Pathol Oral Radiol Endod*, 106(2): 285–93.

Loe, H. (1967). The gingival index, the plaque index and the retention index systems. *J Periodontol*, 36: 610–6.

Ludlow, J.B., Davies-Ludlow, L.E., and White, S.C. (2008). Patient risk related to common dental radiographic examinations: The impact of 2007 International Commission on Radiological Protection recommendations regarding dose calculation. *J Am Dent Assoc*, 139(9): 1237–43.

Ludlow, J.B., Davies-Ludlow, L.E., and Brooks, S.L. (2003). Dosimetry of two extraoral direct digital imaging devices: NewTom cone beam CT and Orthophos Plus DS panoramic unit. *Dentomaxillofac Radiol*, 32: 229–34.

Manson, J.D. (1963). Lamina dura. *Oral Surgery, Oral Medicine, Oral Pathology, Oral Radiology, & Endodontics*, 16: 432–8.

Marmulla, R., et al. (2005). Geometric accuracy of the NewTom 9000 Cone Beam CT. *Dentomaxillofac Radiol*, 34(1): 28–31.

Mattson, J.S., Cerutis, D.R., and Parrish, L.C. (2002). Osteoporosis: A review and its dental implications. *Compend Contin Educ Dent*, 23(11): 1001–4, 1006, 1008 passim; quiz 1014.

Mengel, R., et al. (2005). Digital volume tomography in the diagnosis of periodontal defects: An in vitro study on native pig and human mandibles. *Journal of Periodontology*, 76(5): 665–73.

Misch, K.A., Yi, E.S., and Sarment, D.P. (2006). Accuracy of cone beam computed tomography for periodontal defect measurements. *Journal of Periodontology*, 77(7): 1261–6.

Mol, A. (2004). Imaging methods in periodontology. *Periodontology 2000*, 34: 34–48.

Mol, A., and Balasundaram, A., (2008). In vitro cone beam computed tomography imaging of periodontal bone. *Dentomaxillofac Radiol*, 37(6): 319–24.

Muller, H.P., Eger, T., and Lange, D.E. (1995). Management of furcation-involved teeth: A retrospective analysis. *J Clin Periodontol*, 22(12): 911–7.

Naito, T., Hosokawa, R., and Yokota, M. (1998). Three-dimensional alveolar bone morphology analysis using computed tomography. *Journal of Periodontology*, 69(5): 584–9.

Narai, S., and Nagahata, S. (2003). Effects of alendronate on the removal torque of implants in rats with induced osteoporosis. *Int J Oral Maxillofac Implants*, 18(2): 218–23.

Nicopoulou-Karayianni, K., et al. (2009). Tooth loss and osteoporosis: the OSTEODENT Study. *J Clin Periodontol*, 36(3): 190–7.

Noujeim, M., et al. (2009). Evaluation of high-resolution cone beam computed tomography in the detection of simulated interradicular bone lesions. *Dentomaxillofac Radiol*, 38(3): 156–62.

Oliver, R.C., and Heuer, S.B. (1995). Dental practice patterns. II: Treatment related to oral health status. *Gen Dent*, 43: 170–5.

Ozmeric, N., et al. (2008). Cone-beam computed tomography in assessment of periodontal ligament space: In vitro study on artificial tooth model. *Clin Oral Investig*, 12(3): 233–9.

Palomo, J.M., Rao, P.S., and Hans, M.G. (2008). Influence of CBCT exposure conditions on radiation dose. *Oral Surg Oral Med Oral Pathol Oral Radiol Endod*, 105(6): 773–82.

Pauls, V., and Trott, J.R. (1966). A radiological study of experimentally produced lesions in bone. *Dent Pract Dent Rec*, 16: 254–8.

Pauwels, R., et al. (2012). SEDENTEXCT Project Consortium: Effective dose range for cone beam computed tomography scanners. *Eur J Radiol*, 81(2): 267–71.

Pecoraro, M., et al. (2005). Comparison of observer reliability in assessing alveolar bone height on direct digital and conventional radiographs. *Dentomaxillofac Radiol*, 34: 279–84.

Pepelassi, E., et al. (2011). The relationship between osteoporosis and peridontitis in women aged 45–70 years. *Oral Dis*, E-pub, ahead of print.

Pepelassi, E.A., and Diamanti-Kipioti, A. (1997). Selection of the most accurate method of conventional radiography for the assessment of periodontal osseous destruction. *J Clin Periodontol*, 24: 557–657.

Polson, A.M. (1997). The research team, calibration, and quality assurance in clinical trials in periodontics. *Annals of Periodontology*, 2(1): 75–82.

Preda, L., et al. (1997). Use of spiral computed tomography for multiplanar dental reconstruction. *Dento-Maxillo-Facial Radiology*, 26: 327–31.

Ramadan, A., and Mitchell, D.F. (1962). Roentgenographic study of experimental bone destruction. *Oral Surgery, Oral Medicine, Oral Pathology, Oral Radiology, & Endodontics*, 15: 934–43.

Ramesh, A., et al. (2001). Evaluation of tuned aperture computed tomography (TACT) in the localization of simulated periodontal defects. *Dento-Maxillo-Facial Radiology*, 30(6): 319–24.

Ramesh, A., et al. (2002). Evaluation of tuned-aperture computed tomography in the detection of simulated periodontal defects. *Oral Surgery, Oral Medicine, Oral Pathology, Oral Radiology, & Endodontics*, 93(3): 341–9.

Reddy, M.S. (1997). The use of periodontal probes and radiographs in clinical trials of diagnostic tests. *Ann Periodontol*, 2: 113–22.

Rees, T., Biggs, N.L., and Collins, C.K. (1971). Radiographic interpretation of periodontal osseous defects. *Oral Surgery, Oral Medicine, Oral Pathology, Oral Radiology, & Endodontics*, 2: 141–53.

Ruttimann, U.E., Qi, X.L., and Webber, R.L. (1989). An optimal synthetic aperture for circular tomosynthesis. *Med Phys*, 16: 398–405.

Samarabandu, J., et al. (1994). Algorithm for the automated alignment of radiographs for image substraction. *Oral Surgery, Oral Medicine, Oral Pathology, Oral Radiology, & Endodontics*, 77: 75–9.

Schliephake, H., et al. (2003). Imaging of periimplant bone levels of implants with buccal bone defects. *Clinical Oral Implants Research*, 14(2): 193–200.

Socransky, S.S., et al. (1984). New concepts of destructive periodontal disease. *J Clin Periodontol*, 11: 21–32.

Song, Y.D., Jun, S.H., and Kwon, J.J. (2009). Correlation between bone quality evaluated by cone-beam computerized tomography and implant primary stability. *Int J Oral Maxillofac Implants*, 24(1): 59–64.

Sukovic, P. (2003). Cone beam computed tomography in craniofacial imaging. *Orthod Craniofac Res*, 6(Suppl 1): 31–6; discussion 179–82.

Swoboda, J.R., et al. (2008). Correlates of periodontal decline and biological markers in older adults. *J Periodontol*, 79: 1920–6.

Takane, M., et al. (2010). Clinical application of cone beam computed tomography for ideal absorbable membrane placement in interproximal bone defects. *J Oral Sci*, 52(1): 63–9.

Tugnait, A., Clerehugh, V., and Hirschmann, P.N. (2000). The usefulness of radiographs in diagnosis and management of periodontal diseases: A review. *J Dent*, 28: 219–26.

Tyndall, D.A., and Brooks, S.L. (2000). Selection criteria for dental implant site imaging: A position paper of the American Academy of Oral and Maxillofacial Radiology. *Oral Surgery, Oral Medicine, Oral Pathology, Oral Radiology, & Endodontics*, 89: 630–7.

Vandenberghe, B., et al. (2010). The influence of CBCT exposure parameters on periodontal bone measurements: In-vitro accuracy. *Abstract Book XII European*

Congress of Dento-Maxillo Facial Radiology. Istanbul, Turkey, p. 24.

Vandenberghe, B., Jacobs, R., and Yang, J. (2007a). Diagnostic validity (or acuity) of 2D CCD versus 3D CBCT-images for assessing periodontal breakdown. *Oral Surg Oral Med Oral Pathol Oral Radiol Endod*, 104(3): 395–401.

Vandenberghe, B., Jacobs, R., and Yang, J. (2007b). Topographic assessment of periodontal craters and furcation involvements by using 2D digital images versus 3D cone beam CT: An in-vitro study. *Chin J Dent Res*, 10: 21–9.

Vandenberghe, B., Jacobs, R., and Yang, J. (2008). Detection of periodontal bone loss using digital intra-oral and cone beam computed tomography images: An in vitro assessment of bony and/or infrabony defects. *Dentomaxillofac Radiol*, 37(5): 252–60.

Walter, C., Kaner, D., et al. (2009). Three-dimensional imaging as a pre-operative tool in decision making for furcation surgery. *J Clin Periodontol*, 36(3): 250–7.

Walter, C., Weiger, R., Dietrich, T., et al. (2012). Does three-dimensional imaging offer a financial benefit for treating maxillary molars with furcation involvement? A pilot clinical case series. *Clin Oral Implants Res*, 23(3): 351–8.

Walter, C., Weiger, R., and Zitzmann, N.U. (2010). Accuracy of three-dimensional imaging in assessing maxillary molar furcation involvement. *J Clin Periodontol*, 37(5): 436–41.

Walter, C., Weiger, R., and Zitzmann, N.U. (2011). Periodontal surgery in furcation-involved maxillary molars revisited—An introduction of guidelines for comprehensive treatment. *Clin Oral Investig*, 15(1): 9–20.

Webber, R.L., et al. (1997). Tuned aperture computed tomography (TACT). Theory and application for three-dimensional dento-alveolar imaging. *Dentomaxillofac Radiol*, 26: 53–62.

White, S.C., et al. (2005). Clinical and panoramic predictors of femur bone mineral density. *Osteoporos Int*, 16(3): 339–46.

Wolf, B., von Bethlenfalvy, E., and Hassfeld, S. (2001). Reliability of assessing interproximal bone loss by digital radiography: Intrabony defects. *J Clin Periodontol*, 28: 869–78.

Yang, J., et al. (1999). 2-D and 3-D reconstructions of spiral computed tomography in localization of the inferior alveolar canal for dental implants. *Oral Surgery, Oral Medicine, Oral Pathology, Oral Radiology, & Endodontics*, 87: 369–74.

Index

Page numbers followed by "f" and "t" indicate figures and tables.

Abscesses, 67, 82, 256t
Absorbed dose, 40
Accessory root canals, 225
Accountability, collaborative, 150, 159, 194
Acquisition, defined, 3
Acute otitis media, 81–82
Adenoidal facies, 200
Adenoids, 203–204, 205f
Adenomas, pleomorphic, 70
Adenomatoid odontogenic tumors, 58, 59
Aditus ad antrum, 81
Agenesis, 222
Agger nasi cells, 72, 72f, 75, 77–78
Airway assessment
   arthrides and, 200–201, 200f
   condylysis and, 200f, 201
   facial growth and, 199–200
   imaging protocols and, 198–199
   juvenile arthritis and, 202–203f, 201–206
   orthodontic and orthognathic planning and, 93–94, 94f
   overview of, 197–198, 207–208
   resistance and, 198
ALARA (As Low As Reasonably Achievable)
   principle, 35, 214, 263
Alveolar bone and tooth assessment, 92, 92f
Alveolar bone loss, 253–259, 258f, 259f, 260f, 265–266
Ameloblastic fibromas, 57, 58

Ameloblastomas, 57–58, 57f, 112f, 122
Aneurysmal bone cysts, 58
Angiofibromas. juvenile nasopharyngeal, 70
Angiography, 116, 124
Angles of rotation, 30, 39
Angulation, 256
Ankylosis, 181–182, 182–184f
Anodes, 26, 27
Antrochoanal polyps, 68
Apical periodontitis (AP), 213, 229–230, 241
Application-specific integrated circuits (ASIC), 13
Arthrides, 200–201, 200f
Arthritis, juvenile, 202–203f, 201–206
Artifacts
   beam hardening, 16, 22–23, 220
   common, 20–23, 22f, 23f
   computer-aided surgery and, 96
   cone beam, 14
   metal and, 110, 220
   misregistration, 220
   motion, 220f
   nonuniformity, 20, 22f
   overview of, 220
   partial volume, 220
   ring, 20, 21f
   scatter, 22–23, 110
   streaks, 20, 22, 22f, 220

Cone Beam Computed Tomography: Oral and Maxillofacial Diagnosis and Applications, First Edition. Edited by David Sarment.
© 2014 John Wiley & Sons, Inc. Published 2014 by John Wiley & Sons, Inc.

ASIC. *See* Application-specific integrated circuits
Atherosclerosis, 51
Atomic number, 25
Atoms, 25
Attenuation, 6–7, 220
Atypical odontalgia, 226–227
Auditory canal, external, 85–86, 86t
Aurora, 99
Averaging, 7
Axial plane, 44f

Back projection, 11, 12, 14–15
Background radiation, 33–34, 33f
Basal cell nevus syndrome, 57
Beam hardening artifacts, 16, 22–23, 220
Bifid canals, 135, 135f
Binding energy, 25
Biomarkers, 93
Biphosphonate drugs, 61
Bite registrations, 158, 159, 163
Blur effects, 19–20, 19f
Bohr, Niels, 25
Bone canals, 134
Bone density, 130–132, 132f, 261–263
Bone displacement vectors, 99
Bone grafts. *See* Grafts
Bone reduction guides, 175–176, 176–179f
Bone resorption, 265–266, 265f
Bone window imaging, 9–10, 14, 15f
Bone-supported surgical guides, 168, 171f, 189f
Brachial arch syndromes, 200
Bremsstrahlung photons, 27–28, 28f
Buccal bifurcation cysts, 55
Buccal bone, 136, 138f, 139f, 140, 141, 141f

CAC. *See* Carotid artery calcifications
CAD/CAM
  collaborative accountability and, 159
  imaging protocols and, 159
  overview of, 147–148, 185, 194–195
  prototyping and medical modeling and
    case type patterns and, 150–155
    pretreatment analysis, 149–150, 149t
    stereolithography, 148–149, 148f, 149f, 159
  scanning appliances and, 155–159
  surgical guides and
    bone reduction guides, 175–176, 176–179f
    cutting pathway guides for lateral antroscopy of maxillary sinus, 176, 179–181f
    definition and classification, 161–166
    for extraction of ankylosed teeth, 181–182, 182–184f
    fully integrated, 182, 184–193f
    implant planning and, 129, 138, 141, 142
    implementation into clinical practice, 166–175
    overview, 161

Calcification, 51, 52, 52f
Calcified canals, 233–234
Calcifying epithelial odontogenic tumors, 58
Caldwell-Luc sinus grafting technique, 132, 133–134, 133f
Calibration, 21–22
Canal stenosis, 86
Cancer, radiation-induced, 32–33, 34
Capsules, 46, 47f
Carcinogenesis, 32–33, 34
Carcinomas, 61–62, 70, 87, 204, 208f. *See also* Squamous cell carcinomas
Cardiovascular disease, 241
Carestream Dental 9300 CBCT unit, 148
Carotid arteries, 84
Carotid artery calcifications (CAC), 51–52, 52f
Carotid atheromas, calcified, 51–52, 52f
Carotid canal, 86t
Cartilage, 93
Case type patterns
  I, 149t, 150, 151f
  II and III, 149t, 150–153, 152f, 153f
  IV, 149t, 153–154, 154f
  V, 149t, 154–155, 155f
Cathodes, 26–27, 27f
Cavernous sinus thrombosis, 67
CBCT. *See* Cone beam computed tomography
CCDAP. *See* Chronic continuous dentoalveolar pain
Cemental dysplasia, 50
Cementifying fibroma, 51
Cementoblastoma, 49
Cemento-osseous dysplasia, 50
Cementum, radiopaque lesions and, 48
Central giant cell granulomas (CGCG), 58
Central odontogenic fibromas, 58
Central ossifying fibroma, 51
Cephalometrics, 97–98
CGCG. *See* Central giant cell granulomas
Cherubism, 58–59
Chicken pox, 213
Cholesteatomas, 82–84
Cholesterol granulomas, 84
Chondrosarcomas, 63, 87
Chordomas, 87
Chromosomes, 32
Chronic adhesive sclerosis, 82
Chronic continuous dentoalveolar pain (CCDAP), 226–227
Chronic otitis media, 82
Circular-orbiting cameras, 13f, 14
Clinical attachment measurements, 251
Closest point method, 91, 101, 102f
CMFApp software, 95
Coalescent mastoiditis, 87
Cochlea, 78, 86t
Cochlear implants, 81

Cochlear otosclerosis, 80–81
Coherent scatter, 30, 30f
Collaborative accountability, 150, 159, 194
Collimations, 29–30
Collimators, 5
Color maps, 91, 102, 102f
Co-Me network, 95
Compton scatter, 30–31, 31f
Computer-aided design/computer-aided manufacturing. See CAD/CAM
Computer-aided jaw surgery, 94–100, 95f
Concha bullosa, 54, 71–72, 71f, 204f
Condensing osteitis, 49, 50f
Condylar hypoplasia, 200
Condylar remodeling, 93f
Condylysis, 200f, 201
Cone beam artifacts, 14
Cone beam computed tomography (CBCT), overview of, 3–6, 4f
Continuous exposure, 29
Contrast, 8–9, 9f, 20
Cooling issues, 5
Cortication, 45
Cranial nerves, 86–87
Craniofacial anomalies, 94, 94f
Craters, 252, 256t, 260
C-reactive protein, 93
Crest lines, 97
Cribiform plate, 86
Crista galli, 86
Cross-section views, 44f
CUDA, 14
Cupping, 220
Current, 28–29
Cutting guides, 119, 120f, 124, 176, 179–181f
Cysts
 aneurysmal bone, 58
 buccal bifurcation, 55
 dentigerous, 55, 55f, 59
 jaw, 54–56, 55f, 58
 mucous retention, 67–68, 68f, 68t
 nasopalatine duct, 229
 overview of, 228
 pseudocysts, 56–57, 56f
 radicular, 49, 55, 211, 214
 radiographic diagnosis of, 214
 simple bone, 56, 56f

Deep circumflex iliac artery (DCIA) free flaps, 113
Degenerative joint disease, 200f, 201
Dehiscence of superior semicircular canal, 80
Dehiscences, 80, 257
Dens invaginatus (DI), 222
Dense bone islands, 49–50, 50f, 222–224, 224f

Dental follicles, 59
Dental implants. See Implant placement
Denticles, 48
Dentigerous cysts, 55, 55f, 59
Dentin, 48
Dentition, 3D visualization of, 115–116, 115f
DentoCAT, 3–4, 4f
Dentofacial deformities, 94, 94f
Denture scanning appliances, 149t, 157–158, 158f, 160f
Detector glare, 19
Detector lag, 19
Deterministic effects of ionizing radiation, 31–32
Developmental anomalies, of jaw, 53–54
Deviated nasal septum, 203, 204f
DI. See Dens invaginatus
Digital subtraction radiography, 252
Disinfection, 175
Distraction osteogenesis, 99
DNA, ionizing radiation and, 32
Dolphin Imaging, 95
Drilling guides, 117, 117f
Dual scan protocols, 159, 161f

Ear
 external auditory canal, 85–86, 86t
 inner, 78–81
 middle, 81–85, 84t
Ectopic calcification, 48
Edentulous arch, 141–142
Effective doses, 34–35, 36–37t, 40, 199, 219, 252
Effective treatment, defined, 240
Electromagnetic radiation, 26, 26f
Electromagnetic tracking, 99
Electrons, 25, 27
Enamel, 48
Endodontic treatment
 dentoalveolar trauma, 234–235, 235f, 236f
 differential diagnosis
  anatomic structures hindering performance of task-specific procedures, 227–228
  assessment of nonhealed cases, 229–230
  contradictory or nonspecific signs and symptoms, 226–227
  nonodontogenic lesions, 228
  odontogenic lesions, 228–229
  poorly localized symptoms, 227
  vertical root fractures, 230–233, 232f
 evaluation of anatomy and complex morphology
  additional roots, 225–226
  anomalies, 216f, 222–224
  missed/accessory canals, 225
  root curvatures, 224–225
 implant planning and, 240

Endodontic treatment (*cont'd*)
    implantation vs., 135–136, 136f
    intra- or post-operative assessment of complications
        calcified canals, 233–234
        perforation localization, 234
    limitations of 2D imaging in, 217–218
    limited field of view CBCT in
        advantages of, 214–216
        limitations of, 218–220
    outcome assessment, 240–241
    overview of, 211–214
    overview of applications of CBCT in, 221–222
    presurgical planning, 237–239
    root resorption, 235–237
Endolymphatic duct, 78
Endolymphatic sac tumors, 87
Endoscopy, 70–78
Enostosis, 49–50, 50f, 222–224, 224f
Eosinophilic granulomas, 88
Epitympanum, 81
Equivalent dose, 40
ERR. *See* External root resorption
Esthesioneuroblastomas, 87
Estrogen replacement therapy, 262
Ethmoid foramina, 86
Eustachian canals, 81, 82
Ewing's sarcoma, 63
Exposure, defined, 39–40
Exposure time, 29, 38–39, 38f
External auditory canal, 85, 86
External root resorption (ERR), 236
Extoses, 50, 85
Extractions, 136–137, 181–182, 182–184f

Facial growth, airway and, 199–200
Facial nerve canal, 86t
Fan beam geometries, 4–5
FBP. *See* Filtered back projection
Feldkamp Davis Kress (FDK) algorithm, 11–14, 11f, 12f, 16
Fenestral otosclerosis, 80
Fenestrations, 257
FESS. *See* Functional endoscopic sinus surgery
Fibro cartilage, 93
Fibroma, central ossifying, 51
Fibro-osseous lesions
    of jaw, 48–49, 50–51
    overview of, 228
    of sinuses, 69, 69f
    of skull base, 87
Fibro-osseous sclerosis, 82
Fibrosarcomas, 63
Fibrous dysplasia, 51, 52f, 61, 69, 87
Fibula grafts, 117
Fiduciary markers, 159

Fields of view (FOV). *See also* Limited field of view CBCT
    overview of, 6–7, 6f
    periodontal disease and, 263–264
    radiation risks and, 29–30, 29f, 38, 38f
Filtered back projection (FBP), 11, 15–16
Finite element models, 99
Florid osseous dysplasia (FOD), 50–51, 51f
Focal osteoporotic bone marrow, 54
Focal spot, 27
FOD. *See* Florid osseous dysplasia
Follicular (dentigerous) cysts, 55, 55f, 59
Foramina of Scarpa/Stensen, 229
Fossae of Rosenmuller, 204
Four-dimensional (4D) shape information, 98
FOV. *See* Fields of view
Fractures, 86, 86t, 136, 138f. *See also* Vertical root fractures
Free fibula, 117
Free fibula flaps, 112–113, 113f, 114f, 118f, 122–124
Free vascularized osseous flaps, 112–114, 113f, 114f
Frontal bullar cells, 76–77
Frontal recess cells, 74–77
Frontoethmoid encephaloceles, 70
Full contour scanning appliances, 149t, 155–157, 156f, 157f
Functional endoscopic sinus surgery (FESS), 70–78
Fungal sinusitis, 66
Furcations, 252, 256t, 257, 259–261

Gardner syndrome, 223
Gemination, 222
General purpose graphics processing units (GPGPU), 15
Geometric projections, 10–11, 10f
Giant cell reparative granuloma, 58
Giant cell tumors of skull base, 88
Glomus tumors, 84–85, 87
GPGPU. *See* General purpose graphics processing units
Grafts
    dentition modeling and, 115
    modeling bone and vessels and, 114–115
    overview of, 124
    prefabrication of, 117
    preparation of jaw area, 119–120
    selecting material for, 112–114, 116
    surgery, 120–122
    virtual planning of, 98, 116–119
Granuloma, dental, 49
Granulomas, cholesterol, 84
Ground glass appearance, 51, 69

Haller's cells, 72, 73f
Halos, 46, 47f
Hamartomas, 48
Hemangiomas, 206–207f
Hematopoietic malignancies, 62, 63

Herpes zoster, 213
High tube prolongation, 163f
Hounsfield units (HU), 7
HU. *See* Hounsfield units
Hyperostosis, 78, 208f
Hypopharynx, 197
Hypotympanum, 81

Idiopathic osteosclerosis, 49–50, 50f, 222–224, 224f
Iliac artery flaps, 113
Iliac crest grafts, 110–111, 111f
Image intensity, 7
Image noise, overview of, 18–20
Image quality, 128–130, 164
Image reconstruction
    conventional filtered, 10–14, 10f, 11f, 12–13f, 16f
    defined, 3, 6
    iterative, 14–18, 16f
    overview of, 10
Image registration, 100
Image segmentation, 96–97, 100
Image Took Kit, 96
Imaging protocols, optimization of, 38–39, 38f
Immediate smile model, 182, 190f, 192–193f
Implant placement. *See also* CAD/CAM; Grafts
    anatomic evaluation prior to
        bone density, 130–132, 132f
            mandibles, 134–135
            maxillary sinuses, 132–134
    edentulous arch evaluation and, 141–142
    endodontic treatment vs., 135–136, 136f
    extractions and, 136–157
    image quality and, 128–130
    immediate, 138–140
    maxillofacial reconstructions and, 124
    orthodontic evaluation and, 137–138
    overview of, 127–128, 144
    planning for, 240
    scanning updates and, 142–144
    small, 140–141
Incudomalleolar joint, 79f
Incus, 79f, 81
Ineffective treatment, defined, 240
Inferior alveolar nerve, 239f
Inflammation. *See also* Periodontal disease
    inner ear pathologies and, 78–80
    jaw pathologies and, 49, 53, 54, 59–60
    middle ear pathologies and, 81–82
    sinus pathologies and, 67–68, 68f, 68t, 77
Infrabony defects, 259–261
Infraorbital nerve, 76f
Infrared optical tracking devices, 99
Inner ear, 78–81, 79f, 80f
InstaRecon, Inc., 15, 16–17, 16f, 17f
Interfrontal sinus septal cells, 77

Internal root resorption (IRR), 235–236
Interradicular bone, 136, 140
Invasive fungal sinusitis, 66
Inverting papillomas, 69–70
InVivoDental, 95
Ionization, 25
Ionizing radiation. *See also* X-rays
    biological effects of, 31–33
    Bremsstrahlung photons and, 27–28, 28f
    minimizing exposure to, 35–39
    nature of, 25–26
    risks from CBCT examinations and, 33–34
    X-ray production and, 27f
IRR. *See* Internal root resorption
Ischemia time, 119, 124
ITK-SNAP software, 96, 96f

Jacobson's nerve, 85
Jaw pathologies
    classification of, 47–48
    computer-aided surgery for, 94–100, 95f
    evaluation procedure, 45–47
    overview of CBCT for, 43–44
    protocol for reviewing scan volume, 44–45
    radiolucent lesions
        rapidly growing, 59–63
        slow-growing, 53–59
    radiopaque lesions
        bone tissue lesions, 49–50
        fibro-osseous lesions, 48, 50–51
        miscellaneous, 51–52
        overview of, 48
        tooth tissue lesions, 48–49
    reconstruction after surgery for, 110–112
    role of dentist, 63–64
Jugular bulbs, 84
Jugular foramen, 87
Juvenile arthritis, 202–203f, 201–206
Juvenile nasopharyngeal angiofibromas, 70
Juvenile onset degenerative joint disease, 200f, 201

Keratocystic odontogenic tumors (KOT), 56–57, 56f, 58, 213
Keratosis obturans, 85
Keros classification, 74, 74t, 75f
Kuhn classification, 75, 77t

Labyrinth, 78, 79f, 80f
Labyrinthine fistulas, 84
Labyrinthitis, 78–80
Lamina dura, 251, 261
Lamina papyracea, 74, 75, 76f
Landmark-based measurements, 100–101
Langerhans cell histiocytosis, 88
Lateral periodontal cysts, 55

Lava Chairside Oral Scanner C.O.S., 110, 110f, 117, 122–124
Lenticular process, 81
Lesser sphenoid wings, 86
Limited field of view CBCT, 212f, 214–216, 218–220
Linear nonthreshold (LNT) model, 32–33
Lingual salivary gland depression, 54, 54f, 222
Longitudinal assessments, 93–94, 94f, 100–102, 101f, 102f
Low-contrast detectability, 20
Lymphomas, 70

Malignancies, 61–63, 62f, 70. *See also Specific types*
Malignant otitis externa, 85, 87
Malleus, 79f, 81
Mandibles, 134–135
Mandibular nerves, 134, 135f
Mass tensor models, 99
Mastoiditis, 82, 87
Materialise Dental, 148
Matter, 25, 30–31
Maxilim system, 95
Maxillary sinuses
    augmentation of, 132–134, 142–143, 143f
    cutting guides for lateral antroscopy of, 176, 176–178f
    jaw pathologies and, 47, 47f
Maxillofacial reconstructions
    case report of secondary reconstruction, 122–124
    overview of, 109–110, 110f, 124
    primary reconstruction after tumor ablative surgery, 110–112
    secondary reconstruction of pre-existing defects, 112–122
Measurement noise, defined, 18
Measurements, quantitative, 100–102, 221f, 253–259
Medical Modeling system, 95
Medulla oblongata, 87
Melanoma, sinonasal, 70
Meningiomas, 87
Mesotympanum, 81
Metal, 110, 220
Metastases, of jaw, 52, 61–63
Microdontia taurodontism, 222
Middle ear, 81–85, 84t
Misregistration artifacts, 220
Modulation transfer function (MTF), 20, 21f
Morphometrics, 97–98, 98f
Motion artifacts, 220f
MPR. *See* Multiplanar rendering
MSCT. *See* Multislice computed tomography
MTF. *See* Modulation transfer function
Mucoceles, 67–68, 68t
Mucopyoceles, 68
Mucous retention cysts, 67–68, 68f, 68t
Multilayer mass-spring models, 99
Multimodality registration, 95

Multiplanar rendering (MPR), 7, 8f, 44, 45
Multiple myeloma, 63
Multislice computed tomography (MSCT), 147, 261
Muscular function simulations, 99
Mycetoma, 66
Myringitis, 82, 83f
Myxomas, odontogenic, 57, 58

Nasal mucosal hypertrophy, 204, 205f
Nasal septum, 73
Nasopalatine duct cysts, 229
Nasopharynx, 197, 203–204, 205f
National Alliance of Medical Computing, 101
Necrosis, 61
Necrotic otitis externa, 85, 87
Neoplasms, 81, 84–85, 228–229. *See also Specific types*
Neuromas, 227
Neutrons, 25
NewTom, 39
NIH Visualization Tool Kit, 96
Noise. *See* Image noise; Measurement noise
Nominal tomographic section thickness, 19f, 20
Non-Hodgkin lymphoma, 62f, 63
Nonuniformity artifacts, 20, 22f
Nose, 203, 205f

Obstructive sleep apnea (OSA), 197
Obstructive sleep disordered breathing (OSDB), 197. *See also* Airway assessment
Occipital bone, 86
Occlusal guides, 120–121, 120f
Odontogenic keratocysts, 56–57, 56f, 58, 213
Odontogenic myxomas (OM), 57, 58
Odontomas, 48, 49f, 55f, 57
OF. *See* Ossifying fibromas
Ohm's law, 198
Olfactory fossa, 73–74, 74t, 75f
OM. *See* Odontogenic myxomas
OMC. *See* Osteomeatal complex
Onodi cells, 72, 74f
OpenCL, 14
Operator training, 37–38
Oral pharynx, 206, 206f
Orbital plates, 86
Orbitals, 25
Oropharynx, 197
Orthodontics, 96, 137–138
Orthognathic surgery, 94, 96
Orthopedic corrections, 94
OSA. *See* Obstructive sleep apnea
OSDB. *See* Obstructive sleep disordered breathing
Osseous dysplasia, 50
Ossicles, 81, 86t
Ossifying fibromas (OF), 51, 58, 69
Osteitis, 55f, 213, 229–230, 241

Osteoarthritis, 200f, 201
Osteomas, 69, 69f, 85
Osteomeatal complex (OMC), 70
Osteomyelitis, 52, 60–61, 60f, 82, 87
Osteoneogenesis (hyperostosis), 78, 208f
Osteopetrosis, 52, 87
Osteoplasty, 175, 189f
Osteoporosis, 261–262
Osteoradionecrosis, 61
Osteosarcomas, 52, 61, 63
Osteosclerosis, idiopathic, 49–50, 50f, 222–224, 224f
Osteotomies, virtual, 98–99
Osteotomy techniques, 132–133
Otic capsule, 86
Otitis media, 81–82
Otosclerosis, 80–81, 80f
Outcome assessment, 240–241, 252

Pagetoid appearance, 69
Paget's disease of the bone, 50–51, 61, 80, 87
Palatal mucosa thickness, 265
Panoramic images, 127
Panoramic radiographs, 251
Panoramic reconstructions, 44f, 45, 140, 142f
Papillomas, inverting, 69–70
Paragangliomas, 84–85, 87
Parallel computing, 14–15
Paranasal sinus pathologies
  anatomic variants, 71–74, 72f
  fibro-osseous lesions, 69, 69f
  frontal recess and, 74–77
  functional endoscopic sinus surgery and, 70–78
  inflammatory polyps, mucoceles, mucous retention cysts, 67–68, 68f, 68t
  neoplasms and noninflammatory lesions, 69–70
  overview of, 65–66
  rhinoliths, 70
  silent sinus syndrome, 68
  sinusitis, 66–67, 67f
  Wegener's granulomatosis, 70
Pars flaccida cholesteatomas, 83–84, 83f
Partial volume artifacts, 220
Particulate radiation, 25–26
Perforations, 234
Periapical cemento-osseous dysplasia (PCOD), 50
Periapical cysts, 49, 55, 211, 214
Periapical rarefying osteitis, 213, 229–230, 241
Periapical region, 261
Perilymphatic space, 78
Periodontal cysts, lateral, 55
Periodontal disease
  alveolar bone loss measurement, 253–259, 258f, 259f, 260f
  bone density and, 261–263
  bone tissue lesions and, 49
  future applications of CBCT for, 263–266
  infrabony defects and furcation involvement, 259–261
  landmarks and subjective image analysis, 261
  overview of CBCT for, 253, 254f, 255f, 256t, 266
  prevalence and progression of, 249–250, 250f
  traditional computed tomography for, 252–253
  traditional diagnostic methods for, 250–252
  tuned aperture computed tomography for, 252
Periodontal ligament (PDL), 47, 261
Petrous ridge, 86
Petrous temporal bone, 86
Phantom tooth pain, 226–227
Phantoms, 14, 15f
Photoelectric absorption, 31
Photons, 26, 26f, 28f, 29f
Pindborg tumors, 58
Planning, 168, 169–171f, 194, 237–240
Plasmacytomas, 87
Plenum sphenoidale, 86
Pleomorphic adenomas, 70
Pneumatization, 71–72, 71f, 72f, 73f, 75–77, 77t
Pocket probing depth, 250–251
Poiseuille's law, 198
Polyps, 67–68, 68t, 204, 205f
Polysomnograms, 197
Postcorrection methods, 22f, 23, 23f
Postinflammatory ossicular fixation, 82
Progressive condylar resorption, 200f, 201
Projections, 10–12, 10f, 14–15
Prolongation, 161–162, 163f
ProPlan CMF, 110, 110–111, 116–121
Protective equipment, 39
Protons, 25
Prototyping, rapid, 148–150, 161–162
Provisional restoration scanning appliances, 149t, 158–159
Prussak's space, 84
Pseudocysts, 56–57, 56f
Pulp vitality testing, 59, 213
Pulpal inflammation, 59
Pulsed exposure, 29
Punched out, 45, 46f
Pyogenic sinusitis, 66

Quantitative measurements, 100–102, 221f, 253–259
Quarks, 25

Radiation. *See also* Ionizing radiation
  from 3D CBCT image acquisition, 100
  necrosis from, 61
  overview of, 25
  risks from, 33, 34
  sources of, 33–34, 33f
  units of, 39–40
Radiation dosage, 219. *See also* Effective doses
Radicular cysts, 49, 55, 211, 214

Radiography, 127–128, 251–252, 256t
Rapid prototyping, 148–150, 161–162
RDC/TMD. *See* Research Diagnostic Criteria for Temporomandibular Disorders
Reconstruction grids, 6–7, 6f
Reconstructions. *See* Maxillofacial reconstructions
Regions of interest (ROI), 7, 8f
Rems, 40
Research Diagnostic Criteria for Temporomandibular Disorders (RDC/TMD), 92
Reslicing, 256–257
Resolution, 19–20, 219–220
Resorption, 200f, 201, 235–237, 265–266, 265f
Restorative leadership, 150–159, 194
Retrofenestral otosclerosis, 80–81
Rhabdomyosarcomas, 85
Rhinoliths, 70
Ridge curves, 97
Ring artifacts, 20, 21f
ROI. *See* Regions of interest
Root curvatures, 224–225
Root fractures, vertical, 230–233, 232f
Root perforations, 234
Root resorption, 235–237
Roots, additional, 225–226
Rotating anodes, 27
Rotation angle, 30, 39

Saccule, 78
Safebeam technology, 39
Salivary gland depression, 54, 54f, 222
Sarcomas, 62
SBC. *See* Simple bone cysts
Scala media, 78
Scala tympani, 78
Scalloping, 56
Scan modes, 39
Scanning appliances, 147–148, 149t, 155–159
Scannographic guides, 142, 142f
Scapula grafts, 113–114
Scatter, 22–23, 30–31, 110
Schwannomas, 84–85, 87, 204f
Sclerosing osteitis, 49, 50f
Sclerosis, 45–46
Sclerotic bone masses, 48
SDB. *See* Sleep disordered breathing
Segmentation, 96–97, 100
Selection criteria, 35
Semicircular canals, 78, 80, 86t
Semicircular ducts, 78
Semi-landmarks, 101
Septi, 133
Shape correspondence, 101
Short roots, 222
Sialoliths, submandibular, 51, 52

Sickle cell anemia, 213
Sieverts, 40
Sigmoid sinus thrombosis, 84
Silent sinus syndrome, 68
SimPlant, 95, 110, 115, 148
Simple bone cysts (SBC), 56, 56f
Simulations, 98–99
Single scan protocols, 159, 160f
Sinonasal osteomas, 69
Sinonasal polyps, 68
Sinonasal undifferentiated carcinomas, 87
Sinuses, 93. *See also* Functional endoscopic sinus surgery; Maxillary sinuses; Paranasal sinus pathologies
Sinusitis, 66–67, 67f
Skull base, 85, 86–88
Sleep disordered breathing (SDB), 197. *See also* Airway assessment
Slice sensitivity profiles (SSP), 19–20, 19f
Slicer3, 95
Soft tissue analysis, 264–265, 264f
Soft tissue changes, simulation of, 99
Soft tissue window, 9
Spatial resolution, 19–20, 219–220
SPHARM-PDM framework, 101–102
Sphenoethmoidal recess, 70
Sphenoid bone, 86
Splints, 99
Squamous cell carcinomas, 70, 85, 87, 208f
SSP. *See* Slice sensitivity profiles
Staff training, 37–38
Stafne bone defect, 54, 54f, 222
Standard Model of atoms, 25
Stationary anodes, 27
StealthStation AXIEM, 99
Stereolithography, 148–149, 148f, 149f, 159
Stochastic effects of ionizing radiation, 32–33
Streaks, 20, 22, 22f, 220
Superimposition, 100, 102f
Superior semicircular canal, 80
Supernumerary teeth dentinogenesis imperfecta, 222
Suprabullar cells, 76
Surface-based rendering, 97, 98f, 129, 129f
Surgical guides. *See also* CAD/CAM
 bone reduction guides, 175–176, 176–179f
 cutting pathway guides for lateral antroscopy of maxillary sinus, 176, 179–181f
 definition and classification, 161–166
 for extraction of ankylosed teeth, 181–182, 182–184f
 fully integrated, 182
 implant planning and, 129, 138, 141, 142
 implementation into clinical practice, 166–175
 overview, 161
Surgical simulations, 98–99
SurgiGuide, 148
Syphilitic labyrinthitis, 80

TACT. *See* Tuned aperture computed tomography
Tardieu scanning appliance, 157, 163
Tegmen tympani, 81, 84, 84t
Temporal bone, 78, 86, 86t
Temporomandibular joint (TMJ)
 condylysis and, 200f, 201
 evaluation of, 92–93, 93f
 MPR images and, 45
Tensor-based morphometry, 98f
Three-dimensional (3D) augmented models, 110, 110f
Three-dimensional (3D) volumetric renderings, 44, 44f, 45, 91–92
3dMD Vultus, 95, 199
Threshold dose, 32
Thyroid collars, 39
TMJ. *See* Temporomandibular joint
Tonsilloliths, 51, 52
Tonsils, 206f
Tooth-form scanning appliances, 149t, 155, 156f
Tooth-supported surgical guides, 168–169, 171–172, 172–174f, 185f
Trabecular pattern analysis, 263
Tracking technologies, 99
Training, 37–38
Traumatic bone cysts, 56, 56f
Traumatic injuries, 85–86, 138f, 234–235, 235f, 236f
Treatment planning, 168, 169–171f, 194, 237–240
Tube current, 28–29
Tube voltage, 28
Tuned aperture computed tomography (TACT), 252
Tympanic isthmi, 81
Tympanic membrane, 82, 83, 83f, 84
Tympanosclerosis, 82

UARS. *See* Upper airway resistance syndrome
Ultrasound tracking, 99
Uncinate process, 72, 78
Uniguide, 129–130, 130f
Upper airway resistance syndrome (UARS), 197. *See also* Airway assessment
Utricle, 78

Varicella zoster virus, 213
Vertical root fractures, 230–233, 232f
Vestibular aqueduct, 78, 79f
Vestibule, 86t
Virtual osteotomies, 98–99
Virtual shaping, 110
Vitality testing, 59, 213
Voltage, 28
Volume changes, 100
Volume-based rendering, 97, 98f, 110, 129, 129f, 130f
Voxels, 7, 199, 233, 236–237

Wave theory, 26
Wavelength, 26, 26f
Wegener's granulomatosis, 70

xCAT-ENT, 19f
X-ray beams, 28–29
X-ray tubes, 26–27, 27f
X-rays
 interactions of with matter, 30–31
 nature of, 26, 26f
 parameters of in CBCT units, 23–30
 production of, 26–27

Zygomatic air cell defect, 54